ANNUAL REVIEW *of* DIABETES

2022

THE BEST OF THE

AMERICAN DIABETES ASSOCIATION'S

SCHOLARLY JOURNALS

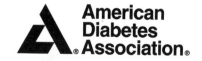

American Diabetes Association®

ANNUAL REVIEW *of* DIABETES
2022

THE BEST OF THE AMERICAN DIABETES ASSOCIATION'S
SCHOLARLY JOURNALS

Printed in the United States of America
1 3 5 7 9 10 8 6 4 2

The suggestions and information contained in this publication are generally consistent with the *Standards of Medical Care in Diabetes* and other policies of the American Diabetes Association, but they do not represent the policy or position of the Association or any of its boards or committees. Reasonable steps have been taken to ensure the accuracy of the information presented. However, the American Diabetes Association cannot ensure the safety or efficacy of any product or service described in this publication. Individuals are advised to consult a physician or other appropriate health care professional before undertaking any diet or exercise program or taking any medication referred to in this publication. Professionals must use and apply their own professional judgment, experience, and training and should not rely solely on the information contained in this publication before prescribing any diet, exercise, or medication. The American Diabetes Association—its officers, directors, employees, volunteers, and members—assumes no responsibility or liability for personal or other injury, loss, or damage that may result from the suggestions or information in this publication. The paper in this publication meets the requirements of the ANSI Standard Z39.48-1992 (permanence of paper).

∞ The paper in this publication meets the requirements of the ANSI Standard Z39.48-1992 (permanence of paper).

American Diabetes Association titles may be purchased for business or promotional use or for special sales. To purchase more than 50 copies of this book at a discount, or for custom editions of this book with your logo, contact the American Diabetes Association at the bulk book sales address below, at booksales@diabetes.org, or by calling 703-299-2046.

American Diabetes Association
Bulk Book Sales
PO Box 7023
Merrifield, Virginia 22116-7023

American Diabetes Association
2451 Crystal Drive, Suite 900
Arlington, Virginia 22202

DOI: 10.2337/9781580408196

ANNUAL REVIEW OF DIABETES 2022

Lifestyle Intervention in Pregnant Women With Obesity Impacts Cord Blood DNA Methylation, Which Associates With Body Composition in the Offspring

Josefine Jönsson,[1] Kristina M. Renault,[2,3] Sonia García-Calzón,[1,4] Alexander Perfilyev,[1] Angela C. Estampador,[5] Kirsten Nørgaard,[6] Mads Vendelbo Lind,[7] Allan Vaag,[6] Line Hjort,[8] Kim F. Michaelsen,[7] Emma Malchau Carlsen,[7,9] Paul W. Franks,[5] and Charlotte Ling[1]

Diabetes 2021;70:854–866 | https://doi.org/10.2337/db20-0487

Maternal obesity may lead to epigenetic alterations in the offspring and might thereby contribute to disease later in life. We investigated whether a lifestyle intervention in pregnant women with obesity is associated with epigenetic variation in cord blood and body composition in the offspring. Genome-wide DNA methylation was analyzed in cord blood from 208 offspring from the Treatment of Obese Pregnant women (TOP)-study, which includes pregnant women with obesity randomized to lifestyle interventions comprised of physical activity with or without dietary advice versus control subjects (standard of care). DNA methylation was altered at 379 sites, annotated to 370 genes, in cord blood from offspring of mothers following a lifestyle intervention versus control subjects (false discovery rate [FDR] <5%) when using the Houseman reference-free method to correct for cell composition, and three of these sites were significant based on Bonferroni correction. These 370 genes are overrepresented in gene ontology terms, including response to fatty acids and adipose tissue development. Offspring of mothers included in a lifestyle intervention were born with more lean mass compared with control subjects. Methylation at 17 sites, annotated to, for example, *DISC1*, *GBX2*, *HERC2*, and *HUWE1*, partially mediates the effect of the lifestyle intervention on lean mass in the offspring (FDR <5%). Moreover, 22 methylation sites were associated with offspring BMI *z* scores during the first 3 years of life ($P < 0.05$). Overall, lifestyle interventions in pregnant women with obesity are associated with epigenetic changes in offspring, potentially influencing the offspring's lean mass and early growth.

Obesity and type 2 diabetes are on the rise worldwide, as is the prevalence of obesity in pregnant women (1). Obesity during pregnancy increases the risk of adverse health outcomes in the offspring, including macrosomia and childhood obesity (2), which might be explained by a metabolically adverse intrauterine environment. The prevalence of childhood obesity, which is associated with an increased risk of adulthood obesity (3), metabolic syndrome (4), and early death (5), more than doubled between 1980 and 2015 (6). Greater increase in weight and height during infancy is associated with greater lean mass and lower risk of the metabolic syndrome in adulthood (7,8). Hence, greater lean mass during infancy might protect against future metabolic disease.

[1]Epigenetics and Diabetes Unit, Department of Clinical Sciences, Lund University Diabetes Centre, Lund University, Scania University Hospital, Malmö, Sweden

[2]Department of Obstetrics and Gynecology, Hvidovre Hospital, University of Copenhagen, Copenhagen, Denmark

[3]Department of Obstetrics, Juliane Marie Centre, Rigshospitalet, University of Copenhagen, Copenhagen, Denmark

[4]Department of Nutrition, Food Sciences and Physiology, University of Navarra, Pamplona, Spain

[5]Genetic and Molecular Epidemiology Unit, Department of Clinical Sciences, Lund University Diabetes Centre, Lund University, Malmö, Sweden

[6]Steno Diabetes Center Copenhagen, Gentofte, Denmark

[7]Department of Nutrition, Exercise and Sports, Faculty of Science, University of Copenhagen, Frederiksberg, Denmark

[8]Department of Obstetrics, Center for Pregnant Women with Diabetes, Rigshospitalet, Copenhagen, Denmark

[9]Department of Pediatrics, Copenhagen University Hospital Hvidovre, Hvidovre, Denmark

Corresponding authors: Josefine Jönsson, josefin.jonsson@med.lu.se, and Charlotte Ling, charlotte.ling@med.lu.se

Received 11 May 2020 and accepted 1 January 2021

This article contains supplementary material online at https://doi.org/10.2337/figshare.13501587.

J.J. and K.M.R. are shared first authors.

P.W.F. and C.L. are shared last authors.

As gestational weight gain (GWG) affects the health of the mother and offspring, the Institute of Medicine recommends women with prepregnancy BMI >30 kg/m^2 to limit their GWG to 5–9 kg (1). We have reported that GWG can be reduced by lifestyle interventions (9) and was positively associated with fat mass in infants born to mothers with obesity (10,11) and with carbohydrate intake in late pregnancy (12). Subsequently, lifestyle interventions might improve the cardiometabolic profile of pregnant mothers with obesity and their offspring.

Epigenetic alterations, such as DNA methylation, may occur following intrauterine perturbations caused by obesity and excess GWG (13,14). DNA methylation regulates gene expression, X-chromosome inactivation, imprinting, and cell differentiation (13). Intrauterine epigenetic alterations may therefore affect future health outcomes in the offspring (15). For example, early maternal exposures such as gestational diabetes, pregestational obesity, and famine were linked to dysregulated gene function in early life by altered DNA methylation (16–19), and dietary interventions during pregnancy impact the offspring epigenome (20). However, to our knowledge, it remains unknown whether interventions in pregnant women with obesity affect the epigenetic pattern in cord blood and whether this is associated with body composition and growth in their offspring.

Our aim was to investigate whether a lifestyle intervention including physical activity with and without advice on a low-energy Mediterranean-style diet in pregnant women with obesity from the Treatment of Obese Pregnant women (TOP)-study (9) is associated with DNA methylation alterations in offspring cord blood. We then tested whether specific epigenetic marks in cord blood are associated with body composition in the offspring at birth and growth during the first 3 years of life.

RESEARCH DESIGN AND METHODS

Design and Clinical Data of the TOP-Study

The TOP-study was approved by the Ethics Committee for the Capital Region of Denmark (January 2009, H-D-2008-119; Hillerød, Denmark) and registered at ClinicalTrials.gov (NCT01345149). Before enrollment, written informed consent was obtained from all participants.

The TOP-study is a randomized controlled trial of 425 pregnant women with obesity including two lifestyle intervention groups—physical activity assessed with pedometer and dietary advice (PA + D) and physical activity assessed with pedometer (PA)—and a control arm receiving standard of care (C) (Fig. 1). The primary end point was to assess the impact of these lifestyle interventions on GWG (9). All participants, including control subjects, had a consultation with a dietitian who recommended a low-energy and low-fat Mediterranean-style diet of 1,200–1,675 kcal, based on Danish national recommendations, and they were encouraged to limit GWG to ≤5 kg. Participants in PA + D had regular contact/visits (every 2 weeks) with an experienced dietitian giving dietary advice and measuring weight. Participants in both PA + D and PA were encouraged to obtain 11,000 steps daily. We based our physical activity recommendation on our previous study of step counts among pregnant women and added 50% to increase physical activity (21). If this was not achievable, they were asked to set their own goal.

Due to participants having miscarriages, withdrawing from the study, and moving from the region, 389 women completed the study (Fig. 1). Maternal age, prepregnancy BMI, maternal educational level, and previous childbirths (parity) were recorded at enrollment (weeks 11–14). Smoking during pregnancy was acquired through medical records, GWG was determined by subtracting self-reported prepregnancy weight with weight measured during weeks 36 and 37, and energy intake was attained from self-administered validated Food Frequency Questionnaires at weeks 11–14 and 36–38. Detailed information on enrollment, conduction of the trial, and clinical measurements is reported elsewhere (9,12).

DXA scans were performed within 48 h of birth to assess offspring body composition. Offspring measurements of interest for this study were: lean mass at birth and growth, in which BMI z scores at birth and at 9, 18, and 36 months of age were used (Fig. 1). Data collection and body composition assessment in the offspring are further described (10,22).

Cord blood was collected from the umbilical vein of the clamped umbilical cord at birth. Samples were immediately frozen (−80°C) and stored in a biobank at Copenhagen University Hospital Hvidovre. Whole-cord blood samples were available for 232 participants (Fig. 1).

DNA Methylation Analyses

Cord blood DNA was extracted using the QIAamp 96 DNA Blood Kit. DNA concentration and purity were determined using NanoDrop (NanoDrop Technologies, Inc.). Eight samples had DNA concentrations that were too low. Bisulfite conversion was performed using the EZ-96 DNA methylation kit (Zymo Research Corporation, Irvine, CA), according to the manufacturer's instructions. Six samples failed bisulfite conversion. DNA methylation was measured using Illumina Infinium HumanMethylation450 BeadChips (Illumina, San Diego, CA), covering 485,577 sites (23). Illumina iScan was used to image the Infinium Human-Methylation450K BeadChips. Three samples were removed due to missing data regarding GWG (a covariate in the methylation model). Preprocessing was performed using R (24) (version 3.5.1), lumi (25), and methylumi (26) packages from Bioconductor. β-Values were calculated as β = intensity of the Methylated allele (M)/(intensity of the Unmethylated allele [U] + intensity of the Methylated allele [M] + 100). A total of 1,739 probes with mean detection P value >0.01, 64 rs probes, 3,089 ch-probes targeting non-CpG sites, 80 Y-chromosome probes, 26,772 cross-reactive probes, and 436 polymorphic probes with a minor allele frequency >0.1 were filtered out (27). Methylation data were obtained for 453,397 probes. For further analyses,

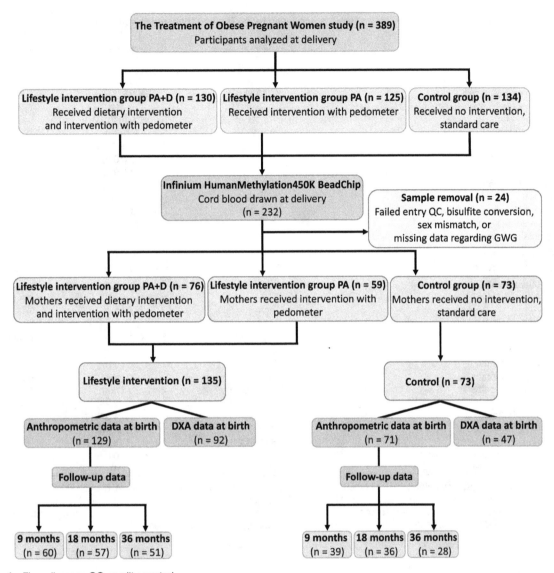

Figure 1—Flow diagram. QC, quality control.

M-values were used, calculated following the formula M = $\log_2(\beta/[1-\beta])$ (28). Background correction and quantile normalization were performed. Beta-Mixture Quantile normalization method (29) was applied. ComBat was applied to correct for batch effects (30,31). Principal component analysis (PCA) before and after applying ComBat ensures that between-array batch effects were removed. Seven participants were further excluded, as these samples clustered to the wrong sex in the PCA. Overall, DNA methylation data were available for 208 participants (Fig. 1 and Table 1). Additional gene annotation was performed using hg38, GENCODE version 22.

Statistical Analyses

We performed a power calculation using R package pwrE-WAS (https://bioconductor.org/packages/devel/bioc/html/pwrEWAS.html). To find 10% difference in methylation between two groups (ratio 1:2) with 75% power, we needed 230 participants. Based on this power calculation, the fact that GWG, the primary end point of the TOP-study, did not differ between the two lifestyle intervention groups and the modest number of samples with cord blood in each lifestyle intervention group, we decided to combine the two lifestyle intervention groups. We subsequently investigated the impact of PA + D together with PA (lifestyle intervention group, $n = 135$) versus C (control group, $n = 73$) on all investigated parameters (Fig. 1).

To test if cord blood DNA methylation is associated with lifestyle intervention assignment, a linear regression model adjusted for maternal age (years), prepregnancy BMI (kilograms per meter squared), GWG (kilograms), gestational age (GA; weeks), and offspring sex was run. Adjustment for cell composition was done using the reference-free method from Houseman et al. (32). We also used the reference-based method to adjust for cell composition (33). We additionally performed linear regression

Table 1—Parental and offspring baseline characteristics according to the lifestyle intervention and control groups for subjects with available cord blood of the TOP-study

	Lifestyle intervention	Control	P value
Maternal characteristics	$n = 135$	$n = 73$	
Maternal age at enrollment (years)*	30.90 (4.30)	31.40 (4.74)	0.440
Prepregnancy BMI (kg/m²)*	34.19 (4.00)	34.36 (3.98)	0.763
Maternal educational level, n (%)†			0.970
Grammar school 10 years	15 (11.1)	6 (8.2)	
Secondary school 12 years	16 (11.9)	9 (12.3)	
Vocational training school	13 (9.6)	6 (8.2)	
Further education 1–2 years	26 (19.3)	12 (16.4)	
Tertiary education 3–4 years (Bachelor level)	46 (34.1)	29 (39.7)	
Advanced education (postgraduate)	18 (13.3)	10 (13.7)	
NA	1 (0.7)	1 (1.4)	
Smoking during pregnancy (yes/no), n (%)†	10 (7.4)	3 (4.1)	0.524
Parity (single/multi), n (%)†	75 (55.6)	39 (53.4)	0.882
Energy intake at enrollment, weeks 11–14 (kJ)‡§	8,019 (2,784)	7,540 (3,246)	0.829
Paternal characteristics	$n = 115$	$n = 65$	
BMI (kg/m²) at enrollment, weeks 11–14*	27.39 (4.51)	27.01 (4.52)	0.585
Offspring characteristics	$n = 135$	$n = 73$	
Sex, n (%)†			0.862
Male	69 (51.1)	39 (53.4)	
Female	66 (48.9)	34 (46.6)	
GA (weeks)*	40.17 (1.23)	40.01 (1.31)	0.393
Weight (g), birth*	3,724 (482)	3,677 (513)	0.515
Weight (kg), 9 months*‖	9.61 (1.03)	9.38 (1.15)	0.299
Weight (kg), 18 months*¶	11.86 (11.83)	11.26 (10.27)	0.014
Weight (kg), 36 months*#	15.30 (18.64)	14.71 (12.97)	0.141
Length (cm), birth***	52.50 (2.17)	52.48 (2.24)	0.958
Length (cm), 9 months*‖	73.14 (2.32)	72.99 (1.97)	0.740
Length (cm), 18 months*††	82.75 (2.87)	82.55 (2.48)	0.724
Height (cm), 36 months*‡‡	96.42 (4.21)	95.95 (3.07)	0.599
Breastfeeding, exclusively (weeks)*§§	10.98 (9.41)	8.38 (10.07)	0.163
Breastfeeding, partially (weeks)*§§	16.30 (11.05)	14.88 (10.71)	0.501

NA, not available. *Mean (SD), two-sided Student t test. †Frequencies, χ^2 test. ‡Median (interquartile range), two-sided Mann-Whitney U test. §Lifestyle intervention, $n = 133$; control, $n = 68$. ‖Lifestyle intervention, $n = 60$; control, $n = 39$. ¶Lifestyle intervention, $n = 58$; control, $n = 36$. #Lifestyle intervention, $n = 51$; control, $n = 29$. **Lifestyle intervention, $n = 129$; control, $n = 71$. ††Lifestyle intervention, $n = 57$; control, $n = 36$. ‡‡Lifestyle intervention, $n = 51$; control, $n = 28$. §§Lifestyle intervention, $n = 77$; control, $n = 42$.

including the same variables as above and calculated principal components (PCs) of the residuals from this model. The top five PCs were then used as covariates to correct for possible inflation, technical variation, and cell type composition.

Linear regression was used to assess whether cord blood DNA methylation (at sites significantly different between lifestyle intervention and control groups) is associated with lean mass at birth. Variables with a $P < 0.25$ in univariate analyses were incorporated in the final regression models (34), which included the following covariates: maternal smoking during pregnancy, GA, and offspring sex as well as factors with putative biological impact on DNA methylation (GWG and prepregnancy BMI). In this linear regression model, lean mass was the dependent variable and DNA methylation of respective site was the independent variable.

To assess if methylation in cord blood (at sites significantly different between the lifestyle intervention and control groups) is associated with growth in the offspring (at birth and at 9, 18, and 36 months of age), linear mixed models (LMMs) for repeated measurements were performed with random intercepts and different fixed slopes of BMI z scores for lifestyle intervention and control groups. BMI z scores, which are weight relative to height and adjusted for age and sex of the child, were calculated according to the World Health Organization using the *anthro* package in R (https://CRAN.R-project.org/package=anthro). Variables with $P < 0.25$ in univariate analyses were incorporated in final models (34). Models were adjusted for maternal education level, maternal smoking during pregnancy, GA, and parity, as well as factors with a likely biological impact on methylation (GWG, prepregnancy BMI, breastfeeding exclusively and partially [weeks], and offspring age at measurement). Association signals for specific methylation sites were considered significant ($P < 0.05$) if the direction of effect in the LMMs was consistent with at least three of the four time points in regular linear regression models.

Spearman correlations between CRP levels in pregnant mothers and cord blood DNA methylation of significant sites were performed. Grubbs test was used to detect outliers.

Table 2—Estimated differences from linear regression models in offspring lean mass and BMI z scores and their associated 95% CIs when comparing lifestyle intervention (n = 92) vs. control (n = 47) groups for subjects with available cord blood of the TOP-study

Phenotype	Estimated difference (95% CI)	P value
Lean mass (g), birth	126.55 (−4.52; 257.62)*	0.058*
Lean mass (%), birth	1.36 (−0.05; 2.77)*	0.059*
Abd. lean mass (g), birth	59.09 (10.53; 107.65)*	0.017*
Abd. lean mass (%), birth	0.88 (0.24; 1.53)*	0.008*
Fat mass (g), birth	51.26 (−19.93; 122.44)*	0.157*
Fat mass (%), birth	1.35 (−0.06; 2.76)*	0.061*
Abd. fat mass (g), birth	6.88 (−3.51; 17.26)*	0.192*
Abd. fat mass (%), birth	0.49 (−0.58; 1.57)*	0.365*
BMI z score, birth[1]	0.15 (−0.14; 0.43)†	0.352†
BMI z score, 9 months[2]	0.31 (−0.14; 0.76)‡	0.315‡
BMI z score, 18 months[3]	0.54 (0.14; 0.93)§	0.006§
BMI z score, 36 months[4]	0.30 (−0.13; 0.74)§	0.169§

[1]Lifestyle intervention, n = 129; control, n = 71. [2]Lifestyle intervention, n = 60; control, n = 39. [3]Lifestyle intervention, n = 57; control, n = 36. [4]Lifestyle intervention, n = 51; control, n = 28. *Adjusted for maternal education level, maternal smoking during pregnancy (yes/no), GWG (in kilograms), prepregnancy BMI, parity (single/multi), GA (in weeks), and offspring sex. †Adjusted for maternal education level, maternal smoking during pregnancy (yes/no), GWG (in kilograms), prepregnancy BMI, parity (single/multi), and GA (in weeks). ‡Adjusted for maternal education level, maternal smoking during pregnancy (yes/no), GWG (in kilograms), prepregnancy BMI, parity (single/multi), GA (in weeks), breastfeeding partially and exclusively, and BMI z score at birth. §Adjusted for maternal education level, maternal smoking during pregnancy (yes/no), GWG (in kilograms), prepregnancy BMI, parity (single/multi), breastfeeding partially and exclusively, and BMI z score at birth.

Statistical analyses were performed using the software R (24) (version 3.6.1) and RStudio (https://www.rstudio.com). Data are presented as mean ± SD, unless stated otherwise. Normalized methylation β-values were used for Spearman correlations and the analyses related to offspring body composition. Unless stated otherwise, models were corrected for multiple testing using false discovery rate (FDR) analysis (Benjamini-Hochberg) in which FDR <5% ($q < 0.05$) was considered significant. Bonferroni multiple-comparison post hoc correction was also used when testing if cord blood DNA methylation is associated with the lifestyle intervention, adjusting the linear model for maternal age, prepregnancy BMI, GWG, GA, and offspring sex.

Gene Ontology Analysis

To analyze possible biological functions of differential DNA methylation found in cord blood, we performed gene ontology (GO) mapping using Generic GO Term Mapper (35) and GO analysis using the gometh function in the missMethyl package (36). For GO mapping, we used Process Ontology in Homo sapiens, GOA slim, the list of the annotated genes, and $P < 0.01$. For GO analysis, we entered a list of the significantly associated methylation sites and removed redundant GO terms using REViGO (37). We allowed for 50% similarity between different GO terms, using Homo sapiens database and SimRel as the semantic similarity measure.

Causal Mediation Analysis

We performed a nonparametric causal mediation analysis, using the mediation R package and default settings (38), to investigate whether DNA methylation of any of the identified 25 sites in cord blood found to be associated with lean mass are part of a pathway through which the lifestyle intervention exerts its effects on lean mass. The effect is estimated for each association between treatment and outcome in participants with different methylation levels. DNA methylation of each respective site was designated as the mediator and lean mass as outcome. The models were adjusted for GWG, maternal BMI, GA, and offspring sex.

DNA Methylation in Muscle and Adipose Tissue

Sites showing differential cord blood methylation from the lifestyle intervention versus control group were also investigated in blood, muscle, and adipose tissue from participants in the Monozygotic Twin cohort. Infinium DNA methylation data from blood, adipose tissue, and muscle of the Monozygotic Twin cohort have been published (39,40). We used Spearman correlations to test whether methylation in blood correlates with methylation in muscle or adipose tissue for sites showing differential DNA methylation in cord blood from the TOP-study.

Data and Resource Availability

DNA methylation data from cord blood of the TOP-study (accession number LUDC2020.08.14) are deposited in the Lund University Diabetes Centre repository (https://www.ludc.lu.se/resources/repository) and are available upon request.

RESULTS

Impact of a Lifestyle Intervention During Pregnancy on DNA Methylation in Cord Blood

To assess if a lifestyle intervention in pregnant mothers with obesity had an effect on the methylome in cord blood, we analyzed DNA methylation in participants of the TOP-

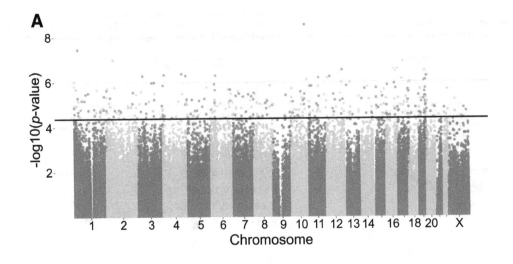

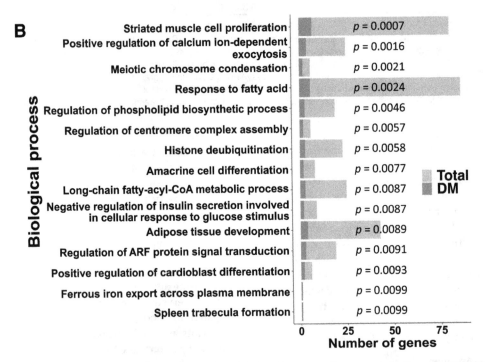

Figure 2—*A*: A Manhattan plot, representing the distribution of methylation sites across the genome, for the association between lifestyle intervention and offspring cord blood DNA methylation, after adjustment for covariates and cell composition adjustment. The black line shows the FDR threshold for multiple testing. Methylation sites that surpassed the FDR threshold ($P < 4.17 \times 10^{-5}$) are highlighted in color (red is hypermethylated and blue is hypomethylated sites in the lifestyle intervention group vs. the control group). *B*: Pathways from GO analysis after removal of redundant GO terms using REViGO ($P < 0.05$). The gray bars indicate the total number of genes in the pathway; the blue bars indicate the number of differently methylated (DM) genes in lifestyle intervention vs. control subjects. Data from *A* are also presented in Supplementary Table 1, and data from *B* are also presented in Supplementary Table 3.

study. Baseline characteristics of pregnant women with obesity included in the lifestyle intervention and control groups of the TOP-study, paternal BMI, as well as for their offspring at birth, are shown in Table 1. At enrollment, there was no difference in energy intake between the lifestyle intervention and control group (Table 1). Mothers in the lifestyle intervention group had a trend toward lower energy intake versus control subjects at weeks 36–38 supporting good adherence to the dietary intervention (Supplementary Fig. 1). During week 17 of pregnancy,

daily step counts were 8,623 ± 2,615 for participants in the lifestyle intervention. As wearing the pedometer was part of the lifestyle intervention, no step counts were available for control subjects. Offspring were similar regarding weight, length, and GA at birth and there were no detectable differences between the groups regarding breastfeeding (Table 1) or BMI *z* scores at birth or 9 or 36 months of age (Table 2).

We next examined if cord blood DNA methylation at individual sites differed between lifestyle intervention and control groups. DNA methylation at 379 sites ($q < 0.05$), as seen in Fig. 2A representing the distribution of methylation sites across the genome, annotated to 370 unique genes, was different between the lifestyle intervention and control groups when adjustment for cell composition was done using the Houseman reference-free method (32) and Benjamini-Hochberg FDR analysis was used to correct for multiple testing (Supplementary Table 1). Three of these sites were significant based on Bonferroni correction. None of these 379 significant sites had been associated with DNA methylation signatures related to cell composition in cord blood, and methylation of 376 of the 379 sites was nominally associated with the lifestyle intervention when adjustment for cell composition was done using the reference-based method with $P = 5.12 \times 10^{-7}$–3×10^{-2} (33) (Supplementary Table 1). Moreover, methylation of 377 out of 379 sites was nominally associated with the lifestyle intervention after adjusting for the first top five PCs of the residuals, $P = 3.08 \times 10^{-9}$–4.7×10^{-2} (Supplementary Table 1). All of these 377 sites had FDR <5% when we performed post hoc Benjamini-Hochberg FDR analysis on 379 sites. The lifestyle intervention was associated with methylation of these sites also when adjusting for fewer covariates and when adjusting for smoking ($P < 0.05$) (Supplementary Table 1), suggesting that these covariates did not substantially influence the association. Moreover, since GWG has been associated with DNA methylation in cord blood (14), we tested if GWG was associated with methylation of the 379 sites. However, no methylation sites were associated with GWG ($q < 0.05$). We also performed a model in which we adjusted for maternal age, maternal BMI, smoking, and GA as well as offspring sex, and then methylation of 377 out of 379 sites was associated with the lifestyle intervention, with $P = 1.3 \times 10^{-8}$–2.4×10^{-4} (Supplementary Table 1).

To understand the biological role of the 370 genes, we used GO Term Mapper and found that ~60% of the genes with differently methylated sites are involved in metabolic processes (Supplementary Table 2). Moreover, performing GO and REViGO analyses, we found 15 biological processes ($P < 0.01$). These include response to fatty acids, adipose tissue development, and negative regulation of insulin secretion involved in cellular response to glucose stimulus (35,37) (Fig. 2B and Supplementary Table 3).

Using the methylation quantitative trait loci (mQTL) database (https://mqtldb.org), we found that cord blood methylation of 110 out of our 379 sites has been associated with single nucleotide polymorphisms (SNPs), so-called mQTLs (Supplementary Table 4). These include cg21753618, which is among the three sites significant based on Bonferroni correction. Several of these sites also appear as mQTLs in peripheral blood in children and their mothers during childhood, adolescence, pregnancy, and middle age (Supplementary Tables 5 and 6). Among these mQTLs, 18 SNPs were associated with disease traits in the genome-wide association studies (GWAS) catalog

(Supplementary Table 4). Moreover, we found that methylation at 56 of the 110 mQTLs are associated with type 2 diabetes, obesity, maternal stress, and sperm viability in previous epigenome-wide association studies (https://bigd.big.ac.cn/ewas/datahub/index) (Supplementary Table 7).

We then tested if SNPs that map to any of the 370 genes included in Supplementary Table 1 have been associated with birth weight, childhood obesity, obesity, adiposity, or type 2 diabetes in published GWAS (41). Sixteen genes annotated to 15 sites (Supplementary Table 8) were linked to SNPs associated with these traits in GWAS: 3 SNPs were associated with adiposity (*MAP2K5*, *MEIS1*, and *IPO9*) (42,43) (downloaded 19 December 2019), 4 with obesity (*MAP2K5*, *PCDH9*, *SCNN1A*, and *TCF4*) (EFO_0001073, downloaded 19 December 2019), 4 genes (*ACSL1*, *HMGA2*, *RPSAP52*, and *SLC9B2*) have SNPs associated with type 2 diabetes (EFO_0001360, downloaded 19 December 2019), and 7 genes (*TENM4*, *HMGA2*, *MAP3K10*, *RB1*, *KLHL29*, *LRIG1*, and *PMFBP1*) have SNPs associated with birth weight (EFO_0004344, downloaded 23 June 2020) (41). None of the discovered genes have SNPs associated with childhood obesity (41,44) (downloaded 22 June 2020). None of these 15 sites were among the 3 significant sites based on Bonferroni correction.

We further examined if our 379 sites were overrepresented within other epigenetic marks such as histone modifications representing active (H3K4me1 and H3K27ac) or inactive (H3K27me3) chromatin. We intersected the position of 379 sites with chromatin immunoprecipitation sequencing data of histone modifications in blood mononuclear cells from the Roadmap Epigenomics Consortium (45). A permutation distribution test using 10,000 permutations showed more significant methylation sites overlapping with H3K4me1 ($P = 0.030$) but not H3K27me3 ($P = 0.356$) and H3K27ac ($P = 0.535$), compared with what would have been expected by chance if all sites on the array were analyzed, indicating an enrichment of enhancer elements in sites differentially methylated in the lifestyle intervention.

We have previously shown that CRP levels were lower in pregnant mothers in lifestyle intervention versus control subjects (46). Therefore, we tested whether CRP levels in pregnant mothers correlated with cord blood methylation of our 379 sites. CRP levels correlated with methylation of two sites: cg17389519, which is annotated to *PTF1A* encoding a transcription factor involved in pancreas and neural tissue development (47), and cg27394563, annotated to *SART3* (Supplementary Fig. 2A and B).

Impact of a Lifestyle Intervention During Pregnancy on Offspring Lean Mass

We proceeded to study the body composition of the offspring (Tables 1 and 2). Offspring to mothers included in the lifestyle intervention group were born with 59 g (95% CI 11; 108) ($P = 0.017$) and 0.88 percentage points (95% CI 0.24; 1.53) ($P = 0.008$) more abdominal lean mass versus control subjects (Fig. 3 and Table 2). We also

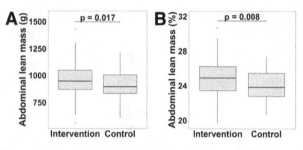

Figure 3—Boxplots are showing abdominal lean mass (g) (*A*) and abdominal lean mass (%) (*B*) in the lifestyle intervention and control groups at birth in median (interquartile range). The *P* values are based on linear regression models adjusted for maternal education level, maternal smoking during pregnancy (yes/no), GWG (kg), pre-pregnancy BMI (kg/m^2), parity (single/multi), GA (weeks), and offspring sex. Data are also presented in Table 2.

observed a trend that offspring of mothers included in the lifestyle intervention group were born with 127 g (95% CI −5; 258) (*P* = 0.058) and 1.36 percentage points (95% CI −0.05; 2.77) (*P* = 0.059) more lean mass versus control subjects (Table 2). At birth, the offspring were similar in size (Tables 1 and 2), indicating that it is the body composition that differs between the groups. We found that offspring of both groups were similar in size at 9 and 36 months of age; however, at 18 months, children from the lifestyle intervention group were larger in size (Tables 1 and 2).

Associations Between DNA Methylation in Cord Blood and Offspring Lean Mass and Growth

Offspring in the lifestyle intervention group had more lean mass at birth and differential cord blood methylation at 379 sites versus control subjects (Table 2 and Supplementary Table 1); thus, we further tested whether there were associations between methylation of these 379 sites and lean mass (percentage) at birth in the offspring. Cord blood methylation of 25 sites was associated with lean mass (*q* < 0.05) (Supplementary Table 9). For the majority of these sites (80%), cord blood methylation levels were higher in the lifestyle intervention group and positively associated with greater lean mass.

We proceeded to assess whether cord blood methylation of the 379 sites was associated with growth over time in the offspring using LMMs and BMI *z* scores at birth and 9, 18, and 36 months of age. We found that methylation of 22 sites was associated with BMI *z* scores (*P* < 0.05). Next, we performed linear regression models to test if methylation at the 379 sites was associated with BMI *z* scores at each time point. The direction of effects for the LMMs was consistent with that for the linear regression models at all time points but for two sites; for these two sites, the direction altered at one time point (Supplementary Table 10). Included within the genes annotated to the 22 sites are *ACSL1*, which is involved in fatty acid β-oxidation and harboring a SNP associated with type 2 diabetes, and *TCF4*, encoding a transcription factor involved in Wnt signaling

and harboring a SNP associated with obesity (EFO_0001073, downloaded 19 December 2019) in GWAS (41) (Supplementary Table 8).

Causal Mediation Analysis

We next used a causal mediation analysis (38) to investigate whether DNA methylation of any of the 25 sites in cord blood found to be associated with lean mass are part of a pathway through which the lifestyle intervention exerts its effects on offspring lean mass. The mediation analysis breaks down the total effect of treatment (lifestyle intervention) on outcome (lean mass) into two parts: first, the indirect effect acting via the mediator of interest (DNA methylation) and second, the direct effect acting directly or via a mediator other than what is under study. The analyses showed that *1*) the lifestyle intervention has an overall effect of β = 1.35 (95% CI −0.092; 2.741) on lean mass, *2*) that effect may operate via an indirect path (indirect effect), possibly through methylation, with a significant average causal mediator effect for 17 methylation sites (*q* < 0.05) (Table 3), and *3*) consequently, the total effect of the lifestyle intervention on lean mass, 32.0–61.8%, is suggested to act via these 17 methylation sites. According to these results, we may call methylation of these sites partial mediators.

Cross-Tissue Methylation of Sites Associated With Lean Mass or Growth

We finally examined whether DNA methylation in blood of the 46 unique sites (one methylation site, cg11594420, overlap) associated with lean mass or growth in the offspring mirrors the methylation pattern in two other tissues of importance for obesity and type 2 diabetes: skeletal muscle and adipose tissue. We used available methylation array data from blood, muscle, and adipose tissue taken from the same individuals (39,40) (Supplementary Table 11). Among these sites, the methylation pattern in blood correlated positively with methylation of four sites in adipose tissue and two sites in muscle (*P* < 0.05) (Supplementary Table 12). Five correlations were nominal and one significant after FDR. These findings suggest that methylation of a few sites may have a biological role in tissues of relevance for obesity and type 2 diabetes.

DISCUSSION

This is, to our knowledge, the first genome-wide epigenetic analysis in cord blood of pregnant women with obesity randomized to a lifestyle intervention including physical activity, with or without a hypocaloric Mediterranean-style diet, versus control subjects receiving standard of care. There are four key findings: first, DNA methylation at individual sites in cord blood differed between lifestyle intervention and control subjects. These sites were annotated to genes overrepresented in relevant GO terms (e.g., response to fatty acids and adipose tissue development). Second, we found that genes linked to SNPs associated

Table 3—Causal mediation analysis on the significant associations between the lifestyle intervention and lean mass–related methylation (CpG) sites as mediators and lean mass (%) as outcome (ACME q value <0.05)

CpG site	Gene	ACME estimate of mediator CpG (95% CI)	ACME q value	ADE estimate (95% CI)	Total effect (95% CI)	Proportion mediated by CpG (%) (95% CI)
cg07405330	MOBP	0.84 (0.35; 1.39)	<0.001	0.52 (−0.84; 1.89)	1.35 (−0.09; 2.74)	0.62 (−0.73; 3.58)
cg06480224	KIAA2012	0.78 (0.19; 1.51)	0.013	0.57 (−0.97; 1.98)	1.35 (−0.09; 2.74)	0.58 (−1.11; 4.27)
cg11612786	AC079135.1;GBX2	0.64 (0.13; 1.38)	0.013	0.71 (−0.66; 2.03)	1.35 (−0.09; 2.74)	0.47 (−0.58; 2.78)
cg20982052		0.53 (0.14; 1.11)	0.013	0.82 (−0.68; 2.18)	1.35 (−0.09; 2.74)	0.39 (−0.62; 2.63)
cg00154557	DSE	0.50 (0.08; 1.08)	0.021	0.86 (−0.64; 2.26)	1.35 (−0.09; 2.74)	0.37 (−0.58; 2.42)
cg13002044	TMEM178B	0.70 (0.14; 1.42)	0.021	0.65 (−0.73; 1.98)	1.35 (−0.09; 2.74)	0.52 (−0.85; 2.87)
cg18088415	LSM2	0.70 (0.19; 1.41)	0.021	0.65 (−0.77; 2.07)	1.35 (−0.09; 2.74)	0.52 (−0.73; 3.42)
cg11594420	TEX101	0.53 (0.10; 1.18)	0.025	0.82 (−0.59; 2.15)	1.35 (−0.09; 2.74)	0.39 (−0.45; 2.84)
cg04678315		0.48 (0.08; 1.02)	0.028	0.87 (−0.56; 2.20)	1.35 (−0.09; 2.74)	0.36 (−0.64; 2.05)
cg08144675		0.70 (0.10; 1.42)	0.032	0.66 (−0.85; 2.20)	1.35 (−0.09; 2.74)	0.52 (−0.98; 3.35)
cg22454673	HERC2	0.63 (0.16; 1.29)	0.032	0.73 (−0.71; 2.18)	1.35 (−0.09; 2.74)	0.46 (−0.77; 3.10)
cg04058675	HUWE1	0.45 (0.08; 1.03)	0.033	0.90 (−0.46; 2.22)	1.35 (−0.09; 2.74)	0.34 (−0.48; 2.09)
cg03190725	RP3-468B3.2	0.54 (0.10; 1.10)	0.035	0.81 (−0.67; 2.19)	1.35 (−0.09; 2.74)	0.40 (−0.65; 2.58)
cg06799721	TARS	0.52 (0.05; 1.27)	0.036	0.84 (−0.54; 2.07)	1.35 (−0.09; 2.74)	0.38 (−0.30; 2.00)
cg15157974	DISC1	0.43 (0.04; 0.96)	0.040	0.92 (−0.50; 2.21)	1.35 (−0.09; 2.74)	0.32 (−0.24; 2.10)
cg26142132	AAT	0.45 (0.06; 0.96)	0.041	0.90 (−0.57; 2.40)	1.35 (−0.09; 2.74)	0.34 (−0.44; 2.26)
cg00354884	ABR	0.53 (0.03; 1.18)	0.047	0.83 (−0.62; 2.17)	1.35 (−0.09; 2.74)	0.39 (−0.45; 2.32)

Models adjusted for GWG (in kilograms), maternal BMI, GA (in weeks), and offspring sex. Based on 139 participants, lifestyle intervention, $n = 92$, and control, $n = 47$. ACME, average causal mediator effect; ADE, average direct effect.

with birth weight, obesity, adiposity, and type 2 diabetes by GWAS have been also annotated to sites that have altered DNA methylation in our study. Additionally, SNPs previously associated with DNA methylation in cord blood of our identified sites were linked to disease traits in the GWAS catalog. Third, offspring to mothers included in the lifestyle intervention were born with more lean mass. Finally, methylation at 17 sites partially mediates the effect of the lifestyle intervention on lean mass in the offspring. Together, these data provide evidence that the presented lifestyle intervention altered the epigenome of genes linked to metabolism and metabolic disease in offspring cord blood from pregnant mothers with obesity.

Previous studies have shown that tissues from people with obesity have different methylation profiles versus lean people (13,16,48); however, DNA methylation can be changed by lifestyle (40,49). Obesity during pregnancy increases the risk of metabolic disease in offspring (2), and obesity in pregnant mothers is associated with epigenetic alterations in cord blood (17). We demonstrate that exercise and healthy diets during pregnancy can change cord blood DNA methylation and that these epigenetic changes took place on genes involved in metabolic processes. It is possible that a healthier lifestyle during pregnancy and the consequential epigenetic changes help enhance the offspring's health later in life. The epigenetic mechanisms linked to exercise and healthy diets in our study seem to be different compared with those previously associated with maternal BMI (17) and gestational diabetes (16,19).

We demonstrate that offspring to mothers in the lifestyle intervention have higher abdominal and a trend toward higher total lean mass versus control subjects. This result indicates a positive effect of the lifestyle intervention on the offspring as they were born with more metabolically active tissue, which might protect against future metabolic diseases. This is supported by studies showing that the body composition of newborns being born small for GA (SGA) differs more in terms of less lean mass than differences in fat mass, compared with appropriate-for-gestational-age newborns (50), and SGA increases the risk of metabolic disease later in life (51). Thereby, suggesting that negative effects of being born SGA could be due to decreased lean mass. Increased muscle mass and higher metabolic activity on the other hand may have beneficial effects on insulin sensitivity and protect from obesity and type 2 diabetes (7). We found associations between cord blood epigenetics and lean mass in the offspring at birth. For the majority of these sites, methylation levels were higher in cord blood of the lifestyle intervention group and positively associated with greater lean mass, and methylation at several sites seems to partially mediate the lifestyle effect on lean mass. Interestingly, the lifestyle intervention group had decreased methylation of SETD3, which encodes a methyltransferase. Hypomethylation of SETD3 correlates with increased expression and, in turn, increased muscle mass (52), which might in part explain the greater lean mass we see in the offspring of the lifestyle intervention group.

Finally, we found that blood-based methylation of sites associated with lean mass or growth in the offspring mirrors methylation patterns in muscle and adipose tissue, tissues of importance for metabolic disease (39,40). These include sites annotated to TCF4 and SYT9 encoding transcription factor 4 and synaptotagmin 9, respectively, which have been implicated in diabetes-related traits (53,54). Although these results are based on nominally significant P values, they give a possible indication that methylation of some identified sites may also have a biological role in tissues of importance for obesity and type 2 diabetes.

Strengths and Limitations

A strength of this study is the randomized design, the high rate of completers in the TOP-study, and the relatively homogenous study population in terms of prepregnancy BMI and ethnicity, which should reduce the risk of bias. A pedometer intervention is an inexpensive method for increasing daily physical activity and can easily be implemented into daily life. Other physical activity interventions often include attendance to classes, which can be difficult to implement. It is also a strength that we used several different methods to adjust the methylation data for cell composition and technical variation, which showed that DNA methylation of a large proportion of the identified sites was associated with the lifestyle intervention independent of the method used, although the strength of the associations was reduced for the reference-based compared with the reference-free method. It is important to adjust cord blood DNA methylation data for cell type composition. For discovery of our significant DNA methylation results, we used the reference-free method developed by Houseman et al. (32) for deconvolving heterogeneous cell mixtures. We then used the reference-based (33) and PCA-based methods to validate our results. These different methods (e.g., reference-based vs. reference-free) have their pros and cons. A reference-based method might provide robust estimations. However, it is usually based on few samples with limited clinical conditions. For umbilical cord blood, there is an available reference of 26 samples (33), which might not be able cover the variance in our data set, as it is eight times larger. In the publication by Houseman et al. (32), they show via a simulation study and several real data analyses that their method can perform as well as or better than methods that make explicit use of reference data sets. They also discuss that this reference-free method may adjust for detailed cell type differences that may be unavailable in existing reference data sets. Additionally, the algorithm estimates the number of cell types, meaning it should also consider the nucleated red blood cells that cord blood contains.

Furthermore, in this study, we used two methods to correct for multiple testing, Benjamini-Hochberg and Bonferroni. However, Bonferroni is known to be too conservative for epigenome-wide association studies since DNA methylation values at nearby probes are known to be correlated and many sites on the array are nonvariable (55,56). The alternative approach, Benjamini-Hochberg adjustment, is potentially a more powerful method identifying the associated sites with the phenotype of interest, but it may also generate some false-positive results. The PCA-based method that we used may, however, reduce false-positive results.

A limitation is that the two lifestyle intervention groups were merged. This was, however, necessary to have sufficient statistical power due to the modest number of samples with cord blood in each group. However, we have shown that lifestyle interventions in the TOP-study were effective and could reduce GWG (9), suggesting that both interventions successfully achieved the main primary end point, thus reducing potential bias when merging them. It should also be noted that the maternal energy intake is self-reported and may infer a type of reporting bias. Nevertheless, the maternal energy intake at late gestation was reduced in the lifestyle intervention group versus control subjects, indicating a successful intervention. Previous dietary analyses of participants in the TOP-study showed that participants having dietary and physical activity intervention changed their dietary composition in a healthier direction (12). Participants in the group only performing physical activity demonstrated a trend toward dietary changes in the same direction (12). This supports the approach of merging the intervention groups.

As in other intervention studies of pregnant women with obesity, it might be a challenge that the intervention intensity was too low, and a high proportion of the participants were noncompliant to the recommended diet and physical activity intervention. Few women achieved the target of the physical activity intervention, possibly indicating that this target was set high for this group and should be revised for future studies.

Of note, the methylation array covers ~2% of sites in the human genome, and it is therefore possible that methylation of additional sites may be associated with the intervention. Future studies are needed to fully understand the biology behind the associations presented in this article and their possible health effects.

In summary, this study demonstrates that a lifestyle intervention in pregnant women with obesity is associated with the cord blood epigenome in offspring. We also provide evidence that epigenetic markers in cord blood associate with lean mass and growth in offspring. These results underline that the intrauterine environment in humans might have the ability to program the epigenome, which in turn may affect metabolism and growth later in life.

Acknowledgments. The authors thank Marlena Maziarz, Department of Clinical Sciences, Lund University/CRC, Skåne University Hospital SUS, Malmö, Sweden, for guidance and expertise in biostatistics and Silja Schrader, Epigenetics and Diabetes Unit, Department of Clinical Sciences, Lund University Diabetes Centre, Lund University, Scania University Hospital, Malmö, Sweden, for help with power calculations. The authors also thank the Danish Diabetes Academy via the Novo Nordisk Foundation for support throughout this project and the National Bioinformatics Infrastructure Sweden, SciLifeLab (Uppsala, Sweden), for the bioinformatics long-term support with Nikolay Oskolkov.

Funding. Sygekassernes Helsefond, Hartmann Fonden, Hvidovre Hospital, and The Danish Council for Strategic Research supported the TOP-study. The work performed by A.C.E. and P.W.F. was supported by grants from the European Foundation for the Study of Diabetes, Vetenskapsrådet, Hjärt-Lungfonden, the H2020 European Research Council (CoG-2015_681742_NASCENT), and Novo Nordisk Fonden. The work performed by J.J., S.G.-C., A.P., and C.L. was supported by grants from the Novo Nordisk Fonden, Vetenskapsrådet, and Region Skåne (ALF), an H2020 European Research Council co-grant (PAINTBOX, number 725840), H2020 Marie Skłodowska-Curie Actions grant agreement 706081 (Epi-Hope), Hjärt-Lungfonden, EXODIAB, Stiftelsen för Strategisk Forskning (IRC15-0067), and Diabetesförbundet. All researchers from Lund University Diabetes Centre were supported by a research center grant from the Swedish Strategic Science Foundation.

Duality of Interest. No potential conflicts of interest relevant to this article were reported.

Author Contributions. J.J. analyzed data, performed the statistical analyses, and drafted and revised the manuscript. K.M.R., A.V., P.W.F., and C.L. designed and planned the current study and participated in drafting the manuscript. K.M.R. and K.N. designed and planned the TOP-study. K.M.R. and E.M.C. conducted the TOP-study and collected data. S.G.-C. participated in analyzing data and drafting the manuscript. A.P. performed DNA methylation analysis. A.C.E. contributed to designing the study and performed statistical analyses. M.V.L. interpreted data and gave statistical support. M.V.L., K.F.M., and E.M.C. collected data on the offspring at follow-up after delivery. L.H. contributed to planning the epigenetic part of the study. E.M.C. analyzed the DXA scans. P.W.F. and C.L. supervised the analyses. All authors reviewed and provided critical comments on the manuscript. J.J. and K.M.R. are the guarantors of this work and, as such, had full access to all the data in the study and take responsibility for the integrity of the data and the accuracy of the data analysis.

References

1. Rasmussen KM, Yaktine AL (Eds). *Weight Gain During Pregnancy: Reexamining the Guidelines*. Washington (DC), National Academies Press, 2009

2. Gu S, An X, Fang L, et al. Risk factors and long-term health consequences of macrosomia: a prospective study in Jiangsu Province, China. J Biomed Res 2012; 26:235–240

3. Simmonds M, Llewellyn A, Owen CG, Woolacott N. Predicting adult obesity from childhood obesity: a systematic review and meta-analysis. Obes Rev 2016; 17:95–107

4. Ervin RB. Prevalence of metabolic syndrome among adults 20 years of age and over, by sex, age, race and ethnicity, and body mass index: United States, 2003-2006. Natl Health Stat Rep 2009;13:1–7

5. Franks PW, Hanson RL, Knowler WC, Sievers ML, Bennett PH, Looker HC. Childhood obesity, other cardiovascular risk factors, and premature death. N Engl J Med 2010;362:485–493

6. Global Burden of Disease Collaborative Network. Global Burden of Disease Study 2015 (GBD 2015) Obesity and Overweight Prevalence 1980-2015, 2017. Institute for Health Metrics and Evaluation. Accessed 11 March 2020. Available from http://ghdx.healthdata.org/record/ihme-data/gbd-2015-obesity-and-overweight-prevalence-1980-2015

7. Kim G, Lee SE, Jun JE, et al. Increase in relative skeletal muscle mass over time and its inverse association with metabolic syndrome development: a 7-year retrospective cohort study. Cardiovasc Diabetol 2018;17:23

8. Bann D, Wills A, Cooper R, et al.; NSHD Scientific and Data Collection Team. Birth weight and growth from infancy to late adolescence in relation to fat and lean mass in early old age: findings from the MRC National Survey of Health and Development. Int J Obes 2014;38:69–75

9. Renault KM, Nørgaard K, Nilas L, et al. The Treatment of Obese Pregnant Women (TOP) study: a randomized controlled trial of the effect of physical activity intervention assessed by pedometer with or without dietary intervention in obese pregnant women. Am J Obstet Gynecol 2014;210:134.e1–134.e9

10. Carlsen EM, Renault KM, Nørgaard K, et al. Newborn regional body composition is influenced by maternal obesity, gestational weight gain and the birthweight standard score. Acta Paediatr 2014;103:939–945

11. Renault KM, Carlsen EM, Nørgaard K, et al. Intake of carbohydrates during pregnancy in obese women is associated with fat mass in the newborn offspring. Am J Clin Nutr 2015;102:1475–1481

12. Renault KM, Carlsen EM, Nørgaard K, et al. Intake of sweets, snacks and soft drinks predicts weight gain in obese pregnant women: detailed analysis of the results of a randomised controlled trial. PLoS One 2015;10: e0133041

13. Ling C, Rönn T. Epigenetics in human obesity and type 2 diabetes. Cell Metab 2019;29:1028–1044

14. Morales E, Groom A, Lawlor DA, Relton CL. DNA methylation signatures in cord blood associated with maternal gestational weight gain: results from the ALSPAC cohort. BMC Res Notes 2014;7:278

15. Jørgensen SW, Brøns C, Bluck L, et al. Metabolic response to 36 hours of fasting in young men born small vs appropriate for gestational age. Diabetologia 2015;58:178–187

16. Hjort L, Martino D, Grunnet LG, et al. Gestational diabetes and maternal obesity are associated with epigenome-wide methylation changes in children. JCI Insight 2018;3:e122572

17. Sharp GC, Salas LA, Monnereau C, et al. Maternal BMI at the start of pregnancy and offspring epigenome-wide DNA methylation: findings from the pregnancy and childhood epigenetics (PACE) consortium. Hum Mol Genet 2017; 26:4067–4085

18. Heijmans BT, Tobi EW, Stein AD, et al. Persistent epigenetic differences associated with prenatal exposure to famine in humans. Proc Natl Acad Sci U S A 2008;105:17046–17049

19. Howe CG, Cox B, Fore R, et al. Maternal gestational diabetes mellitus and newborn DNA methylation: findings from the pregnancy and childhood epigenetics consortium. Diabetes Care 2020;43:98–105

20. Geraghty AA, Sexton-Oates A, O'Brien EC, et al. A low glycaemic index diet in pregnancy induces DNA methylation variation in blood of newborns: results from the ROLO randomised controlled trial. Nutrients 2018;10:455

21. Renault K, Nørgaard K, Andreasen KR, Secher NJ, Nilas L. Physical activity during pregnancy in obese and normal-weight women as assessed by pedometer. Acta Obstet Gynecol Scand 2010;89:956–961

22. Ejlerskov KT, Christensen LB, Ritz C, Jensen SM, Mølgaard C, Michaelsen KF. The impact of early growth patterns and infant feeding on body composition at 3 years of age. Br J Nutr 2015;114:316–327

23. Bibikova M, Barnes B, Tsan C, et al. High density DNA methylation array with single CpG site resolution. Genomics 2011;98:288–295

24. R Core Team. A language and environment for statistical computing version 3.6.1. Vienna, Austria, R Foundation for Statistical Computing, 2019

25. Du P, Kibbe WA, Lin SM. lumi: a pipeline for processing Illumina microarray. Bioinformatics 2008;24:1547–1548

26. Davis S, Du P, Bilke S, Triche T Jr., Bootwalla M. methylumi: Handle Illumina methylation data. R package version 2.28.0, Bioconductor, 2018

27. McCartney DL, Walker RM, Morris SW, McIntosh AM, Porteous DJ, Evans KL. Identification of polymorphic and off-target probe binding sites on the Illumina Infinium MethylationEPIC BeadChip. Genom Data 2016;9:22–24

28. Du P, Zhang X, Huang CC, et al. Comparison of Beta-value and M-value methods for quantifying methylation levels by microarray analysis. BMC Bioinformatics 2010;11:587

29. Teschendorff AE, Marabita F, Lechner M, et al. A beta-mixture quantile normalization method for correcting probe design bias in Illumina Infinium 450 k DNA methylation data. Bioinformatics 2013;29:189–196

30. Johnson WE, Li C, Rabinovic A. Adjusting batch effects in microarray expression data using empirical Bayes methods. Biostatistics 2007;8:118–127

31. Leek JT, Johnson WE, Parker HS, Jaffe AE, Storey JD. The sva package for removing batch effects and other unwanted variation in high-throughput experiments. Bioinformatics 2012;28:882–883

32. Houseman EA, Molitor J, Marsit CJ. Reference-free cell mixture adjustments in analysis of DNA methylation data. Bioinformatics 2014;30:1431–1439

33. Gervin K, Salas LA, Bakulski KM, et al. Systematic evaluation and validation of reference and library selection methods for deconvolution of cord blood DNA methylation data. Clin Epigenetics 2019;11:125

34. Bursac Z, Gauss CH, Williams DK, Hosmer DW. Purposeful selection of variables in logistic regression. Source Code Biol Med 2008;3:17

35. Boyle EI, Weng S, Gollub J, et al. GO:TermFinder: open source software for accessing Gene Ontology information and finding significantly enriched Gene Ontology terms associated with a list of genes. Bioinformatics 2004;20:3710–3715

36. Phipson B, Maksimovic J, Oshlack A. missMethyl: an R package for analyzing data from Illumina's HumanMethylation450 platform. Bioinformatics 2016;32: 286–288

37. Supek F, Bošnjak M, Škunca N, Šmuc T. REVIGO summarizes and visualizes long lists of gene ontology terms. PLoS One 2011;6:e21800

38. Tingley D, Yamamoto T, Hirose K, Keele L, Imai K. mediation: R package for causal mediation analysis. J Stat Softw 2014;59:38

39. Nilsson E, Jansson PA, Perfilyev A, et al. Altered DNA methylation and differential expression of genes influencing metabolism and inflammation in adipose tissue from subjects with type 2 diabetes. Diabetes 2014;63:2962–2976

40. Nitert MD, Dayeh T, Volkov P, et al. Impact of an exercise intervention on DNA methylation in skeletal muscle from first-degree relatives of patients with type 2 diabetes. Diabetes 2012;61:3322–3332

41. Buniello A, MacArthur JAL, Cerezo M, et al. The NHGRI-EBI GWAS Catalog of published genome-wide association studies, targeted arrays and summary statistics 2019. Nucleic Acids Res 2019;47:D1005–D1012

42. Graff M, Scott RA, Justice AE, et al.; CHARGE Consortium; EPIC-InterAct Consortium; PAGE Consortium. Genome-wide physical activity interactions in adiposity: a meta-analysis of 200,452 adults. PLoS Genet 2017;13: e1006528

43. Karlsson T, Rask-Andersen M, Pan G, et al. Contribution of genetics to visceral adiposity and its relation to cardiovascular and metabolic disease. Nat Med 2019;25:1390–1395

44. Bradfield JP, Vogelezang S, Felix JF, et al.; Early Growth Genetics Consortium. A trans-ancestral meta-analysis of genome-wide association studies reveals loci associated with childhood obesity. Hum Mol Genet 2019;28:3327–3338

45. Kundaje A, Meuleman W, Ernst J, et al.; Roadmap Epigenomics Consortium. Integrative analysis of 111 reference human epigenomes. Nature 2015;518:317–330

46. Renault KM, Carlsen EM, Hædersdal S, et al. Impact of lifestyle intervention for obese women during pregnancy on maternal metabolic and inflammatory markers. Int J Obes 2017;41:598–605

47. Jin K, Xiang M. Transcription factor Ptf1a in development, diseases and reprogramming. Cell Mol Life Sci 2019;76:921–940

48. Davegårdh C, Broholm C, Perfilyev A, et al. Abnormal epigenetic changes during differentiation of human skeletal muscle stem cells from obese subjects. BMC Med 2017;15:39

49. Perfilyev A, Dahlman I, Gillberg L, et al. Impact of polyunsaturated and saturated fat overfeeding on the DNA-methylation pattern in human adipose tissue: a randomized controlled trial. Am J Clin Nutr 2017;105:991–1000

50. Hediger ML, Overpeck MD, Kuczmarski RJ, McGlynn A, Maurer KR, Davis WW. Muscularity and fatness of infants and young children born small- or large-for-gestational-age. Pediatrics 1998;102:E60

51. Hattersley AT, Tooke JE. The fetal insulin hypothesis: an alternative explanation of the association of low birthweight with diabetes and vascular disease. Lancet 1999;353:1789–1792

52. Seaborne RA, Strauss J, Cocks M, et al. Human skeletal muscle possesses an epigenetic memory of hypertrophy. Sci Rep 2018;8:1898

53. Wei H, Qu H, Wang H, et al. 1,25-Dihydroxyvitamin-D3 prevents the development of diabetic cardiomyopathy in type 1 diabetic rats by enhancing

autophagy via inhibiting the β-catenin/TCF4/GSK-3β/mTOR pathway. J Steroid Biochem Mol Biol 2017;168:71–90

54.　Shim YJ, Kim JE, Hwang SK, et al. Identification of candidate gene variants in Korean MODY families by whole-exome sequencing. Horm Res Paediatr 2015;83: 242–251

55.　Mansell G, Gorrie-Stone TJ, Bao Y, et al. Guidance for DNA methylation studies: statistical insights from the Illumina EPIC array. BMC Genomics 2019;20: 366

56.　Saffari A, Silver MJ, Zavattari P, et al. Estimation of a significance threshold for epigenome-wide association studies. Genet Epidemiol 2018;42:20–33

Pathogenesis Study Based on High-Throughput Single-Cell Sequencing Analysis Reveals Novel Transcriptional Landscape and Heterogeneity of Retinal Cells in Type 2 Diabetic Mice

Tian Niu, Junwei Fang, Xin Shi, Mengya Zhao, Xindan Xing, Yihan Wang, Shaopin Zhu, and Kun Liu

Diabetes 2021;70:1185–1197 | *https://doi.org/10.2337/db20-0839*

Diabetic retinopathy (DR) is the leading cause of acquired blindness in middle-aged people. The complex pathology of DR is difficult to dissect, given the convoluted cytoarchitecture of the retina. Here, we performed single-cell RNA sequencing (scRNA-seq) of retina from a model of type 2 diabetes, induced in leptin receptor–deficient (*db/db*) and control *db/m* mice, with the aim of elucidating the factors mediating the pathogenesis of DR. We identified 11 cell types and determined cell-type-specific expression of DR-associated loci via genome-wide association study (GWAS)-based enrichment analysis. DR also impacted cell-type-specific genes and altered cell-cell communication. Based on the scRNA-seq results, retinaldehyde-binding protein 1 (RLBP1) was investigated as a promising therapeutic target for DR. Retinal RLBP1 expression was decreased in diabetes, and its overexpression in Müller glia mitigated DR-associated neurovascular degeneration. These data provide a detailed analysis of the retina under diabetic and normal conditions, revealing new insights into pathogenic factors that may be targeted to treat DR and related dysfunctions.

Diabetic retinopathy (DR) is the leading cause of acquired blindness in middle-aged people and imparts a substantial burden on global public health resources (1). Although commonly regarded as a microvascular complication of diabetes, neurodegeneration is now recognized to precede any microvascular dysfunction (2).

Intraocular DR treatment strategies aim to alleviate microvascular complications and focus on advanced-stage disease (3). However, laser therapy primarily preserves useful vision, and reversal of vision loss is uncommon. Although anti–vascular endothelial growth factor (VEGF) treatment is a mainstream treatment strategy for macular edema or proliferative DR (PDR), it is not universally available, and some patients become resistant after long-term administration (4). Intravitreal steroid use causes considerable side effects, such as glaucoma and cataracts, whereas vitrectomy alleviates severe complications (5). As existing therapies exclusively target advanced DR with permanent vision damage, strategies for prevention and early intervention are urgently required.

Transcriptomic profiling of the aqueous humor, vitreous humor, and retinal tissue has provided insight into the large-scale genomic changes that occur during DR pathogenesis and can help identify biomarkers and therapeutic targets (6–8). Nevertheless, the retina is a complex tissue with several cell types. Existing DR transcriptomic profiles are basced on heterogeneous mixtures of cells, concealing crucial information regarding vulnerable cell types. Single-cell RNA sequencing (scRNA-seq) is an unbiased and powerful method for characterizing different cell types in complex tissues in the contexts of health and disease (9).

As 90% of diabetes cases are cases of type 2 diabetes, we used a mouse model of type 2 diabetes induced by leptin receptor deficiency (10,11), and we performed high-resolution scRNA-seq to capture diabetes-induced gene alterations in

Department of Ophthalmology, Shanghai General Hospital, Shanghai Jiao Tong University School of Medicine; National Clinical Research Center for Eye Diseases; Shanghai Key Laboratory of Ocular Fundus Diseases; Shanghai Engineering Center for Visual Science and Photo Medicine; and Shanghai Engineering Center for Precise Diagnosis and Treatment of Eye Diseases, Shanghai, China

Corresponding author: Kun Liu, drliukun@sjtu.edu.cn

Received 15 August 2020 and accepted 26 February 2021

This article contains supplementary material online at https://doi.org/10.2337/figshare.14120015.

T.N. and J.F. contributed equally to the study.

thousands of individual retinal cells, providing novel insights regarding the cellular and molecular alterations of various retinal cell types in DR.

RESEARCH DESIGN AND METHODS

Animals

All animal studies were approved by the Shanghai Jiao Tong University School of Medicine Animal Care and Use Committee and performed according to the guidelines of the Association for Research in Vision and Ophthalmology in the Statement for the Use of Animals in Ophthalmic and Visual Research. Male homozygous *db/db* mice (BKS.Cg-Dock7m$^{+/+}$ Leprdb/J) and *db/m* (Dock7m$^{+/+}$ Leprdb) heterozygotes from the same colony were purchased from The Jackson Laboratory (Bar Harbor, ME) and housed in a pathogen-free environment with a 12-h light/dark cycle at 22 ± 1°C with free access to food and water.

After the mice were fasted for 6 h, body weights and tail blood glucose levels were monitored monthly from 2 to 8 months of age. For glucose tolerance tests, mice were fasted overnight before being administered 2 g/kg body weight glucose i.p., and tail blood glucose levels were measured 0, 15, 30, 60, 90, and 120 min later with a glucometer. The area under the curve was calculated at 2 and 8 months of age.

Study Design: Experiment 1

Retinal Cell Dissection and Dissociation

Three *db/m* and *db/db* mice each were sacrificed at 8 months of age. One eye from each mouse was used for scRNA-seq, and the other was used for generation of retinal cryosections. The globes were removed and dissected in DMEM (Thermo Fisher Scientific, Waltham, MA) on ice. Retinal tissues were dissociated with use of the Worthington Papain Dissociation System (Worthington, Lakewood, NJ). Briefly, retinal samples were shredded with scalpels and digested in Earle's balanced salt solution containing papain (20 units/mL) and DNAse I (2,000 units/mL) for 20 min at 37°C. Dissociation was stopped with ovomucoid. Intact cells were separated on a single-step discontinuous density gradient and resuspended in Earle's balanced salt solution with 10% FBS.

scRNA-seq

Retinal cell suspensions were loaded on the Chromium Single Cell Controller Instrument (10x Genomics) for generation of single-cell gel beads in emulsion. For scRNA-seq, libraries were prepared with a Chromium Single Cell 5' Reagent Kit, version 3, according to the manufacturer's protocol. Sequencing was performed on an Illumina HiSeq X Ten System and 150–base pair paired-end reads were generated. One full lane was used per sample, with approximately >90% sequencing saturation.

scRNA-seq Data Preprocessing and Quality Control

The Cell Ranger software pipeline (version 3.0.0) from 10x Genomics was used to demultiplex cellular barcodes, map reads to the genome and transcriptome (with use of the STAR aligner), and down-sample reads as required for generation of normalized aggregate data across samples, to produce a matrix of gene counts versus cells. We processed the unique molecular identifier count matrix using the R package Seurat (version 2.3.4). To remove low-quality cells and likely multiple captures (a major concern in microdroplet-based experiments), we retained the cells with >200 genes and <8,000 genes; >400 unique molecular identifiers and <20% mitochondrial RNA. Library size normalization on the filtered matrix was performed in Seurat to obtain normalized counts.

Identification of Cell Clusters

The top variable genes between single cells were identified with the method described by Macosko et al. (12). Briefly, principal components analysis was performed with the variably expressed genes, and the top 25 principal components were applied for cell clustering with use of a graph-based clustering approach at a resolution of 0.2. We performed *t*-distributed stochastic neighbor embedding (*t*-SNE) with the same number of principal components and default parameters to visualize the clustering results. These steps were performed in R with the Seurat package. Comparison with canonic cell type markers indicated that the 17 clusters identified corresponded to 11 cell types.

GWAS Analysis

Single nucleotide polymorphism–trait associations were downloaded on 9 December 2020 from the NHGRI-EBI GWAS Catalog for the traits (13). Heat maps were generated with R. Calculated module scores were calculated for gene expression programs in cell types with use of the AddModuleScore function in Seurat.

Cell-Cell Gene Coexpression Analysis

To quantify alterations in cell-cell communication in the retina during diabetes, we used CellPhoneDB (v2.0) to identify biologically relevant interacting ligand-receptor partners in the scRNA-seq data (14). We defined a ligand or receptor as "expressed" in a particular cell type if 10% of the cells of that type had nonzero read counts for the gene encoding the ligand/receptor. To define cell-cell communication networks, we linked any two cell types where the ligand and receptor were expressed in the former and latter cell types, respectively. For each receptor-ligand pair in the cell-cell communication, we computed the Spearman correlation coefficient between the mean $\log_2$(normalized data + 1) ligand gene expression in the ligand-expressing cell and the logit-transformed proportions of the receptor-expressing cell across samples.

Identification of Retinal Differentially Expressed Genes Between db/m and db/db Mice

Differentially expressed genes (DEGs) were identified with use of the FindMarkers function (test.use = bimod) in Seurat. P value <0.05 and $|\log_2\text{fold change}| > 0.26$ was set as the threshold for significantly differential expression. Heat maps, volcano plots, and violin plots were generated with R. DEGs were enriched for their involvement in various biological pathways with use of KEGG (Kyoto Encyclopedia of Genes and Genomes) Pathway Enrichment.

Study Design: Experiment 2

Adeno-Associated Virus Vector Preparation and Injection

Müller glia-specific viruses were constructed with the Müller glia-specific adeno-associated virus (AAV) serotype shH10Y and a ubiquitous synthetic cytomegalovirus promoter (15). AAV vectors expressing either retinaldehyde-binding protein 1 (RLBP1) (ShH10Y.RLBP1) or GFP (ShH10Y.GFP) were used. The animals were randomly divided into four groups: untreated *db/m* mice, untreated *db/db* mice, *db/db* mice treated with intravitreal ShH10Y.RLBP1, and *db/db* mice treated with intravitreal ShH10Y.GFP. Intravitreal injection of corresponding virus with 4 μL/eye was performed in the mice at 4 months of age. Untreated mice received equal amounts of PBS. The retinas were harvested at 8 months of age. For determination of the transfection efficiency, cryosections were generated from the retinas of *db/db* mice injected with ShH10Y.GFP.

Immunofluorescence, Western blot, ELISA, electroretinogram, TUNEL assays, trypsin digest for retinal vascular architecture, and detection of vascular permeability are described in Supplementary Materials.

Statistical Analyses

Data were analyzed with GraphPad Prism 8.4.0 (GraphPad Software, San Diego, CA) and are presented as the mean ± SD. Normality was analyzed with the Kolmogorov-Smirnov test. Statistical differences between two groups were compared with unpaired two-tailed Student t test, and those between multiple groups were examined with ANOVA with a Bonferroni correction. $P < 0.05$ was considered statistically significant.

Data and Resource Availability

The data sets have been deposited into National Center for Biotechnology Information Sequence Read Archive (SRA) database under accession number PRJNA653629. All other data generated during the current study are available from the corresponding author upon reasonable request.

RESULTS

Identification of Retinal Cell Types

The experimental set consisted of retina cells from three control (*db/m*) and three diabetic (*db/db*) mice. Their fasting body weights and blood glucose levels were measured monthly from 2 to 8 months of age (Supplementary Table 1). All mice underwent glucose tolerance tests at 2 and 8 months of age, and their glycemic responses at these time points are shown in Supplementary Fig. 1A and B. At 2 months of age, *db/db* mice already displayed glucose intolerance, as shown by the increased area under the glycemic curve in comparison with that for control mice ($P < 0.001$ [Supplementary Fig. 1C]). The tendency for glucose intolerance in *db/db* mice continued to increase until 8 months of age ($P < 0.001$ [Supplementary Fig. 1C]). Isolated retinas from control and diabetic mice were dissociated into single-cell suspensions. After scRNA-seq and quality control filters, 34,010 and 51,558 retinal cells derived from control and diabetic mice were sequenced, respectively. The cells were classified into 17 transcriptionally distinct clusters (Fig. 1A). Based on the expression of well-established markers, we determined cell identifiers such as rods [rhodopsin (Rho) and G protein subunit α transducin 1 (Gnat1)], cone bipolar cells [secretagogin (Scgn)], rod bipolar cells [Sebox], Müller glia [glutamate-ammonia ligase (Glul) and RLBP1], amacrine cells [solute carrier family 32 member 1 (Slc32a1) and glutamate decarboxylase 1 (Gad1)], retinal ganglion cells [RGCs] [POU class 4 homeobox 1 (Pou4f1) and synuclein γ (Sncg)], cones [opsin 1 (cone pigments) medium-wave-sensitive (color blindness, deutan) (Opn1mw) and opsin 1 (cone pigments) short-wave-sensitive (color blindness, tritan) (Opn1sw)], microglia [allograft inflammatory factor 1 (Aif1) and C-X3-C motif chemokine receptor 1 (Cx3cr1)], vascular endothelial cells [cadherin 5 (Cdh5) and platelet and endothelial cell adhesion molecule 1 (Pecam1)], pericytes [potassium voltage-gated channel subfamily J member 8 (Kcnj8) and platelet-derived growth factor receptor β (Pdgfrb)], and horizontal cells [LIM homeobox 1 (Lhx1)] (16,17) (Fig. 1B and C and Supplementary Fig. 3). The cell clusters were not due to batch or technical effects (Supplementary Fig. 2).

Retinal Cell Types Vulnerable to DR and Cell-Type-Specific Expression of DR-Associated Risk Loci

To determine which retinal cell types are vulnerable to DR, we compared the proportions of various cell clusters in the retinas of diabetic and control mice (Fig. 1D). Moreover, genetic variants have been reproducibly linked to DR through population-based GWAS (13). To uncover potential links between the identified cell clusters and DR and PDR, we quantified the overlap between candidate loci from GWAS and the expression signatures of the retinal cell clusters in *db/m* and *db/db* mice (Fig. 2A and B). For example, acid-sensing ion channel 5 expression increased in cluster 3 but decreased in clusters 1 and 9. In summary, our

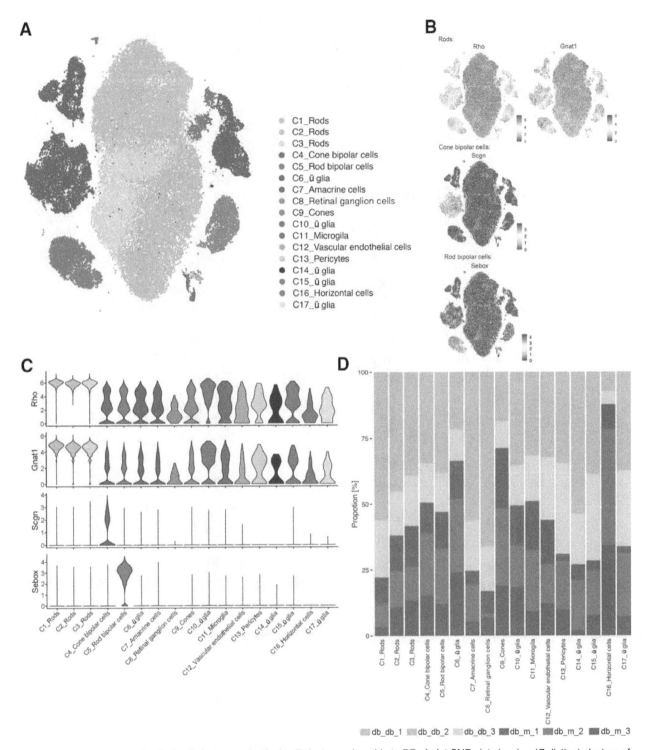

Figure 1—Determination of retinal cell clusters and retinal cell clusters vulnerable to DR. *A*: A *t*-SNE plot showing 17 distinct clusters of retina cells. Each colored dot represents a cell. *B*: *t*-SNE plots showing expression of known cell markers. *C*: Violin plots for visualizing well-established marker genes used to identify clusters. *D*: Bar graphs show the percentages of cells from each mouse assigned to each cell cluster. Cells were obtained from the retinas of *db/m* and *db/db* mice (*n* = 3 each).

single retinal cell sequencing data set can be used to identify the cell types relevant to DR and PDR (Supplementary Fig. 4). Rods, rod bipolar cells, cones, and vascular endothelial cells were the most intimate relative of PDR risk. Furthermore, among Müller glia clusters, cluster 6 was more strongly linked to retinal changes between *db/m* and *db/db* mice than the others.

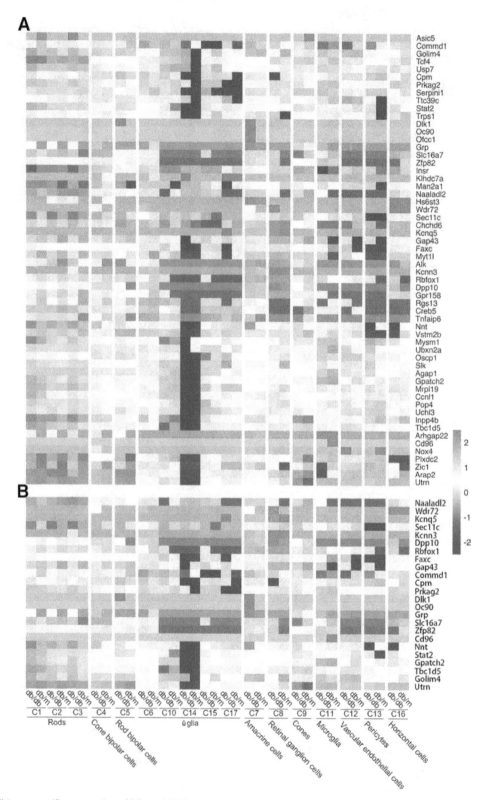

Figure 2—Cell-type-specific expression of DR- and PDR-associated risk loci. *A*: Heat map of the cell cluster–specific expression of genes reported in DR-related GWAS analyses in the retina of *db/m* mice or *db/db* mice. *B*: Heat map of the cell cluster–specific expression of genes reported in PDR-related GWAS analyses in the retina of *db/m* mice or *db/db* mice. The color gradient denotes average expression per cell.

DR Alters Retinal Cell-Cell Communication

To diagram the wiring of cell-cell interactions more generally between diabetic and control mice, we mapped receptor-ligand pairs onto cell types to construct a putative cell-cell communication across disease states (Fig. 3A). The most active cell types in both states were RGCs, vascular endothelial cells, and Müller glia. Furthermore, microglial activity was increased in the retinal cell-cell communication networks of *db/db* mice in comparison with those of *db/m* mice. Conversely, other cell types presented decreased activity.

Specific receptor-ligand interactions also changed between control and diabetic mice. The full data set of ligand-receptor partners between clusters is available upon request. We hypothesized that changes in the proportions of cell types could be explained by shifts in genes that are involved in cell-cell interaction and expressed by other cell types. To test this, we examined all cell subset pairs for each receptor-ligand partner: whether the ligand's expression level in one cell subset was associated with the proportions of the cell subset expressing its receptor (including autocrine communication). For instance, VEGFA upregulation by RGCs, rods, and cones during diabetes is correlated with decreased proportions of Müller glia, which express its receptor VEGFR2 that is encoded by kdr (Fig. 3B) (Spearman's ρ = –0.26, –0.77, and –0.20, respectively). Additionally, the frequency of Müller glia, which express ephb1, was correlated with the expression by RGCs of efnb3 (Fig. 3B) (Spearman's ρ = 0.99).

Identification of Genes Associated With DR Vulnerability

In contrast to bulk tissue gene expression, we used scRNA-seq for gene expression analysis, with the expectation that genomic information in individual cell types would help elucidate the mechanisms of DR pathology that might be hidden in bulk analysis. To

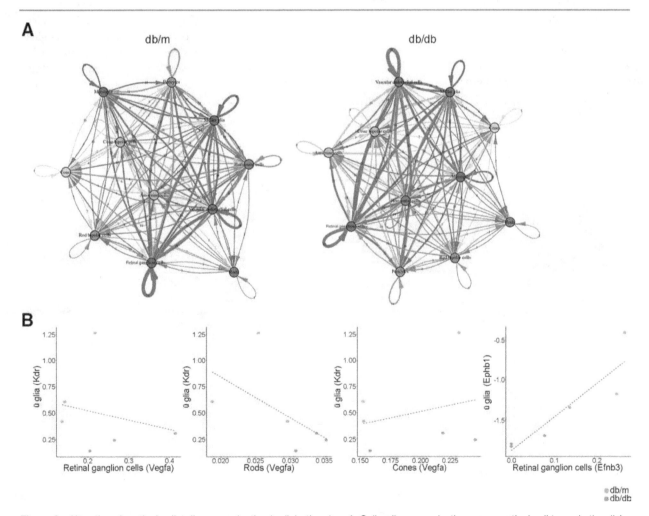

Figure 3—Alterations in retinal cell-cell communication in diabetic mice. *A*: Cell-cell communication among retinal cell types in the *db/m* and *db/db* groups. Arrow color corresponds to the ligand source, and the numbers indicate the quantity of detected ligand-receptor pairs between the indicated cell types. *B*: Each panel shows the mean expression level of the ligand in one cell type (*x*-axis) and the logit-transformed proportion of the cell type expressing the receptor (*y*-axis) in each sample for a pair of cells connected by a receptor-ligand interaction. Dashed line represents the best linear fit.

identify cell-specific genes that may contribute to DR pathogenesis, we determined the top 25 up- and down-regulated genes between diabetic and control retinal cells in each cell type (Fig. 4, Supplementary Fig. 5). There were several DEGs identified as multi-cell type (Fig. 5A). In comparison with their levels in control retinas, fos, madd, and pttg1 were upregulated in multiple cell types. Notably, the expression of RLBP1, which encodes CRALBP, was reduced in Müller glia but increased in several other retinal cell types in diabetic mice in comparison with that in control mice. In addition to these relatively universal DEGs, cell-type-specific DEGs could serve as selective therapeutic targets to alleviate or normalize specific pathological abnormalities of DR (Fig. 5B). For example, calcium voltage-gated channel subunit α1 H, encoded by CACNA1H, was downregulated in cone bipolar cells during DR. DEGs were used for analysis of functional enrichment with KEGG. The top 30 most significantly enriched KEGG pathways were exhibited in different cell types (Supplementary Fig. 6).

RLBP1 Promotes Restoration of DR

Targeting pan-retinal DEGs may offer more comprehensive and stronger therapeutic effects by normalizing multiple retinal cell types. Several DEGs were identified in multi-cell type affected by diabetes, including RLBP1,

which has been widely studied in the context of autosomal recessive retinal diseases. Mutations in human *RLBP1* can cause retinitis punctata albescens, Newfoundland rod-cone dystrophy, autosomal recessive retinitis pigmentosa, and Bothnia dystrophy (18). However, little is known regarding its role in DR, possibly because previous bulk measurements could not distinguish changes in RLBP1, which is downregulated in DR Müller glia but upregulated in other retinal cell types.

We hypothesized that upregulated RLBP1 expression in the Müller glia could serve as a target to mitigate neurovascular degeneration in DR. To our knowledge, we first confirmed the significant downregulation of CRALBP in diabetic retinal tissue using immunofluorescence staining and Western blotting (Fig. 6A and B). After verifying that intravitreal AAV injection efficiently delivered the transgenes to the Müller glia (via the Müller glia–specific ShH10Y.GFP [15] [Fig. 6C]), we used the AAV vectors to express RLBP1 specifically in the Müller glia of *db/db* mice and recorded the fasting body weights and blood glucose levels of all four groups (Supplementary Table 2). We also examined whether RLBP1 overexpression could affect glial dysfunction and proinflammatory cytokine induction. Glial responses were assessed with the gliotic marker GFAP. As shown in Fig. 6D, GFAP expression was limited in astrocytes and in the end feet of Müller glia in the retinas of db/m (control) mice. However, GFAP expression in

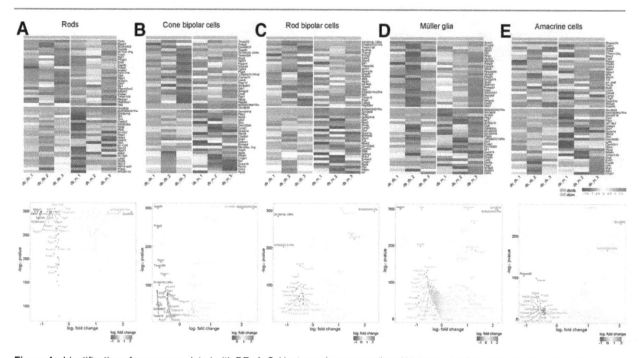

Figure 4—Identification of genes associated with DR. *A–C*: Heat map (upper panel) and Volcano plot (lower panel) of dysregulated genes in the rods (*A*), cone bipolar cells (*B*), rod bipolar cells (*C*), Müller glia (*D*), and amacrine cells (*E*) of *db/db* mice. Data of top 50 dysregulated genes (25 upregulated and 25 downregulated) were *z* normalized for heat map visualization. Each column represents an individual sample from the *db/m* or *db/db* groups. Volcano plot of dysregulated genes at *P* < 0.05 and a fold change of above 1.2 or below −1.2. The top 50 DEGs are labeled.

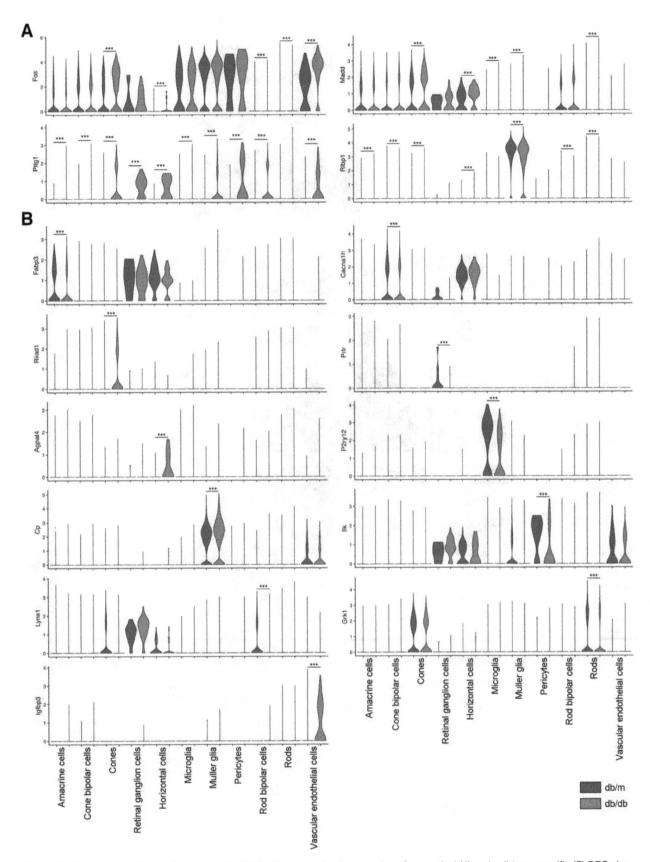

Figure 5—Pan-retinal and top cell-type-specific DEGs. The normalized expression of pan-retinal (A) and cell-type-specific (B) DEGs between *db/m* and *db/db* samples is displayed in violin plots. Single cells from *db/m* and *db/db* samples are indicated by blue and red plots, respectively. ***$P < 0.001$.

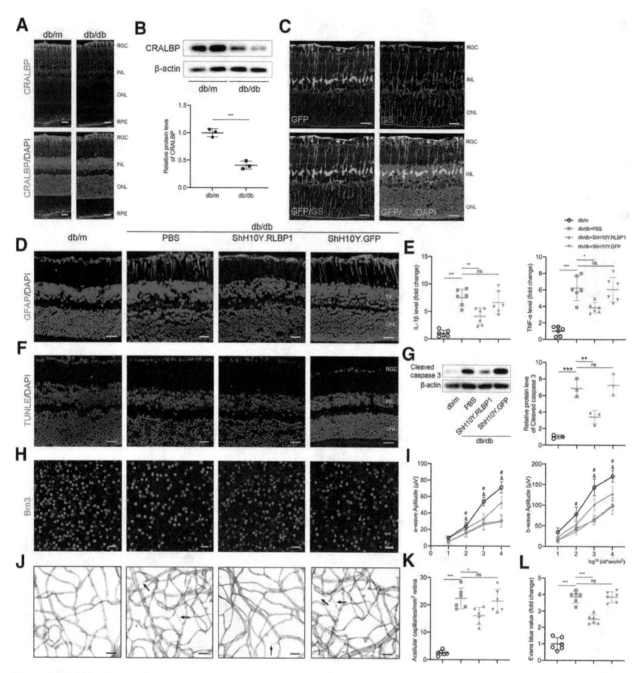

Figure 6—RLBP1 mitigates diabetic retinal neurovascular disease. *A*: Fluorescent images of retinas stained for CRALBP (red). *B*: The expression levels of CRALBP in retinas were measured by Western blotting; β-actin was used as a loading control (upper panel). The band densities were assessed with ImageJ software, and CRALBP expression levels are represented as their ratios to β-actin (lower panel). *C*: Retinal cryosections from 8-month-old *db/db* mice intravitreally injected with ShH10Y.GFP at 4 months old. GS, Müller glia marker (red). *D–L*: Comparison of *db/m* mice and *db/db* mice that received intravitreal injection of PBS, ShH10Y.RLBP1, or ShH10Y.GFP. *D*: GFAP staining of retinal cross sections (red). *E*: The expression level of IL-1β (left panel) and TNF-α (right panel) in retinal tissue. *F*: TUNEL-positive cells in retinal cross sections (red). *G*: The expression levels of cleaved caspase 3 in retinas were measured by Western blotting; β-actin was used as a loading control (left panel). The band densities were assessed with ImageJ software, and cleaved caspase 3 expression levels are represented as their ratios to β-actin (right panel). *H*: Brn3 staining of retinal flat mount (red). *I*: Amplitudes of the a-wave (left panel) and b-wave (right panel) under different background illuminance conditions. *J*: Trypsin-digested retinas. Arrows indicate acellular capillaries. *K*: Enumeration of acellular capillaries per mm² retinal area. *L*: Quantification of retinal vascular permeability with Evans blue technique. Nuclei were counterstained with DAPI (blue). Scale bar, 25 μm. Data represent the mean ± SD (n = 6). GCL, ganglion cell layer; INL, inner nuclear layer; ONL, outer nuclear layer. *P < 0.05, **P < 0.01, ***P < 0.001; ns, nonsignificant. #P < 0.05, *db/db* mice that received intravitreal injection of PBS vs. *db/m* mice. &P < 0.05, *db/db* mice that received intravitreal injection of ShH10Y.RLBP1 vs. PBS.

untreated *db/db* mice was detected in the cell processes of the Müller glia, indicating their activation or damage (Fig. 6*D*). However, *db/db* mice intravitreally injected with ShH10Y.RLBP1 displayed decreased upregulation of GFAP in the astrocytes and Müller glia (Fig. 6*D*). Moreover, diabetes led to increased expression of IL-1β ($P < 0.001$ [Fig. 6*E*]) and TNF-α ($P < 0.001$ [Fig. 6*E*]), whereas overexpressing RLBP1 resulted in downregulating these cytokines among *db/db* mice ($P < 0.01$ and 0.05 [Fig. 6*E*]). Furthermore, the number of TUNEL-positive cells, indicating DNA strand breaks, was significantly increased in the retinas of untreated *db/db* mice compared with that in the retinas of *db/m* mice (Fig. 6*F*). In *db/db* mice injected with ShH10Y.RLBP1, the number of TUNEL-positive cells in retinas significantly decreased compared with that in *db/db* mice administered PBS (Fig. 6*F*). In evaluation of neuronal dysfunction, RGC-specific marker Brn3 revealed significant attenuation in RGCs of untreated *db/db* mice in comparison with *db/m* mice (Fig. 6*H*). However, *db/db* mice intravitreally injected with ShH10Y.RLBP1 displayed increased RGCs in comparison with *db/db* mice intravitreally injected with PBS (Fig. 6*H*). In addition, the amplitudes of both a- and b-waves increased in a light intensity–dependent manner in the *db/m* mice. However, a- and b-waves were significantly decreased in the *db/db* mice that were intravitreally injected with PBS in comparison with the *db/m* mice from the second data point to the fourth data point. Compared with treatment with PBS, intravitreal injection of ShH10Y.RLBP1 significantly reduced attenuation of a- and b-wave amplitudes (Fig. 6*I*). At the 2nd, 3rd, and 4th a-wave data points, there were significant increases in the ShH10Y.RLBP1-treated group compared with the PBS-treated group. Moreover, at the 3rd and 4th b-wave data point, there was a significant increase in the ShH10Y.RLBP1-treated group in comparison with the PBS-treated group. We next assessed the impact of RLBP1 on DR vasculopathy by examining acellular capillaries (Fig. 6*J*). As expected, *db/db* mice that were administered PBS had significantly increased numbers of retinal acellular capillaries in comparison with *db/m* mice ($P < 0.001$ [Fig. 6*K*]), whereas *db/db* mice that were intravitreally injected ShH10Y.RLBP1 had a significantly decreased number of retinal acellular capillaries in comparison with those injected with PBS ($P < 0.05$ [Fig. 6*K*]). Evans blue was used to determine the extent of blood-retinal barrier (BRB) permeability. BRB breakdown and increased vascular permeability were observed in *db/db* mice that were intravitreally injected with PBS relative to *db/m* mice ($P < 0.001$ [Fig. 6*L*]). *db/db* mice with RLBP1 overexpression exhibited a significant decrease in vascular permeability in comparison with *db/db* mice that were intravitreally injected with PBS ($P < 0.001$ [Fig. 6*L*]). However, there were no significant differences in the indicators between *db/db* mice injected with PBS and ShH10Y.GFP (Fig. 6*D–L*).

DISCUSSION

Here, we described high-throughput parallel scRNA-seq analysis of retinal cells from control and diabetic mice. This enabled the characterization of genes as cell-specific markers within the complex retinal cytoarchitecture and identified genes whose expression is significantly changed in diabetes, thus providing a rich resource for the study of DR pathogenesis. Viewed holistically, our analyses of changes in cell proportions, cell-cell communication, and gene expression indicate that most retinal cell types demonstrate various degrees of sensitivity to DR.

GWAS have identified genomic loci associated with various human phenotypes; however, the specific cellular mechanisms behind these disease associations remain largely unknown. Exploring the cell-type-specific expression of DR-associated risk loci can provide deeper understanding of DR pathogenesis. Müller glia cluster 6, as well as all clusters containing rods, rod bipolar cells, cones, and vascular endothelial cells, was the most intimate relative in PDR, indicating that they may play greater roles in the disease process.

With in-depth pathological studies and improved retinal imaging to conceptualize DR, it has been found that the retinal dysfunction induced by diabetes may be viewed as an impairment in the retinal neurovascular unit. The retinal neurovascular unit contains the physical and biochemical relationship among neural cell types, glial cells, professional immune cells, and vascular cells (19). This prompted us to consider DR as a whole, with a focus on cell-cell interactions. In comparison with *db/m* mice, microglial activity in retinal cell-cell communication was increased in *db/db* mice, probably due to their diabetes-induced activation and consequent migration from the inner retinal layers into the outer plexiform and photoreceptor layers (20). However, other cell types showed decreased activity, possibly because of impaired morphology and function. Importantly, retinal neurodegeneration precedes microvascular changes in DR (21). As the Müller glia are the only cells that span the entire retina, with intimate contacts with other retinal cell types, and VEGFR2-mediated Müller cell survival is vital for retinal neuron viability in diabetes (22), we studied the association between the proportion of Müller cells expressing VEGFR2 and neurons expressing VEGF. As shown in our results, the proportion of Müller glia that expresses VEGFR2 decreased with the VEGF upregulation of RGCs, rods, and cones during diabetes. Thus, we speculate that increased VEGF expression in neurons leads to decreased Müller glia expressing VEGFR2. We also observed some ligand-receptor interactions that were altered in diabetes that may improve our understanding of DR pathogenesis. For instance, signaling between erythropoietin-producing human hepatocellular (Eph) receptors and Eph family receptor–interacting (ephrins) proteins was active in retinal tissue both among several cell types and in autocrine loops in single cell types. The Eph receptor/ephrin system controls cell fate and is typically mediated via contact-dependent intercellular communication. It has a number of roles in both development and adulthood (23,24). In retinal development, Eph receptors and ephrins participate in retinotectal mapping. They also contribute to retinal neovascularization via Eph receptor A2/ephrin A1 signaling in endothelial cells and via RGC apoptosis via Eph receptor B/ephrin B signaling in Müller glia (25,26). Based on our result, the lesser the expression of ephrin B3 (EFNB3) in RGCs, the lower the proportions of Müller glia that express EPH receptor B1 (EPHB1). This may indicate a cascade between RGCs and Müller glia via Eph receptor B/ephrin B signaling. Other Eph receptors/ephrins have not been extensively researched in retinopathy, and our study reveals their new roles in DR. Eph receptor A4 (EPHA4) affects ischemic brain injury by controlling astrocyte glutamate uptake capacity, preventing glutamate excitotoxicity, mediating neuroinflammation and tissue damage in traumatic brain injury, and promoting glial scarring after ischemic stroke (27–29). Analogously, glutamate excitotoxicity, reactive gliosis, and neuroinflammation are characteristic retinal neurodegeneration phenotypes of DR (30). Thus, the role of EPHA4 in DR should be examined further.

Single-cell data were essential for prioritization of the numerous promising therapeutic targets in the diverse cell types. There are some cell-type-specific DEGs, such as purinergic receptor P2Y12 (P2RY12). P2RY12, which was decreased in retina during diabetes in this study, is a marker in homeostatic microglia, which was lost in active and slowly expanding lesions (31). In central nervous system, microglia are resident immune cells, including the retina, and are vital for the homeostatic maintenance of the nervous and retinal microenvironment (32). Recently, microglia were proven to be essential for initiating the infiltration of immune cells in experimental autoimmune uveoretinitis (EAU) murine model (33). Microglia-Müller glia or retinal pigment epithelial (RPE) cells cross talk drives inflammation and destroy BRB in DR (34,35). Hence, it seems that future studies on P2RY12 in microglia may be valuable. Additionally, connective tissue growth factor (CTGF) is a major contributor to fibrotic responses in DR. CTGF was only significantly increased in Müller glia in our study, suggesting that these cells are the major source of CTGF in DR. DEG enrichment analysis also revealed significant pathways and gene sets that changed in different cell types with diabetes. For instance, mitophagy-related genes were strongly enriched in RGCs, consistent with results from studies on cell differentiation and glaucoma (36–38). This indicates that further research into RGC mitophagy is needed to shed light on DR pathogenesis and provide novel treatment strategies.

Pan-retinal DEGs were identified in multi-cell types. Notably, RLBP1 one of the most robust DEGs across retinal cell types, exhibited opposing trends between the Müller glia and other retinal cell types. Müller glia form the supporting architectural structure across the entire thickness of the retina and can be viewed as the core of the retinal neurovascular unit, as they provide an anatomical connection between retinal blood vessels and neurons (19). The three primary functions of Müller glia are 1) uptake and recycling of retinoic acid compounds, neurotransmitters, and ions; 2) blood flow regulation and BRB maintenance; and 3) control of retinal metabolism and nutrients. Müller glia play a noteworthy role in DR, causing chronic inflammation, apoptosis, vascular leakage, and neovascularization (39). After selectively overexpressing RLBP1 in diabetic Müller glia, we observed decreased gliosis and protected retinal capillaries and neurons. RLBP1 is an 11-*cis*-retinoid-binding protein that is abundantly expressed in both RPE cells and Müller glia and is vital for the retinal visual cycle. Phototransduction is triggered when the 11-*cis*-retinal chromophore of a photopigment molecule in the outer segment of a vertebrate rod or cone captures a photon and is isomerized to its all-*trans* form. Regeneration of light detection requires reconverting the "bleached" all-*trans* retinal back into a light-sensitive 11-*cis* retinal (40). In RPE cells, RLBP1 contributes 11-*cis*-retinal to rods and cones, while cones also depend on an 11-*cis* chromophore present in Müller glia, which explains the characteristic rapid dark adaptation and saturation resistance of cones (41). Accumulating evidence suggests that visual dysfunction and retinal neurodegeneration precede retinal microvascular degeneration (21). Impaired retinoid metabolism during diabetes is characterized by 11-*cis*-retinal deficiency, resulting in increased unbound opsin that constitutively activates the phototransduction cascade, causing photoreceptor damage and exaggerating oxidative stress (42). As 11-*cis*-retinal is highly unstable, Malechka et al. (42) showed that the administration of the relatively stable 11-*cis*-retinal isomer 9-*cis*-retinal to a model of type 1 diabetes rescued visual pigment formation and decreased oxidative stress and retinal neuron apoptosis. How RLBP1 overexpression in Müller glia alleviates diabetes-driven retinal neurovascular degeneration remains a matter of speculation; however, it is possible that the normalization of retinoid metabolism results in decreased oxidation stress and apoptosis, while maintaining Müller glia homeostasis to benefit the entire retina.

Our study has limitations. Because of the differences between mouse and human retinas, mouse models only partially recapitulate the pathological complexity of patients with DR, and further research will be necessary to translate this information in humans. In addition, retinal scRNA-seq at different time points of *db/db* mice should be added for full understanding of the occurrence and development of the disease. Another challenge is the accurate detection of rare cell types using scRNA-seq. Distinguishing rare cell types from massive scRNA-seq data sets and building their precise signatures are challenging tasks (43), and estimating rare cell proportions is particularly difficult with small sample sizes because of increased stochasticity. We hope to further improve on the detection accuracy of rare cell types in future studies.

To summarize, this study identified DR-associated genes, cell-cell communication pathways, and retinal cell types, laying the foundation for further DR pathogenesis studies and for the development of novel treatment strategies for DR and related disorders.

Acknowledgments. The authors thank OE Biotech Co., Ltd (Shanghai, China) for providing single-cell RNA-seq.

Funding. This work was supported by grants from the National Key R&D Program of China (grant 2016YFC0904800 and 2019YFC0840607), National Science and Technology Major Project of China (grant 2017ZX09304010), National Natural Science Foundation of China (81870667 and 81800799), Shanghai Medical Excellent Discipline Leader Program (2017BR056), and Shanghai Municipal Education Commission–Gaofeng Clinical Medicine Grant Support Program (20161426).

The funding organizations had no roles in the design, conduct, analysis, or publication of this study.

Duality of Interest. No potential conflicts of interest relevant to this article were reported.

Author Contributions. T.N. and K.L. designed the research. T.N., X.S., M.Z., and Y.W. performed the research. J.F., X.X., and Y.W. analyzed the data. T.N., S.Z., and K.L. wrote and revised the manuscript. K.L. obtained funding and supervised the study, and all authors read and approved the final manuscript. K.K. is the guarantor of this work and, as such, had full access to all the data in the study and takes responsibility for the integrity of the data and the accuracy of the data analysis.

References

1. Ting DS, Cheung GC, Wong TY. Diabetic retinopathy: global prevalence, major risk factors, screening practices and public health challenges: a review. Clin Exp Ophthalmol 2016;44:260–277

2. Gardner TW, Davila JR. The neurovascular unit and the pathophysiologic basis of diabetic retinopathy. Graefes Arch Clin Exp Ophthalmol 2017;255:1–6

3. Stitt AW, Curtis TM, Chen M, et al. The progress in understanding and treatment of diabetic retinopathy. Prog Retin Eye Res 2016;51:156–186

4. Ciulla TA, Hussain RM, Ciulla LM, Sink B, Harris A. Ranibizumab for diabetic macular edema refractory to multiple prior treatments. Retina 2016;36:1292–1297

5. Wong TY, Cheung CM, Larsen M, Sharma S, Simó R. Diabetic retinopathy. Nat Rev Dis Primers 2016;2:16012

6. Chen S, Yuan M, Liu Y, et al. Landscape of microRNA in the aqueous humour of proliferative diabetic retinopathy as assessed by next-generation sequencing. Clin Exp Ophthalmol 2019;47:925–936

7. He M, Wang W, Yu H, et al. Comparison of expression profiling of circular RNAs in vitreous humour between diabetic retinopathy and non-diabetes mellitus patients. Acta Diabetol 2020;57:479–489

8. Kandpal RP, Rajasimha HK, Brooks MJ, et al. Transcriptome analysis using next generation sequencing reveals molecular signatures of diabetic retinopathy and efficacy of candidate drugs. Mol Vis 2012;18:1123–1146

9. Heng JS, Rattner A, Stein-O'Brien GL, et al. Hypoxia tolerance in the Norrin-deficient retina and the chronically hypoxic brain studied at single-cell resolution. Proc Natl Acad Sci U S A 2019;116:9103–9114

10. Zheng Y, Ley SH, Hu FB. Global aetiology and epidemiology of type 2 diabetes mellitus and its complications. Nat Rev Endocrinol 2018;14:88–98

11. Olivares AM, Althoff K, Chen GF, et al. Animal models of diabetic retinopathy. Curr Diab Rep 2017;17:93

12. Macosko EZ, Basu A, Satija R, et al. Highly parallel genome-wide expression profiling of individual cells using nanoliter droplets. Cell 2015;161:1202–1214

13. Buniello A, MacArthur JAL, Cerezo M, et al. The NHGRI-EBI GWAS Catalog of published genome-wide association studies, targeted arrays and summary statistics 2019. Nucleic Acids Res 2019;47:D1005–D1012

14. Efremova M, Vento-Tormo M, Teichmann SA, Vento-Tormo R. CellPhoneDB: inferring cell-cell communication from combined expression of multi-subunit ligand-receptor complexes. Nat Protoc 2020;15:1484–1506

15. Pellissier LP, Hoek RM, Vos RM, et al. Specific tools for targeting and expression in Müller glial cells. Mol Ther Methods Clin Dev 2014;1:14009

16. Pauly D, Agarwal D, Dana N, et al. Cell-type-specific complement expression in the healthy and diseased retina. Cell Rep 2019;29:2835–2848.e4

17. Yan W, Laboulaye MA, Tran NM, Whitney IE, Benhar I, Sanes JR. Mouse retinal cell atlas: molecular identification of over sixty amacrine cell types. J Neurosci 2020;40:5177–5195

18. Xue Y, Shen SQ, Jui J, et al. CRALBP supports the mammalian retinal visual cycle and cone vision. J Clin Invest 2015;125:727–738

19. Duh EJ, Sun JK, Stitt AW. Diabetic retinopathy: current understanding, mechanisms, and treatment strategies. JCI Insight 2017;2:e93751

20. Altmann C, Schmidt MHH. The role of microglia in diabetic retinopathy: inflammation, microvasculature defects and neurodegeneration. Int J Mol Sci 2018;19:110

21. Sohn EH, van Dijk HW, Jiao C, et al. Retinal neurodegeneration may precede microvascular changes characteristic of diabetic retinopathy in diabetes mellitus. Proc Natl Acad Sci U S A 2016;113:E2655–E2664

22. S, Dong S, Zhu M, et al. Müller glia are a major cellular source of survival signals for retinal neurons in diabetes. Diabetes 2015;64:3554–3563

23. Pasquale EB. Eph-ephrin bidirectional signaling in physiology and disease. Cell 2008;133:38–52

24. Malik VA, Di Benedetto B. The blood-brain barrier and the EphR/ephrin system: perspectives on a link between neurovascular and neuropsychiatric disorders. Front Mol Neurosci 2018;11:127

25. Ojima T, Takagi H, Suzuma K, et al. EphrinA1 inhibits vascular endothelial growth factor-induced intracellular signaling and suppresses retinal neovascularization and blood-retinal barrier breakdown. Am J Pathol 2006;168:331–339

26. Liu ST, Zhong SM, Li XY, et al. EphrinB/EphB forward signaling in Müller cells causes apoptosis of retinal ganglion cells by increasing tumor necrosis factor alpha production in rat experimental glaucomatous model. Acta Neuropathol Commun 2018;6:111

27. Yang J, Luo X, Huang X, Ning Q, Xie M, Wang W. Ephrin-A3 reverse signaling regulates hippocampal neuronal damage and astrocytic glutamate transport after transient global ischemia. J Neurochem 2014;131:383–394

28. Kowalski EA, Chen J, Hazy A, et al. Peripheral loss of EphA4 ameliorates TBI-induced neuroinflammation and tissue damage. J Neuroinflammation 2019;16:210

29. Goldshmit Y, Bourne J. Upregulation of EphA4 on astrocytes potentially mediates astrocytic gliosis after cortical lesion in the marmoset monkey. J Neurotrauma 2010;27:1321–1332

30. Araszkiewicz A, Zozulinska-Ziolkiewicz D. Retinal neurodegeneration in the course of diabetes-pathogenesis and clinical perspective. Curr Neuropharmacol 2016;14:805–809

31. Zrzavy T, Hametner S, Wimmer I, Butovsky O, Weiner HL, Lassmann H. Loss of 'homeostatic' microglia and patterns of their activation in active multiple sclerosis. Brain 2017;140:1900–1913

32. Ginhoux F, Greter M, Leboeuf M, et al. Fate mapping analysis reveals that adult microglia derive from primitive macrophages. Science 2010;330:841–845

33. Okunuki Y, Mukai R, Nakao T, et al. Retinal microglia initiate neuroinflammation in ocular autoimmunity. Proc Natl Acad Sci U S A 2019;116:9989–9998

34. Portillo JC, Lopez Corcino Y, Miao Y, et al. CD40 in retinal Müller cells induces P2X7-dependent cytokine expression in macrophages/microglia in diabetic mice and development of early experimental diabetic retinopathy. Diabetes 2017;66:483–493

35. Jo DH, Yun JH, Cho CS, Kim JH, Kim JH, Cho CH. Interaction between microglia and retinal pigment epithelial cells determines the integrity of outer blood-retinal barrier in diabetic retinopathy. Glia 2019;67:321–331

36. Esteban-Martínez L, Sierra-Filardi E, McGreal RS, et al. Programmed mitophagy is essential for the glycolytic switch during cell differentiation. EMBO J 2017;36:1688–1706

37. Hass DT, Barnstable CJ. Mitochondrial uncoupling protein 2 knock-out promotes mitophagy to decrease retinal ganglion cell death in a mouse model of glaucoma. J Neurosci 2019;39:3582–3596

38. Rosignol I, Villarejo-Zori B, Teresak P, et al. The *mito*-QC reporter for quantitative mitophagy assessment in primary retinal ganglion cells and experimental glaucoma models. Int J Mol Sci 2020;21:1882

39. Subirada PV, Paz MC, Ridano ME, et al. A journey into the retina: Müller glia commanding survival and death. Eur J Neurosci 2018;47: 1429–1443

40. Saari JC. Vitamin A metabolism in rod and cone visual cycles. Annu Rev Nutr 2012;32:125–145

41. Sato S, Kefalov VJ. cis retinol oxidation regulates photoreceptor access to the retina visual cycle and cone pigment regeneration. J Physiol 2016;594: 6753–6765

42. Malechka VV, Moiseyev G, Takahashi Y, Shin Y, Ma JX. Impaired rhodopsin generation in the rat model of diabetic retinopathy. Am J Pathol 2017;187:2222–2231

43. Grün D, van Oudenaarden A. Design and analysis of single-cell sequencing experiments. Cell 2015;163:799–810

Genetic Evidence for Different Adiposity Phenotypes and Their Opposing Influences on Ectopic Fat and Risk of Cardiometabolic Disease

Susan Martin,[1] Madeleine Cule,[2] Nicolas Basty,[3] Jessica Tyrrell,[1] Robin N. Beaumont,[1] Andrew R. Wood,[1] Timothy M. Frayling,[1] Elena Sorokin,[2] Brandon Whitcher,[3] Yi Liu,[2] Jimmy D. Bell,[3] E. Louise Thomas,[3] and Hanieh Yaghootkar[1,3]

Diabetes 2021;70:1843–1856 | https://doi.org/10.2337/db21-0129

To understand the causal role of adiposity and ectopic fat in type 2 diabetes and cardiometabolic diseases, we aimed to identify two clusters of adiposity genetic variants: one with "adverse" metabolic effects (UFA) and the other with, paradoxically, "favorable" metabolic effects (FA). We performed a multivariate genome-wide association study using body fat percentage and metabolic biomarkers from UK Biobank and identified 38 UFA and 36 FA variants. Adiposity-increasing alleles were associated with an adverse metabolic profile, higher risk of disease, higher CRP, and higher fat in subcutaneous and visceral adipose tissue, liver, and pancreas for UFA and a favorable metabolic profile, lower risk of disease, higher CRP and higher subcutaneous adipose tissue but lower liver fat for FA. We detected no sexual dimorphism. The Mendelian randomization studies provided evidence for a risk-increasing effect of UFA and protective effect of FA for type 2 diabetes, heart disease, hypertension, stroke, nonalcoholic fatty liver disease, and polycystic ovary syndrome. FA is distinct from UFA by its association with lower liver fat and protection from cardiometabolic diseases; it was not associated with visceral or pancreatic fat. Understanding the difference in FA and UFA may lead to new insights in preventing, predicting, and treating cardiometabolic diseases.

Obesity is a significant risk factor for various conditions including type 2 diabetes, heart disease, and hypertension—a cluster of events often referred to as the metabolic syndrome (1). However, in the general population, ~15–40% of individuals categorized as obese do not present any obesity-related metabolic conditions or diseases and are "metabolically benign" at the specific time point of measurement, supporting the existence of metabolically benign obesity (2,3).

Previously we showed that a genetic predisposition to storing excess fat in subcutaneous adipose tissue (SAT) is associated with a reduced propensity to store fat in the liver, consequently reducing risk of disease (4). The identification of "favorable adiposity" variants, with their adiposity-increasing alleles paradoxically associated with lower risk of type 2 diabetes, heart disease, and hypertension (4–7), provided genetic evidence for the paradox of metabolically benign obesity. These genetic findings suggest that there are at least two types of variants associated with higher adiposity: one with favorable metabolic profile (favorable adiposity [FA]) and the other with an unfavorable metabolic profile (unfavorable adiposity [UFA]).

Although our previous studies suggested an important role for liver fat, we have been unable to determine whether pancreatic fat deposition or liver and pancreas volumes were similarly implicated due to lack of data, and it has not been possible to investigate mechanisms imposed by each variant individually. Clarification of the underlying pathophysiologic mechanisms that link adiposity to higher risk of type 2 diabetes and other cardiometabolic disease is

[1]Genetics of Complex Traits, University of Exeter Medical School, University of Exeter, Royal Devon & Exeter Hospital, Exeter, U.K.
[2]Calico Life Sciences LLC, South San Francisco, CA
[3]Research Centre for Optimal Health, School of Life Sciences, University of Westminster, London, U.K.

Corresponding author: Hanieh Yaghootkar, h.yaghootkar@exeter.ac.uk

Received 11 February 2021 and accepted 6 May 2021

This article contains supplementary material online at https://doi.org/10.2337/figshare.14555463.

S.M., M.C., E.L.T., and H.Y. contributed equally.

critical to understanding disease progression and remission, especially given the rising prevalence of obesity and the rapid rise of type 2 diabetes in an aging population. The availability of both metabolic markers and MRI scan data in the UK Biobank (8) has enabled us to test in more detail the characteristics of adiposity variants and the role of ectopic fat in disease mechanism.

In this study, we focused on how higher adiposity is associated with ectopic fat, metabolic derangements, and cardiometabolic risk. Specifically, we aimed to 1) identify distinct clusters of FA and UFA variants, 2) investigate the relation between FA and UFA variants and ectopic fat deposition in the liver and pancreas, 3) examine how FA and UFA variants are associated with circulating markers of inflammation, 4) determine whether sexual dimorphism is a factor in the association between the clusters and metabolic biomarkers, fat distribution, and disease risk; and 5) use Mendelian randomization (MR) to determine the potential causal role of "favorable" and "unfavorable" adiposity in different components of metabolic syndrome.

RESEARCH DESIGN AND METHODS

Discovery Data Set—UK Biobank

UK Biobank recruited >500,000 individuals aged 37–73 years (99.5% were between 40 and 69 years of age) between 2006 and 2010 from across the U.K. (8) (Supplementary Table 1). The UK Biobank has approval from the North West Multicenter Research Ethics Committee (https://www.ukbiobank.ac.uk/ethics/), and these ethics regulations cover the work in this study. Written informed consent was obtained from all participants.

The steps performed to identify variants associated with adiposity but with different effects on metabolic traits are outlined in Supplementary Fig. 1 and, briefly, are as follows.

Step 1: Genetic Variants Associated With Both Body Fat Percentage and Composite Metabolic Biomarkers

We performed a multivariate genome-wide association study (GWAS) of relevant metabolic biomarkers that were available in individuals of European ancestry from the UK Biobank, including HDL cholesterol (HDL) ($n = 392,965$), sex hormone–binding globulin (SHBG) ($n = 389,354$), triglycerides ($n = 429,011$), AST ($n = 427,778$), and ALT ($n = 429,203$), using BOLT-LMM v2.3.4 (9) and metaCCA software (10) as described previously (4). Specifically, metaCCA uses canonical correlation analysis to identify the maximal correlation coefficient between genome-wide genetic variants and a linear combination of the above phenotypes, based on the computed phenotype-phenotype Pearson correlation matrix. We chose these specific metabolic biomarkers to be consistent with our previous approach (4). These biomarkers are used to discriminate between three monogenic forms of insulin resistance: lipodystrophy (disorders of fat storage), monogenic obesity, and insulin signaling defects (6,11).

We identified 254 variants at $P < 5 \times 10^{-8}$ associated with both our univariate GWAS of body fat percentage ($n = 620$ variants previously published [4]) and our composite metabolic phenotype as estimated by the above multivariate GWAS model. This represents an increase in 221 signals compared with the 33 previously reported using a similar approach (4). This increase was largely attributable to the availability of the metabolic biomarkers in 451,099 individuals of European ancestry from UK Biobank, whereas previous studies were limited to smaller separate data (e.g., 100,000 with HDL and triglycerides, 21,800 with SHBG, and 55,500 with ALT).

Step 2: Classification of Adiposity Variants

We applied a k-means algorithm on the 254 variants and their effects on the values of the six phenotypes from the first step and used the parameter k = 3 to group them into FA and UFA. We considered a third cluster of "conflicting" to group any variants that do not belong to the FA or UFA clusters and did not pursue these variants in the rest of the analyses to minimize false discovery. Within UFA and FA clusters, we inspected whether the loci are driven by colocalization of signals from a combination of traits or represent a strong univariate signal.

Step 3: Validation of FA and UFA Variants

To validate FA and UFA variants, we assessed their effects on risk of type 2 diabetes using data from GWAS of 31 studies, excluding UK Biobank, which included 55,005 case and 400,308 control subjects of European ancestry (12). We expected to observe adiposity-increasing alleles as associated with lower risk of type 2 diabetes for FA variants and higher risk of type 2 diabetes for UFA variants.

Imaging Study

A subcohort of 100,000 subjects were selected for the imaging enhancement of the UK Biobank, currently at 49,938. Abdominal MRI scans were obtained with a MAGNETOM Aera 1.5T scanner (software version *syngo* MR D13) (Siemens Healthineers, Erlangen, Germany) (13). Image-derived phenotypes were generated from the three-dimensional Dixon neck-to-knee acquisition, the high-resolution T1-weighted three-dimensional pancreas acquisition, and liver and pancreas single-slice multiecho acquisitions. Images for this study were obtained through UK Biobank application no. 44584. Following automated preprocessing of the different sequences, volumes of organs of interest (including the liver, pancreas, and SAT and visceral adipose tissue [VAT]) were segmented using convolutional neural networks (14). Fat content of the liver and pancreas was obtained from the multiecho acquisitions after preprocessing where the proton density fat fraction was estimated (15).

GWAS of Imaging-Derived Phenotypes

We used the UK Biobank Imputed Genotypes v3 (16), excluding single nucleotide polymorphisms with minor allele frequency <1% and imputation quality <0.9. We excluded participants not recorded as European, exhibiting sex chromosome aneuploidy, with a discrepancy between genetic and self-reported sex, heterozygosity outliers, and genotype call rate outliers. We used BOLT-LMM (9) v2.3.2 to conduct the genetic association study. We included age at imaging visit, age squared, sex, imaging center, and genotyping batch as fixed-effects covariates, in addition to scan date scaled and scan time scaled and genetic relatedness derived from genotyped single nucleotide polymorphisms as a random effect to control for population structure and relatedness. We performed GWAS for VAT ($n = 32,859$), SAT ($n = 32,859$), VAT-to-SAT ratio ($n = 32,859$), pancreatic fat ($n = 24,673$), liver fat ($n = 32,655$), pancreas volume ($n = 31,758$) and liver volume ($n = 32,859$) (Supplementary Table 1).

Replication Data Set

To replicate the effect of FA and UFA variants on measures of adiposity, metabolic biomarkers, and C-reactive protein (CRP), we used summary statistics from published GWAS, which were independent of UK Biobank (Supplementary Table 1). To replicate the effects on subcutaneous and ectopic fat, we used data from a combined multiethnic sample size–weighted fixed-effects meta-analysis of SAT ($n = 18,247$), VAT ($n = 18,332$), VAT-to-SAT ratio ($n = 18,191$), and pericardial adipose tissue ($n = 12,204$) measured by computed tomography (CT) or MRI (17) (Supplementary Table 1).

Genetic Score Analysis

We studied the association of individual variants and of genetic scores with cardiometabolic traits and diseases in the UK Biobank using our GWAS results. We performed GWAS with BOLT-LMM to account for population structure and relatedness using covariates such as age, sex, genotyping platform, and study center in the model. For genetic score analysis, we used the inverse variance–weighted method (IVW), assigning a weight of 1 to each variant. This method approximates the association of an unweighted genetic score (18).

MR Studies

We investigated the causal associations between FA and UFA using FA and UFA clusters as instruments and six cardiometabolic disease outcomes (type 2 diabetes, heart disease, hypertension, stroke, nonalcoholic fatty liver disease [NAFLD], and polycystic ovary syndrome [PCOS]) by performing two-sample MR analysis (19). We used IVW as our main analysis and MR-Egger and weighted median as sensitivity analyses in order to detect unidentified pleiotropy of our genetic instruments. We used two sources of data: FinnGen GWAS summary results (20) and published GWAS of the same diseases, excluding UK Biobank to separate it from our discovery data set and allow us to run two-sample MR (Supplementary Table 1). We

performed MR within each data source and then meta-analyzed the results across the two data sets using a random-effects model with the R package metafor (21). We ran the same models in UK Biobank data for comparison. For more information on definition of diseases and ICD codes, please see Supplementary Material.

Tissue Enrichment Analyses

We used DEPICT (Data-Driven Expression-Prioritized Integration for Complex Traits) v.1 rel194 β (22) to identify tissues and cells in which the genes from associated loci are highly expressed. Using 37,427 human Affymetrix HGU133a2.0 platform microarrays, DEPICT assesses whether genes at the relevant loci are highly expressed in any of the 209 tissues, cell types, and physiological systems annotated by Medical Subject Headings (MeSH).

Data and Resource Availability

The data sets analyzed during the current study are available from FinnGen (20) and the relevant published GWAS (Supplementary Table 1). The data that support the findings of this study are available from UK Biobank, but restrictions apply to the availability of these data, which were used under license for the current study (UK Biobank project application nos. 9072, 9055, and 44584) and therefore are not publicly available. No applicable resources were generated or analyzed during the current study.

RESULTS

Clusters of Adiposity Variants

Among 254 variants associated (at $P < 5 \times 10^{-8}$) with both body fat percentage (4) and a composite metabolic phenotype, we identified two distinct clusters of adiposity variants: 1) 38 variants grouped as UFA and 2) 36 variants grouped as FA (Supplementary Tables 2–4 and Supplementary Fig. 2). UFA genetic score was associated with higher body fat percentage and higher BMI and an adverse metabolic profile including lower HDL and SHBG and higher triglycerides, ALT, and AST. FA genetic score was also associated with higher body fat percentage and BMI but, in contrast, a favorable metabolic profile including higher HDL and SHBG and lower triglycerides, ALT, and AST (Table 1 and Fig. 1A). There was no sex difference in the association of FA and UFA genetic scores with adiposity measures or biomarkers at the multiple testing–corrected significance threshold (0.05 of 44 tests = 0.0011) (Supplementary Table 5 and Supplementary Fig. 3). The association between UFA adiposity-increasing alleles and an adverse metabolic profile and FA adiposity-increasing alleles and a favorable metabolic profile was replicated in independent published GWAS of these biomarkers (Supplementary Table 6).

The mean (SD) UFA and FA genetic scores in the UK Biobank were 36.99 (3.83) and 37.32 (3.75) respectively. The distributions of UFA and FA genetic scores among the UK Biobank participants with and without type 2

Table 1—Sex-combined effects of FA and UFA genetic scores on BMI, biomarkers, MRI-derived measures of fat distribution, and cardiometabolic diseases

Outcome	UFA		FA	
	Effect (95% CI)	P	Effect (95% CI)	P
BMI (SD)	1.27 (1.01, 1.53)	4E−22	0.67 (0.50, 0.84)	3E−15
HDL (SD)	−0.64 (−0.89, −0.40)	2E−7	1.26 (0.96, 1.56)	3E−16
SHBG (SD)	−0.47 (−0.62, −0.32)	1E−9	1.10 (0.44, 1.76)	0.001
Triglycerides (SD)	0.49 (0.34, 0.64)	7E−11	−1.54 (−1.92, −1.15)	4E−15
ALT (SD)	0.45 (0.36, 0.54)	4E−21	−0.90 (−1.12, −0.69)	6E−17
AST (SD)	0.35 (0.19, 0.50)	1E−5	−0.54 (−0.71, −0.36)	2E−9
CRP (SD)	0.52 (0.38, 0.65)	3E−14	0.30 (0.09, 0.51)	0.005
SAT (SD)	1.09 (0.87, 1.31)	1E−22	0.96 (0.74, 1.18)	1E−17
VAT (SD)	0.56 (0.41, 0.72)	2E−12	−0.02 (-0.35, 0.31)	0.92
VAT-to-SAT ratio (SD)	−0.34 (−0.50, −0.18)	3E−5	−0.85 (−1.16, −0.53)	1E−7
Liver fat (SD)	0.46 (0.30, 0.63)	2E−8	−0.72 (−1.01, −0.43)	9E−7
Pancreas fat (SD)	0.52 (0.36, 0.69)	7E−10	0.16 (-0.20, 0.51)	0.38
Liver volume (SD)	0.64 (0.44, 0.85)	3E−10	−0.43 (−0.73, −0.13)	0.006
Pancreas volume (SD)	0.06 (−0.15, 0.28)	0.57	−0.46 (−0.76, −0.15)	0.003
Type 2 diabetes (OR)	1.06 (1.04, 1.07)	6E−16	0.93 (0.91, 0.96)	2E−9
Heart disease (OR)	1.05 (1.03, 1.07)	2E−7	0.94 (0.92, 0.97)	3E−5
Hypertension (OR)	1.13 (1.08, 1.18)	4E−8	0.90 (0.85, 0.95)	0.0001
Stroke (OR)	1.01 (1.01, 1.02)	0.0005	0.99 (0.98, 1.00)	0.17
Fatty liver disease (OR)	1.01 (1.00, 1.01)	0.004	0.99 (0.98, 0.999)	0.03
PCOS (OR)	1.01 (1.00, 1.01)	7E−5	0.995 (0.99, 0.999)	0.02

Effects are shown per 1-SD-higher body fat percentage as estimated by "favorable adiposity" and "unfavorable adiposity" genetic scores using data from UK Biobank. ASAT, abdominal SAT; VATSAT, VAT-to-SAT ratio.

diabetes are shown in Supplementary Fig. 4. The UFA and FA variants explained 0.6% and 0.2% variance in body fat percentage in the UK Biobank, respectively.

We used data from the latest GWAS of type 2 diabetes excluding UK Biobank (12) to validate the paradoxical association between the adiposity-increasing alleles at FA and UFA variants and risk of type 2 diabetes. Among 38 UFA variants, 33 adiposity-increasing alleles were correlated with higher risk of type 2 diabetes ($P_{\text{two-tailed binomial}}$ = 4E−6), with 24 at $P < 0.05$. Among 36 FA variants, all adiposity-increasing alleles were correlated with lower risk of type 2 diabetes ($P_{\text{two-tailed binomial}}$ = 3E−11), including 23 variants at $P < 0.05$ (Fig. 2). This paradoxical association was consistent with the pattern of association with type 2 diabetes with use of data from the UK Biobank (Supplementary Fig. 5).

To explore whether the UFA and FA variants represent biologically meaningful entities, we searched whether genes at the relevant loci were enriched for expression in certain tissues or pathways. FA variants were enriched (at

false discovery rate <5%) in adipocyte-related cells and tissues and in physiological systems labeled as "digestive" (small intestine, esophagus, pancreas, upper gastrointestinal tract, and ileum) and "cardiovascular" (arteries), while UFA variants were enriched in mesenchymal stem cells and in physiological systems labeled as cardiovascular (aortic valve, heart valves) (Fig. 3 and Supplementary Tables 7 and 8).

Association With MRI-Derived Measures of Abdominal Fat Distribution

To investigate the relation between UFA and FA variants and abdominal fat distribution, we looked at the effect of FA and UFA variants on SAT, VAT, and ectopic fat in the liver and pancreas in addition to liver and pancreas volume in 32,859 individuals of European ancestry from the UK Biobank. While both UFA and FA genetic scores were associated with higher SAT with similar effect size, UFA score was associated with higher liver and pancreatic fat, higher VAT, and increased liver volume, but FA score was

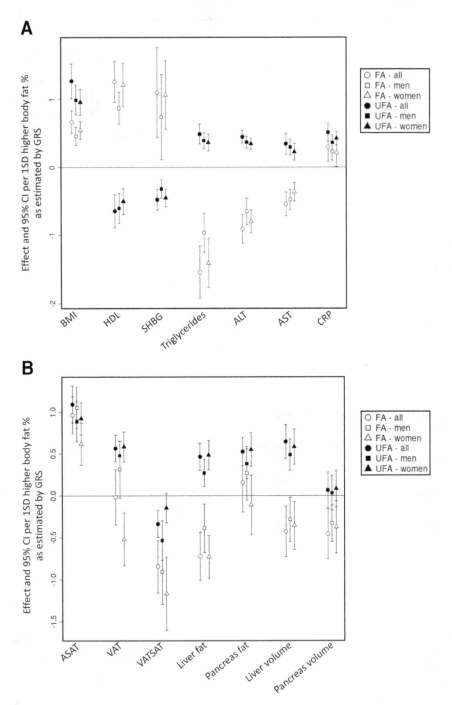

Figure 1—The sex-combined and sex-specific effects and 95% CIs per 1-SD-higher body fat percentage as estimated by FA and UFA genetic scores for measures of adiposity and biomarkers (*A*), MRI-derived measures of fat distribution (*B*), and cardiometabolic diseases in UK Biobank (*C*). ASAT, abdominal SAT; CRP, C-reactive protein; GRS, genetic risk score; VATSAT, VAT-to-SAT ratio.

associated with lower liver fat and smaller liver and pancreas volume and had no effect on pancreatic fat (Table 1 and Fig. 1*B*). Both UFA and FA genetic scores were associated with lower VAT-to-SAT ratio.

We replicated these associations using independent data from the published GWAS of abdominal fat as measured by

CT or MRI in up to 18,332 individuals for some of the measured phenotypes. UFA genetic score was associated with higher SAT (*P* = 3E−8), higher VAT (*P* = 6E−7), and higher pericardial adipose tissue (*P* = 0.003) but had no effect on VAT-to-SAT ratio (*P* = 0.70), while FA genetic score was associated with higher SAT (*P* = 6E−6) and lower VAT-to-SAT ratio

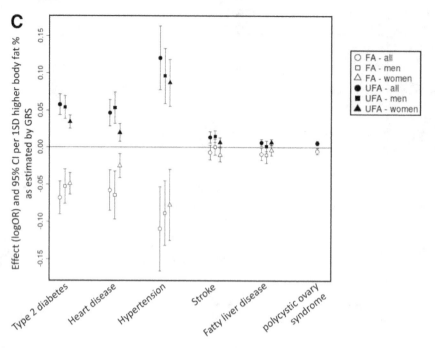

Figure 1—Continued.

($P = $ 2E$-$6) and had no effect on VAT ($P = 0.92$) or pericardial adipose tissue ($P = 0.50$) (Supplementary Table 6).

There was no sex difference in the association between FA and UFA clusters and MRI-derived measures of fat distribution at the multiple testing–corrected significance threshold except for VAT, where FA score was associated with higher VAT in men versus lower VAT in women ($P_{\text{difference}} = 0.0006$ [Supplementary Table 5 and Supplementary Fig. 3]).

With the data from the UK Biobank MRI subcohort, among 38 UFA variants, adiposity-increasing alleles at 31 variants ($P_{\text{two-tailed binomial}} = 0.0001$) were correlated with higher ectopic liver fat, including 7 variants with $P < 0.05$ (Supplementary Fig. 6), and 31 adiposity-increasing alleles were correlated with higher pancreatic fat ($P_{\text{two-tailed binomial}} = 0.0001$), including 7 variants at $P < 0.05$ (Supplementary Fig. 7). Of the 36 FA variants, 29 adiposity-increasing alleles were correlated with lower liver fat ($P_{\text{two-tailed binomial}} = 0.0003$), including 9 variants at $P < 0.05$ (Supplementary Fig. 6). FA variants had a mixed effect on pancreatic fat, as only 14 adiposity-increasing alleles were correlated with lower pancreatic fat ($P_{\text{two-tailed binomial}} = 0.24$), including two alleles associated with higher and two with lower pancreatic fat at $P < 0.05$ (Supplementary Fig. 7).

Results on interesting individual FA variants with paradoxical effects where adiposity-increasing alleles are associated with lower risk of type 2 diabetes (from UK Biobank–independent GWAS) and lower liver fat (from the UK Biobank) at $P < 0.05$ are illustrated as forest plots in Supplementary Fig. 8. These include eight variants:

rs4684847 (*PPARG*), rs12130231 (*LYPLAL1/SLC30A10*), rs11664106 (*EMILIN2*), rs13389219 (*GRB14/COBLL1*), rs2943653 (*NYAP2/IRS1*), rs30351 (*ANKRD55*), rs4450871 (*CYTL1*), and rs7133378 (*DNAH10*). Among these variants, the FA alleles at only two variants were associated with pancreatic fat at $P < 0.05$: near *GRB14*, with lower pancreatic fat, and near *PPARG*, with higher pancreatic fat.

Association With CRP Levels

To understand the role of inflammation in the mechanisms that link higher adiposity to risk of cardiometabolic disease, we looked at the association between FA and UFA variants and CRP levels as an inflammatory marker. In the UK Biobank, both UFA and FA genetic scores were associated with higher CRP (Table 1 and Fig. 1A). These associations were replicated using an independent GWAS of CRP (23) (Supplementary Table 6). There was no sex difference in the association between UFA and FA variants and CRP levels (Supplementary Table 5 and Supplementary Fig. 3). Of 38 UFA adiposity-increasing alleles, 35 ($P_{\text{two-tailed binomial}} = $ 7E$-$8) and, of 36 FA adiposity-increasing alleles, 27 ($P_{\text{two-tailed binomial}} = 0.004$) were correlated with higher CRP, including 32 and 15 variants with $P < 0.05$, respectively (Supplementary Fig. 9). To further understand the role of higher adiposity on the association between UFA and FA genetic scores and higher CRP, we ran our statistical models, but we additionally adjusted for BMI or body fat percentage. This adjustment removed the association with higher CRP for both genetic scores, indicating that the effect was mediated by higher adiposity (Supplementary Table 9).

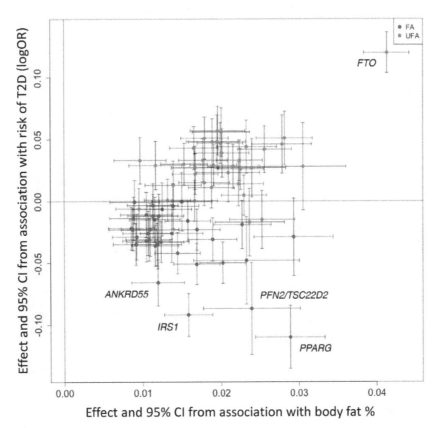

Figure 2—Adiposity-increasing alleles were correlated with lower risk of type 2 diabetes for all 36 FA variants, and 33 adiposity-increasing alleles of 38 UFA variants were correlated with higher risk of type 2 diabetes. Effects on *x*-axis are from the GWAS of body fat percentage in UK Biobank and on *y*-axis from the GWAS of type 2 diabetes published by Mahajan et al. (12) excluding data from UK Biobank. OR, odds ratio.

Association With Cardiometabolic Disease Risk

For UK Biobank data, UFA genetic score was associated with higher risk of type 2 diabetes ($P = 6E-16$), heart disease ($P = 2E-7$), hypertension ($P = 4E-8$), stroke ($P = 0.0005$), fatty liver disease ($P = 0.004$), and PCOS ($P = 7E-5$) (Table 1 and Fig. 1*C*). In contrast, FA genetic score was associated with lower risk of type 2 diabetes ($P = 2E-9$), heart disease ($P = 3E-5$), hypertension ($P = 0.0001$), fatty liver disease ($P = 0.03$), and PCOS ($P = 0.02$) (Table 1 and Fig. 1*C*). These findings were replicated with use of UK Biobank–independent GWAS data (Supplementary Table 6). There was no sex difference in the association of UFA and FA clusters with risk of disease at the multiple testing–corrected significance threshold (Supplementary Table 5 and Supplementary Fig. 3).

To understand the causal nature of these associations, we took an MR approach and used two UK Biobank–independent data sets (published GWAS and FinnGen). A 1-SD-higher genetically instrumented UFA was associated with higher risk of type 2 diabetes (IVW odds ratio 5.50 [95% CI 4.29, 7.05]; $P = 4E-41$), heart disease (1.66 [1.08, 2.54]; $P = 0.02$), hypertension (3.03 [2.18, 4.22]; $P = 5E-11$), stroke (1.43 [1.23, 1.67]; $P = 3E-6$), NAFLD (3.70 [1.22, 11.17]; $P = 0.02$), and PCOS (7.13 [3.66,

13.90]; $P = 8E-9$) (Table 2, Fig. 4, and Supplementary Table 10). In contrast, a 1-SD-higher genetically instrumented FA was associated with lower risk of type 2 diabetes (0.11 [0.08, 0.16]; $P = 4E-33$), heart disease (0.34 [0.25, 0.47]; $P = 2E-11$), hypertension (0.34 [0.21, 0.55]; $P = 1E-5$), stroke (0.65 [0.52, 0.83]; $P = 0.0004$), and NAFLD (0.14 [0.03, 0.79]; $P = 0.03$). There was a trend toward an association with lower odds of PCOS (0.51 [0.21, 1.23]; $P = 0.13$) but with wider CIs due to smaller sample size in the UK Biobank–independent GWAS (Table 2, Fig. 4, and Supplementary Table 10).

DISCUSSION

In this study, we used a unique genetic approach to understand the role of body adiposity in relation to the fat content and volumes of the liver and pancreas, as well as pathogenicity of cardiometabolic disease. We have identified two distinct clusters of variants associated with higher adiposity: one with a favorable metabolic profile (FA), consisting of 36 variants, and the other with an unfavorable metabolic profile (UFA), which included 38 variants. Although the adiposity-increasing alleles in both clusters are associated with increased SAT, the FA alleles are specifically associated with a lower liver fat and appear

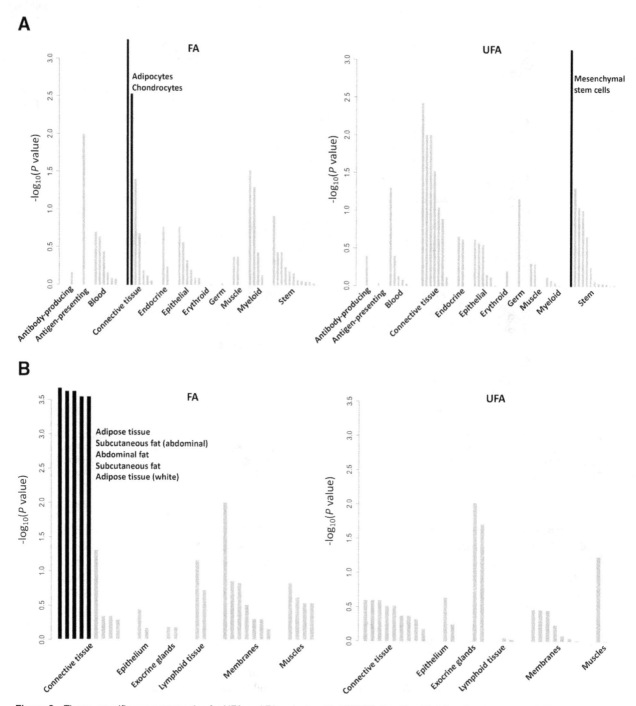

Figure 3—Tissue-specific gene expression for UFA and FA variants with DEPICT. Results with false discovery rate <0.05 are highlighted in black. Results are grouped by type and ordered by -log10(P-value) within cell types (A), tissues (B), and specific systems (C) (details in Supplementary Tables 7 and 8).

to provide protection against risk of cardiometabolic diseases, whereas the UFA alleles are associated with higher deposition of all fat depots including liver, pancreas, and visceral fat and are associated with higher risk of cardiometabolic disease.

The results of our genetic analysis support the observations from phenotyping studies that have proposed different obesity phenotypes related to the distribution of body fat (24,25). The two adiposity phenotypes that we have described in the current study highlight the role of SAT as a metabolic sink in obesity. In FA, this metabolic sink can accommodate excess triglycerides to specifically protect the liver from ectopic fat accumulation and prevent or delay pathogenic processes; in UFA, the excess

C

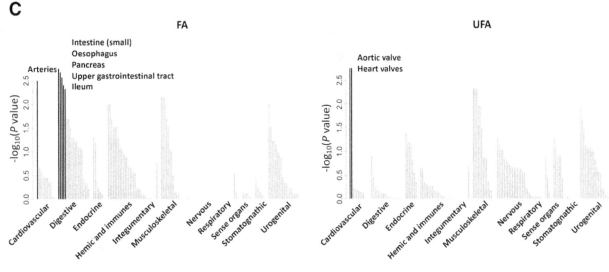

Figure 3—Continued.

triglycerides appear to exceed the capacity of the SAT metabolic sink and are consequently being deposited in alternate sites, including the VAT depot, liver, pancreas, and pericardial adipose tissue (26).

Our data, consistent with previous findings, provide evidence that accumulation of fat in the liver, which is an organ integral to glucose, insulin, and metabolism, directly contributes to the development of metabolic derangements associated with higher adiposity (27,28). Using a small subset of FA variants and a limited sample size with MRI scans (n = 9,510), we previously showed that FA alleles were associated with lower ectopic liver fat in women but not men (4). The availability of MRI scans of liver fat in 32,859 UK Biobank participants allowed us to demonstrate that there is no sex-specific association with liver fat. However, both FA and UFA variants had a greater overall effect on liver fat in women than men, which could indicate the confounding effects of other factors in the measured liver fat in men. The association of both FA and UFA clusters with, respectively, smaller and

bigger liver size is most likely biased by the accumulation of liver fat (29).

The pattern of association between FA and UFA variants and MRI-derived measures of ectopic fat can help with understanding the role of each ectopic fat depot in the pathophysiology of cardiometabolic diseases. While the FA cluster is associated with lower ectopic liver fat, it has no effect on VAT. This is consistent with previous studies showing the effect of thiazolidinediones, a class of medicines that improve insulin sensitivity, on promotion of differentiation of new adipocytes in SAT without changing VAT (30). In the light of strong association between VAT and development of metabolic dysfunction (31), our data suggest that VAT may reflect the ectopic fat deposition in the liver (r between the two measures = 0.5 [14]) but itself may not be causally related to the development of cardiometabolic diseases. The sex-specific association between the FA cluster and lower VAT in women and higher VAT in men is also consistent with the more general sex-specific pattern of VAT distribution

Table 2—IVW two-sample MR meta-analysis of cardiometabolic diseases from published GWAS and FinnGen for FA and UFA clusters

Outcome	FA				UFA			
	OR	Lower 95% CI	Upper 95% CI	P	OR	Lower 95% CI	Upper 95% CI	P
Type 2 diabetes	0.11	0.08	0.16	4E−33	5.50	4.29	7.05	4E−41
Heart disease	0.34	0.25	0.47	2E−11	1.66	1.08	2.54	0.02
Hypertension	0.34	0.21	0.55	1E−05	3.03	2.18	4.22	5E−11
Stroke	0.65	0.52	0.83	0.0004	1.43	1.23	1.67	3E−06
NAFLD	0.14	0.03	0.79	0.03	3.70	1.22	11.17	0.02
PCOS	0.51	0.21	1.23	0.13	7.13	3.66	13.90	8E−09

OR, odds ratio.

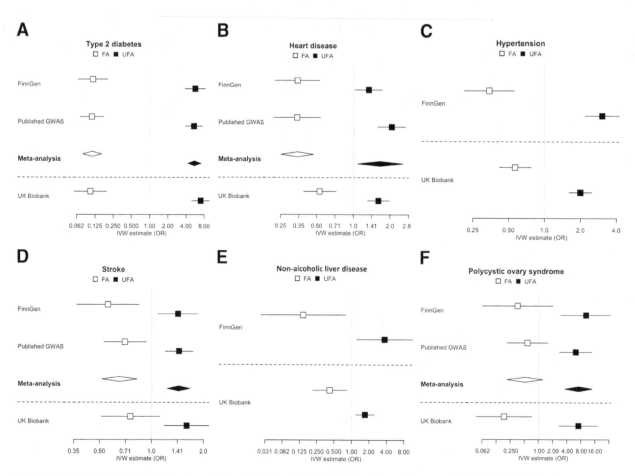

Figure 4—The IVW two-sample MR meta-analysis of published GWAS and FinnGen and one-sample MR of UK Biobank for FA and UFA clusters on risk of disease. The error bars and width of diamonds represent the 95% CIs of the IVW estimates in odds ratio (OR) per SD change in genetically determined FA and UFA.

as previously shown by genetic studies of waist-to-hip ratio (WHR) (32). Furthermore, while FA alleles are associated with lower VAT in women and higher VAT in men, they are associated with protection from cardiometabolic diseases with similar effect size between men and women.

Although the UFA cluster was associated with higher pancreatic fat, we did not detect any association between the FA cluster and this fat depot. FA variants individually had a mixed effect on pancreatic fat with the FA allele near *PPARG*, which is the most prominent example of FA variants mimicking the effect of thiazolidinediones, being associated with higher pancreatic fat. The role of pancreatic fat in the pathogenicity of type 2 diabetes is currently not clear-cut. Although many cross-sectional studies have reported higher pancreatic fat in subjects with type 2 diabetes compared with age-matched control subjects (33–36), there are conflicting views regarding whether pancreatic fat is itself a driver of type 2 diabetes, with some studies showing no association between type 2 diabetes and pancreatic fat using either CT or histology at autopsy (37–40). Moreover, a recent study testing the so-called "twin cycle model" (liver and pancreatic fat) before

and after the onset of type 2 diabetes showed that liver fat was the main mediator associated with glycemic control (41). Furthermore, a recent genetic study of pancreatic fat and liver fat in the UK Biobank showed that genetic variants associated with pancreatic fat did not have a significant impact on metabolic disease (14), suggesting that pancreatic fat has no direct role in pathogenicity of type 2 diabetes and other metabolic disease. Longitudinal imaging studies of individuals prior to and after clinical disease onset in addition to MR studies of pancreatic fat in type 2 diabetes and other metabolic diseases will help to unravel the cause and consequence of this relationship.

The FA cluster was associated with a smaller pancreas volume, whereas the UFA cluster had no association with pancreas volume. Studies of individuals with type 2 diabetes using CT or ultrasound have shown 7–33% lower pancreas volume compared with that of control subjects (39,42–44). Given that only 1–2% of the adult pancreas is composed of endocrine islets, changes in exocrine cell number may contribute more to lower pancreas volume as shown in studies of type 1 diabetes (45). Since insulin also acts as a growth stimulation hormone and maintains tissue mass (46,47), a decline in pancreas size in diabetes could be due to a loss of the trophic effect of insulin on exocrine cells (48,49). We previously showed that variants associated with FA are associated with lower fasting insulin levels (4–6), which could explain why the FA cluster was associated with a smaller pancreas volume.

Subclinical inflammation is another factor that has been shown to be associated with components of metabolic syndrome and vascular disease (50–54). Our data provided no evidence for any direct role of CRP in mechanisms that link FA and UFA clusters to, respectively, lower and higher risk of disease, since both clusters were associated with higher CRP levels, consistent with the findings of the largest MR study of CRP and risk of metabolic disease (23). We observed that the association between FA and UFA genetic scores and higher CRP levels disappeared after adjustment for adiposity (BMI or body fat percentage), indicating that their effect on higher CRP was mediated by higher adiposity. This pattern of association could suggest that higher CRP levels are secondary to higher adiposity. Data on other markers of inflammation, including tumor necrosis factor-α and interleukin-6, could clarify further the role of inflammation in cardiometabolic disease mechanisms.

Our tissue enrichment analysis provided further evidence that UFA and FA are biologically two different subtypes of adiposity. FA loci were enriched for genes expressed in adipose tissue and adipocytes, while UFA loci were enriched for genes expressed in mesenchymal stem cells. The enrichment of genes in adipose-related tissues and cells was previously shown for loci associated with WHR (55) in contrast to BMI loci enriched in the central nervous system (56). However, this is the first time mesenchymal stem cells have been highlighted in tissue enrichment analysis to be associated with adiposity. Mesenchymal stem cells are major sources of adipocyte generation, and in addition to adipose tissue, they also exist in skeletal muscle, the liver, and pancreas, which could suggest that they are responsible for ectopic fat formation in these organs (57,58). Further experiments and data are necessary to determine the relationship between mesenchymal stem cells and ectopic lipid accumulation.

There have been few approaches to identify variants associated with FA and UFA using different combinations of traits. Winkler et al. (59) used 159 variants associated with BMI, WHR, or WHR adjusted for BMI and described 24 FA variants as those associated with both lower WHR and higher BMI and 82 UFA variants as those associated with both higher WHR and higher BMI. Pigeyre et al. (60) used polygenic correlation between BMI and type 2 diabetes to identify genetic regions where BMI-increasing effect was linked to a corresponding increase, decrease, or neutral effect on type 2 diabetes risk. Our FA and UFA variants that overlap with these studies are listed in Supplementary Table 11. The main difference between

our approach and these two studies is that they have started with variants associated with BMI or WHR as measures of adiposity. Recent studies have demonstrated that BMI is a poor proxy for body adiposity (61), particularly at an individual level, providing limited insight into body fat distribution, VAT, or nonadipose deposition of fat (25). For example, only 7 and 12 of 36 FA variants are associated with BMI and WHR, respectively. Similarly, while UFA variants are enriched for BMI variants, 7 variants are not associated with BMI and only 14 of 38 UFA variants are associated with WHR (Supplementary Fig. 10). Furthermore, using only BMI and type 2 diabetes to identify variants with opposite effects can induce index event bias (62), e.g., TCF7L2 (60).

There are several limitations to our study. First, we did not have independent studies to replicate the association with liver and pancreas fat and volume measurements. However, we used the largest data set on MRI phenotypes available from the UK Biobank, with 32,859 samples, and replicated the association with some fat depots available from a published GWAS (17). Second, our study population was limited to Europeans only; it is unclear how our findings can be generalized to other populations and whether they can explain the excess risk of cardiometabolic disease in non-Europeans (63). Third, we lacked data on ectopic fat accumulation in muscle in our samples; future studies of MRI-derived muscle fat in the UK Biobank will enable the role of this ectopic fat in the pathophysiology of cardiometabolic disease to be investigated. Fourth, lower-body subcutaneous fat mass in the gluteofemoral or leg region has previously been associated favorably with obesity-related cardiometabolic diseases (64). It would also have been of interest to study whether the FA cluster is protective of cardiometabolic diseases, particularly via increasing gluteofemoral and leg fat mass. Fifth, we used ALT and AST in our discovery pipeline to identify FA and UFA variants, which could have biased our findings toward those variants that influence liver fat more than pancreatic fat. Finally, in comparison with our previous study (4), we did not have fasting insulin and adiponectin in our composite metabolic phenotype, since these two biomarkers are not available in the UK Biobank. However, our 36 FA variants include all 14 variants previously identified as FA (4) and the comparison of the multivariate GWAS P values for these variants (Supplementary Fig. 11) indicates additional power gained in the current study largely attributable to the availability of other metabolic biomarkers in 451,099 individuals in a single cohort, the UK Biobank.

One of the major strengths of this study was the unique approach to understanding different mechanisms underlying the association between adiposity and risk of cardiometabolic diseases. This unique approach is coupled with gold standard measurements of organ volume and content from MRI scans for understanding the role of different fat depots in pathogenicity. The availability of the

UK Biobank made it possible to study the sex-specific effects of our variants against metabolic biomarkers, MRI measures of fat distribution and ectopic fat, and risk of disease. We used the largest published GWAS and Finn-Gen study and independently replicated our results against risk of disease and performed MR studies. Unlike previous studies that examined the role of ectopic fat and pancreas size in small groups of participants categorized by diabetes status, we investigated the role of these phenotypes in a population-based study of 32,859 participants, which minimizes the effect of confounding factors and statistical bias. Finally, our sets of FA and UFA variants provide two important genetic instruments for any MR study to examine the causal role of adiposity on risk of disease uncoupled from its metabolic effect.

Conclusion

This study provides genetic evidence for two types of adiposity: one coupled with a favorable metabolic profile and the other with an unfavorable profile. Both FA and UFA variants were associated with higher CRP levels. We demonstrated that reduced liver fat, but not VAT or pancreatic fat, is on the pathway that links FA to lower risk of diseases related to metabolic syndrome. We determined no sexual dimorphism in the way the FA and UFA variants are associated with metabolic profile, abdominal fat distribution, and risk of disease. Future MR, longitudinal, and independent studies are required to elucidate whether higher pancreatic fat and smaller pancreas volume are a consequence of the ongoing pathological processes or causal of cardiometabolic disease outcomes. Better understanding of the difference between FA and UFA may lead to new insights in preventing and predicting, and treating people who suffer from, cardiometabolic diseases.

Acknowledgments. This research has been conducted using data from the UK Biobank resource and carried out under UK Biobank project application numbers 9072, 9055, and 44584. UK Biobank protocols were approved by the National Research Ethics Service Committee. The authors acknowledge the participants and investigators of the FinnGen study. The authors thank Amoolya Singh and Kevin Wright, Calico Life Sciences LLC, for their feedback on the manuscript. The authors would like to acknowledge the use of the University of Exeter High-Performance Computing (HPC) facility in carrying out this work. We acknowledge use of high-performance computing funded by an MRC Clinical Research Infrastructure award (MRC Grant: MR/M008924/1).

Funding. S.M. is funded by the Medical Research Council. H.Y. is funded by a Diabetes UK RD Lawrence fellowship (17/0005594). J.T. is supported by an Academy of Medical Sciences (AMS) Springboard Award, which is supported by the AMS, the Wellcome Trust, the Global Challenges Research Fund, the U.K. Government Department of Business, Energy & Industrial Strategy, the British Heart Foundation, and Diabetes UK (SBF004\1079).

Duality of Interest. M.C., E.S., and Y.L. are employees of Calico Life Sciences LLC. M.C., E.S., and Y.L. are funded by Calico Life Sciences LLC. No other potential conflicts of interest relevant to this article were reported.

The funders had no role in the design and conduct of the study; collection, management, analysis, and interpretation of the data; preparation, review, or approval of the manuscript; and decision to submit the manuscript for publication.

Authors Contributions. S.M. performed the statistical analyses. S.M. and H.Y. designed the study and wrote the first draft of the manuscript. N.B., B.W., Y.L., J.D.B., and E.L.T. created the MRI-derived phenotypes and contributed to the writing of the manuscript. M.C. and E.S. performed the GWAS of MRI-derived phenotypes. J.T., R.N.B., A.R.W., and T.M.F. contributed to the analysis of biomarkers from the UK Biobank. H.Y. is the guarantor of this work and, as such, had full access to all the data in the study and takes responsibility for the integrity of the data and the accuracy of the data analysis.

References

1. Lindsay RS, Howard BV. Cardiovascular risk associated with the metabolic syndrome. Curr Diab Rep 2004;4:63–68
2. Stefan N, Kantartzis K, Machann J, et al. Identification and characterization of metabolically benign obesity in humans. Arch Intern Med 2008;168:1609–1616
3. Primeau V, Coderre L, Karelis AD, et al. Characterizing the profile of obese patients who are metabolically healthy. Int J Obes 2011;35:971–981
4. Ji Y, Yiorkas AM, Frau F, et al. Genome-wide and abdominal MRI data provide evidence that a genetically determined favorable adiposity phenotype is characterized by lower ectopic liver fat and lower risk of type 2 diabetes, heart disease, and hypertension. Diabetes 2019;68:207–219
5. Yaghootkar H, Lotta LA, Tyrrell J, et al. Genetic evidence for a link between favorable adiposity and lower risk of type 2 diabetes, hypertension, and heart disease. Diabetes 2016;65:2448–2460
6. Yaghootkar H, Scott RA, White CC, et al. Genetic evidence for a normal-weight "metabolically obese" phenotype linking insulin resistance, hypertension, coronary artery disease, and type 2 diabetes. Diabetes 2014;63:4369–4377
7. Lotta LA, Gulati P, Day FR, et al.; EPIC-InterAct Consortium; Cambridge FPLD1 Consortium. Integrative genomic analysis implicates limited peripheral adipose storage capacity in the pathogenesis of human insulin resistance. Nat Genet 2017;49:17–26
8. Collins R. What makes UK Biobank special? Lancet 2012;379:1173–1174
9. Loh PR, Tucker G, Bulik-Sullivan BK, et al. Efficient Bayesian mixed-model analysis increases association power in large cohorts. Nat Genet 2015;47:284–290
10. Cichonska A, Rousu J, Marttinen P, et al. metaCCA: summary statistics-based multivariate meta-analysis of genome-wide association studies using canonical correlation analysis. Bioinformatics 2016;32:1981–1989
11. Semple RK, Savage DB, Cochran EK, Gorden P, O'Rahilly S. Genetic syndromes of severe insulin resistance. Endocr Rev 2011;32:498–514
12. Mahajan A, Taliun D, Thurner M, et al. Fine-mapping type 2 diabetes loci to single-variant resolution using high-density imputation and islet-specific epigenome maps. Nat Genet 2018;50:1505–1513
13. Littlejohns TJ, Holliday J, Gibson LM, et al. The UK Biobank imaging enhancement of 100,000 participants: rationale, data collection, management and future directions. Nat Commun 2020;11:2624
14. Liu Y, Basty N, Whitcher B, Bell JD, Sorokin EP, van Bruggen N, Thomas EL, Cule M. Genetic architecture of 11 organ traits derived from abdominal MRI using deep learning. Elife. 2021 Jun 15:10:e65554
15. Bydder M, Ghodrati V, Gao Y, Robson MD, Yang Y, Hu P. Constraints in estimating the proton density fat fraction. Magn Reson Imaging 2020;66:1–8
16. Bycroft C, Freeman C, Petkova D, et al. The UK Biobank resource with deep phenotyping and genomic data. Nature 2018;562:203–209
17. Chu AY, Deng X, Fisher VA, et al. Multiethnic genome-wide meta-analysis of ectopic fat depots identifies loci associated with adipocyte development and differentiation. Nat Genet 2017;49:125–130
18. Burgess S, Butterworth A, Thompson SG. Mendelian randomization analysis with multiple genetic variants using summarized data. Genet Epidemiol 2013;37:658–665

19. Pierce BL, Burgess S. Efficient design for Mendelian randomization studies: subsample and 2-sample instrumental variable estimators. Am J Epidemiol 2013;178:1177–1184

20. FinnGen documentation of R4 release, 2020. Available from https://finngen.gitbook.io/documentation/releases

21. Viechtbauer W. Conducting meta-analyses in R with the metafor package. J Stat Softw 2010;36:1–48

22. Pers TH, Karjalainen JM, Chan Y, et al.; Genetic Investigation of ANthropometric Traits (GIANT) Consortium. Biological interpretation of genome-wide association studies using predicted gene functions. Nat Commun 2015;6:5890

23. Ligthart S, Vaez A, Võsa U, et al.; LifeLines Cohort Study; CHARGE Inflammation Working Group. Genome analyses of >200,000 individuals identify 58 loci for chronic inflammation and highlight pathways that link inflammation and complex disorders. Am J Hum Genet 2018;103:691–706

24. O'Donovan G, Thomas EL, McCarthy JP, et al. Fat distribution in men of different waist girth, fitness level and exercise habit. Int J Obes 2009;33:1356–1362

25. Thomas EL, Frost G, Taylor-Robinson SD, Bell JD. Excess body fat in obese and normal-weight subjects. Nutr Res Rev 2012;25:150–161

26. Unger RH. Minireview: weapons of lean body mass destruction: the role of ectopic lipids in the metabolic syndrome. Endocrinology 2003;144:5159–5165

27. Krssak M, Falk Petersen K, Dresner A, et al. Intramyocellular lipid concentrations are correlated with insulin sensitivity in humans: a ^{1}H NMR spectroscopy study. Diabetologia 1999;42:113–116

28. Fabbrini E, Magkos F, Mohammed BS, et al. Intrahepatic fat, not visceral fat, is linked with metabolic complications of obesity. Proc Natl Acad Sci USA 2009;106:15430–15435

29. Kromrey ML, Ittermann T, vWahsen C, et al. Reference values of liver volume in Caucasian population and factors influencing liver size. Eur J Radiol 2018;106:32–37

30. Adams M, Montague CT, Prins JB, et al. Activators of peroxisome proliferator-activated receptor gamma have depot-specific effects on human preadipocyte differentiation. J Clin Invest 1997;100:3149–3153

31. Lee JJ, Pedley A, Hoffmann U, Massaro JM, Levy D, Long MT. Visceral and intrahepatic fat are associated with cardiometabolic risk factors above other ectopic fat depots: the Framingham Heart Study. Am J Med 2018;131:684–692.e12

32. Pulit SL, Stoneman C, Morris AP, et al.; GIANT Consortium. Meta-analysis of genome-wide association studies for body fat distribution in 694 649 individuals of European ancestry. Hum Mol Genet 2019;28:166–174

33. Tushuizen ME, Bunck MC, Pouwels PJ, et al. Pancreatic fat content and beta-cell function in men with and without type 2 diabetes. Diabetes Care 2007;30:2916–2921

34. Lingvay I, Esser V, Legendre JL, et al. Noninvasive quantification of pancreatic fat in humans. J Clin Endocrinol Metab 2009;94:4070–4076

35. Steven S, Hollingsworth KG, Small PK, et al. Weight loss decreases excess pancreatic triacylglycerol specifically in type 2 diabetes. Diabetes Care 2016;39:158–165

36. Wang CY, Ou HY, Chen MF, Chang TC, Chang CJ. Enigmatic ectopic fat: prevalence of nonalcoholic fatty pancreas disease and its associated factors in a Chinese population. J Am Heart Assoc 2014;3:e000297

37. Clark A, Wells CA, Buley ID, et al. Islet amyloid, increased A-cells, reduced B-cells and exocrine fibrosis: quantitative changes in the pancreas in type 2 diabetes. Diabetes Res 1988;9:151–159

38. Gilbeau JP, Poncelet V, Libon E, Derue G, Heller FR. The density, contour, and thickness of the pancreas in diabetics: CT findings in 57 patients. AJR Am J Roentgenol 1992;159:527–531

39. Saisho Y, Butler AE, Meier JJ, et al. Pancreas volumes in humans from birth to age one hundred taking into account sex, obesity, and presence of type-2 diabetes. Clin Anat 2007;20:933–942

40. Yamazaki H, Tsuboya T, Katanuma A, et al. Lack of independent association between fatty pancreas and incidence of type 2 diabetes: 5-year Japanese cohort study. Diabetes Care 2016;39:1677–1683

41. Koivula RW, Atabaki-Pasdar N, Giordano GN, et al.; IMI DIRECT Consortium. The role of physical activity in metabolic homeostasis before and after the onset of type 2 diabetes: an IMI DIRECT study. Diabetologia 2020;63:744–756

42. Alzaid A, Aideyan O, Nawaz S. The size of the pancreas in diabetes mellitus. Diabet Med 1993;10:759–763

43. Lim S, Bae JH, Chun EJ, et al. Differences in pancreatic volume, fat content, and fat density measured by multidetector-row computed tomography according to the duration of diabetes. Acta Diabetol 2014;51:739–748

44. Macauley M, Percival K, Thelwall PE, Hollingsworth KG, Taylor R. Altered volume, morphology and composition of the pancreas in type 2 diabetes. PLoS One 2015;10:e0126825

45. Wright JJ, Saunders DC, Dai C, et al. Decreased pancreatic acinar cell number in type 1 diabetes. Diabetologia 2020;63:1418–1423

46. Adler G, Kern HF. Regulation of exocrine pancreatic secretory process by insulin in vivo. Horm Metab Res 1975;7:290–296

47. Mössner J, Logsdon CD, Williams JA, Goldfine ID. Insulin, via its own receptor, regulates growth and amylase synthesis in pancreatic acinar AR42J cells. Diabetes 1985;34:891–897

48. Henderson JR, Daniel PM, Fraser PA. The pancreas as a single organ: the influence of the endocrine upon the exocrine part of the gland. Gut 1981;22:158–167

49. Kusmartseva I, Beery M, Hiller H, et al. Temporal analysis of amylase expression in control, autoantibody-positive, and type 1 diabetes pancreatic tissues. Diabetes 2020;69:60–66

50. Libby P. Inflammation in atherosclerosis. Arterioscler Thromb Vasc Biol 2012;32:2045–2051

51. Schmidt MI, Duncan BB, Sharrett AR, et al. Markers of inflammation and prediction of diabetes mellitus in adults (Atherosclerosis Risk in Communities study): a cohort study. Lancet 1999;353:1649–1652

52. Festa A, D'Agostino R Jr, Tracy RP; Insulin Resistance Atherosclerosis Study. Elevated levels of acute-phase proteins and plasminogen activator inhibitor-1 predict the development of type 2 diabetes: the insulin resistance atherosclerosis study. Diabetes 2002;51:1131–1137

53. Hundal RS, Petersen KF, Mayerson AB, et al. Mechanism by which high-dose aspirin improves glucose metabolism in type 2 diabetes. J Clin Invest 2002;109:1321–1326

54. Pickup JC. Inflammation and activated innate immunity in the pathogenesis of type 2 diabetes. Diabetes Care 2004;27:813–823

55. Shungin D, Winkler TW, Croteau-Chonka DC, et al.; ADIPOGen Consortium; CARDIOGRAMplusC4D Consortium; CKDGen Consortium; GEFOS Consortium; GENIE Consortium; GLGC; ICBP; International Endogene Consortium; LifeLines Cohort Study; MAGIC Investigators; MuTHER Consortium; PAGE Consortium; ReproGen Consortium. New genetic loci link adipose and insulin biology to body fat distribution. Nature 2015;518:187–196

56. Locke AE, Kahali B, Berndt SI, et al.; LifeLines Cohort Study; ADIPOGen Consortium; AGEN-BMI Working Group; CARDIOGRAMplusC4D Consortium; CKDGen Consortium; GLGC; ICBP; MAGIC Investigators; MuTHER Consortium; MIGen Consortium; PAGE Consortium; ReproGen Consortium; GENIE Consortium; International Endogene Consortium. Genetic studies of body mass index yield new insights for obesity biology. Nature 2015;518:197–206

57. Uezumi A, Fukada S, Yamamoto N, Takeda S, Tsuchida K. Mesenchymal progenitors distinct from satellite cells contribute to ectopic fat cell formation in skeletal muscle. Nat Cell Biol 2010;12:143–152

58. Matsushita K, Dzau VJ. Mesenchymal stem cells in obesity: insights for translational applications. Lab Invest 2017;97:1158–1166

59. Winkler TW, Günther F, Höllerer S, et al.; A joint view on genetic variants for adiposity differentiates subtypes with distinct metabolic implications. Nat Commun. 2018;9(1):1946

60. Pigeyre M, Sjaarda J, Mao S, et al. Identification of novel causal blood biomarkers linking metabolically favorable adiposity with type 2 diabetes risk. Diabetes Care 2019;42:1800–1808

61. Nuttall FQ. Body mass index: obesity, BMI, and health: a critical review. Nutr Today 2015;50:117–128

62. Yaghootkar H, Bancks MP, Jones SE, et al. Quantifying the extent to which index event biases influence large genetic association studies. Hum Mol Genet 2017;26:1018–1030

63. Yaghootkar H, Whitcher B, Bell JD, Thomas EL. Ethnic differences in adiposity and diabetes risk - insights from genetic studies. J Intern Med 2020;288:271–283

64. Stefan N. Causes, consequences, and treatment of metabolically unhealthy fat distribution. Lancet Diabetes Endocrinol 2020;8:616–627

Role of the Neutral Amino Acid Transporter SLC7A10 in Adipocyte Lipid Storage, Obesity, and Insulin Resistance

Regine Å. Jersin,[1,2] Divya Sri Priyanka Tallapragada,[1,2] André Madsen,[1,2] Linn Skartveit,[1,2] Even Fjære,[3] Adrian McCann,[4] Laurence Dyer,[1,2] Aron Willems,[1,2] Jan-Inge Bjune,[1,2] Mona S. Bjune,[1,2] Villy Våge,[2,5] Hans Jørgen Nielsen,[6] Håvard Luong Thorsen,[7] Bjørn Gunnar Nedrebø,[1,8] Christian Busch,[9] Vidar M. Steen,[10,11] Matthias Blüher,[12] Peter Jacobson,[13] Per-Arne Svensson,[13] Johan Fernø,[1,2] Mikael Rydén,[14] Peter Arner,[14] Ottar Nygård,[1,15] Melina Claussnitzer,[1,16,17] Ståle Ellingsen,[3,18] Lise Madsen,[3,19] Jørn V. Sagen,[1,2,20] Gunnar Mellgren,[1,2] and Simon N. Dankel[1,2]

Diabetes 2021;70:680–695 | https://doi.org/10.2337/db20-0096

Elucidation of mechanisms that govern lipid storage, oxidative stress, and insulin resistance may lead to improved therapeutic options for type 2 diabetes and other obesity-related diseases. Here, we find that adipose expression of the small neutral amino acid transporter SLC7A10, also known as alanine-serine-cysteine transporter-1 (ASC-1), shows strong inverse correlates with visceral adiposity, insulin resistance, and adipocyte hypertrophy across multiple cohorts. Concordantly, loss of Slc7a10 function in zebrafish in vivo accelerates diet-induced body weight gain and adipocyte enlargement. Mechanistically, SLC7A10 inhibition in human and murine adipocytes decreases adipocyte serine uptake and total glutathione levels and promotes reactive oxygen species (ROS) generation. Conversely, SLC7A10 overexpression decreases ROS generation and increases mitochondrial respiratory capacity. RNA sequencing revealed consistent changes in gene expression between human adipocytes and zebrafish visceral adipose tissue following loss of SLC7A10, e.g., upregulation of *SCD* (lipid storage) and downregulation of *CPT1A* (lipid oxidation). Interestingly, ROS scavenger reduced lipid accumulation and attenuated the lipid-storing effect of SLC7A10 inhibition. These data uncover adipocyte SLC7A10 as a novel important regulator of adipocyte resilience to nutrient and oxidative stress, in part by enhancing glutathione levels and mitochondrial respiration, conducive to decreased ROS generation, lipid accumulation, adipocyte hypertrophy, insulin resistance, and type 2 diabetes.

Adipocyte hypertrophy in both subcutaneous (SC) and visceral white adipose tissue (AT) is strongly associated with whole-body insulin resistance, with or without obesity and AT inflammation (1,2), and with fatty liver, dyslipidemia, impaired mitochondrial function, and reduced insulin-stimulated

[1]Mohn Nutrition Research Laboratory, Department of Clinical Science, University of Bergen, Bergen, Norway
[2]Hormone Laboratory, Haukeland University Hospital, Bergen, Norway
[3]Institute of Marine Research, Bergen, Norway
[4]Bevital A/S, Laboratoriebygget, Bergen, Norway
[5]Center of Health Research, Førde Hospital Trust, Førde, Norway
[6]Department of Surgery, Voss Hospital, Bergen Health Trust, Voss, Norway
[7]Department of Surgery, Haugesund Hospital, Haugesund, Norway
[8]Department of Medicine, Haugesund Hospital, Haugesund, Norway
[9]Plastikkirurg1 AS, Bergen, Norway
[10]NORMENT, K.G. Jebsen Center for Psychosis Research, Department of Clinical Science, University of Bergen, Bergen, Norway
[11]Dr. E. Martens Research Group for Biological Psychiatry, Department of Medical Genetics, Haukeland University Hospital, Bergen, Norway
[12]Clinic for Endocrinology and Nephrology, Medical Research Center, Leipzig, Germany
[13]Institute of Medicine, The Sahlgrenska Academy at the University of Gothenburg, Gothenburg, Sweden
[14]Department of Medicine (H7), Karolinska Institutet, Karolinska University Hospital, Huddinge, Stockholm, Sweden
[15]Department of Heart Disease, Haukeland University Hospital, Bergen, Norway
[16]Broad Institute of MIT and Harvard, Cambridge, MA
[17]Department of Medicine, Beth Israel Deaconess Medical Center, Harvard Medical School, Boston, MA
[18]Department of Biological Sciences, University of Bergen, Bergen, Norway
[19]Department of Biology, University of Copenhagen, Copenhagen, Denmark
[20]Bergen Stem Cell Consortium, Haukeland University Hospital, Bergen, Norway

Corresponding author: Simon N. Dankel, simon.dankel@uib.no

Received 30 January 2020 and accepted 14 December 2020

This article contains supplementary material online at https://doi.org/10.2337/figshare.13377155.

glucose uptake in adipocytes (3). Experimental impairment of mitochondrial respiration and increased reactive oxygen species (ROS) generation in adipocytes reduce adipocyte insulin sensitivity (4), and the extent of mitochondrial dysfunction determines the severity of insulin resistance and type 2 diabetes (5). However, the molecular mechanisms that promote adipocyte hypertrophy and insulin resistance remain incompletely understood, and we urgently need new potential treatment targets.

SLC7A10, also known as alanine-serine-cysteine transporter-1 (ASC-1), has sodium-independent activity and high affinity for the small neutral amino acids (AAs) glycine, L-alanine, L-threonine, L-cysteine, L-serine, and D-serine (6,7). SLC7A10 is highly expressed in certain regions of the brain and is being explored as a therapeutic target in neuropsychiatric disorders (e.g., schizophrenia) (8).

A previous report showed selective expression of SLC7A10 in white but not beige or brown adipocytes, with fivefold higher expression in AT compared with the highest expressing parts of the brain, and diminished expression in other tissues (9). However, the possible role of SLC7A10 in metabolic regulation has not been explored.

While AAs known to be transported by SLC7A10 in the brain, e.g., serine, glycine, and cysteine, have central roles in one-carbon metabolism, the methionine cycle, glutathione synthesis, and redox balance (6,7,10,11), the AAs carried by SLC7A10 in adipocytes and the consequent metabolic effects are unknown. By transcriptome screens and interrogation of several human obesity cohorts along with functional experiments, we here uncover SLC7A10 as an important novel regulator of core metabolic functions in white adipocytes, providing new insight into the development of obesity and insulin resistance.

RESEARCH DESIGN AND METHODS

Human Cohorts and Samples
Anthropometric data are summarized in Table 1 (seven cohorts).

RNA and Gene Expression Analyses
Whole AT was homogenized or fractionated into isolated adipocytes or stromal vascular fraction (SVF), and RNA was purified, as described previously (12). Global gene expression in whole AT was measured by microarrays as described previously for the biliopancreatic diversion (BDP)-Fat cohort (13), Sib Pair cohort (14), very low calorie diet (VLCD) study (baseline data) (15) and RIKEN cohort (16). Quantitative PCR (qPCR) was performed with SYBR Green dye following cDNA synthesis with a high-capacity cDNA reverse transcription kit (Applied Biosystems) (Supplementary Table 1).

Human Cell Cultures

Primary Human Adipocyte Cultures
Human liposuction aspirates from the abdomen and flanks were collected with informed consent from donors undergoing cosmetic surgery at Aleris medical center and Plastikkirurg1. The donors comprised 18 women and 1 man between 21 and 68 years of age (mean ± SD age 46.3 ± 12.4 years) and with BMI between 24.3 and 32.8 kg/m^2 (27.9 ± 2.7 kg/m^2), all free of diabetes and otherwise healthy (Supplementary Table 2).

Isolation and Culturing of Human SVF
The SVF from SC AT was isolated as previously described (17) with some modifications. Briefly, Krebs-Ringer phosphate buffer containing Liberase Blendzyme 3 (Roche) and DNase was added to the liposuction aspirate. Following a 1-h incubation at 37°C, the digested fat tissue was filtered, washed with 0.9% NaCl, and centrifugated. Red blood cells were lysed (NH$_4$Cl [155 mmol/L], K$_2$HPO$_4$ [5.7 mmol/L], and EDTA [0.1 mmol/L]). Preadipocytes were seeded and cultured in GlutaMAX DMEM (Thermo Fisher Scientific) supplemented with 10% FBS and 50 μg/mL gentamicin (Sigma-Aldrich) and grown at 37°C with 5% CO$_2$. The following day, differentiation of primary human adipose cells (human adipose stromal cells [hASCs]) was induced by supplementing of the culture medium with 33 μmol/L biotin, 1 nmol/L triiodothyronine, 17 μmol/L DL-pantothenate, 10 μg/mL transferrin, 66 nmol/L insulin, 100 nmol/L cortisol, 15 mmol/L HEPES, and 10 μmol/L rosiglitazone. Rosiglitazone was discontinued after 6 days, and terminal differentiation was defined at 12–13 days.

Mouse Cell Cultures and Primary Cells
3T3-L1 mouse preadipocytes were cultured and differentiated as described previously (18).

SLC7A10 Inhibitors
BMS-466442 (AOBIOUS), referred to as SLC7A10 inhibitor 1 (19), and Lu AE00527, referred to as SLC7A10 inhibitor 2 (20), were used to inhibit SLC7A10 function in in vitro cell culture experiments at a standard final concentration of 10 μmol/L. The latter inhibitor was provided by H. Lundbeck A/S (Valby, Denmark).

Gene Expression Analysis
Total RNA from human and mouse cell cultures was isolated with RNeasy kit (QIAGEN) and quality checked by QIAxpert spectrophotometer (QIAGEN) prior to cDNA synthesis with 200 ng RNA input with use of a high-capacity cDNA reverse transcription kit (Applied Biosystems). cDNA was analyzed by LightCycler 480 (Roche) quantitative real-time PCR with SYBR Green dye (Roche) and target primers (Supplementary Table 1). Relative mRNA expression was determined by standard curves and normalized to a reference gene (HPRT or Rps13). Prior to RNA sequencing (RNA-seq), samples were DNase treated and RNA integrity number (>9) was confirmed by Bioanalyzer (Agilent). cDNA libraries were generated with a TruSeq Stranded mRNA Library Prep kit and sequenced by Illumina HiSeq 4000. Reads were mapped against the

Table 1—Overview of the analyzed human cohorts

Cohort and adiposity	n	% male	Age (years)	BMI (kg/m²)	WHR	% with T2D	Tissue	Expression	Figure/data set
BPD-Fat									
Obese	12	25	40.4 ± 12.5	51.5 ± 4.9	n/a	42	SC/OM	Illumina	Supplementary Table 4
Post–1 year	12	25	42.2 ± 11.7	32.9 ± 5.6	n/a	0	SC		
Sib Pair, nonobese/obese	88	47	65.9 ± 6.7	29.3 ± 5.5	0.94 ± 0.08	18	SC	Affymetrix	Fig. 1E and Supplementary Table 4
VLCD, obese	24	75	48.3 ± 10.4	37.6 ± 4.9	1.02 ± 0.08	29	SC	Affymetrix	Fig. 1E and Supplementary Fig. 1B
ADIPO									
Obese	12	33	43.1 ± 10.4	43.8 ± 5.4	n/a	17	SC/OM[a]	Illumina	Fig. 1A and C
Lean	12	42	43.5 ± 12.1	22.8 ± 2.2	0.89 ± 0.06	0	SC[a]	Illumina	Supplementary Table 4
WNOB									
Obese	324	21	40.4 ± 12.5	42.4 ± 5.4	n/a	21	SC/OM	qPCR	Fig. 1B
Post–1 year	137		42.6 ± 11.8	28.9 ± 5.2	n/a	0	SC	qPCR	
Nonobese	59	82	49.1 ± 16.5	24.7 ± 3.1	n/a	0	SC	qPCR	
ISO									
Obese, IR	40	50	51.5 ± 9.7	45.5 ± 1.4	n/a	0	SC/OM	qPCR	Fig. 1D
Obese, IS	40	50	51.4 ± 9.6	45.1 ± 1.8	n/a	0	SC/OM	qPCR	
RIKEN, nonobese/obese	56	0	42.9 ± 12.0	33.1 ± 9.9	0.93 ± 0.08	0	SC[b]	Affymetrix	Fig. 1E and Supplementary Fig. 1A

IR, insulin resistant; IS, insulin sensitive; post–1 year, 1 year after bariatric surgery; T2D, type 2 diabetes. [a]SLC7A10 expression was measured in isolated adipocytes and SVF. [b]SLC7A10 expression was measured in isolated adipocytes.

human genome (GrCH38) with use of HISAT (version 2.1.0), tabulated by featureCounts (version 1.5.2), and analyzed with DESeq2 (version 1.22.2).

Coexpression, Gene Ontology, and Pathway Analysis

Coexpression analysis was performed based on global gene expression data for human adipocytes isolated directly from biopsies of 12 lean and 12 obese patients (ADIPO cohort). Pearson correlation coefficients were calculated for correlations between *SLC7A10* mRNA and all other transcripts globally ($\sim$47,000 probes, including 21,000 individual genes) across the 24 patients. Genes with correlation coefficients $\beta > 0.65$ or $\beta < -0.65$ were analyzed with the PANTHER Gene List Analysis tool (http://www.pantherdb.org/) for performance of a statistical overrepresentation test (binomial statistics, Bonferroni corrected for multiple testing). RNA-seq results from hASCs were analyzed by PANTHER (v.14.0), using Fisher exact test (21).

Transfection

Transfection with mouse Slc7a10 expression plasmid was performed with the transfection reagent TransIT-L1, following the manufacturer's protocol (Mirus Bio LCC). Slc7a10 plasmid (2.0 μg) or empty vector was used per milliliter of medium (Supplementary Table 3).

Western Blotting

Cells were lysed in radioimmunoprecipitation assay buffer (Thermo Fisher Scientific) containing EDTA-free protease inhibitor cocktail (Roche) and PhosphoStop (Sigma-Aldrich). Protein content in the lysates was determined with DC Protein Assay (Bio-Rad Laboratories), loaded onto 4–20% TGX Gels (Bio-Rad Laboratories) and subjected to SDS-PAGE prior to transfer to nitrocellulose membrane. Membranes were developed with Femto solution (Thermo Fisher Scientific), and target protein amount relative to endogenous control was quantified by densitometry.

AA Quantification

Extracellular (medium) AA concentrations were assayed by gas chromatography–tandem mass spectrometry (GC-MS/MS) (Agilent) (22). Flux was calculated based on AA concentration in unconditioned and conditioned medium.

Radiolabeled AA Uptake Assays

AA uptake was measured in sodium-free assay buffer, as described previously (19), with use of unlabeled controls (D- or L-serine, final concentration 10 mmol/L) and stock solutions of D-[^{3}H]-serine (15 Ci/mmol) and L-[^{14}C]-serine (100 mCi/mmol) (PerkinElmer). Sample radioactivity was measured as 5-min averaged counts per minute (CPM) (QuantaSmart software).

Mitochondrial Respiration Assay

Cellular respiration was measured by the Seahorse XF Cell Mito Stress Test kit and XF96 Analyzer (Agilent). Preadipocytes were seeded in gelatin-coated (0.1% w/v) microplates and differentiated. Cells were washed and treated in XF base medium supplemented with L-glutamine (2 mmol/L), sodium pyruvate (2 mmol/L), and glucose (10 mmol/L) and incubated in a CO_2-free incubator for 1 h. Oxygen consumption rate (OCR) data were normalized to numbers of cells per well, measured by Hoechst staining.

Lipid Staining

Lipid accumulation was assessed by oil red O (ORO) staining as described previously (23).

Radiolabeled Glucose Uptake Assays

Adipocytes were washed with PBS and incubated overnight in glucose-reduced DMEM with or without treatment. Subsequently, cells were starved in glucose-free medium with or without treatment for 2.5 h. Insulin (final concentration 10 nmol/L) was added to indicated wells for 30 min prior to the assay. Deoxy-D-[^{14}C]-glucose (57.7 mCi/mmol) (PerkinElmer) was added for 30 min and incubated at 37°C. Cells were placed on ice and washed, and lysates were collected in Ultima Gold fluid cartridges (PerkinElmer). Isotope retention in lysate was measured as 5-min averaged CPM (QuantaSmart software) in a scintillation counter.

ROS Assay

Adipocytes were incubated for 30 min with or without 5 μmol/L CM-H2DCFDA as described previously (24). Cells were washed and incubated in Krebs-Ringer bicarbonate buffer or sodium-free assay buffer, with indicated compounds, followed by measurement of fluorescent emission of oxidized H2DCFDA probe (538 nm following 485 nm excitation) with a SpectraMax Gemini EM (Molecular Devices) plate reader at 37°C.

Glutathione Assay

Total glutathione was measured with the GSH/GSSG-Glo Assay (Promega) according to the manufacturer's protocol. Briefly, cells were lysed with glutathione lysis reagent and incubated in luciferin generation reagent for 30 min at room temperature. Samples were incubated for 15 min following addition of luciferin detection reagent. Luminescence was measured with FLUOstar OPTIMA EM (Thermo Fisher Scientific).

In Vivo Zebrafish Model

Heterozygous Slc7a10b loss-of-function *Danio rerio* (zebrafish) were obtained from The Zebrafish Model Organism Database (ZFIN) (genomic feature sa15382) and crossed for obtaining homozygote and wild-type (WT) zebrafish.

Genotyping

Genomic DNA was extracted from caudal fin biopsies of mature zebrafish with a DNeasy kit (QIAGEN). For genotyping, a 298 base pair (bp) region of the *Slc7a10b* gene containing the intron splice site A→T mutation was amplified by PCR with Platinum Taq High Fidelity DNA Polymerase (Invitrogen) and the flanking primers 5′-TCGCCTA CTTCTCCTCCATG-3′ (forward) and 5′-TTCCCAAGTCCTCC

TGATGC-3′ (reverse). Samples were subjected to endonuclease digestion with use of the restriction enzyme AccI (New England Biolabs) prior to band separation by agarose gel electrophoresis. Genotypes were determined based on signature fragment digestion of the PCR product where the A→T mutation abolished the AccI recognition cleavage site.

Selection and Genomic Features

The ZFIN genomic feature sa15382 zebrafish used in this study exhibited a point mutation in the conserved 3′ splice site between exons 6 and 7 in the *Slc7a10b* gene (ENS-DART00000073398.5). This A→T mutation disrupts the dinucleotide splice site, and the intron between exon 6 and 7 is not spliced during maturation of the mRNA. Thus, the mRNA length is increased and the Slc7a10b protein product is inactive. Heterozygous larvae were raised and bred for obtaining zebrafish homozygous for this mutation. Due to the large variation in body weight between male and female zebrafish in a pilot study, the overfeeding study was performed with male zebrafish.

Husbandry

Four-month-old male zebrafish were housed in 3-L tanks (on average 20 per tank) with a recirculating system (Aquatic Habitats; Pentair AES) at $28.5 \pm 1°C$ (mean $\pm$ SD) and pH 7.51 ± 0.3 (mean $\pm$ SD), with 10% daily water exchange, electrical conductivity 500 ± 50 μs, and a 14-h light and 10-h dark circadian cycle. Zebrafish were fed 8.2 mg Gemma Micro 500 (Skretting) per day, divided over three time points (at 8:00 A.M., noon, and 4:00 P.M.), in addition to freshly hatched *Artemia* (three drops of a 24-h *Artemia* culture) once per day. Gemma Micro 500, which the zebrafish were fed under both normal and overfeeding conditions, consisted of fishmeal, lecithin, wheat gluten, zebrafish oil, vitamins and mineral premixes, and betaine, containing 59% (w/w) protein sources and 14% (w/w) lipids (containing 14% n-3 fatty acids).

Overfeeding

Three adult zebrafish were held per 1.5-L tank, in total 33 WT and 39 loss-of-function zebrafish. For weight gain, 12.3 mg feed per zebrafish per day (50% more feed than normal) was given for the first 3 weeks and 16.4 mg (100% more feed than normal) for the last 5 weeks of the overfeeding study. The circulation system was turned off for 5 min before and 30 min after each feeding, allowing consumption of all supplied food. Zebrafish were otherwise fed as under normal conditions (described above).

Measuring and Weighing

Zebrafish length and weight were recorded at the start and the end of the study, while weight was also measured after 3 and 6 weeks. Since it was not feasible to control the feed intake of each individual fish, we combined recorded data and tissue samples from the three zebrafish in each tank to obtain an average for each tank. Before handling, each zebrafish was sedated with 75–200 mg/L Tricain mesylate (Pharmaq).

Sample Collection and RNA Sequencing

After sacrifice, tissue biopsies from three zebrafish in each tank were pooled together and snap frozen in liquid nitrogen. Adipose and liver biopsies were fixed in 4% (v/v) paraformaldehyde in 0.1 mol/L phosphate buffer for 12 h and paraffin embedded after gradual dehydration as described previously (25). Slice sections of 5 μm were stained with hematoxylin-eosin, and adipocyte size was analyzed and quantified with ImageJ open-source software as previously described (18). RNA was isolated from visceral AT (VAT) of WT and Slc7a10b mutant zebrafish and cDNA libraries were generated for RNA-seq in the same way as described for human adipose cultures. Sample reads were mapped against the zebrafish genome (GRCz10) with HISAT (version 2.05), tabulated by featureCounts (version 1.5.2), and analyzed with DESeq2 (version 1.22.1).

Statistics

Differences between groups in human cohort data were analyzed with paired *t* test, one- or two-way ANOVA, and are presented as means $\pm$ SD. For Pearson correlation and multiple regression analyses, adjustments for BMI and sex are indicated. Differences between groups in cell culture experiments were assessed using with two-tailed unpaired Student *t* test or one-way ANOVA with Dunnett or Sidak correction for multiple comparisons. Sample data from empirical experiments were assumed to be normally distributed, and results are presented as means $\pm$ SD, except for the Seahorse data, which are presented as geometric means $\pm$ 95% CI. All data were plotted as box and whisker plots, with Tukey's method to detect and remove outliers. Statistical significance was calculated in GraphPad or with the R Bioconductor package limma (v3.34.9). Statistical details and the number of biological samples (*n*) for all experiments are provided in the figure legends. For cell experiments, *n* annotates the number of parallel wells per treatment. For zebrafish samples, *n* annotates the number of zebrafish per treatment. For qPCR data, *n* annotates either the number of patients or the number of wells in a cell experiment.

Study Approval

All human samples analyzed in the current study were obtained with written informed consent, and approval was given by the respective regional ethics committees (REC) (2010/502 and 2010/3405, REC West Norway; Dnr 721-96 and S 172-02, REC in Gothenburg, Sweden; 2009/1881-31/1, 2011/1002-31/1, and 2015/530-32, Committee of Ethics at Karolinska Institutet; and the Ethics Committee of the University of Leipzig, Leipzig, Germany).

Zebrafish were raised and cared for according to the Norwegian Animal Welfare Act guidelines, and all experiments after 5 days postfertilization were approved by the Norwegian Food Safety Authority (FOTS identifier 9199).

Data and Resource Availability

Data sets generated and/or analyzed during the current study are available from the corresponding author upon reasonable request. In addition, the RNA-seq data sets in this publication have been deposited in the National Center for Biotechnology Information (NCBI) Gene Expression Omnibus (GEO) (26) and are accessible through GEO Series accession number GSE135156.

RESULTS

Implication of Adipocyte *SLC7A10* in Abdominal Adiposity and Insulin Resistance

In transcriptome screens of adipose samples from people at the peak of extreme obesity (BPD-Fat cohort [Table 1]), we prioritized candidate genes with concomitant differential expression in two separate disease-relevant comparisons of adipose function: VAT (omental [OM]) and abdominal SC AT in extreme obesity, and before and after profound fat loss (SC AT from the same patients). This combined transcriptome screen identified 65 genes with both depot- and fat loss–dependent expression (fold change ≥1.5 and *q* value <0.01 cutoffs in both analyses) (Supplementary Table 4). Further supporting a role for many of these genes in insulin resistance, we found strong significant correlations for 27 of the 65 genes (42%) with waist-to-hip ratio (WHR) adjusted for BMI and sex, in a second cohort of 88 people (Sib Pair cohort) (14) (Supplementary Table 4). Among these genes, only five (8%) showed inverse correlations with WHR, four of which displayed highest expression in OM AT and upregulation in SC AT after profound fat loss (*CIDEA*, *SLC7A10*, *GPD1L*, and *HOXA5*) (Supplementary Table 4). Among the 27 candidates, we additionally prioritized genes with high expression in adipocytes specifically, based on a cohort containing isolated adipocytes and SVF (ADIPO cohort). Calculation of adipocyte–to–SVF expression ratios revealed *CIDEA* and *SLC7A10* as standout candidates with similar expression profiles (Fig. 1*A*). While previous studies have investigated functional roles of CIDEA in adipocytes (27), there is a paucity of functional data on adipocyte SLC7A10.

qPCR analysis of a larger cohort of people with severe obesity (Western Norway Obesity Biobank [WNOB] cohort) confirmed the adipose depot- and fat loss–dependent expression pattern of *SLC7A10* (Fig. 1*B*). *SLC7A10* mRNA was also higher in OM compared with SC samples in both isolated adipocytes and SVF (ADIPO cohort) but with diminished expression in SVF (Fig. 1*C*). Consistent with increased SC *SLC7A10* expression after surgery-induced fat loss (Fig. 1*C*), SC adipocytes and SVF from lean people showed higher expression than samples from those with obesity (Fig. 1*C*). Furthermore, insulin-resistant obese (IRO) patients showed lower *SLC7A10* mRNA compared with BMI-matched insulin-sensitive obese (ISO) patients (28) in SC as well as OM fat (ISO cohort) (Fig. 1*D*). Consistently, SC whole tissue *SLC7A10* mRNA levels showed strong inverse correlations with HOMA of insulin resistance, triacylglycerol levels, SC adipocyte volume, WHR, and visceral fat volume (Fig. 1*E* and Supplementary Fig. 1). On the other hand, SC *SLC7A10* mRNA showed positive

correlations with SC adipocyte number and SC abdominal fat mass with adjustment for BMI and sex (Fig. 1*E* and Supplementary Fig. 1). Finally, comparing patients with and without type 2 diabetes in the WNOB morbid obesity cohort, we observed decreased *SLC7A10* mRNA expression in OM as well as SC postsurgery AT (Fig. 1*F*).

Loss of Slc7a10b Function in Zebrafish Causes Body Weight Gain and Visceral Adipocyte Hypertrophy

To determine a potential causal role for SLC7A10 in the regulation of fat storage and adipose metabolism, we obtained zebrafish containing a splice site (loss-of-function) mutation in intron 6 of *Slc7a10* isoform b. After 2 months of overfeeding, the knockout zebrafish had on average gained 38% more body weight than their WT counterparts (Fig. 2*A*). Assessing AT morphology, we observed on average 49% larger adipocytes in the loss-of-function zebrafish compared with WT (Fig. 2*B* and *C*). Histological analyses of liver, which may reveal altered morphology related to impaired fatty acid oxidation (i.e., fatty liver), showed no apparent differences in cell size and lipid droplet formation between the Slc7a10b loss-of-function and WT zebrafish (Fig. 2*C*).

SLC7A10 Is Upregulated in Mature Adipocytes and Regulates Lipid Metabolism

We consequently explored mechanisms of the fat accretion by studying direct effects of altered SLC7A10 function in adipocytes. In differentiated mouse 3T3-L1 adipocytes and primary hASCs, SLC7A10 showed a marked increased mRNA and protein expression (Fig. 3*A–D*). To study the consequence of decreased SLC7A10 function in adipocytes, we inhibited SLC7A10 using the selective inhibitors BMS-466442 (SLC7A10 inhibitor 1) (19,29) or Lu AE00527 (SLC7A10 inhibitor 2) (20) during differentiation and observed increased lipid accumulation in 3T3-L1s (Fig. 3*E*) as well as hASCs (Fig. 3*F*) in comparison with controls.

Adipose SLC7A10 Impairment Affects Energy Metabolic Pathways

To systematically explore SLC7A10-dependent metabolic processes, we first correlated mRNA levels of *SLC7A10* and other genes in a global transcriptome analysis of adipocytes isolated directly from human SC fat biopsies (ADIPO cohort). By performing gene ontology (GO) analysis, we found that genes antiexpressed to *SLC7A10* (113 unique genes [Supplementary Table 5]) mapped primarily to cellular/developmental processes and protein transport (Fig. 4*A*) and genes coexpressed (323 unique genes [Supplementary Table 5]) mapped to lipid metabolic processes and oxidative phosphorylation (Fig. 4*A*). Moreover, RNA-seq in SLC7A10 inhibitor–treated primary human adipocytes revealed a profound transcriptome effect (Supplementary Fig. 2*A–C*). Among 862 significantly downregulated genes, GO analysis revealed an enrichment of genes involved in biological processes such as immune response,

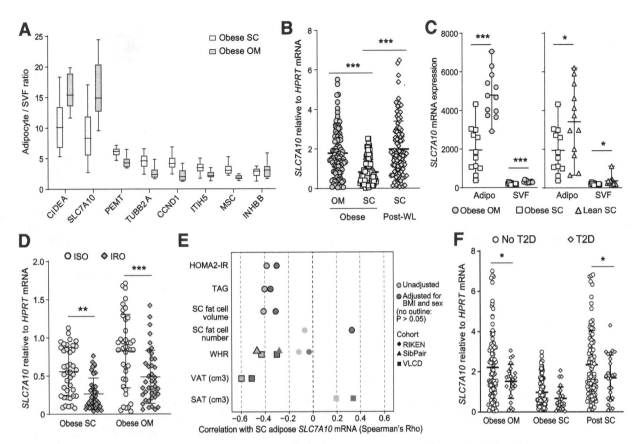

Figure 1—*SLC7A10* mRNA expression is high in VAT and correlates inversely with obesity and insulin resistance. *SLC7A10* mRNA expression was measured in human visceral (OM) and SC adipose samples by microarrays or by qPCR (calculated relative to *HPRT* mRNA). *A*: Adipocytes and SVF were isolated from OM and SC ATs of people with severe obesity (*n* = 12) (ADIPO cohort). *SLC7A10* mRNA expression was measured by Illumina microarrays, and genes enriched in the adipocyte fraction relative to SVF are shown. Data are presented as median ± interquartile range. *B*: *SLC7A10* mRNA was measured by qPCR in OM and SC ATs collected from people with morbid obesity (BMI ≥40 kg/m², or >35 kg/m² with at least one obesity-related health condition) and SC AT collected 1 year after profound fat loss following bariatric surgery from the same subjects (Post-WL) (*n* = 101 pairs). Data are presented as mean ± SD. *C*: Adipocytes and SVF were isolated from OM and SC ATs of lean people (*n* = 12) and people with severe adiposity (*n* = 12) (ADIPO cohort). *SLC7A10* mRNA expression was measured by Illumina microarrays. Data are presented as means ± SD. *D*: *SLC7A10* mRNA was measured by qPCR in OM and SC AT in insulin sensitive obese (ISO) and insulin resistant obese (IRO) people (n=40 each) from the ISO cohort, where insulin resistance was measured by hyperinsulinemic-euglycemic clamp. Data are presented as means ± SD. *E*: Correlations of SC AT *SLC7A10* mRNA with clinical parameters in the RIKEN (*n* = 56), VLCD (*n* = 24), and Sib Pair (*n* = 88) cohorts, calculated as Spearman ρ with and without adjustment. Data are adjusted for BMI and sex for Sib Pair and VLCD cohorts and for BMI for the RIKEN cohort. Symbols outlined in bold indicate statistical significance. *F*: *SLC7A10* mRNA was measured in OM (*n* = 88), SC (*n* = 81), and post–weight loss SC (*n* = 88) ATs of obese people without diabetes and in OM (*n* = 22), SC (*n* = 23), and post–weight loss SC (*n* = 24) ATs of obese people with diabetes in the WNOB cohort. Data are presented as mean ± SD. *P < 0.05. **P < 0.01. ***P < 0.001. Post SC, post–weight loss SC; T2D, type 2 diabetes; TAG, triacylglycerol.

inflammation, extracellular matrix organization, and cell differentiation (Supplementary Fig. 2D). Among 1,113 significantly upregulated genes, there were striking enrichments for the isopentenyl diphosphate biosynthetic process (26 fold), NADPH regeneration (26 fold), pentose phosphate shunt (26 fold), triglyceride biosynthetic process (9.3 fold), and glutathione metabolic processes (8.2 fold) (Supplementary Fig. 2D), indicating mechanisms that fueled lipid storage. Additionally, by pathway analysis we found a marked enrichment of genes involved in ATP synthesis (16 fold), tricarboxylic acid cycle (13 fold), and cholesterol biosynthesis (12 fold) among upregulated genes, and in, for example, glycolysis and angiogenesis for the downregulated genes (Fig. 4B and C).

Global gene expression in VAT from Slc7a10b loss-of-function and WT zebrafish was also assayed by RNA-seq. We visualization of RNA-seq reads we identified the expected mutation in the splice site of exon 6 (Supplementary Fig. 3A). Of note, mutants exhibited increased mRNA levels of the defective *Slc7a10b* (Supplementary Fig. 3B), compensatory to the impaired splicing and function. Before further analysis, we removed outliers using multidimensional scaling plots (Supplementary Fig. 3C) and excluded samples that differed significantly from the others in the expression of immediate-early stress-responsive genes (Supplementary Fig. 3D). RNA-seq revealed 1,736 differentially expressed genes in the *Slc7a10b* loss-of-function zebrafish, including 880 upregulated

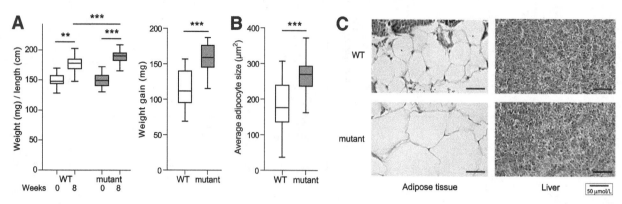

Figure 2—Loss of SLC7A10 function in zebrafish in vivo causes body weight gain and visceral adipocyte hypertrophy. Four-month-old WT and Slc7a10b loss-of-function mutant male zebrafish were fed 50–100% more than their regular feed for 8 weeks. Body weight and length were recorded at start and end, and weight, length, and adipose morphology were assessed after sacrifice. VAT from three zebrafish housed in the same tank during overfeeding was pooled, and RNA was isolated. *A*: Body weight and length were measured before and after overfeeding of the zebrafish. Data are presented as mean ± SD (WT [*n* = 31] and loss of function [*n* = 36]). *B* and *C*: VAT and liver tissue were fixed, sectioned (5 μm), and stained with hematoxylin-eosin for morphological analyses. Adipocyte size was analyzed and quantified using ImageJ, and average adipocyte size was calculated for each section (WT [*n* = 27] and loss-of-function mutant [*n* = 29]). Pictures representative of the group averages are shown. **P < 0.01. ***P < 0.001.

and 856 downregulated transcripts. The loss of function caused a particularly striking upregulation of *Urahb*, which encodes an enzyme that regulates degradation of uric acid to (S)-allantoin (Supplementary Fig. 4*A* and *B*), a product of purine nucleotide degradation and a marker of oxidative stress in most nonhuman mammals. Consistently, metabolism of urate, purine nucleobase, and hydrogen peroxide (H_2O_2) were among the most affected biological processes in the zebrafish VAT, together with oxygen transport, AA metabolism, lipoprotein remodeling, and lipid and citrate transport (Supplementary Fig. 4*B*). The RNA-seq analysis for SLC7A10 inhibition in the differentiating hASCs largely supported an effect on these processes, including steroid biosynthesis and oxidation-reduction process (Supplementary Fig. 5*A*). A total of 121 of the 216 GO terms identified in the zebrafish data set overlapped with the human data set. While genes in some terms showed directionality opposite that of expression, several of the most significant terms in zebrafish showed the same directionality in human cells (Supplementary Fig. 5*A*). From the 444 differentially expressed genes in the zebrafish data set, 26 genes overlapped with the human data set, of which 17 were regulated in the same direction. Among these were *SLC7A10* (reflecting a compensatory upregulation), *SCD* (a marker of nutritionally regulated lipid storage), *HSD17B10* (an isoleucine-catabolizing enzyme), *PKM* and *PC* (related to pyruvate metabolism and glyceroneogenesis which provides glycerol for lipid storage), and *CPT1A* (rate limiting for mitochondrial lipid β-oxidation) (Supplementary Fig. 5*B*).

In accordance with the transcriptome changes indicating effects on mitochondrial function, SLC7A10 inhibition for 24 h decreased basal respiration, ATP synthesis,

maximal consumption rate, and spare respiratory capacity by up to 50% in murine (Supplementary Fig. 6*A* and *B*) and primary human adipocytes (Fig. 5*A*), with detectable effects after 2 h inhibition. Exposure to SLC7A10 inhibitor 2 (Lu) reproduced the suppression of maximal respiration and spare respiratory capacity (Fig. 5*B*). Conversely, overexpressing *Slc7a10* (Supplementary Fig. 6*C*) in murine fat cells increased these measures along with basal respiration and ATP synthesis (Fig. 5*C*).

SLC7A10 Transports Serine in Adipocytes

To examine the mechanism by which SLC7A10 modulates adipocyte metabolism, we tested the effect of SLC7A10 inhibition on the flux of neutral AAs, some of which are direct precursors of glutathione (e.g., cysteine, glycine, and serine) (6,7). SLC7A10 impairment strongly increased medium concentrations of serine from around day 8 of human adipocyte differentiation, while concentrations of other SLC7A10-linked neutral AAs showed only minor effects (Fig. 6*A* and Supplementary Fig. 7*A*). We confirmed the reduction in serine influx in response to SLC7A10 inhibition in cultured adipocytes from four independent donors (Supplementary Fig. 7*B*). Additionally, with use of radiolabeled AAs in sodium-free conditions, SLC7A10 inhibition reduced uptake of D-serine (Fig. 6*B* and Supplementary Fig. 7*C*) and L-serine in adipocytes (Supplementary Fig. 7*C* and *D*). The primary effect on serine transport is consistent with an important role for this AA in lipid synthesis, antioxidant regeneration, tricarboxylic acid cycle, glycolysis, and oxidative phosphorylation, in part because serine serves as a key methyl donor that controls biosynthesis and regeneration of ATP, NADPH, purines, glutathione, and other molecules through one-carbon metabolism (11) (Fig. 6*C*).

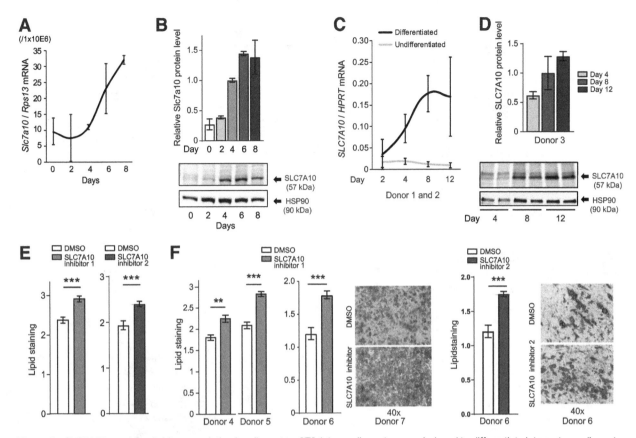

Figure 3—SLC7A10 regulates lipid accumulation in adipocytes. 3T3-L1 preadipocytes were induced to differentiate into mature adipocytes and harvested every 2nd day throughout differentiation. Cultured primary hASCs were induced to differentiate into mature adipocytes and harvested every 2nd or 4th day throughout differentiation. Lipid accumulation was measured by ORO lipid staining. *A–D*: mRNA expression of 3T3-L1 *Slc7a10* was quantified by qPCR, relative to *Rps13* expression (*n* = 3). mRNA expression of *SLC7A10* from hASC cultures was measured by combining the expression profiles of differentiating fat cells from two people (n = 2, donors 1 and 2) and quantified relative to *HPRT* mRNA expression. For Western blotting, a representative expression profile is shown (*n* = 2 replicates, for both 3T3-L1 and donor 3) and protein expression was calculated relative to HSP90. Protein (20 and 30 μg per well) was loaded for 3T3-L1 and hASCs, respectively, and the following antibodies were used: HSP90 (1:1,000, cat. no. 4874; Cell Signaling Technology), SLC7A10 (1:500, cat. no. sc-292032; Santa Cruz Biotechnology), horseradish peroxidase goat anti-rabbit IgG (1:10,000, cat. no. 3546; Thermo Fisher Scientific), and horseradish peroxidase goat anti-mouse IgG (1:7,500, cat. no. 554002; BD Biosciences). Data are presented as means ± SD. *E* and *F*: SLC7A10 inhibition throughout differentiation of 3T3-L1s (days 2–8) and hASC cultures (days 3–12) increased lipid accumulation as measured by ORO lipid staining. SLC7A10 inhibitors 1 and 2 were used at a final concentration of 10 μmol/L. Data for 3T3-L1s and representative hASC cultures (n = 4, donors 4, 5, 6, and 7) are shown (*n* = 3–6 replicate wells). Data are presented as means ± SD. **P < 0.01. ***P < 0.001.

SLC7A10 Modulates Glutathione Levels, ROS Generation, and Insulin-Stimulated Glucose Uptake in Adipocytes

The effects of SLC7A10 inhibition on several genes in NADPH- and glutathione-related metabolism (Fig. 6*D*) prompted us to examine whether SLC7A10 affects cellular glutathione levels. SLC7A10 impairment decreased total glutathione levels detected after only 15–45 min inhibition in murine and human adipocytes (Fig. 6*E* and *F*). The decrease was confirmed with inhibitor 2, albeit not significant in the human adipocytes (Fig. 6*E* and *F*), while SLC7A10 overexpression in 3T3-L1 adipocytes increased total glutathione levels (Fig. 6*G*). Consistently, intracellular ROS levels increased progressively after 20 min of SLC7A10 inhibition in 3T3-L1 adipocytes (Fig. 6*H*) and after 60 min in mature human adipocytes (Fig. 6*I*), while SLC7A10 overexpression reduced ROS generation (Fig.

6*J*). Interestingly, when treating SLC7A10-inhibited adipocytes with the ROS scavenger N-acetyl-L-cysteine (Nac), we observed a 50–70% reduction in lipid accumulation (Fig. 6*K*), indicating that ROS generation may have partially mediated the lipid-storing effect of reduced SLC7A10 activity. On the other hand, this partial reversal of SLC7A10 inhibitor–dependent lipid accumulation by Nac was not clear upon prolonged stimulation with insulin, which increased lipid accumulation to a degree similar to that with SLC7A10 inhibition (Fig. 6*K*). These data suggest that the lipid-storing effects of SLC7A10 impairment might at least partially involve increased levels of ROS, whereas the effects of insulin may largely occur independent of ROS generation.

Finally, we tested whether reduced SLC7A10 activity also affects insulin-stimulated glucose uptake. Inhibition of SLC7A10 diminished insulin-stimulated glucose uptake

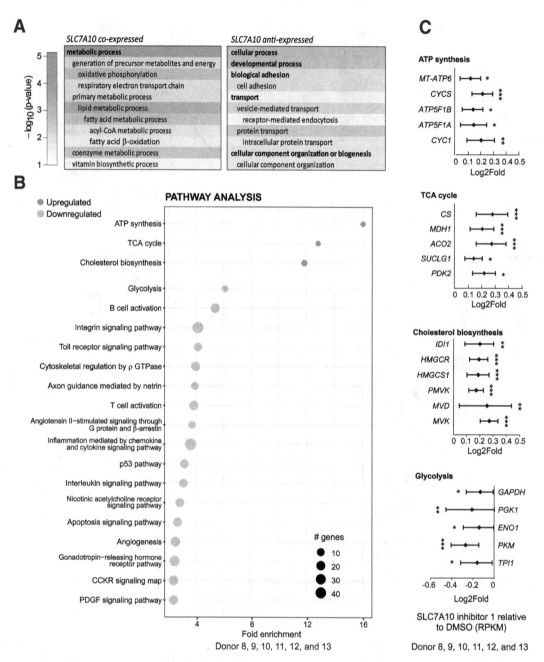

Figure 4—SLC7A10 inhibition strongly affects genes related to energy metabolism in adipocytes. SLC7A10-associated gene expression patterns were analyzed in mature adipocytes isolated from SC AT (*A*) and in cultured primary hASCs treated with DMSO or SLC7A10 inhibitor 1 from day 7 to 8 during adipogenic differentiation (*B* and *C*). *A*: Mature adipocytes were isolated from biopsies of people with a BMI between 18 and 45 kg/m^2 (*n* = 24, ADIPO cohort). Global gene expression was profiled by Illumina microarrays. Genes across the genome that were co- or antiexpressed with *SLC7A10* (Pearson correlation β > 0.65) were subjected to PANTHER GO analysis. The biological processes most enriched with *SLC7A10*-correlated genes are shown, with indication of enrichment *P* values by the color scale. *B* and *C*: hASCs were obtained from abdominal SC AT (*n* = 6, donors 8–13), differentiated for 8 days, and treated with DMSO or SLC7A10 inhibitor 1 for 24 h from day 7 to 8. GO terms were analyzed by PANTHER following RNA-seq. Up- and downregulated pathways are shown here with enrichment visualized on the *x*-axis, while the number of genes found in each pathway is shown by the size of the circle. Relative gene expression between SLC7A10 inhibitor 1 and DMSO-treated hASCs is depicted for genes in the top up- and downregulated pathways (*C*). Data are presented as mean ± SD. **P* < 0.05. **P < 0.01. ***P < 0.001. RPKM, reads per kilobase per million mapped reads.

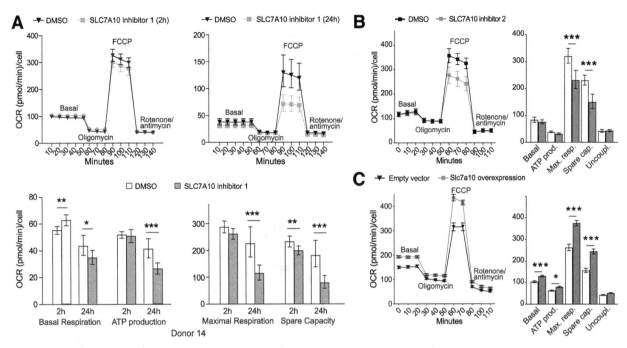

Figure 5—SLC7A10 stimulates adipocyte mitochondrial respiratory capacity. hASCs and 3T3-L1 preadipocytes were differentiated for 12 and 8 days, respectively, and treated for 2–24 h prior to respiration measurements. OCR and respiratory capacity in live adipocytes were measured by the Seahorse XF Cell Mito Stress Test assay. OCR was measured under basal conditions and after sequential addition of the following compounds at indicated final concentrations: oligomycin (3 μmol/L), carbonyl cyanide 4-(trifluoromethoxy) phenylhydrazone (FCCP) (1.5 μmol/L), rotenone (1 μmol/L), and antimycin A (1 μmol/L). Outliers were removed based on a whisker Tukey test of the OCR data for each time point in each well, before basal respiration, ATP production (ATP prod.), maximal respiration (Max. resp.), spare respiratory capacity (Spare cap.) and uncoupling (Uncoupl.) were calculated according to the manufacturer's protocol. Results are presented as geometric means ± 95% CI (n = 12–44 replicate wells in a 96-well plate). *A*: hASCs (donor 14) were differentiated until day 11 and treated with DMSO or SLC7A10 inhibitor 1 for 2 or 24 h. *B*: 3T3-L1 preadipocytes were differentiated until day 8 and treated with DMSO or SLC7A10 inhibitor 2 for 24 h from day 7 to 8. *C*: 3T3-L1 preadipocytes were induced to differentiate and transfected with an expression plasmid encoding Slc7a10 or empty vector on days 2, 4, and 6, before analysis on day 8. *P < 0.05. **P < 0.01. ***P < 0.001.

in mouse and human adipocytes (Fig. 7A and B), supporting that SLC7A10 directly modulates adipocyte insulin sensitivity.

DISCUSSION

We here identified SLC7A10 as a novel facilitator of serine uptake in adipocytes, and that this function may buffer against oxidative stress, lipid accumulation, insulin resistance and dyslipidemia. Our data show that pharmacological inhibition of SLC7A10 in adipocytes decreases glutathione levels (within minutes), increases ROS generation (within an hour), decreases mitochondrial respiratory capacity (within hours) and promotes lipid accumulation (within days). SLC7A10 inhibition also decreases insulin-stimulated glucose uptake. Furthermore, SLC7A10 overexpression showed inverse effects, suggesting that SLC7A10 activation may improve important metabolic functions in adipocytes, potentially counteracting development of obesity and insulin resistance. The overfeeding experiments in zebrafish support that functional impairment of SLC7A10 increases body weight and adipocyte size in vivo.

Our clinical cohort data reveal consistent inverse correlations between adipose *SLC7A10* mRNA expression and

several key features of insulin resistance, including WHR, adipocyte hypertrophy, visceral fat mass, triacylglycerol, and HOMA of insulin resistance after adjustment for BMI and sex, further underscored by increased *SLC7A10* mRNA in people with insulin sensitive compared with insulin resistant obesity. SC adipose *SLC7A10* was previously shown to have a strong heritable expression ($h^2 = 0.79$), to be lower in people carrying type 2 diabetes risk variants in the *KLF14* locus, and to correlate negatively with metabolic traits linked to disease risk (30).

The potential clinical relevance of SLC7A10 in adipocyte metabolism is further supported by previously unconnected lines of evidence from other studies. Firstly, a metabolomics study found reduced uptake of serine in VAT from people with severe obesity compared with nonobese participants (31). Secondly, total glutathione levels are higher in OM than SC AT of lean individuals, and altered glutathione synthesis in adipocytes affects insulin sensitivity (32,33). Moreover, total glutathione levels are reduced in AT of people with obesity compared with lean people (34), in line with the pattern of *SLC7A10* expression reported here. Thirdly, SC AT in obesity and type 2 diabetes exhibits increased mitochondrial ROS levels, e.g., H_2O_2, combined with reduced expression of antioxidant enzymes

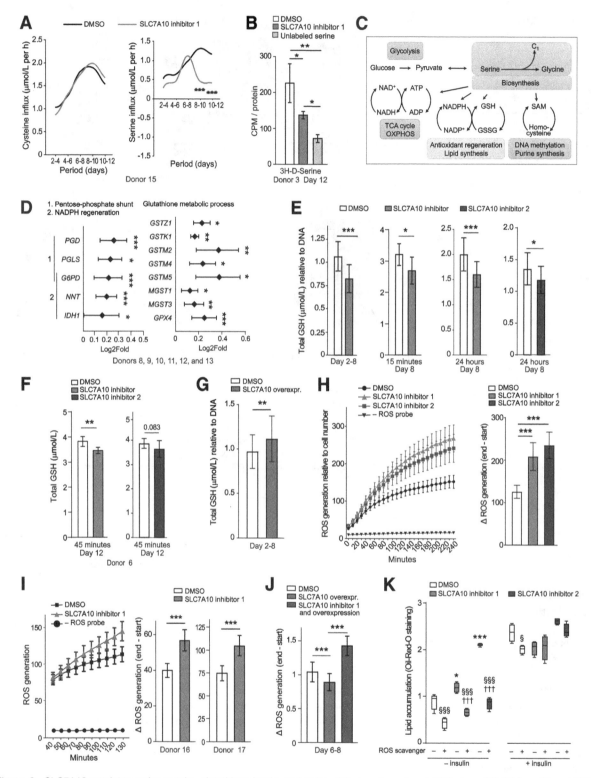

Figure 6—SLC7A10 regulates serine uptake, glutathione levels, and redox state in adipocytes. hASCs from SC AT (*n* = 6) and 3T3-L1 preadipocytes were cultured, differentiated, and treated with DMSO or SLC7A10 inhibitors or transfected with Slc7a10 expression plasmid. Total glutathione (GSH) levels were measured with a glutathione probe coupled to a luciferase reaction (*E–G*). ROS generation was measured by an ROS probe detected by a laser plate reader (*H–J*), and lipid accumulation was measured by ORO (*K*). Fluxes of small neutral AAs in cultured hASCs in response to the selective SLC7A10 inhibitor 1 (10 μmol/L) were assessed by measurement of changes in medium concentrations by GC-MS/MS (*A*) and by radiometric assays (*B*). *A*: AA flux in cultured hASCs throughout adipogenic differentiation were assessed based on the AA concentrations in unconditioned medium and change in concentrations upon cell culture during 48-h periods. Data for the mean of two replicate wells from a representative experiment are shown (donor 4). *B*: Cultured hASCs were washed three times using sodium-free assay buffer (120 mmol/L choline chloride, 25 mmol/L triethylammonium bicarbonate, 1.5 mmol/L KCl, 1.2 mmol/L CaCl2, 1.2 mmol/L MgCl2, 1.2 mmol/L KH2PO4, 10 mmol/L glucose, 10 mmol/L HEPES, and 5.5 mmol/L glucose, adjusted to pH 7.4 and sterile

(35). A recent report showed 46% higher H_2O_2 levels in visceral fat of men with central obesity compared with lean men and positive correlations of the adipose H_2O_2 concentrations with insulin resistance (36). Importantly, recent studies suggest that oxidative stress in adipocytes is not only a consequence of metabolic disease but also a cause (37) and that elevated intracellular ROS levels in adipocytes might contribute to adipocyte dysfunction, increased fat storage, and insulin resistance (24,38). Taken together, our study points to SLC7A10 as a potential candidate for therapeutic intervention to mitigate oxidative stress and unhealthy lipid storage in adipocytes.

In line with our experimental data linking reduced SLC7A10 function to increased lipid accumulation via decreased glutathione levels and elevated ROS, glutathione depletion has been found to promote adipogenesis in 3T3-L1 adipocytes (39). Although a recent study in 3T3-L1 adipocytes found that long-term treatment with the ROS scavenger Nac increased ROS levels (40), others found that Nac treatment decreased ROS levels (as expected), while increasing oxygen consumption, decreasing body fat in mice in vivo (41), and inhibiting insulin-stimulated lipid accumulation in 3T3-L1 adipocytes (42), in line with our data. ROS can modulate intracellular signaling and a transient increase in ROS levels can promote adipocyte differentiation (38,43), while sustained elevation of cellular ROS levels has been linked to adipocyte lipid storage (24), also observed in microorganisms (44). Our data show a clear positive relationship between ROS levels and lipid accumulation, in contrast to a recent study in mice where

increased mitochondrial levels of the H_2O_2-hydrolyzing enzyme catalase were associated with reduced ROS and increased adiposity, adipocyte size, and adipose glyceroneogenic and lipogenic gene expression (45). Another study also found reduced body weight with increased ROS levels in AT with aging (46). A possible explanation for these inconsistent results might be the specific metabolic contexts and distinct effects of specific sources of ROS on glyceroneogenesis and lipid accumulation, which requires further investigation.

It is possible that inhibition of SLC7A10 and the concomitant increase in ROS levels promoted lipid storage in our study, at least in part, by reducing mitochondrial respiratory capacity. A recent study in SC and visceral human adipose–derived stem cells linked high ROS generation to decreased mitochondrial respiration (47), and increased ROS generation in epididymal fat has been shown to precede lowered mitochondrial biogenesis in nutritionally challenged mice (48). Additionally, elevated mitochondrial and extracellular ROS concentrations have been shown to inhibit mitochondrial respiration and to cause mitochondrial dysfunction in cultured 3T3-L1 and primary rat adipocytes (24,41). Recent studies also showed that ROS can impair insulin-dependent glucose uptake (4,49), in line with the SLC7A10-dependent phenotype we observed.

While our data indicate that altered serine uptake mediated the lipid-storing effects of impaired SLC7A10 function, effects of serine on adipocyte metabolism and mechanisms regulating adipocyte serine flux are largely unknown. Serine is vital in maintenance of mitochondrial

filtered) and treated with SLC7A10 inhibitor 1 for 30 min. Unlabeled D-serine was added to designated wells (as positive control) before radioactive-labeled (1 μmol/L) 3H-D-serine was added to all wells. Following incubation at 37°C for 30 min, assays were stopped by placing of cells on ice and washing three times with ice-cold assay buffer. Cells were lysed and loaded in Ultima Gold fluid cartridges (PerkinElmer), and isotope retention (CPM) in cell lysates was quantified with a TRI-CARB 4910TR Scintillation Counter (PerkinElmer). CPM values were normalized to protein content in a corresponding sample by use of DC Protein Assay (Bio-Rad Laboratories) ($n = 4$–6, donor 3). Data are presented as means ± SD. *C*: Summary figure of serine-dependent processes and metabolic pathways (based on Newman and Maddocks) (11). Serine is important for several metabolic pathways and processes, such as oxidative phosphorylation (OXPHOS), and is also a precursor for biosynthesis of molecules such as methyl groups, purines, and glutathione. *D*: Gene expression measured by RNA-seq showed an enrichment of genes involved in the pentose phosphate shunt, NADPH regeneration, and glutathione metabolic processes ($n = 6$ individuals, donors 8–13). Data are presented as means ± SD. *E–F*: 3T3-L1 preadipocytes and hASCs (donor 6) were induced to differentiate to days 8 and 12, respectively. Total glutathione following treatment with DMSO or SLC7A10 inhibitors 1 and 2 (10 μmol/L) for 15 min or 24 h (3T3-L1s) and 45 min (hASCs) ($n = 10$–22 replicate wells), by the GSH/GSSG-Glo Assay (Promega), which uses a glutathione probe activated by a luciferase reaction. Data are presented as means ± SD. *G*: 3T3-L1 preadipocytes were induced to differentiate and transfected with Slc7a10 expression plasmid or empty vector on every 2nd day of differentiation (days 2, 4, and 6). Total glutathione was measured on day 8 as described above ($n = 37$–39). Data are presented as means ± SD. *H–I*: 3T3-L1 preadipocytes and hASCs (donors 16, 17) were induced to differentiate until day 8 and day 12, respectively, and treated with DMSO or SLC7A10 inhibitors 1 and 2 (10 μmol/L) immediately before the assay. ROS generation was measured with the fluorescent probe CM-H2DCFDA (Thermo Fisher Scientific). Cells treated without ROS probe served as negative control. The time course for a representative experiment is shown (donor 17), together with change in ROS generation from start to end ($n = 11$ replicate wells in 96-well plates). Data are presented as mean ± SD. *J*: 3T3-L1 preadipocytes were induced to differentiate and Slc7a10 was overexpressed (overexpr.) (1 μg/mL or 3 μg/mL) for 48 h (days 6–8) with the transfection reagent TransIT-LT1, and additionally cells were treated with DMSO or SLC7A10 inhibitor 1 for 48 h (days 6–8). ROS generation was measured on day 8 as described above. Change in ROS generation from start to end is shown here ($n = 11$ replicate wells in 96-well plates). Data are presented as means ± SD. *K*: 3T3-L1 preadipocytes were induced to differentiate and treated with DMSO or SLC7A10 inhibitors 1 and 2 every 2nd day during differentiation from day 2 to 8 with and without ROS scavenger Nac (10 mmol/L) (Sigma-Aldrich) and with and without insulin (1 μg/mL) from day 4 to 8. Lipid accumulation was measured by ORO lipid staining ($n = 3$). Data are presented as means ± SD. *$P < 0.05$, **$P < 0.01$, ***$P < 0.001$ (comparing DMSO and SLC7A10 inhibitor without ROS scavenger Nac). §$P < 0.05$, §§§$P < 0.001$ (comparing with/without ROS scavenger Nac). †††$P < 0.001$ (comparing DMSO and SLC7A10 inhibitor with ROS scavenger Nac). TCA cycle, tricarboxylic acid cycle.

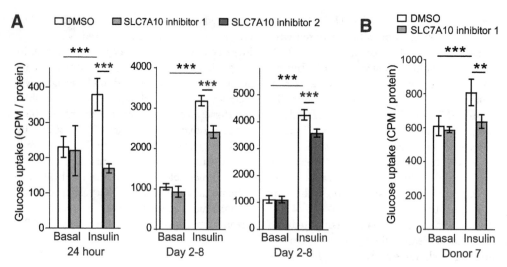

Figure 7—SLC7A10 inhibition decreases insulin-stimulated glucose uptake. Glucose uptake was assessed by radiometric assay in cultured 3T3-L1 preadipocytes (A) or hASCs (B) induced to differentiate for 8 and 12 days, respectively. 3T3-L1s were treated with DMSO or SLC7A10 inhibitors 1 and 2 (10 μmol/L) for either 24 h (days 2–8) or from day 2 to 8, and hASCs (donor 7) were treated with DMSO or SLC7A10 inhibitor 1 (10 μmol/L) for 24 h (days 11–12). Insulin (final concentration 10 nmol/L) was added 30 min prior to the assay, and deoxy-D-[14C]-glucose was added for 30 min. Glucose uptake was measured with a scintillation counter ($n = 6$ replicate wells in 12-well plates). Data are presented as means ± SD. **$P < 0.01$. ***$P < 0.001$.

respiration (50,51), and both imported and de novo synthesized serine play a role in protein, lipid, and purine metabolism (11). In mouse embryonic fibroblasts lacking the first enzyme in de novo serine synthesis, external L-serine depletion increased formation of specific sphingolipids (52), and serine supplementation in mice reduced hepatic ROS levels, ameliorating alcoholic fatty liver by supporting glutathione levels (53,54).

Our study has limitations. The SLC7A10 inhibitors BMS-466442 and Lu AE00527 have been used to study functions of SLC7A10 in the brain and show high selectivity (19,20,29,55). However, we cannot entirely rule out nonspecific effects, even though overexpression of SLC7A10 showed inverse effects compared with loss of SLC7A10 function in adipocyte cultures. Previous studies have shown the utility of zebrafish for investigating AT biology and the dynamics of obesity and type 2 diabetes development (56,57), and they share common obesity-related pathophysiological pathways with mammals (58). Nonetheless, future studies should perform adipocyte-selective *Slc7a10* manipulation, e.g., by overexpression in mice, to determine the degree to which maintained Slc7a10 activity can prevent and reverse obesity and systemic insulin resistance. Additionally, further studies are needed for determination of whether loss of SLC7A10 activity directly in visceral fat, where *SLC7A10* mRNA is twofold higher than in SC fat, might render this depot particularly vulnerable to adipocyte hypertrophy and metabolic dysfunction.

In conclusion, our study has identified *SLC7A10* as a novel gene involved in the regulation of adipocyte energy metabolism, ROS generation, and lipid accumulation,

implicating novel adipocyte pathways linked to serine transport in obesity and insulin resistance.

Acknowledgments. The authors thank Olivera Bozickovic, Margit Solsvik, Iren Drange Hjellestad, and Novin Balafkan at the University of Bergen and Haukeland University Hospital and Øyvind Reinshol at the Institute of Marine Research (technical assistance); personnel at Voss Hospital, Haugesund Hospital, and Haraldsplass Deaconess Hospital, Bergen, Norway (sample collection); and Per Magne Ueland, University of Bergen, for reviewing the manuscript. The Genomics Core Facility (GCF) at the University of Bergen, which is part of the NorSeq consortium, provided services on microarray and RNA-seq global gene expression profiling.

Funding. This project is supported by the Research Council of Norway (263124/F20), K.G. Jebsen Center for Diabetes Research, Western Norway Regional Health Authority, and the Norwegian Diabetes Association, Norway. GCF is supported in part by major grants from the Norwegian Research Council (grant 245979/F50) and the Trond Mohn Foundation (TMS) (Bergens Forskningsstiftelse). The authors also thank Kenneth Vielsted Christensen at H. Lundbeck A/S for providing the SLC7A10 inhibitor Lu AE00527.

Duality of Interest. This project is also supported by Novo Nordisk Scandinavia AS. No other potential conflicts of interest relevant to this article were reported.

Author Contributions. R.Å.J. and S.N.D. designed the study, carried out experiments, analyzed and interpreted the results, and wrote the manuscript. D.S.P.T. and A.M. helped carry out experiments, analyze and interpret data, and write the manuscript. L.S., L.D., A.W., J.-I.B., and M.S.B. assisted with experiments and data analysis. R.Å.J., E.F., L.M., and S.E. performed the zebrafish feeding experiment. A.M. performed metabolomics analyses. V.V., H.J.N., B.G.N., and C.B. planned and carried out collection of AT and clinical data. M.B., P.J., P.-A.S., M.R., P.A., O.N., and M.C. provided and analyzed cohort data. V.M.S. helped design and support the transcriptome analyses. J.F., J.V.S., G.M., and S.N.D. facilitated the laboratory work and collection and analyses of cohort samples. All authors reviewed and approved the final version of the manuscript. S.N.D. is the guarantor of this work and, as such, had full access to all the data in the study and takes responsibility for the integrity of the data and the accuracy of the data analysis.

References

1. Acosta JR, Douagi I, Andersson DP, et al. Increased fat cell size: a major phenotype of subcutaneous white adipose tissue in non-obese individuals with type 2 diabetes. Diabetologia 2016;59:560–570

2. Kim JI, Huh JY, Sohn JH, et al. Lipid-overloaded enlarged adipocytes provoke insulin resistance independent of inflammation. Mol Cell Biol 2015;35:1686–1699

3. Heinonen S, Saarinen L, Naukkarinen J, et al. Adipocyte morphology and implications for metabolic derangements in acquired obesity. Int J Obes 2014;38:1423–1431

4. Wang C-H, Wang C-C, Huang H-C, Wei Y-H. Mitochondrial dysfunction leads to impairment of insulin sensitivity and adiponectin secretion in adipocytes. FEBS J 2013;280:1039–1050

5. Szendroedi J, Phielix E, Roden M. The role of mitochondria in insulin resistance and type 2 diabetes mellitus. Nat Rev Endocrinol 2012;8:92–103

6. Fukasawa Y, Segawa H, Kim JY, et al. Identification and characterization of a Na(+)-independent neutral amino acid transporter that associates with the 4F2 heavy chain and exhibits substrate selectivity for small neutral D- and L-amino acids. J Biol Chem 2000;275:9690–9698

7. Nakauchi J, Matsuo H, Kim DK, et al. Cloning and characterization of a human brain Na(+)-independent transporter for small neutral amino acids that transports D-serine with high affinity. Neurosci Lett 2000;287:231–235

8. Rosenberg D, Artoul S, Segal AC, et al. Neuronal D-serine and glycine release via the Asc-1 transporter regulates NMDA receptor-dependent synaptic activity. J Neurosci 2013;33:3533–3544

9. Ussar S, Lee KY, Dankel SN, et al. ASC-1, PAT2, and P2RX5 are cell surface markers for white, beige, and brown adipocytes. Sci Transl Med 2014;6:247ra103

10. Yang M, Vousden KH. Serine and one-carbon metabolism in cancer. Nat Rev Cancer 2016;16:650–662

11. Newman AC, Maddocks ODK. Serine and functional metabolites in cancer. Trends Cell Biol 2017;27:645–657

12. Veum VL, Dankel SN, Gjerde J, et al. The nuclear receptors NUR77, NURR1 and NOR1 in obesity and during fat loss. Int J Obes 2012;36:1195–1202

13. Dankel SN, Fadnes DJ, Stavrum A-K, et al. Switch from stress response to homeobox transcription factors in adipose tissue after profound fat loss. PLoS One 2010;5:e11033

14. Ahlin S, Sjöholm K, Jacobson P, et al. Macrophage gene expression in adipose tissue is associated with insulin sensitivity and serum lipid levels independent of obesity. Obesity (Silver Spring) 2013;21:E571–E576

15. Saiki A, Olsson M, Jernås M, et al. Tenomodulin is highly expressed in adipose tissue, increased in obesity, and down-regulated during diet-induced weight loss. J Clin Endocrinol Metab 2009;94:3987–3994

16. Arner E, Mejhert N, Kulyté A, et al. Adipose tissue microRNAs as regulators of CCL2 production in human obesity. Diabetes 2012;61:1986–1993

17. Lee M-J, Fried SK. Optimal protocol for the differentiation and metabolic analysis of human adipose stromal cells. Methods Enzymol 2014;538:49–65

18. Dankel SN, Degerud EM, Borkowski K, et al. Weight cycling promotes fat gain and altered clock gene expression in adipose tissue in C57BL/6J mice. Am J Physiol Endocrinol Metab 2014;306:E210–E224

19. Brown JM, Hunihan L, Prack MM, et al. In vitro characterization of a small molecule inhibitor of the alanine serine cysteine transporter -1 (SLC7A10). J Neurochem 2014;129:275–283

20. Sason H, Billard JM, Smith GP, et al. Asc-1 transporter regulation of synaptic activity via the tonic release of D-serine in the forebrain. Cereb Cortex 2017;27:1573–1587

21. Mi H, Muruganujan A, Huang X, et al. Protocol update for large-scale genome and gene function analysis with the PANTHER classification system (v.14.0). Nat Protoc 2019;14:703–721

22. Midttun Ø, McCann A, Aarseth O, et al. Combined measurement of 6 fat-soluble vitamins and 26 water-soluble functional vitamin markers and amino acids in 50 μL of serum or plasma by high-throughput mass spectrometry. Anal Chem 2016;88:10427–10436

23. Bjune J-I, Dyer L, Røsland GV, et al. The homeobox factor Irx3 maintains adipogenic identity. Metabolism 2019;103:154014

24. Jones AR IV, Meshulam T, Oliveira MF, Burritt N, Corkey BE. Extracellular redox regulation of intracellular reactive oxygen generation, mitochondrial function and lipid turnover in cultured human adipocytes. PLoS One 2016;11:e0164011

25. Cinti S, Zingaretti MC, Cancello R, Ceresi E, Ferrara P. Morphologic techniques for the study of brown adipose tissue and white adipose tissue. Methods Mol Biol 2001;155:21–51

26. Edgar R, Domrachev M, Lash AE. Gene Expression Omnibus: NCBI gene expression and hybridization array data repository. Nucleic Acids Res 2002;30:207–210

27. Puri V, Ranjit S, Konda S, et al. Cidea is associated with lipid droplets and insulin sensitivity in humans. Proc Natl Acad Sci U S A 2008;105:7833–7838

28. Klöting N, Fasshauer M, Dietrich A, et al. Insulin-sensitive obesity. Am J Physiol Endocrinol Metab 2010;299:E506–E515

29. Torrecillas IR, Conde-Ceide S, de Lucas AI, et al. Inhibition of the alanine-serine-cysteine-1 transporter by BMS-466442. ACS Chem Neurosci 2019;10:2510–2517

30. Small KS, Hedman ÅK, Grundberg E, et al.; GIANT Consortium; MAGIC Investigators; DIAGRAM Consortium; MuTHER Consortium. Identification of an imprinted master trans regulator at the KLF14 locus related to multiple metabolic phenotypes. Nat Genet 2011;43:561–564

31. Hanzu FA, Vinaixa M, Papageorgiou A, et al. Obesity rather than regional fat depots marks the metabolomic pattern of adipose tissue: an untargeted metabolomic approach. Obesity (Silver Spring) 2014;22:698–704

32. Achari AE, Jain SK. L-cysteine supplementation increases insulin sensitivity mediated by upregulation of GSH and adiponectin in high glucose treated 3T3-L1 adipocytes. Arch Biochem Biophys 2017;630:54–65

33. Kobayashi H, Matsuda M, Fukuhara A, Komuro R, Shimomura I. Dysregulated glutathione metabolism links to impaired insulin action in adipocytes. Am J Physiol Endocrinol Metab 2009;296:E1326–E1334

34. Jankovic A, Korac A, Srdic-Galic B, et al. Differences in the redox status of human visceral and subcutaneous adipose tissues–relationships to obesity and metabolic risk. Metabolism 2014;63:661–671

35. Chattopadhyay M, Khemka VK, Chatterjee G, Ganguly A, Mukhopadhyay S, Chakrabarti S. Enhanced ROS production and oxidative damage in subcutaneous white adipose tissue mitochondria in obese and type 2 diabetes subjects. Mol Cell Biochem 2015;399:95–103

36. Akl MG, Fawzy E, Deif M, Farouk A, Elshorbagy AK. Perturbed adipose tissue hydrogen peroxide metabolism in centrally obese men: association with insulin resistance. PLoS One 2017;12:e0177268

37. Maslov LN, Naryzhnaya NV, Boshchenko AA, Popov SV, Ivanov VV, Oeltgen PR. Is oxidative stress of adipocytes a cause or a consequence of the metabolic syndrome? J Clin Transl Endocrinol 2018;15:1–5

38. Castro JP, Grune T, Speckmann B. The two faces of reactive oxygen species (ROS) in adipocyte function and dysfunction. Biol Chem 2016;397:709–724

39. Vigilanza P, Aquilano K, Baldelli S, Rotilio G, Ciriolo MR. Modulation of intracellular glutathione affects adipogenesis in 3T3-L1 cells. J Cell Physiol 2011;226:2016–2024

40. Peris E, Micallef P, Paul A, et al. Antioxidant treatment induces reductive stress associated with mitochondrial dysfunction in adipocytes. J Biol Chem 2019;294:2340–2352

41. Wang T, Si Y, Shirihai OS, et al. Respiration in adipocytes is inhibited by reactive oxygen species. Obesity (Silver Spring) 2010;18:1493–1502

42. Kim J-H, Park S-J, Kim B, Choe Y-G, Lee D-S. Insulin-stimulated lipid accumulation is inhibited by ROS-scavenging chemicals, but not by the Drp1 inhibitor Mdivi-1. PLoS One 2017;12:e0185764

43. Tormos KV, Anso E, Hamanaka RB, et al. Mitochondrial complex III ROS regulate adipocyte differentiation. Cell Metab 2011;14:537–544

44. Shi K, Gao Z, Shi T-Q, et al. Reactive oxygen species-mediated cellular stress response and lipid accumulation in oleaginous microorganisms: the state of the art and future perspectives. Front Microbiol 2017;8:793

45. Townsend LK, Weber AJ, Barbeau PA, Holloway GP, Wright DC. Reactive oxygen species-dependent regulation of pyruvate dehydrogenase kinase-4 in white adipose tissue. Am J Physiol Cell Physiol 2020;318:C137–C149

46. Findeisen HM, Pearson KJ, Gizard F, et al. Oxidative stress accumulates in adipose tissue during aging and inhibits adipogenesis. PLoS One 2011;6: e18532

47. Sriram S, Yuan C, Chakraborty S, et al. Oxidative stress mediates depot-specific functional differences of human adipose-derived stem cells. Stem Cell Res Ther 2019;10:141

48. Wang PW, Kuo HM, Huang HT, et al. Biphasic response of mitochondrial biogenesis to oxidative stress in visceral fat of diet-induced obesity mice. Antioxid Redox Signal 2014;20:2572–2588

49. Liemburg-Apers DC, Willems PHGM, Koopman WJH, Grefte S. Interactions between mitochondrial reactive oxygen species and cellular glucose metabolism. Arch Toxicol 2015;89:1209–1226

50. Lucas S, Chen G, Aras S, Wang J. Serine catabolism is essential to maintain mitochondrial respiration in mammalian cells. Life Sci Alliance 2018;1: e201800036

51. Gao X, Lee K, Reid MA, et al. Serine availability influences mitochondrial dynamics and function through lipid metabolism. Cell Rep 2018;22:3507–3520

52. Esaki K, Sayano T, Sonoda C, et al. L-serine deficiency elicits intracellular accumulation of cytotoxic deoxysphingolipids and lipid body formation. J Biol Chem 2015;290:14595–14609

53. Zhou X, He L, Wu C, Zhang Y, Wu X, Yin Y. Serine alleviates oxidative stress via supporting glutathione synthesis and methionine cycle in mice. Mol Nutr Food Res 2017;61:1700262

54. Sim W-C, Yin H-Q, Choi H-S, et al. L-serine supplementation attenuates alcoholic fatty liver by enhancing homocysteine metabolism in mice and rats. J Nutr 2015;145:260–267

55. Mikou A, Cabayé A, Goupil A, Bertrand HO, Mothet JP, Acher FC. Asc-1 transporter (SLC7A10): homology models and molecular dynamics insights into the first steps of the transport mechanism. Sci Rep 2020;10:3731

56. Den Broeder MJ, Kopylova VA, Kamminga LM, Legler J. Zebrafish as a model to study the role of peroxisome proliferating-activated receptors in adipogenesis and obesity. PPAR Res 2015;2015:358029

57. Zang L, Shimada Y, Nishimura N. Development of a novel zebrafish model for type 2 diabetes mellitus. Sci Rep 2017;7:1461

58. Oka T, Nishimura Y, Zang L, et al. Diet-induced obesity in zebrafish shares common pathophysiological pathways with mammalian obesity. BMC Physiol 2010;10:21

LTB$_4$-Driven Inflammation and Increased Expression of *ALOX5/ACE2* During Severe COVID-19 in Individuals With Diabetes

Icaro Bonyek-Silva,[1,2] Antônio Fernando Araújo Machado,[3] Thiago Cerqueira-Silva,[1,2] Sara Nunes,[1,2] Márcio Rivison Silva Cruz,[3,4] Jéssica Silva,[1,2] Reinan Lima Santos,[1,5] Aldina Barral,[1,2,6] Pablo Rafael Silveira Oliveira,[7] Ricardo Khouri,[1,2] C. Henrique Serezani,[8] Cláudia Brodskyn,[1,2,6] Juliana Ribeiro Caldas,[3,4,9,10] Manoel Barral-Netto,[1,2,6] Viviane Boaventura,[1,2] and Natalia Machado Tavares[1,2,6]

Diabetes 2021;70:2120–2130 | https://doi.org/10.2337/db20-1260

Diabetes is a known risk factor for severe coronavirus disease 2019 (COVID-19), the disease caused by the new coronavirus severe acute respiratory syndrome coronavirus 2 (SARS-CoV-2). However, there is a lack of knowledge about the mechanisms involved in the evolution of COVID-19 in individuals with diabetes. We aimed to evaluate whether the chronic low-grade inflammation of diabetes could play a role in the development of severe COVID-19. We collected clinical data and blood samples of patients with and without diabetes hospitalized for COVID-19. Plasma samples were used to measure inflammatory mediators and peripheral blood mononuclear cells, for gene expression analysis of the SARS-CoV-2 main receptor system (*ACE2/TMPRSS2*), and for the main molecule of the leukotriene B$_4$ (LTB$_4$) pathway (*ALOX5*). We found that diabetes activates the LTB$_4$ pathway and that during COVID-19 it increases *ACE2/TMPRSS2* as well as *ALOX5* expression. Diabetes was also associated with COVID-19–related disorders, such as reduced oxygen saturation as measured by pulse oximetry/fraction of inspired oxygen (FiO$_2$) and arterial partial pressure of oxygen/FiO$_2$ levels, and increased disease duration. In addition, the expressions of *ACE2* and *ALOX5* are positively correlated, with increased expression in patients with diabetes and COVID-19 requiring intensive care assistance. We confirmed these molecular results at the protein level, where plasma LTB$_4$ is significantly increased in individuals with diabetes. In addition, IL-6 serum levels are increased only in individuals with diabetes requiring intensive care assistance. Together, these results indicate that LTB$_4$ and IL-6 systemic levels, as well as *ACE2/ALOX5* blood expression, could be early markers of severe COVID-19 in individuals with diabetes.

As of 17 May 2021, >162 million confirmed cases of coronavirus disease 19 (COVID-19) and >3.3 million deaths worldwide from the pandemic had been recorded (1). The disease is caused by the new severe acute respiratory syndrome coronavirus 2 (SARS-CoV-2) that emerged in China and rapidly spread around the world (2). Estimates indicate that ~80% of infected individuals are asymptomatic or develop mild symptoms. The other 20% can develop moderate to severe disease, occasionally

---

[1]Gonçalo Moniz Institute, Oswaldo Cruz Foundation, Salvador, Bahia, Brazil
[2]Medical School, Federal University of Bahia, Salvador, Bahia, Brazil
[3]Salvador University, Salvador, Bahia, Brazil
[4]Critical Care Unit, Ernesto Simões Filho Hospital, Salvador, Bahia, Brazil
[5]Pharmacy School, Federal University of Bahia, Salvador, Bahia, Brazil
[6]Institute of Investigation in Immunology, National Institute of Science and Technology, São Paulo, São Paulo, Brazil
[7]Institute of Biological Sciences, Federal University of Bahia, Salvador, Bahia, Brazil
[8]Division of Infectious Diseases, Department of Medicine, Vanderbilt University Medical Center, Nashville, TN
[9]Critical Care Unit, São Rafael Hospital–Rede d'Or, Salvador, Bahia, Brazil
[10]Bahiana School of Medicine and Public Health, Salvador, Bahia, Brazil

Corresponding author: Natalia Machado Tavares, natalia.tavares@fiocruz.br

V.B. and N.M.T. contributed equally to this work.

Received 15 December 2020 and accepted 10 June 2021

This article contains supplementary material online at https://doi.org/10.2337/figshare.14770662.

This article is part of a special article collection available at https://diabetes.diabetesjournals.org/collection/diabetes-and-COVID19-articles.

requiring medical assistance due to acute respiratory disease and pneumonia, burdening health care systems (3,4). Risk factors in developing severe COVID-19 include, among others, hypertension, age, obesity, and diabetes (5–9). Individuals with diabetes are at high risk of developing severe COVID-19 as accounted for by their high rates of intensive care unit (ICU) admission and death (7).

Considering that 463 million people live with diabetes worldwide (10) and that COVID-19 is a highly transmissible disease, the need for identification of mechanisms that prevent infection in this population is urgent (6,7). As seen in multiple infectious diseases, including COVID-19, infection-induced inflammatory response can result in a cytokine storm, recruiting cells to infected tissues and establishing a proinflammatory feedback loop. This uncontrolled inflammation causes multiorgan damage, especially of the heart, liver, and kidneys, with high risk of death (11). Although several reports have described cytokines and chemokines involved in the inflammatory storm during COVID-19 (11,12), studies on lipid mediators of inflammation and their roles in this new disease are scarce.

Eicosanoids are potent lipid mediators produced by arachidonic acid metabolism, found in cell surface, that signals many biological processes, including inflammation and immune responses (13). Some classes of eicosanoids, especially leukotrienes, have been associated with the pathogenesis of respiratory disease (14,15). We and others have already shown increased levels of leukotriene B_4 (LTB_4) in diabetes, which is associated with inflammation, compromised wound healing, insulin resistance, and susceptibility to infections (16–20). LTB_4 is a product of the action of 5-lipoxygenase (5-LO) (encoded by the arachidonate 5-lipoxygenase [*ALOX5*] gene) and its activating protein FLAP (encoded by *ALOX5AP* gene) that are rapidly produced after several stimuli, mainly by neutrophils and monocytes/macrophages. After its release, LTB_4 can be signaled in an autocrine or paracrine manner by different cell types through the leukotriene receptor (encoded by the *LTB4R* gene), triggering an increase in chemotaxis and inflammatory exacerbation (18,21–23). In the current study, we sought to evaluate whether LTB_4 plays a role in the severity of COVID-19 in individuals with diabetes.

RESEARCH DESIGN AND METHODS
Ethics Statement
This study followed the principles specified in the Declaration of Helsinki. The Institutional Board for Ethics in Human Research at the Gonçalo Moniz Institute (Oswaldo Cruz Foundation) and Irmã Dulce Social Works approved this study (protocol numbers CAAE 36199820.6.0000.0040 and 33366020.5.0000.0047, respectively). Participants gave informed consent previous to any data and sample collection.

Acquisition of Microarray Data Set
Diabetes is considered a risk factor for complicated acute respiratory syndrome caused by SARS-CoV-2 infection (5,7). Given the lack of data on the mechanisms that drive these complications, we sought to analyze public transcriptome data of peripheral blood mononuclear cells (PBMCs) from individuals with diabetes. Microarray analysis was performed from a search of the National Center for Biotechnology Information Gene Expression Omnibus (GEO) database using the terms "diabetes" and "human." Among the data sets found, we selected the data set with GEO accession number GSE95849 that was done on Phalanx Human lncRNA OneArray v1_mRNA (GPL22448) platform (24). This data set compared six samples of PBMCs from healthy control subjects (individuals with normal glucose tolerance and without a family history of diabetes or chronic diseases) and six samples from individuals with diabetes. The criteria for including individuals in the diabetes group were fasting plasma glucose ≥7 mmol/L, 2-h plasma glucose after oral glucose tolerance test ≥11.1 mmol/L, or use of glucose-lowering drugs or physician-diagnosed diabetes. Differentially expressed genes (DEGs) were considered when the fold change ranged from −2.0 to 2.0 with a false discovery rate–adjusted $P < 0.05$.

Detection of Metabolic Network in Diseases and Pathway Enrichment Analysis
Metabolic networks (compound-reaction-enzyme-gene) were found based on the expression of significantly modulated genes in comparisons of healthy control subjects with individuals with diabetes. We used MetDisease version 1.1.0 in Cytoscape 3.7.2 software (Cytoscape Consortium, San Diego, CA) to build disease-based metabolite networks according to the Kyoto Encyclopedia of Genes and Genomes (KEGG). Next, data were further filtered to retain disease Medical Subject Headings terms relevant to reported clinical COVID-19 manifestations, such as pneumonia, respiratory distress syndrome (adult), acute lung injury, and inflammation. Matched metabolites found in these conditions were clustered using a Venn diagram to find common molecules.

The identification of enriched pathways was based on genes and compounds using the integrated KEGG and Edinburgh Human Metabolic Network (EHMN) databases stored at the National Center for Biotechnology Information. Canonical pathways were detected by MetScape version 3.1.3 in the Cytoscape 3.7.2 software using significantly modulated genes between healthy control subjects and individuals with diabetes.

Study Design, Cohort Definition, and Clinical Data
Patients were admitted with confirmed diagnosis of COVID-19 at Ernesto Simões Filho General Hospital, Salvador, Bahia, Brazil. A convenience sample of 53 patients were enrolled in this study (24 without diabetes [the non-DM group: NDM] and 29 with diabetes [the diabetes

mellitus group: DM]). This sample size considered a 95% CI (two-sided), and the power estimated for each parameter measured, using Epi Info software, was >80%. All groups were matched for sex, age, and hospitalization type (i.e., clinical beds [CBs], ICU). According to the Brazilian Diabetes Society guidelines, 2019–2020 (25), the diagnosis of diabetes was confirmed by HbA_{1c} levels measured during hospitalization. Patients with HbA_{1c} ≥6.5% (48 mmol/mol) and a medical history of insulin use were considered to have diabetes. The NDM group included individuals with HbA_{1c} ≤6.4% (46 mmol/mol) who were not considered to have diabetes or prediabetes (without the need for insulin during hospitalization). Comorbidity data were collected according to medical records. The study included patients with a positive diagnosis of COVID-19 based on positive molecular test (quantitative real-time PCR), serology or tomography results for or clinical history of COVID-19. Patients who did not agree to sign the free and informed consent, were pregnant, had symptoms for ≥14 days, and had been in the hospital for >48 h were excluded. Clinical data from all patients, obtained from medical records, are shown in Table 1.

Sample Collection

Blood samples from all patients were collected at admission by venipuncture using tubes with heparin. Plasma was separated (to quantify inflammatory mediators), and PBMCs (to analyze gene expression) were purified using Histopaque-1077 (Sigma-Aldrich, St. Louis, MO).

Analysis of Gene Expression in PBMCs

Total RNA was extracted from PBMCs using miRNeasy Mini Kit (QIAGEN, Hilden, Germany) according to the manufacturer's guidelines. Relative expression of *ALOX5* (assay identifier [ID] Hs.PT.56a.28007202.g); *ACE2* (assay ID Hs.PT.58.27645939); transmembrane serine protease 2 (*TMPRSS2*) (assay ID Hs.PT.58.4661363); furin, paired basic amino acid cleaving enzyme (*FURIN*) (assay ID Hs.PT.58.1294 962), and basigin (*CD147*) (assay ID Hs.PT.56a.39293590.g) were analyzed. After RNA quantification and quality analysis by spectrophotometry, cDNA synthesis was performed using the SuperScript III Reverse Transcriptase Kit (Invitrogen, Carlsbad, CA). Then, cDNA was amplified by quantitative real-time PCR using the SYBR Green PCR Master Mix (Thermo Fisher Scientific, Waltham, MA). Relative gene expression is shown as the fold change between the NDM and DM groups using the $2^{-\Delta\Delta CT}$ method [$\Delta\Delta Ct = \Delta Ct$ (target DM) – mean ΔCt (target NDM), where $\Delta Ct = Ct$ (gene of interest) – Ct (housekeeping gene)]. To identify the distribution within the control group (NDM), we applied $\Delta\Delta Ct = \Delta Ct$ (target NDM) – mean ΔCt (target NDM), with $\Delta Ct = Ct$ (gene of interest) – Ct (housekeeping gene). β-Actin was the housekeeping gene (*ACTB*) (assay ID Hs.PT.39a.22214847). All primers were purchased from Integrated DNA Technologies (Coralville, IA).

Quantification of Inflammatory Mediators

Based on the inflammatory profile already described in the literature for diabetes and COVID-19 (6,8,26), serum levels of TNF-α, IL-6, and IL-1β cytokines

Table 1—Characteristics of individuals hospitalized because of complications of COVID-19, Salvador, Bahia, Brazil, 2020 (N = 53)

	NDM	DM	P
Patients, *n*	24	29	
Male sex, *n* (%)	15 (62.5)	16 (55)	0.59
Age (years), median (min–max)	59 (27–88)	59 (43–93)	0.12
HbA_{1c}, median (min–max)			<0.0001
%	5.6 (4.5–6.3)	7.9 (6.5–12.9)	
mmol/mol	38 (26–45)	63 (48–117)	
Comorbidities, *n/N* (%)			
Obesity	3/18 (16.6)	7/21 (33.3)	0.23
Dyslipidemia	3/13 (23.0)	3/11 (27.2)	0.99
Liver disease	1/22 (4.5)	0/24 (0.0)	0.47
Kidney disease	8/24 (33.3)	5/27 (18.5)	0.22
COPD	3/16 (18.7)	3/14 (21.4)	0.99
HAS	9/24 (37.5)	22/26 (84.6)	0.001
Symptoms, *n/N* (%)			
Fever	12/19 (63.1.0)	14/21 (66.6)	0.99
Cough	16/23 (69.5.5)	16/22 (72.7)	0.81
Dyspnea	13/22 (59.0)	22/24 (91.6)	0.01
Expectoration	1/17 (5.8)	3/16 (18.7)	0.33
COVID-19 confirmed, *n/N* (%)	18/21 (85.7)	26/27 (96.3)	0.30

HAS, systemic arterial hypertension; min–max, minimum to maximum; *n/N* positive number/valid number.

(Invitrogen) were evaluated using sandwich ELISAs. LTB$_4$ levels were determined by Competition ELISA Kit (Cayman Chemical, Ann Arbor, MI), considering the manufacturer's instructions.

Statistical Analysis

The Benjamini-Hochberg method was used to control false discovery rate in evaluation of DEGs from the GEO transcriptome data set. For variables with normal distribution, we used Student t test (two groups) and one-way ANOVA test followed by Tukey post hoc test (three or more groups). For nonnormal distribution, we used Mann-Whitney test (two groups), Kruskal-Wallis with Dunn posttest (three or more groups), and Spearman test for correlation analysis. Symptom and comorbidity analyses were performed using χ^2 or Fisher exact test. All tests were conducted using GraphPad Prism 7 software (GraphPad Software, San Diego, CA). Differences were considered statistically significant when $P < 0.05$ or adjusted $P < 0.05$ for DEGs and multiple comparisons.

Data and Resource Availability

The public data set analyzed during the current study is available in GEO under accession number GSE95849 (https://www.ncbi.nlm.nih.gov/geo/query/acc.cgi?acc=GSE95 849). The data sets generated during the current study are not publicly available but can be made available by the corresponding author upon request.

RESULTS

LTB$_4$ Signaling Activated in Individuals With Diabetes Is Similar to That Found in Respiratory Disorders

Initially, we found that 3,585 genes were significantly modulated when comparing cells from individuals with or without diabetes. Of these, 3,405 were upregulated, and 180 were downregulated in individuals with diabetes (Fig. 1A).

Next, we searched for disorders associated with these DEGs by detecting molecule networks. We focused on conditions related to severe COVID-19, such as pneumonia, severe acute respiratory syndrome, and acute lung injury; we also focused on inflammation. Interestingly, we found only two molecules in common among these conditions: carbon dioxide and the lipid mediator LTB$_4$ (Fig. 1B).

We further searched for signaling pathways associated with these DEGs, and among 61 routes found, the LTB$_4$ pathway was at a central position within the network (Fig. 1C). Next, we assessed the expression of molecules crucial for LTB$_4$ production, such as the ALOX5 gene (which encodes the 5-LO enzyme that converts arachidonic acid into leukotrienes), ALOX5AP (the 5-LO–activating protein), and LTB4R (the LTB$_4$ receptor) in this data set. We found increased expression of all evaluated genes in the PBMCs from DM compared with NDM (Fig. 1D). Together, these findings indicate that LTB$_4$ is a

potential target to study mechanisms under complicated COVID-19 in individuals with diabetes.

Increased Expression of ALOX5 and ACE2/TMPRSS2 in PBMCs From DM and NDM Patients With COVID-19

The expression of SARS-CoV-2 receptors (27) and the inflammatory response (11) are related to the complications found in COVID-19. We then assessed the expression of ALOX5 (which encodes for the 5-LO enzyme) and ACE2/TMPRSS2, FURIN, and CD147 (surface molecules used by SARS-CoV-2 to invade human cells). The results showed a significant increase in the expression of ALOX5 (Fig. 2A) and ACE2/TMPRSS2 (Fig. 2B and C) in PBMCs from COVID-19 in DM compared with NDM. The increase in ALOX5, ACE2, and TMPRSS2 was also preliminarily assessed in the tracheal secretion of the NDM and DM groups with COVID-19 under mechanical ventilation. Despite the small sample size, we observed a trend toward increased expression, indicating that blood cells mirror the immune response in the lungs ($P = 0.055$) (Supplementary Fig. 1). These findings confirm our previous result (from public transcriptome data), showing that ALOX5 expression is increased in diabetes (Fig. 1D). Such findings support the possible role of 5-LO in the chronic low-grade inflammation observed in LTB$_4$ pathway–induced diabetes, rendering individuals with diabetes more prone to infections (19,21). We also found increased expressions of the SARS-CoV-2 main receptor system ACE2 and TMPRSS2 in the PBMCs from individuals in the DM group, suggesting that immune cells that will fight the infection are more prone to viral invasion.

Expression of ALOX5 Correlates With That of ACE2 in PBMCs From DM Patients With COVID-19

ACE2 expression is crucial for cell invasion and progression in COVID-19 (11,27). Therefore, we investigated whether the expression of ALOX could be correlated with ACE2 expression. First, we correlated ALOX5 with ACE2/TMPRSS2 (summarized in the correlation matrix [Fig. 3A]) separately between the DM and NDM groups. We found a positive correlation between ACE2 and TMPRSS2 in both groups since these molecules act together during viral invasion (11) (Fig. 3B and C). However, the correlation between ALOX5 and ACE2 was only present in the DM group (Fig. 3D and Supplementary Fig. 2), suggesting that cells that have high levels of ALOX5 also have increased ACE2 expression in the DM group.

Next, we evaluated whether ALOX5 and ACE2 expressions are correlated with the clinical evolution of COVID-19. First, we compared the need for ICU admission between the DM and NDM groups stratified by the expression levels of ALOX5 and ACE2. The results showed that individuals in the DM group with higher levels of ACE2 (Fig. 3E) and ALOX5 (Fig. 3F) required ICU care more frequently than those with low expression of these genes, but no difference was found with the gene expression of TMPRSS2 (Fig. 3G). Together, these findings

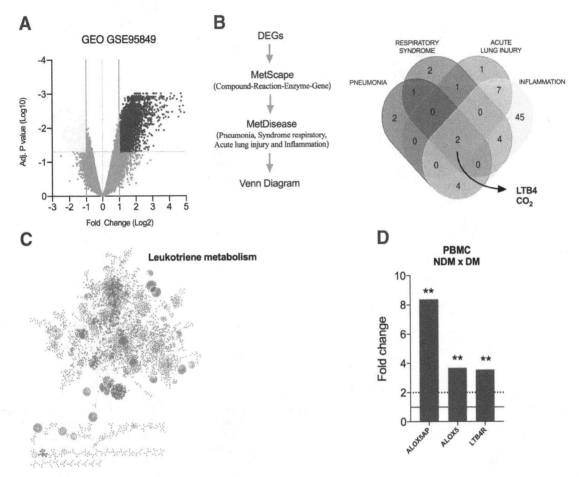

Figure 1—Upregulation of LTB$_4$ signaling in individuals in the DM group. *A*: Volcano plot with DEGs (blue, upregulated genes; yellow, downregulated genes) in PBMCs from DM patients vs. NDM patients. *B*: Workflow to identify molecules associated with inflammation and respiratory disorders based on gene expression shown in A and the resulting Venn diagram showing molecules in common among pneumonia, respiratory syndrome, acute lung injury, and inflammation. *C*: Enriched pathways raised from DEG analyses of PBMCs from DM patients vs. NDM patients, highlighting in red the central position of leukotriene metabolism among pathways. *D*: Fold change of genes involved with LTB$_4$ production (*ALOX5AP* and *ALOX5*) and signaling (*LTB4R*) in PBMCs of DM vs. NDM patients. Dotted line = cutoff point for a DEG; solid line = average of the control group. Data are medians. **$P < 0.01$. Adj., adjusted.

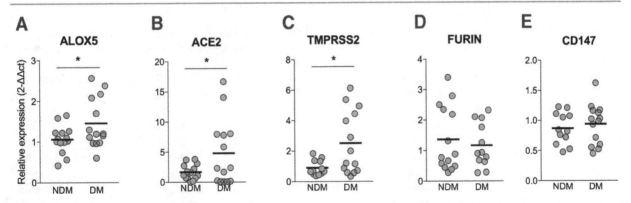

Figure 2—Increased expression of ALOX5 and ACE2/TMPRSS2 receptor system for SARS-CoV-2 infection in individuals with COVID-19 in the DM group. Expressions of *ALOX5* (*A*), *ACE2* (*B*), *TMPRSS2* (*C*), *FURIN* (*D*), and *CD147* (*E*) in PBMCs from DM and NDM patients. Data are means. *$P < 0.05$, **$P < 0.01$.

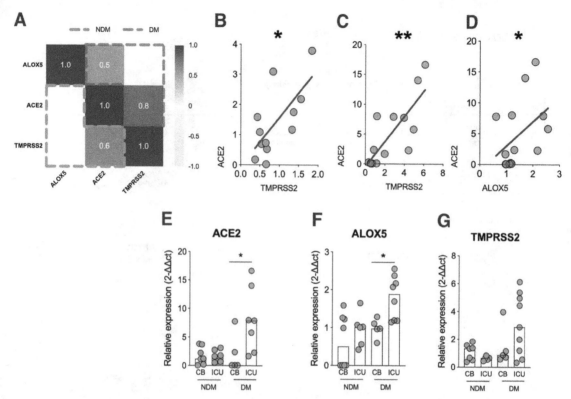

Figure 3—ALOX5 expression positively correlates with ACE2 expression in individuals with diabetes and COVID-19, and this is associated with an increased rate in ICU admissions. *A*: Correlation matrix between *ALOX5* and *ACE2/TMPRSS2* expression in PBMCs from DM (red) and NDM (gray) patients. *B*: Correlation analysis between ACE2 and TMPRSS2 expressions in PBMCs of NDM (*B*) and DM (*C*) individuals with COVID-19. *D*: Correlation analysis between *ALOX5* and *ACE2* expression in PBMCs from DM patients. *E* to *G*: Hospitalization type among DM or NDM individuals with COVID-19 based on the expression of *ACE2*, *ALOX5* and *TMPRSS2*. Data are medians. Spearman *r* correlation. **P* < 0.05, ***P* < 0.01.

indicate that the increased expressions of *ALOX5* and *ACE2* in blood cells from individuals with diabetes are associated with more severe conditions of COVID-19, requiring ICU care.

Increased Systemic Levels of LTB$_4$ in DM Patients With COVID-19

The cytokine storm described in COVID-19 is characterized by several inflammatory mediators. However, the role of lipid mediators in this context is still unknown (11). We measured the levels of inflammatory cytokines (IL-6, TNF-α, and IL-1β) and a lipid mediator of inflammation (LTB$_4$) in the plasma of individuals with and without diabetes and COVID-19. The results showed a significant increase of LTB$_4$ levels in the sera of individuals in the DM group (Fig. 4*A*). No statistical differences in the levels of IL-6 (Fig. 4*B*), TNF-α (Fig. 4*C*), or IL-1β (Supplementary Fig. 3) were found in comparisons of the DM and NDM groups. Supplementary Fig. 4 shows the production of these inflammatory mediators individually for each patient in the NDM and DM groups.

We further detailed the production of LTB$_4$, IL-6, and TNF-α between the NDM and DM groups based on the hospitalization type. No differences were found for LTB$_4$

and TNF-α production (Fig. 4*D* and *F*). With regard to IL-6 production, in the DM group, there was a significant increase in ICU admissions compared with CB admissions (Fig. 4*E*). Together, these findings indicate the predominance of LTB$_4$ production in the DM group compared with the NDM group. Moreover, IL-6 production seems to be an indicator for COVID-19 severity (hospitalization type) in the DM group.

ALOX5 Expression, Involved in LTB$_4$ Synthesis, Was Correlated With Clinical Outcomes of COVID-19 in the DM Group

Despite studies reporting diabetes as a risk factor for COVID-19, few explored the mechanisms related to these patients' worse prognosis (7,28,29). We compared LTB$_4$ signaling in patients with different clinical outcomes associated with COVID-19. In an analysis of days spent in the hospital (Fig. 5*A*) and death rate (Fig. 5*B*), we found no difference between the NDM and DM groups. However, there was a significantly longer disease duration (the period between symptom onset and disease outcome [death or hospital discharge]) in the DM group (Fig. 5*C*). These data suggest that individuals with diabetes develop COVID-19 symptoms for prolonged periods, possibly due to the low-

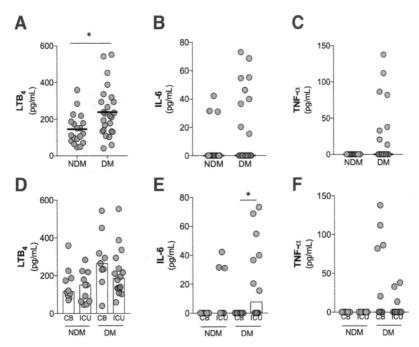

Figure 4—Increased systemic levels of LTB$_4$ in patients in the DM group, with COVID-19. Levels of LTB4 (*A*), IL-6 (*B*), and TNF-α (*C*) in plasma samples from DM and NDM patients affected by COVID-19. Plasma levels of LTB4 (*D*), IL-6 (*E*), and TNF-α (*F*) in NDM and DM patients with COVID-19 categorized by hospitalization type: clinical beds (CB) or intensive care units (ICU). Data are means. *$P < 0.05$.

grade inflammation already present in these individuals even in the absence of an infectious agent. Furthermore, the pulmonary condition in the DM group was more severe than in the NDM group, measured by oxygen saturation by pulse oximetry (SpO$_2$)–to–fraction of inspired oxygen (FiO$_2$) ratio (Fig. 5*D*), arterial partial pressure of oxygen (PaO$_2$)–to–FiO$_2$ ratio (Fig. 5*E*), and O$_2$ saturation (Supplementary Fig. 5) at the moment of admission to the hospital. For both parameters, individuals in the DM group arrived at the hospital in a more critical condition.

Finally, we correlated these clinical aspects with LTB$_4$ production and *ALOX5* and *ACE2* expression in all

individuals (Fig. 6*A*). The results show a positive correlation between LTB$_4$ and *ALOX5*, as expected, since the 5-LO enzyme produces LTB$_4$ ($r = 0.5$) (Supplementary Fig. 6*A*). We found that *ALOX5* negatively correlates with the worse pulmonary condition, such as SpO$_2$-to-FiO$_2$ ratio ($r = -0.6$) and PaO$_2$-to-FiO$_2$ ratio ($r = -0.9$) (Fig. 6*B* and *C*). In addition, we found that patients with a low SpO$_2$-to-FiO$_2$ ratio and increased production of IL-6 had a longer hospital stay for COVID-19 (Fig. 6*D*).

Taken together, these results show that patients with COVID-19 and diabetes develop a more pronounced systemic inflammatory response with the predominance of

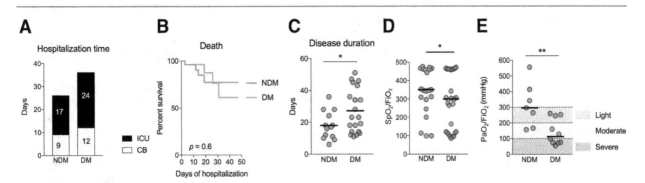

Figure 5—Diabetes induces greater severity of COVID-19. *A*: Number of days that NDM and DM patients remained hospitalized in CBs or the ICU because of COVID-19. *B*: Survival curves of NDM and DM patients hospitalized for COVID-19. *C*: Disease duration measured from the onset of symptoms to hospital discharge for NDM and DM patients with COVID-19. *D*: O$_2$ saturation of NDM and DM patients with COVID-19. *E*: Degree of lung injury in NDM and DM patients with COVID-19. Data are medians in *A*, *B*, and *D* and means in *C*. *$P < 0.05$, **$P < 0.01$.

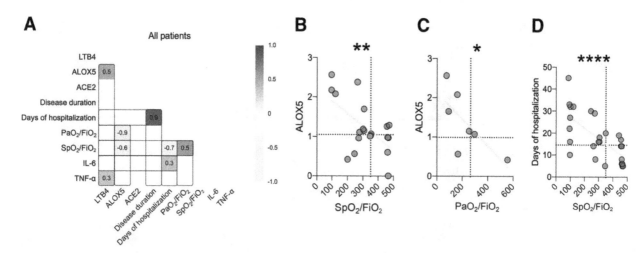

Figure 6—ALOX5 plays a role in the severity of COVID-19 in individuals with diabetes. *A*: Correlation matrix among genes, inflammatory parameters, and clinical outcome changes found in all patients with COVID-19. *B* and *C*: Dispersion of values with all patients between the correlation of ALOX5 with SpO$_2$-to-FiO$_2$ and PaO$_2$-to-FiO$_2$ ratios. *D*: Correlation between oxygen saturation and days of hospitalization. Dotted lines = median of the NDM group. Spearman *r* correlation. *$P < 0.05$, **$P < 0.01$, ****$P < 0.0001$.

LTB$_4$ and increased expression of SARS-CoV-2 receptor system *ACE2/TMPRSS2*. These individuals more frequently require critical care due to lung injury, suggesting that LTB$_4$ signaling could be a mediator produced by individuals with diabetes that increases the risk for severe COVID-19.

DISCUSSION

As SARS-CoV-2 emerged and spread globally, identifying mechanisms involved in severe COVID-19 and its risk factors became crucial for improving disease management. Diabetes is considered a risk factor for severe COVID-19 (5,7,28), but the mechanisms under these complications remain unknown. Inflammation associates with severe COVID-19 (18,21,22), and LTB$_4$ drives the chronic low-grade inflammation observed in experimental models of diabetes, while its role is not fully elucidated in humans with diabetes (17–19,21,30–32). The current study shows that individuals with diabetes and COVID-19 have increased expression of genes from the LTB$_4$ pathway in blood cells. During COVID-19, the expression of *ACE2* and *TMPRSS2*, which encode the main receptor system for SARS-CoV-2 cell invasion, are also increased in PBMCs of individuals with diabetes. Moreover, the increased expression of *ALOX5* correlates with *ACE2*, which was present in patients with critical conditions requiring intensive care.

As revealed by pathway analysis, LTB$_4$ is critical in several physiological disorders (observed in severe COVID-19), including inflammation and respiratory complications such as pneumonia, respiratory distress syndrome, and acute lung injury (11,28). LTB$_4$ is also an essential molecule in diabetes pathogenesis. Several studies with experimental models have indicated that LTB$_4$ dictates the chronic low-grade inflammation in diabetes, rendering mice more prone to infections (17,19,33). Our group previously showed that increased production of LTB$_4$ induced by diabetes alters the outcome of cutaneous leishmaniasis (17). Another study showed that LTB$_4$ is associated with pulmonary complications, such as pneumonia, acute lung injury, acute respiratory distress syndrome (ARDS), and respiratory failure (15,34,35).

The interaction between SARS-CoV-2 and host cells involves several molecules, such as ACE2 and TMPRSS2 that interact with the viral spike protein (11,36,37). High glucose concentrations increase the expression of *ACE2* and SARS-CoV-2 viral load in human monocytes (27). A meta-analysis revealed an increase of *ACE2* expression in the lungs of patients with comorbidities, including diabetes (5), and another study showed an increase in the ACE2 protein in the lungs of individuals with diabetes (38). Besides the expression of ACE2 in the lungs, monocytes and lymphocytes are crucial for the COVID-19 immunopathogenesis (5,11,12,27,36). Our data show that *ACE2* and *TMPRSS2* expression are increased in PBMCs of individuals with diabetes and COVID-19, which can be related to a greater susceptibility to SARS-CoV-2 infection (27,38).

Additionally, *ALOX5* expression positively correlates with *ACE2*, and ICU admission is associated with increased *ALOX5/ACE2* expression in patients with diabetes and COVID-19. The interaction between the LTB$_4$ and ACE2 pathways is still unknown, but the positive independent regulation of these genes in monocytes can influence the process of inflammation and infection, respectively (21,27). During SARS-CoV-2 infection, mononuclear cells are recruited to the lung tissue, where they probably contribute to the control of infection and the healing process but also cause cause tissue damage (11).

In the current study, individuals in the DM group with COVID-19, age and sex matched to individuals in the NDM group with COVID-19, had a higher frequency of dyspnea, which is in agreement with data from Wuhan, China (7). Hypertension is more frequent in patients with diabetes and patients with COVID-19 and is a known risk factor for severe COVID-19 (7,38). According to previous studies, diabetes and hypertension are frequent in patients with COVID-19 and may play a role in increased death rates (6,7,39). In our study, mortality rates were similar between patients with COVID-19 with or without diabetes, but the disease severity is more pronounced in those with diabetes. Although our cohort shows no difference in obese individuals between the NDM and DM groups, the influence of weight differences between the groups should not be excluded, since obesity was determined only by medical observation.

The cytokine storm contributes to mortality in $\sim$28% of fatal COVID-19 cases (11). This condition encompasses several cytokines and chemokines, such as IL-1β, IL-6, IFN-γ, MCP-1, CCL2, CXCL10, and TNF-α (11,28). The IL-6 cytokine is one of the most related to the severity of COVID-19, and as in previous studies, our findings demonstrate this association in the context of COVID-19 in individuals with diabetes (6,8,26). However, knowledge is lacking about the implications of lipid mediators in the inflammatory response during COVID-19. LTB$_4$ is a potent inducer of inflammatory cytokines, including those of the cytokine storm, which may drive COVID-19 severity (16,21). Bronchoalveolar lavage fluid exhibited high levels of LTB$_4$ in an experimental model of acute lung injury (34). LTB$_4$ plays a significant role in the chronic obstructive pulmonary disease (COPD), and individuals with severe COPD have high levels of LTB$_4$ in exhaled air; such levels correlate with disease severity (14). LTB$_4$ levels better correlate with lung injury severity and clinical outcomes in ARDS than several other eicosanoids (35).

The number of patients with severe COVID-19 who require ICU care is a challenge for health care systems worldwide. Individuals with ARDS exhibit three to five times more LTB$_4$ levels than control subjects (40). The role of LTB$_4$ in the outcome of lung diseases is associated with neutrophil tissue infiltration, a condition present in COVID-19 (12). Our group has recently shown that LTB$_4$ is involved in the activation of pathogen-induced inflammasomes (18). A recent preliminary study associated the activation of inflammasomes in the lungs of patients with COVID-19 with a worse disease prognosis (41).

The Randomized Evaluation of COVID-19 Therapy (RECOVERY) study showed that dexamethasone slightly reduced death rates among patients with COVID-19 requiring invasive mechanical ventilation or oxygen therapy (42). Additionally, montelukast, a leukotriene antagonist, is proposed for the prophylaxis of COVID-19 symptoms (43). Together, these studies suggested strategies to treat COVID-19 that, directly or indirectly, act through eicosanoids. Our results confirm that LTB$_4$ signaling is a crucial branch of the inflammatory response observed in COVID-19 and reinforces the possibility of its inhibition in clinical practice.

Several studies reported the association of diabetes and increased COVID-19 death rates (4,5,19,22), whereas others did not find such an association with disease severity (4,5,33). We have not found a direct association between diabetes and mortality rates in our cohort. The participants in the DM group in this study developed severe forms of COVID-19, requiring ICU hospitalization, but their disease evolution seemed similar to that of patients in the NDM group. On the other hand, we found a significantly longer disease duration in DM patients with COVID-19. The disease duration refers to the period between the onset of symptoms until the patient's discharge or death, indicating that patients with diabetes experience COVID-19 symptoms for prolonged periods.

Although we have not found a direct association between systemic levels of LTB$_4$ and a worse COVID-19 prognosis in individuals with diabetes, our findings show that patients with COVID-19 and diabetes more frequently present reduced SpO$_2$-to-FiO$_2$ and PaO$_2$-to-FiO$_2$ ratios that correlate with ALOX5 expression in the blood. The dissociation between the expression of the *ALOX5* gene and its metabolic product may be due to different sources of LTB$_4$ detected in the bloodstream. Different immune cell types are able to produce LTB$_4$, such as neutrophils (14), a cell type not represented in our sample of mononuclear cells. LTB$_4$ is also locally produced at the site of infection caused by different agents (17–19,44) and has been associated with increased lung injury in experimental models (34). Our results add a new player to the inflammation panorama of COVID-19, suggesting that circulating mononuclear cells already present a proinflammatory profile that, once recruited to the lung, may amplify local inflammation and tissue injury. Further studies are necessary to confirm pulmonary production of LTB$_4$ and its role in COVID-19 outcomes.

In summary, our findings show that diabetes induces a proinflammatory profile on circulating immune cells with increased expression of *ACE2* and *ALOX5* genes, rendering these cells more prone to SARS-CoV-2 invasion. Together, our data reveal a potential role of LTB$_4$ in COVID-19, which is poorly explored, and open new ways to study implications and applications of this mediator in SARS-CoV-2 infection. Furthermore, we found that IL-6, a known cytokine for COVID-19 severity, is also a potential indicator in individuals with diabetes in need of intensive care.

Acknowledgments. The authors thank the developers of the MetScape and MetDisease software for making it possible to analyze the data in a more integrated way, Dr. Manuela da Silva Solcà (Federal University of

Bahia) for help in the construction of the table, and the health professionals who participated directly and indirectly in the care of patients.

Funding. This work was supported by the Inova Fiocruz/Fundação Oswaldo Cruz to N.M.T. (VPPCB-005-FIO-20-2-75), Coordenação de Aperfeiçoamento de Pessoal de Nível Superior–Brazil (CAPES) under Finance Code 001 to I.B.-S., S.N., and J.S., Conselho Nacional de Desenvolvimento Científico e Tecnológico–Brazil (CNPq) (to I.B.-S., S.N., A.B., C.B., and M.B.-N.), and National Institutes of Health grants R01HL124159-01, DK122147-01A1 and AI149207A (to C.H.S.).

Duality of Interest. No potential conflicts of interest relevant to this article were reported.

Author Contributions. I.B.-S., A.F.A.M., T.C.-S., S.N., and H.S contributed to the acquisition of the data or the analysis and interpretation of information. I.B.-S., T.C.-S., S.N., R.L.S., A.B., P.R.S.O., R.K., C.B., M.B.-N., V.B., and N.M.T. contributed to the writing of the manuscript or had substantial involvement in its revision before submission. I.B.-S., S.N., and J.S. conducted the processing of biological samples in the laboratory. I.B.-S., V.B., and N.M.T. were involved in the conception, hypotheses delineation, and design of the study. A.F.A.M., M.R.S.C., and J.R.C. conducted the medical care of the research participants. N.M.T. is the guarantor of this work and, as such, had full access to all the data in the study and takes responsibility for the integrity of the data and the accuracy of the data analysis.

References

1. World Health Organization. WHO Coronavirus (COVID-19) Dashboard. Accessed 17 May 2021. Available from https://covid19.who.int

2. Zhou P, Yang X-L, Wang X-G, et al. A pneumonia outbreak associated with a new coronavirus of probable bat origin. Nature 2020;579:270–273

3. Guan WJ, Ni ZY, Hu Y, et al.; China Medical Treatment Expert Group for Covid-19. Clinical characteristics of coronavirus disease 2019 in China. N Engl J Med 2020;382:1708–1720

4. Wang D, Hu B, Hu C, et al. Clinical characteristics of 138 hospitalized patients with 2019 novel coronavirus-infected pneumonia in Wuhan, China. JAMA 2020;323:1061–1069

5. Pinto BGG, Oliveira AER, Singh Y, et al. ACE2 expression is increased in the lungs of patients with comorbidities associated with severe COVID-19. J Infect Dis 2020;222:556–563

6. Sardu C, D'Onofrio N, Balestrieri ML, et al. Outcomes in patients with hyperglycemia affected by COVID-19: can we do more on glycemic control? Diabetes Care 2020;43:1408–1415

7. Shi Q, Zhang X, Jiang F, et al. Clinical characteristics and risk factors for mortality of COVID-19 patients with diabetes in Wuhan, China: a two-center, retrospective study. Diabetes Care 2020;43:1382–1391

8. Li X, Xu S, Yu M, et al. Risk factors for severity and mortality in adult COVID-19 inpatients in Wuhan. J Allergy Clin Immunol 2020;146:110–118

9. Richardson S, Hirsch JS, Narasimhan M, et al.; the Northwell COVID-19 Research Consortium. Presenting characteristics, comorbidities, and outcomes among 5700 patients hospitalized with COVID-19 in the New York City area. JAMA 2020;323:2052–2059

10. International Diabetes Federation. IDF Diabetes Atlas-2019. Brussels, Belgium, International Diabetes Federation, 2019

11. Tay MZ, Poh CM, Rénia L, MacAry PA, Ng LFP. The trinity of COVID-19: immunity, inflammation and intervention. Nat Rev Immunol 2020;20:363–374

12. Zhang B, Zhou X, Qiu Y, et al. Clinical characteristics of 82 cases of death from COVID-19. PloS One 2020;15:e0235458

13. Peters-Golden M, Henderson WR Jr. Leukotrienes. N Engl J Med 2007;357:1841–1854

14. Biernacki WA, Kharitonov SA, Barnes PJ. Increased leukotriene B4 and 8-isoprostane in exhaled breath condensate of patients with exacerbations of COPD. Thorax 2003;58:294–298

15. Auner B, Geiger EV, Henrich D, Lehnert M, Marzi I, Relja B. Circulating leukotriene B4 identifies respiratory complications after trauma. Mediators Inflamm 2012;2012:536156

16. Serezani CH, Lewis C, Jancar S, Peters-Golden M. Leukotriene B4 amplifies NF-κB activation in mouse macrophages by reducing SOCS1 inhibition of MyD88 expression. J Clin Invest 2011;121:671–682

17. Bonyek-Silva I, Nunes S, Santos RLS, et al. Unbalanced production of LTB$_4$/PGE$_2$ driven by diabetes increases susceptibility to cutaneous leishmaniasis. Emerg Microbes Infect 2020;9:1275–1286

18. Salina ACG, Brandt SL, Klopfenstein N, et al. Leukotriene B$_4$ licenses inflammasome activation to enhance skin host defense. Proc Natl Acad Sci U S A 2020;117:30619–30627

19. Brandt SL, Wang S, Dejani NN, et al. Excessive localized leukotriene B4 levels dictate poor skin host defense in diabetic mice. JCI Insight 2018;3:120220

20. Li P, Oh DY, Bandyopadhyay G, et al. LTB4 promotes insulin resistance in obese mice by acting on macrophages, hepatocytes and myocytes. Nat Med 2015;21:239–247

21. Brandt SL, Serezani CH. Too much of a good thing: how modulating LTB$_4$ actions restore host defense in homeostasis or disease. Semin Immunol 2016;33:37–43

22. Afonso PV, Janka-Junttila M, Lee YJ, et al. LTB4 is a signal-relay molecule during neutrophil chemotaxis. Dev Cell 2012;22:1079–1091

23. Morato CI, da Silva IA Jr, Borges AF, et al. Essential role of leukotriene B4 on Leishmania (Viannia) braziliensis killing by human macrophages. Microbes Infect 2014;16:945–953

24. Luo L, Zhou WH, Cai JJ, et al. Gene expression profiling identifies downregulation of the neurotrophin-MAPK signaling pathway in female diabetic peripheral neuropathy patients. J Diabetes Res. 2017;2017:8103904

25. Lyra R, Oliveira M, Lins D, et al. Diabetes Mellitus Tipo 1 e Tipo 2. Vol. 5. São Paulo, Brazil, Sociedade Brasileira de Diabetes, 2020, pp. 709–717

26. Han H, Ma Q, Li C, et al. Profiling serum cytokines in COVID-19 patients reveals IL-6 and IL-10 are disease severity predictors. Emerg Microbes Infect 2020;9:1123–1130

27. Codo AC, Davanzo GG, de Brito Monteiro L, et al. Elevated glucose levels favor SARS-CoV-2 infection and monocyte response through a HIF-1α/glycolysis dependent axis. Cell Metab 2020;32:437–446.e5

28. Muniyappa R, Gubbi S. COVID-19 pandemic, coronaviruses, and diabetes mellitus. Am J Physiol Endocrinol Metab 2020;318:E736–E741

29. Rao S, Lau A, So HC. Exploring diseases/traits and blood proteins causally related to expression of ACE2, the putative receptor of SARS-CoV-2: a mendelian randomization analysis highlights tentative relevance of diabetes-related traits. Diabetes Care 2020;43:1416–1426

30. Zhang Y, Olson RM, Brown CR. Macrophage LTB4 drives efficient phagocytosis of Borrelia burgdorferi via BLT1 or BLT2. J Lipid Res 2017;58:494–503

31. Filgueiras LR, Serezani CH, Jancar S. Leukotriene B4 as a potential therapeutic target for the treatment of metabolic disorders. Front Immunol 2015;6:515

32. Das UN. Is there a role for bioactive lipids in the pathobiology of diabetes mellitus? Front Endocrinol (Lausanne) 2017;8:182

33. Filgueiras LR, Brandt SL, Wang S, et al. Leukotriene B4-mediated sterile inflammation promotes susceptibility to sepsis in a mouse model of type 1 diabetes. Sci Signal 2015;8:ra10

34. Eun JC, Moore EE, Mauchley DC, et al. The 5-lipoxygenase pathway is required for acute lung injury following hemorrhagic shock. Shock 2012;37:599–604

35. Masclans JR, Sabater J, Sacanell J, et al. Possible prognostic value of leukotriene B(4) in acute respiratory distress syndrome. Respir Care 2007;52:1695–1700

36. Radzikowska U, Ding M, Tan G, et al. Distribution of ACE2, CD147, CD26, and other SARS-CoV-2 associated molecules in tissues and immune cells in health and in asthma, COPD, obesity, hypertension, and COVID-19 risk factors. Allergy 2020;75:2829–2845

37. Ing P, Bello I, Areiza M, Oliver J. SARS-CoV-2 invades host cells via a novel route: CD147-spike protein Ke. J Chem Inf Model 2020;53:45–50

38. Wijnant SRA, Jacobs M, Van Eeckhoutte HP, et al. Expression of ACE2, the SARS-CoV-2 receptor, in lung tissue of patients with type 2 diabetes. Diabetes 2020;69:2691–2699

39. Mudatsir M, Fajar JK, Wulandari L, et al. Predictors of COVID-19 severity: a systematic review and meta-analysis. F1000Res 2020;2019:1107

40. Davis JM, Yurt RW, Barie PS, et al. Leukotriene B4 generation in patients with established pulmonary failure. Arch Surg 1989;124:1451–1455

41. Rodrigues TS, de Sá KSG, Ishimoto AY, et al. Inflammasomes are activated in response to SARS-CoV-2 infection and are associated with COVID-19 severity in patients. J Exp Med 2021;218:e20201707

42. The RECOVERY Collaborative Group. Dexamethasone in hospitalized patients with COVID-19: preliminary report. Drug Ther Bull 2020; 58:133

43. Sanghai N, Tranmer GK. Taming the cytokine storm: repurposing montelukast for the attenuation and prophylaxis of severe COVID-19 symptoms. Drug Discov Today 2020;25:2076–2079

44. Serezani CH, Perrela JH, Russo M, Peters-Golden M, Jancar S. Leukotrienes are essential for the control of Leishmania amazonensis infection and contribute to strain variation in susceptibility. J Immunol 2006;177: 3201–3208

MEK/ERK Signaling in β-Cells Bifunctionally Regulates β-Cell Mass and Glucose-Stimulated Insulin Secretion Response to Maintain Glucose Homeostasis

Yoshiko Matsumoto Ikushima,[1] Motoharu Awazawa,[1] Naoki Kobayashi,[1] Sho Osonoi,[2] Seiichi Takemiya,[1] Hiroshi Kobayashi,[3] Hirotsugu Suwanai,[4] Yuichi Morimoto,[5,6] Kotaro Soeda,[1] Jun Adachi,[7] Masafumi Muratani,[8] Jean Charron,[9] Hiroki Mizukami,[2] Noriko Takahashi,[10] and Kohjiro Ueki[1,11]

Diabetes 2021;70:1519–1535 | https://doi.org/10.2337/db20-1295

In diabetic pathology, insufficiency in β-cell mass, unable to meet peripheral insulin demand, and functional defects of individual β-cells in production of insulin are often concurrently observed, collectively causing hyperglycemia. Here we show that the phosphorylation of ERK1/2 is significantly decreased in the islets of *db/db* mice as well as in those of a cohort of subjects with type 2 diabetes. In mice with abrogation of ERK signaling in pancreatic β-cells through deletion of *Mek1* and *Mek2*, glucose intolerance aggravates under high-fat diet–feeding conditions due to insufficient insulin production with lower β-cell proliferation and reduced β-cell mass, while in individual β-cells dampening of the number of insulin exocytosis events is observed, with the molecules involved in insulin exocytosis being less phosphorylated. These data reveal bifunctional roles for MEK/ERK signaling in β-cells for glucose homeostasis, i.e., in regulating β-cell mass as well as in controlling insulin exocytosis in individual β-cells, thus providing not only a novel perspective for the understanding of diabetes pathophysiology but also a potential clue for new drug development for diabetes treatment.

The insulin secretion capacity of pancreas is determined by the amount of β-cells and the function of individual β-cell in secretion of insulin, both of which could be affected by various factors in the pathogenesis of diabetes (1,2). Mitogen-activated protein kinase (MAPK) kinase (MEK)/extracellular signal–regulated kinase (ERK) signaling is involved in many cellular functions including cell growth and survival and cellular differentiation (3). In mammals, the MEK/ERK pathway involves the kinases ERK1 (*Mapk3*) and ERK2 (*Mapk1*) and the MAPK kinases MEK1 (*Map2k1*) and MEK2 (*Map2k2*). At present, ERK1 and ERK2 are the only known substrates of MEK1 and MEK2 (4), whose functions are known to be redundant, consistent with the high homology in their amino acid sequences (5).

The MEK/ERK signaling pathway is activated by multiple upstream stimuli including insulin (6), and our group,

[1]Department of Molecular Diabetic Medicine, Diabetes Research Center, Research Institute, National Center for Global Health and Medicine, Tokyo, Japan

[2]Department of Pathology and Molecular Medicine, Hirosaki University Graduate School of Medicine, Hirosaki, Japan

[3]Department of Stem Cell Biology, Research Institute, National Center for Global Health and Medicine, Tokyo, Japan

[4]Department of Diabetes, Metabolism and Endocrinology, Tokyo Medical University, Tokyo, Japan

[5]Laboratory of Structural Physiology, Center for Disease Biology and Integrative Medicine, Faculty of Medicine, The University of Tokyo, Tokyo, Japan

[6]International Research Center for Neurointelligence (WPI-IRCN), University of Tokyo Institutes for Advanced Study (UTIAS), The University of Tokyo, Tokyo, Japan

[7]Laboratory of Proteome Research, Laboratory of Proteomics for Drug Discovery, Center for Drug Design Research, National Institutes of Biomedical Innovation, Health and Nutrition, Osaka, Japan

[8]Department of Genome Biology, Faculty of Medicine, University of Tsukuba, Tsukuba, Japan

[9]Centre de Recherche sur le Cancer de l'Université Laval, L'Hôtel-Dieu de Québec, Quebec City, Quebec, Canada

[10]Department of Physiology, Kitasato University School of Medicine, Sagamihara, Japan

[11]Department of Molecular Diabetology, Graduate School of Medicine, The University of Tokyo, Tokyo, Japan

Corresponding author: Kohjiro Ueki, uekik@ri.ncgm.go.jp

Received 6 January 2021 and accepted 23 April 2021

This article contains supplementary material online at https://doi.org/10.2337/figshare.14473791.

as well as others, has demonstrated a significant role that the insulin signaling pathway plays in β-cells in the pathophysiological regulation of glucose metabolism (7). The MEK/ERK signaling pathway could also be activated by other hormones such as glucagon and growth factors including insulin-like growth factor 1 and platelet-derived growth factor—or by environmental stress as well (6,8,9). Besides, glucose and other nutrients may provoke MEK/ERK signaling activation in cultured β-cell lines, where glucose is proposed to stimulate MEK/ERK signaling in both insulin receptor–dependent and –independent fashions (8,10). While MEK/ERK signaling has been extensively studied in numerous models and its significant roles for β-cell physiology have been proposed (9,11), a systematic in vivo assessment of the roles that MEK/ERK signaling plays in β-cells for glucose metabolism has not been conducted.

Here we have performed in vivo assessments of the significance of MEK/ERK signaling in β-cells, which is downregulated in diabetic mice and in humans with diabetes. Studies using β-cell–specific *Mek1/2*-deficient mice and phosphoproteomics analyses of their islets and cultured β-cells have revealed that MEK/ERK signaling is required for β-cell mass regulation and plays a role in exocytosis of insulin granules, suggesting that MEK/ERK signaling plays roles in both the quantitative and the qualitative control of pancreatic β-cells.

RESEARCH DESIGN AND METHODS

Human Subjects

Autopsied pancreatic tissues from 13 subjects without diabetes and those from 5 subjects with type 2 diabetes were evaluated. Clinical data are briefly summarized in Supplementary Table 1. All patients were autopsied within 5 h of death for avoidance of autolytic changes in pancreas. Excised body of the pancreas was fixed with 10% neutral buffered formalin and embedded in paraffin (FFPE). Snap-frozen pancreas was also prepared for phosphorylated (phospho)-ERK immunofluorescence. The use of pancreatic tissue was approved by the ethics committee of the Hirosaki University Graduate School of Medicine (approval no. 2017-121).

Animals

Male *db/db* mice, *misty/misty* mice, and C57BL/6J mice were purchased from CLEA Japan. For preparation of DIO mice, C57BL/6J mice were assigned either a high-fat diet (HFD) (HFD32; CLEA Japan) or a low-fat diet (a normal chow diet [NCD], CE-2; CLEA Japan) at 5 weeks of age. Genetically engineered mice used in this study are presented in Table 1. β-Cell–specific *Mek1* deletion was conducted by crossing of *Mek1*-floxed mice with *MIP-Cre/ERT* mice and intraperitoneal injection of tamoxifen (Tmx) (100 mg/kg body wt for five consecutive days) (Sigma-Aldrich) at 6 weeks of age. For *Mek1* and *Mek2* abrogation in β-cells, *MIP-Cre/ERT* mice were crossed with

mice homozygous for *Mek1*-floxed alleles on a systemic *Mek2*-knockout background, with Cre induction by Tmx at 6 weeks of age (*MIP-Cre/ERT$^+$/Mek1$^{f/f}$/Mek2$^{ko/ko}$* [Tmx$^+$]: hereafter referred to as β*Mek1/2DKO* mice). The offspring were obtained by crossing of *MIP-Cre/ERT$^+$/Mek1$^{f/f}$* mice with *Mek1$^{f/f}$* mice or by crossing of *MIP-Cre/ERT$^+$/Mek1$^{f/f}$/Mek2$^{ko/ko}$* mice with *Mek1$^{f/f}$/Mek2$^{ko/ko}$* mice, and these mice were maintained in their respective closed colonies on a 129/SvEv/C57BL/6JJcl mixed background. As it has already been suggested that the expression of human growth hormone (hGH) in *MIP-Cre/ERT* construct itself may affect β-cell homeostasis (12,13), we used littermates of the same genotype injected with vehicle (corn oil) (*MIP-CreERT$^+$/Mek1$^{f/f}$/Mek2$^{ko/ko}$* [Tmx$^-$]: hereafter referred to as Tmx$^-$ controls) as the experimental controls. All the experiments were conducted after >4 weeks' washout period following Tmx administration. HFD feeding was started 2 weeks after the last intraperitoneal injection of Tmx. Animal care and experimentations were approved by the Animal Care and Use Committee of the National Center for Global Health and Medicine.

Cell Line

MIN6 clone 4 (MINcl4) β-cell line (14) was maintained in DMEM containing 25 mmol/L glucose, 15% FBS, 0.07 mmol/L 2-mercaptoethanol, 100 units/mL penicillin, and 0.05 mg/mL streptomycin in humidified 5% CO_2 at 37°C.

Metabolic Studies

Insulin tolerance tests, glucose tolerance tests (GTTs), and the measurements of plasma insulin levels on a glucose challenge were conducted as previously described (15). Blood glucose levels were measured with Glutest Neo alpha or Glutest Mint (Sanwa Kagaku Kenkyusho). Plasma insulin levels were measured with Morinaga Mouse Insulin ELISA kits and Morinaga Ultra Sensitive Mouse Insulin ELISA kits (Morinaga Institute of Biological Science, Inc.). For estimation of insulin clearance, mice were intraperitoneally injected with human insulin (Eli Lilly) (1.0 units/kg body wt) and blood samples were collected at the indicated time points. Plasma human insulin levels were measured with a human insulin–specific ELISA kit (Mercodia).

Islet Isolation

Pancreas was perfused with Liberase TL (Roche) solution and subsequently digested for 24 min at 37°C as previously described (15). Islets were picked manually, washed with PBS, and immediately used for further experiments or maintained in recovery media (16).

Immunoblotting

MINcl4 cells and freshly isolated islets were lysed by sonication in buffer A (17). Other tissues were

Table 1—The mouse lines, antibodies used for immunoblotting and immunostaining, and primers and probes used for quantitative RT-PCR analyses

Resource	Source	Identifier	Dilution
Mouse lines			
BKS.Cg-+ $Lepr^{db}$/+ $Lepr^{db}$/Jcl	CLEA Japan	N/A	
BKS.Cg-m+/m+/Jcl	CLEA Japan	N/A	
C57BL/6JJcl	CLEA Japan	N/A	
MIP-CreERT (B6.Cg-Tg(Ins1-cre/ERT)1Lphi/J)	The Jackson Laboratory	024709 (49)	
$Mek2^{ko/ko}$	Laboratory of Charron J (50)	N/A	
$Mek1^{f/f}$	Laboratory of Charron J (51)	N/A	
Antibodies			
For immunoblotting			
Rabbit anti-ERK1/2	Cell Signaling Technology	9102S	1:1,000
Rabbit anti–phospho-ERK1/2	Cell Signaling Technology	9101S	1:1,000
Rabbit anti-MEK1	Cell Signaling Technology	9146S	1:1,000
Rabbit anti-MEK2	Cell Signaling Technology	9147S	1:1,000
Rabbit anti–phospho-MEK1/2	Cell Signaling Technology	9154S	1:1,000
Rabbit anti-AKT	Cell Signaling Technology	4691S	1:1,000
Rabbit anti–phospho-AKT	Cell Signaling Technology	9271S	1:1,000
Mouse anti-ACTB	Sigma-Aldrich	A2228	1:5,000
For immunostaining			
Rabbit anti-Ki67	NeoMarkers	RM-9106-S0	1:500
Guinea pig anti-insulin	DAKO	A0564	1:300
Guinea pig anti-Gcg	DAKO	A0565	1:200
Rabbit anti-MEK1	Abcam	ab32091	1:150
Rabbit anti-SOX9	Millipore	AB5535-250G	1:100
Mouse anti-NGN3	Developmental Studies Hybridoma Bank	F25A1B3	1:100
Rabbit anti-insulin	Abcam	ab181547	1:5,000
Mouse anti–phospho-ERK1/2	Santa Cruz Biotechnology	sc-7383	1:1,000
Primers and probes for quantitative RT-PCR analyses			
Ccnd1	ABI	Mm00432359_m1	
Ccnd2	ABI	Mm00438070_m1	
Ccnd3	ABI	Mm01612362_m1	
Ccne1	ABI	Mm01266311_m1	
Cdkn1a (p21)	ABI	Mm00432448_m1	
Gcg	ABI	Mm00801714_m1	
Arx	Integrated DNA Technologies	Mm.PT.58.31593773	
Stx1a	ABI	Mm00444008_m1	
Rab27a	ABI	Mm00469997_m1	
Vamp2	ABI	Mm00494118_g1	
Snap25	ABI	Mm00456921_m1	
Itpr3	ABI	Mm01306070_m1	
Rab37	ABI	Mm00445351_m1	
Pclo	ABI	Mm00465330_m1	
Sytl4	ABI	Mm00489110_m1	
Rims2	ABI	Mm01158145_m1	

homogenized in homogenization buffer (17). The samples were prepared by heating at 100°C with Laemmli buffer for 5 min and subjected to immunoblotting with use of antibodies listed in Table 1. Primary antibodies were diluted in 2.5% BSA in Tris-buffered saline with Tween, except for MEK1, MEK2, phospho-MEK1/2, and phospho-AKT antibodies, where Can Get Signal Solution 1 (TOYOBO) was used for dilution. The blots were developed with use of Chemi-Lumi One L (Nacalai Tesque) or BM Chemiluminescence Western Blotting Substrate (POD) (Roche). The band intensity was quantified with Image Lab (Bio-Rad Laboratories).

Immunostaining and Morphometric Analysis of Human Subjects

Several consecutive 4-μm-thick sections were obtained from FFPE specimens. The proportion of β-cell area relative to total pancreatic parenchymal area (β-cell volume density [$V_β$]) was determined by insulin immunostaining (Abcam) with the point-counting method on at least 2,000 islets in each subject captured with Axio Imager A1 (Carl Zeiss) as previously described (18,19). For phospho-ERK immunofluorescence, 7-μm-thick frozen sections were incubated with primary antibodies for insulin (Abcam) and phospho-ERK (Santa Cruz Biotechnology), followed by incubation with Alexa Fluor 594– and Alexa

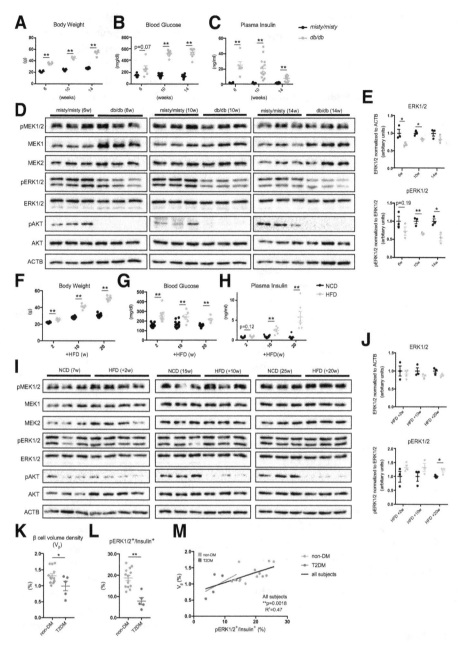

Figure 1—ERK phosphorylation was attenuated in the islets of *db/db* mice but was maintained in those of DIO mice. *A–C*: Profiles of *db/db* and *misty/misty* mice at 6, 10, and 14 weeks (w) of age: body weight (*A*), blood glucose levels (*B*), and plasma insulin concentrations (*C*). **$P < 0.01$, $n = 6$–15. All data are represented as mean ± SEM. *D*: Immunoblots of proteins of interest in the islets of 6-, 10-, and 14-week-old *db/db* mice and *misty/misty* mice. *E*: Levels of ERK and pERK as quantified in the immunoblots. *$P < 0.05$, **$P < 0.01$, $n = 3$. All data are represented as mean ± SEM. *F–H*: Profiles of DIO mice fed HFD for 2, 10, and 20 weeks and the age-matched control mice on NCD; body weight (*F*), blood glucose levels (*G*), and plasma insulin concentrations (*H*). **$P < 0.01$, $n = 6$–13. All data are represented as mean ± SEM. *I*: Immunoblots of proteins of interest in the islets of DIO mice fed HFD for 2, 10, and 20 weeks and age-matched control mice fed NCD. *J*: Levels of ERK and phospho-ERK as quantified in the immunoblots. *$P < 0.05$, $n = 3$–4. All data are represented as mean ± SEM. *K*: V_β in the subjects with (T2DM) or without (non-DM) type 2 diabetes. *$P < 0.05$, $n = 5$–13. All data are represented as mean ± SEM. *L*: Quantified proportions of phospho-ERK1/2$^+$ cells in insulin$^+$ cells in the subjects with or without type 2 diabetes. **$P < 0.01$, $n = 5$–13. All data are represented as mean ± SEM. *M*: Relation between the proportion of phospho-ERK1/2$^+$ cells in insulin$^+$ cells and the V_β in the subjects with or without type 2 diabetes. Note that the regression line for those without diabetes and that for all subjects were almost indistinguishable. $y = 0.03126x + 0.7314$, **$P = 0.0018$, $R^2 = 0.47$ for all subjects; $y = 0.02959x + 0.7572$, $P = 0.052$, $R^2 = 0.30$ for subjects without diabetes; and $y = 0.05306x + 0.5734$, $P = 0.29$, $R^2 = 0.36$ for subjects with type 2 diabetes. $n = 5$, type 2 diabetes; $n = 13$, no diabetes. See also Supplementary Fig. 1 and Supplementary Table 1. p, phosphorylated.

Fluor 488–conjugated secondary antibodies (Invitrogen). Immunofluorescence images were captured at ×40 magnification with the BZ-X700 (KEYENCE). All morphometric analyses were performed in a blinded manner.

Immunostaining and Morphometric Analysis of Mouse Samples

The adult mice were perfused with PBS and 4% paraformaldehyde (PFA) under anesthesia. Resected mouse pancreases were further fixed in 4% PFA overnight and embedded in paraffin. Embryonic pancreases from mouse embryos (embryonic day 14.5) were fixed in 4% PFA and embedded in paraffin. Paraffin sections (3 μm) were deparaffined and autoclaved in 0.01 mol/L citrate buffer (pH 6.0) for antigen retrieval. For MEK1, NGN3, and SOX9 staining, sections were additionally incubated in 0.1% Triton X-100 for permeabilization after antigen retrieval. Sections were stained with antibodies listed in Table 1 and subsequently incubated with Alexa Fluor 594– and Alexa Fluor 488–conjugated secondary antibodies (Invitrogen), except for the MEK1 staining, where EnVision+ System- HRP Labeled Polymer Anti-rabbit (Dako) was used as a secondary antibody and DAB Peroxidase Substrate Kit ImmPACT (Vector Labs) was used for visualization. Counterstain was conducted with hematoxylin-eosin. The TUNEL staining was performed with an In Situ Cell Death Detection Kit (Roche). Images were obtained with the BZ-X700 (KEYENCE) and analyzed with Analysis Application Hybrid Cell Count (KEYENCE).

RNA Sequence Analysis

Total RNA was isolated from isolated islets with TRIZOL reagent (Invitrogen). Sample preparation and RNA sequencing were performed as previously described (20). FASTQ files were imported to CLC Genomics Workbench (CLC-GW) (version 10.1.1; QIAGEN). Reads were mapped to the mouse reference genome (mm10) and quantified for the annotated 49,585-gene set provided by CLC-GW.

Quantitative RT-PCR Analysis

Total RNA was extracted by RNeasy Mini Kit (QIAGEN), followed by reverse transcription with a high-capacity cDNA reverse transcription kit (Applied Biosystems [ABI]). Quantitative RT-PCR was performed by ABI StepOnePlus with use of KAPA PROBE FAST qPCR Master Mix (2X) ABI Prism (Kapa Biosystems). Gene expression levels were normalized to the expression of cyclophilin A *(CypA)* in each sample. The primer sequences for *CypA* are as follows: F, GGTCCTGGCATCTTGTCCAT, and R, CAGTCTTGGCAGTGCAGATAAAA. Other primers and probes, purchased from ABI and Integrated DNA Technologies, are listed in Table 1.

Two-Photon Excitation Imaging

Two-photon imaging of the islets was performed with an inverted laser-scanning microscope (IX81; Olympus) with 60X oil immersion objective lens (1.2 numerical aperture)

at the wavelength of 830 nm as previously described (21). Glucose-stimulated exocytotic events of insulin granules were detected with extracellular polar tracer, sulforhodamine B (Thermo Fisher Scientific), counted in a region of interest (typically 3,200–4,500 μm^2) and normalized to an area of 800 μm^2. The acetoxymethyl esters of the Ca^{2+} indicators, Fura-2 (Thermo Fisher Scientific), as well as those of the caged-Ca^{2+} compound NP-EGTA (Thermo Fisher Scientific) were loaded to the islets as previously described (22). The intensity of Fura-2 poststimulation fluorescence (*F*) was analyzed in the cytoplasm and normalized by the resting fluorescence (F_0). Photolysis of NP-EGTA was induced with a brief flash (1.0 s) of a mercury lamp (model IX-RFC; Olympus).

Phosphoproteomics Analysis for Isolated Islets and MINcl4 Cells

Isolated islets were placed in recovery media for 2 h in humidified 5% CO_2 at 37°C (16). The islets were lysed by sonication in buffer A. Islets (500–1,000) were pooled to make one sample. MINcl4 cells were maintained in Krebs-Ringer bicarbonate buffer (KRBB) (15) with 0.2% BSA supplemented with 2.8 mmol/L glucose for 2 h at 37°C. Thirty minutes before glucose stimulation, U0126 (10 μmol/L) or vehicle (0.1% DMSO) was added to the buffer. The cells were then stimulated for 5 min by 2.8 mmol/L or 22.2 mmol/L glucose with U0126 (10 μmol/L) or vehicle (0.1% DMSO). After glucose stimulation, MINcl4 cells were lysed in buffer A. Lysates of islets or MINcl4 cells were boiled, sonicated, and subjected to reduction, alkylation, and digestion with trypsin and Lys-C (23). Phosphopeptides were enriched by a Fe-IMAC/C18 StageTip and labeled by TMT 10plex reagent. Labeled phosphopeptides were fractionated into seven fractions (24). The phosphoproteomics analysis was conducted with Q Exactive Plus (Thermo Fisher Scientific). Phosphopeptide identification was carried out with MaxQuant. The settings of liquid chromatography–tandem mass spectrometry and database search were performed according to the methodology of a previous phosphoproteomics study (23).

Statistical Analyses

Statistical significance was determined by an unpaired two-tailed Student *t* test, one-way ANOVA with the Tukey multiple comparisons test, and two-way ANOVA with the Sidak multiple comparisons test and with the Tukey multiple comparisons test, with use of GraphPad Prism, version 7 (GraphPad).

Data and Resource Availability

RNA-sequencing data generated and analyzed during the current study are available in DDBJ repository with accession code E-GEAD-385. Phosphoproteomics data generated and analyzed during the current study are available in jPOSTrepo and can be accessed with accession code JPST001021. No applicable resources were generated or analyzed during the current study.

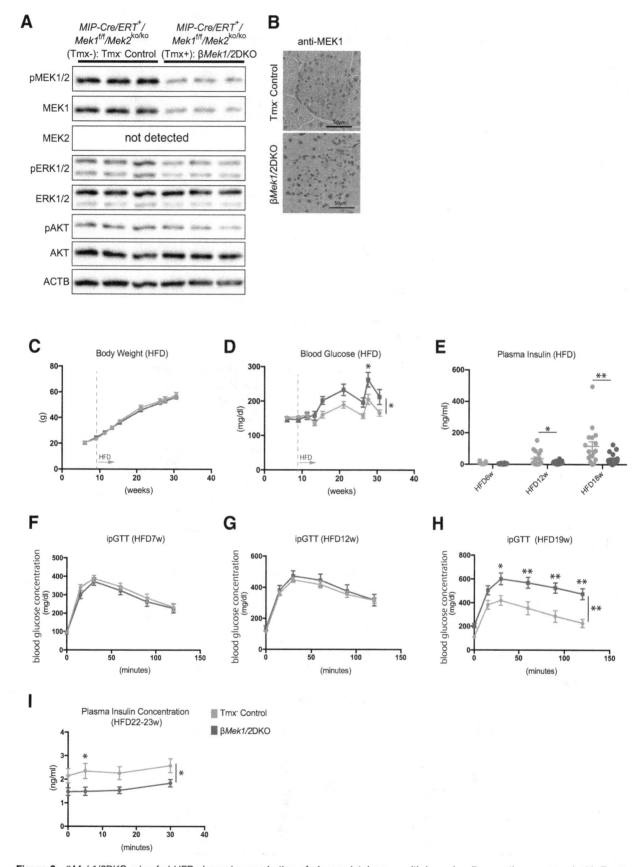

Figure 2—β*Mek1/2*DKO mice fed HFD showed exacerbation of glucose intolerance with lower insulin secretion compared with Tmx⁻ control mice. *A*: Immunoblots of proteins of interest in the islets of 14-week-old *MIP-Cre/ERT⁺/Mek1^{f/f}/Mek2^{ko/ko}* mice with or without

RESULTS

MEK/ERK Phosphorylation Was Reduced in the Islets of *db/db* Mice but Remained Unchanged Under HFD Conditions

We first investigated the two different obese animal models, namely, *db/db* mice (25) and DIO mice (26). The *db/db* mice showed marked hyperinsulinemia at 6 weeks of age compared with the lean *misty/misty* control mice, and thereafter their circulating insulin levels declined and hyperglycemia developed (27) (Fig. 1A–C), while the plasma insulin levels continuously increased in the DIO mice, with their hyperglycemia being only mild for up to 20 weeks of HFD feeding (Fig. 1F–H). Interestingly, unlike the levels of Akt phosphorylation, which were significantly lower in the islets of both of the obese models compared with their controls (15) (Fig. 1D and I and Supplementary Fig. 1A and B), the levels of MEK1/2 and ERK1/2 phosphorylation were significantly lower in the *db/db* mouse islets (Fig. 1D and E and Supplementary Fig. 1A), while those in the DIO mouse islets were maintained or even higher compared with their controls (Fig. 1I and J and Supplementary Fig. 1B). These results prompted us to hypothesize that maintained MEK/ERK signaling would be necessary for the compensatory β-cell adaptation in insulin resistance.

On the other hand, a cohort of patients with nonobese type 2 diabetes (Supplementary Table 1), showing a smaller proportion of β-cell area relative to the total pancreatic parenchymal area (V_β) (19) (Fig. 1K), exhibited a significantly lower proportion of phospho-ERK1/2$^+$ cells in insulin$^+$ cells compared with the subjects without diabetes (Fig. 1L and Supplementary Fig. 1C), with a strong correlation observed between V_β and the proportion of phospho-ERK1/2$^+$ cells in insulin$^+$ cells (Fig. 1M). These data suggested a possibility that MEK/ERK signaling could be involved in the regulation of β-cell mass under nondiabetic conditions and also in the pathogenesis of a certain type of diabetes in humans.

β*Mek1/2*DKO Mice Exhibited Glucose Intolerance With Lower Insulin Secretion Under HFD Conditions

To assess the role of MEK/ERK signaling in vivo, we created a mouse model with defective pancreatic β-cell MEK/ERK signaling by targeting MEK1 and MEK2, the upstream kinases responsible for ERK1 and ERK2

phosphorylation (28). While the mice with β-cell–specific *Mek1* deletion or those with systemic *Mek2* deletion did not exhibit complete abrogation of ERK1/2 phosphorylation in the islets (Supplementary Fig. 2A and B), consistent with the functional redundancy of MEK1 and MEK2 as previously reported (5), β*Mek1/2*DKO mice showed robust reductions in the levels of MEK1 protein expression as well as those of MEK1/2 and ERK1/2 phosphorylation in the islets compared with the Tmx$^-$ control mice (Fig. 2A and B and Supplementary Fig. 2C). The levels of MEK1 protein expression remained unchanged in the liver, muscle, epididymal white adipose tissue, and hypothalamus (Supplementary Fig. 2D).

To clarify the significance of MEK/ERK signaling in β-cells in diet-induced obesity, we fed β*Mek1/2*DKO mice with HFD and investigated their metabolic phenotypes. While the body weight gain was similar between the DIO β*Mek1/2*DKO mice and the Tmx$^-$ control DIO mice, the DIO β*Mek1/2*DKO mice showed higher blood glucose levels with ad libitum status (Fig. 2C and D) with significantly lower plasma insulin levels (Fig. 2E) than the Tmx$^-$ controls at 12 weeks or 18 weeks of HFD feeding. The DIO β*Mek1/2*DKO mice showed higher plasma glucose levels during a GTT than the Tmx$^-$ controls, as they developed obesity after 19 weeks of HFD feeding (Fig. 2F–H). The DIO β*Mek1/2*DKO mice also showed a moderate but significant decrease in plasma insulin levels on a glucose challenge than the Tmx$^-$ controls at 22–23 weeks of HFD feeding (Fig. 2I), while there was no difference between the groups in their blood glucose levels during insulin tolerance tests (Supplementary Fig. 2E–G). We found no metabolic differences among *Mek2*$^{ko/ko}$, *Mek2*$^{wt/ko}$, and *Mek2*$^{wt/wt}$ (Supplementary Fig. 3A–I) or between the *Mek1*$^{f/f}$/*Mek2*$^{ko/ko}$ mice injected with Tmx and those injected with vehicle (corn oil) (Supplementary Fig. 4A–I) under HFD conditions. Taken together, these data indicated that *Mek1/2* deletion in β-cells exacerbated glucose intolerance with lower insulin secretion under HFD feeding conditions.

β*Mek1/2*DKO Mice Had Smaller β-Cell Mass Than Tmx$^-$ Controls

Next, we histologically assessed the islets of DIO β*Mek1/2*DKO mice. In parallel with the results of GTTs, we observed a significantly smaller proportion of insulin$^+$ islet

Tmx injection (β*Mek1/2*DKO and Tmx$^-$ control mice). B: Immunohistochemistry staining with an MEK1-specific antibody of the pancreatic sections from 15-week-old β*Mek1/2*DKO and Tmx$^-$ control mice. Scale bar, 50 μm. C and D: Profiles of β*Mek1/2*DKO and Tmx$^-$ control mice fed HFD; body weight (C) blood glucose levels (D). *P < 0.05, n = 10. All data are represented as mean ± SEM. E: Plasma insulin concentrations in β*Mek1/2*DKO and Tmx$^-$ control mice fed HFD. *P < 0.05, **P < 0.01, n = 17–18. All data are represented as mean ± SEM. F–H: Blood glucose levels after intraperitoneal injection of glucose (1.0 g/kg body wt) in β*Mek1/2*DKO and Tmx$^-$ control mice fed HFD for 7 weeks (F), 12 weeks (G), and 19 weeks (H). **P < 0.01, n = 7–10. All data are represented as mean ± SEM. I: Plasma insulin concentrations after intraperitoneal injection of glucose (3.0 g/kg body wt) in β*Mek1/2*DKO and Tmx$^-$ control mice fed HFD for 22–23 weeks. *P < 0.05, n = 22–25. All data are represented as mean ± SEM. See also Supplementary Figs. 2–4. p, phosphorylated.

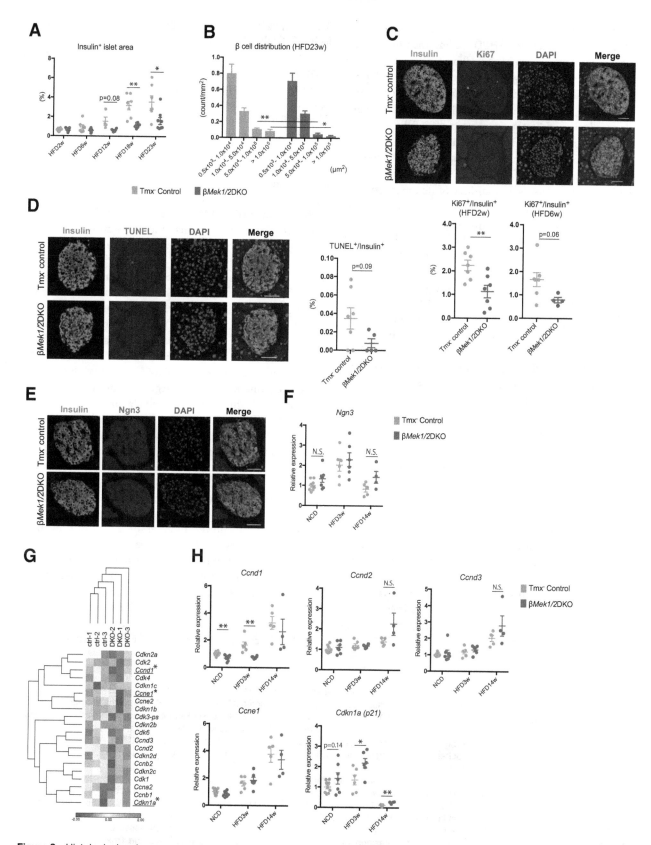

Figure 3—Histological and gene expression analyses of islets from β*Mek1/2*DKO mice fed HFD. *A*: Proportion of insulin⁺ islet area in the whole pancreas as assessed using anti-insulin antibody- and DAPI-stained pancreas sections from β*Mek1/2*DKO and Tmx⁻ control mice fed HFD for the indicated period of weeks (w). Four whole pancreatic sections per animal (400 μm apart) were analyzed. *P < 0.05, **P < 0.01, n = 4–8. All data are represented as mean ± SEM. *B*: The number of islets with a cross-sectional area of interest in the pancreas

area in the total pancreatic area in the βMek1/2DKO mice at 18 and 23 weeks of HFD feeding than in the DIO Tmx⁻ control mice (Fig. 3A), which was accounted for by the lower number of large islets their size >5 × 10⁴ μm² when normalized to the total pancreatic area (Fig. 3B). Furthermore, the proportion of Ki67⁺ cells in insulin⁺ cells was lower, while the proportion of TUNEL⁺ cells in insulin⁺ cells also tended to be lower, in the islets of DIO βMek1/2DKO mice than in those of DIO Tmx⁻ control animals (Fig. 3C and D). We found neither Ngn3⁺ cells (Ngn3ʰⁱ) in the islets as an indicator of de-differentiation of β-cells (29) in DIO βMek1/2DKO mice at 18 weeks of HFD feeding nor significant difference in Ngn3 mRNA expression levels between the DIO βMek1/2DKO and DIO Tmx⁻ control mouse islets (Fig. 3E and F and Supplementary Fig. 5A). The islets of DIO βMek1/2DKO mice showed a significantly higher ratio of glucagon (Gcg)⁺ area to insulin⁺ area and tended to show higher levels of Gcg and Aristaless-related homeobox (Arx) mRNA expression than those of Tmx⁻ control islets (Supplementary Fig. 5B and C). However, the extent of increase in these α-cell markers was reciprocal to the extent of reduction in the insulin⁺ islet area, suggesting that transdifferentiation of β-cells into α-cells was unlikely to account for the mechanism of lower insulin⁺ islet area observed in the DIO βMek1/2DKO mouse islets. Thus, these data indicated that the lower insulin secretion in the DIO βMek1/2DKO mice was associated with smaller β-cell mass accompanied by decreased β-cell proliferation compared with that in the Tmx⁻ control mice. Consistently with the decreased β-cell proliferation in the DIO βMek1/2DKO mice, RNA-sequencing and real-time PCR analyses revealed that the expression of cyclin D1 (Ccnd1) was lower, and that of cyclin-dependent kinase inhibitor 1a (Cdkn1a, p21) higher, in DIO βMek1/2DKO islets than in those of Tmx⁻ controls after as early as 3 weeks of HFD feeding (Fig. 3G and H). These data suggested that Mek1/2 abrogation in β-cells led to dysregulated expressions of cell cycle regulatory genes.

The Regulation of Insulin Exocytosis Was Impaired in the β-Cells of DIO βMek1/2DKO Mice

The levels of insulin secretion are determined by both the total amount of pancreatic β-cells and the insulin-secretion capacity of individual pancreatic β-cells (1,2). To assess the insulin-secretion capacity of β-cells in DIO βMek1/2DKO mice, we conducted two-photon excitation imaging analyses of the islets, which allowed for assessment of insulin granule exocytotic events and Ca²⁺ influx on a single-cell basis (21,30). There was a trend toward lower number of exocytotic events associated with high-glucose stimulation in the DIO βMek1/2DKO mouse islets within 10 min (Fig. 4A), suggesting that the β-cells of the DIO βMek1/2DKO mice may have impairment in their glucose-stimulated insulin secretion (GSIS) response. The insulin content normalized by the number of islets or islet DNA contents were comparable between the DIO βMek1/2DKO islets and Tmx⁻ control islets (Supplementary Fig. 6A–C). The assessments of individual β-cells for Ca²⁺ influx revealed that the levels of Ca²⁺ influx on glucose stimulation were comparable between the β-cells of DIO βMek1/2DKO mice and those of Tmx⁻ controls (Fig. 4B), while the same extent of a large and rapid increase in Ca²⁺ influx induced by photolysis of a caged-Ca²⁺ compound (Fig. 4C) (22) led to a markedly lower number of exocytotic events in the βMek1/2DKO mouse islets in comparison with Tmx⁻ controls (Fig. 4D).

βMek1/2DKO Mice Fed NCD Showed Impaired Insulin Secretion

Interestingly, the lower number of exocytotic events was clearly observed after glucose stimulation in the β-cells of lean βMek1/2DKO mice fed NCD (Fig. 5A). The insulin contents normalized by the number of islets or islet DNA contents were comparable between the DIO βMek1/2DKO islets and Tmx⁻ control islets (Supplementary Fig. 6D–F). Also, the βMek1/2DKO and Tmx⁻ control mouse islets were comparable in

sections from βMek1/2DKO and Tmx⁻ control mice fed HFD for 23 weeks (HFD23w). *P < 0.05, **P < 0.01, n = 7–8. All data are represented as mean ± SEM. C: Immunohistochemistry (IHC) staining with an insulin-specific antibody (red), a Ki67-specific antibody (green), and DAPI (blue) of pancreatic sections from βMek1/2DKO and Tmx⁻ control mice fed HFD for 6 weeks (upper) and quantified proportions of Ki67⁺ cells in insulin⁺ cells for βMek1/2DKO and Tmx⁻ control mice fed HFD for 2 weeks and 6 weeks; **P = 0.01, n = 4–7 (lower). The number of Ki67⁺insulin⁺ cells was manually counted in at least 800 insulin⁺ β-cells per animal. Scale bar, 50 μm. All data are represented as mean ± SEM. D: Immunohistochemistry staining with an insulin-specific antibody (red), TUNEL staining (green), and DAPI (blue) of pancreatic sections from βMek1/2DKO and Tmx⁻ control mice fed HFD for 6 weeks (left) and quantified proportions of TUNEL⁺ cells in insulin⁺ cells; n = 5–7 (right). The number of TUNEL⁺insulin⁺ cells was manually counted in at least 1,400 insulin⁺ β-cells per animal. Scale bar, 50 μm. All data are represented as mean ± SEM. E: Immunohistochemistry staining with an insulin-specific antibody (red), an Ngn3-specific antibody (green), and DAPI (blue) of pancreatic sections from βMek1/2DKO and Tmx⁻ control fed HFD for 18 weeks. Scale bar, 50 μm. F: Levels of Ngn3 expression in the islets from βMek1/2DKO and Tmx⁻ control mice fed NCD or HFD for indicated periods. n = 4–9. All data are represented as mean ± SEM. G: Expression profiles of cell cycle–related genes as assessed by RNA-sequencing analyses (z scores). Genes with significantly altered expression values (P value <0.05) between βMek1/2DKO and Tmx⁻ control islets are indicated with an asterisk and underbar. H: Levels of expression of genes of interest in the islets from βMek1/2DKO and Tmx⁻ control mice fed NCD or HFD for indicated periods. *P = 0.05, **P = 0.01, n = 4–9. All data are represented as mean ± SEM. See also Supplementary Fig. 5.

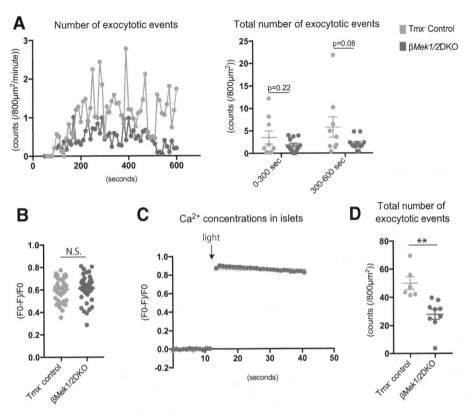

Figure 4—The number of glucose-stimulated exocytotic events was lower in the β-cells from βMek1/2DKO mice fed HFD compared with Tmx⁻ controls. A: Average number of glucose-stimulated exocytotic events in the islets from βMek1/2DKO and Tmx⁻ control mice fed HFD for 24 weeks, as normalized to an arbitrary area (800 μm²) of islets (left), and the total number of exocytotic events occurring within 0–5 min and 5–10 min of glucose stimulation (right). n = 9 islets from one Tmx⁻ control mouse and 12 islets from two βMek1/2DKO mice. All data are represented as mean ± SEM. B: Glucose-stimulated Ca^{2+} influx as measured on a single–β-cell basis by the Ca^{2+} indicator Fura-2. Maximum rates of change in $(F_0 - F)/F_0$ are shown. Fura-2 F values were normalized by their respective F_0 values. n = 44 regions of interest for four islets from two Tmx⁻ control mice and 40 regions of interest for four islets from two βMek1/2DKO mice. All data are represented as mean ± SEM. C: Alteration of cytosolic Ca^{2+} concentrations provoked by photolysis of a caged-Ca^{2+} compound in the islets of βMek1/2DKO and Tmx⁻ control mice fed HFD for 24 weeks. The average of six ROI from one Tmx⁻ control islet and the average of seven ROI from one βMek1/2DKO islet are shown. D: Total number of exocytotic events occurring in the islets on caged Ca^{2+} stimulation, as normalized to an arbitrary area (800 μm²) of islets. *$P < 0.01$, n = 6 islets from two Tmx⁻ control mice and 9 islets from two βMek1/2DKO mice. All data are represented as mean ± SEM. See also Supplementary Fig. 6.

their ATP production on high-glucose stimulation (Fig. 5B). The glucose-stimulated Ca^{2+} influx was slightly lower in the β-cells of βMek1/2DKO mice than that in Tmx⁻ control mice (Fig. 5C), while the provoked Ca^{2+} influx again led to markedly fewer events of exocytosis in βMek1/2DKO mouse islets than in those of Tmx⁻ controls (Fig. 5D and E). The NCD-fed βMek1/2DKO mice also showed a moderate but significant decrease in plasma insulin levels on a glucose challenge at 12 weeks of age than the Tmx⁻ control mice, while otherwise no metabolic differences were observed between the groups (Fig. 5F–K and Supplementary Fig. 7A). Plasma human insulin levels after human insulin injection were comparable between the groups, suggesting that insulin clearance was not affected in βMek1/2DKO mice (Supplementary Fig. 7B). Immunohistochemistry analyses showed that the islet areas were comparable between βMek1/2DKO mice and Tmx⁻ controls at a younger

age and were different only at 23 weeks of age, with a lower distribution of larger islets seen in βMek1/2DKO mice than in Tmx⁻ controls (Supplementary Fig. 7C and D). We again ruled out the possible impact of Mek2 deletion alone or Tmx injection per se on the difference in plasma insulin levels on a glucose challenge (Supplementary Fig. 7E–O). Collectively these data suggested that MEK/ERK signaling could play significant roles in the regulation of insulin exocytosis in pancreatic β-cells.

Phosphoproteomic Analyses Revealed Altered Phosphorylated Protein Levels in βMek1/2DKO Mouse Islets Compared With Those of Tmx⁻ Control Mice

We next explored the molecular mechanism(s) whereby Mek1/2 abrogation led to a lower number of exocytotic events in β-cells. First, in order to assess the downstream targets of MEK/ERK signaling in β-cells, we compared phosphoproteome of βMek1/2DKO mouse islets versus

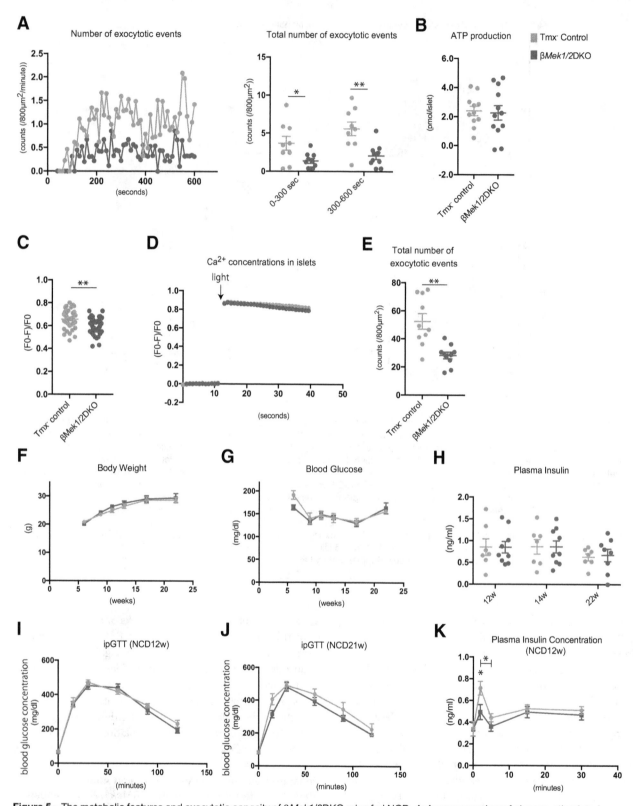

Figure 5—The metabolic features and exocytotic capacity of β*Mek1/2*DKO mice fed NCD. *A*: Average number of glucose-stimulated exocytotic events of islets of 15-week-old β*Mek1/2*DKO and Tmx⁻ control mice fed NCD, as normalized to an arbitrary area (800 μm²) of islets (left), and total number of exocytotic events occurring within 0–5 min and 5–10 min of glucose stimulation (right). *P < 0.05, **P < 0.01, *n* = 9 islets from two Tmx⁻ control mice and 10 islets from two β*Mek1/2*DKO mice. All data are represented as mean ± SEM. *B*: ATP production per isolated islet of β*Mek1/2*DKO and Tmx⁻ control mice on NCD after incubation with 22.2 mmol/L glucose. A total of 40 islets of equivalent size per mouse were divided into two groups and maintained in KRBB with 0.2% BSA supplemented with 2.8 mmol/L glucose for 30 min at 37°C. Subsequently, the islets were incubated for 30 minutes in KRBB with 0.2% BSA containing either 2.8 mmol/L glucose

those of Tmx⁻ control mice fed NCD (Fig. 6A). We identified 10,886 phosphosites in 3,718 proteins (Fig. 6B and C). In gene ontology (GO) analyses (31), the genes with the GO term "insulin secretion" were highly enriched in the 190 molecules harboring the 241 sites that were phosphorylated at significantly lower levels in βMek1/2DKO mouse islets than in the Tmx⁻ control mouse islets (P value <0.05, fold change < −1.5) (Fig. 6D), with the phosphorylation sites of exocytosis-regulating proteins SNAP25, PCLO, ITPR3, RAB37, SYTL4, and RIMS2 being significantly less phosphorylated (Fig. 6E). Gene expression analysis showed no differences between the groups in these molecules and those established to be involved in exocytosis of insulin granules such as STX1A, VAMP2, or a dock protein, RAB27A (32) (Supplementary Fig. 8A). In addition, the genes with GO terms related to cytoskeleton were highly enriched in the less phosphorylated proteins in βMek1/2DKO mouse islets compared with Tmx⁻ controls (Fig. 6D and Supplementary Fig. 8B), among which molecules, such as MARCKS, MAPT, and MAP2, have been reported to be involved in exocytosis of insulin or other secretory granules (33–35). Thus, these results suggested the possibility that the MEK/ERK pathway regulated insulin secretion through dynamic changes in phosphorylation status of exocytosis-regulating molecules including cytoskeleton–related molecules in pancreatic β-cells.

Acute Stimulation by Glucose Dynamically Changed Phosphorylation Status of Cytoskeleton–Related Proteins Through MEK/ERK Signaling in MINcl4 Cells

Finally, we attempted to elucidate the possible upstream signaling responsible for MEK/ERK activation in β-cells. According to previous reports, glucose stimulation of β-cells causes phosphorylation of ERK1/2 in minutes (10,36), as we confirmed in the MINcl4 β-cell line (Fig. 7A). Moreover, pretreatment of MINcl4 cells with MEK inhibitor U0126 led to a decrease in their GSIS response (Fig. 7B), as already reported (37). Collectively with the results from our in vivo models, these data prompted us to hypothesize that glucose stimulation activated MEK/ERK signaling, which in turn caused phosphorylation of GSIS-related molecules and thereby impinged on GSIS response. To test the hypothesis, we compared phosphoproteomic profiles of MINcl4 cells cultured in low concentration of glucose (LG) with those stimulated with 22.2 mmol/L glucose for 5 min in absence or presence of U0126 (HG or HGi) (Fig. 7C). We identified 12,168 phosphosites in 3,589 proteins in total (Fig. 7D). GO analyses of the 282 molecules harboring the 373 sites that were phosphorylated at significantly higher levels in HG condition than in LG condition (P value <0.05, fold change >1.5) demonstrated that the MAPK signaling pathway was a main signaling pathway regulated by acute glucose stimulation (Fig. 7E and Supplementary Fig. 9A). A total of 155 phosphosites were phosphorylated at significantly higher levels in HG condition in comparison with both LG and HGi conditions (P value <0.05) (Fig. 7F). We considered them as the phosphosites regulated by glucose stimulation in a MEK/ERK signaling–dependent manner, which included ERK1^{T203}, ERK1^{Y205}, ERK2^{T183}, and ERK2^{Y185} residues (Fig. 7G). GO analyses of the 112 molecules harboring these 155 phosphosites showed high enrichment of GO terms related to cytoskeleton (Fig. 7F and Supplementary Fig. 9B). Between the phosphosites showing less phosphorylation in the βMek1/2DKO islets than in the Tmx⁻ control mouse islets (P value < 0.05) and those showing higher phosphorylation in HG condition in comparison with LG and HGi conditions in MINcl4 cell (P value < 0.05), we found in common 21 sites of 15 proteins (Fig. 7H and Supplementary Table 2). Collectively, these data suggested that glucose was a potential stimulant causing MEK/ERK-mediated phospholyrations in β-cells, which could regulate GSIS response.

DISCUSSION

To date, several genetic factors have been suggested to cause maladaptation of β-cells leading to insufficient insulin production in the pathogenesis of diabetes, while its exact molecular mechanisms remain unclear (2).

---

or 22.2 mmol/L glucose. ATP concentration was measured with use of ATPlite (PerkinElmer). Differences between the values of ATP content per islet incubated in 2.8 mmol/L glucose condition and those in 22.2 mmol/L glucose condition are defined as ATP production. **$P <$ 0.01, n = 11–12. All data are represented as means ± SEM. C: Glucose-stimulated Ca²⁺ influx as measured on a single–β-cell basis with the Ca²⁺ indicator Fura-2. Maximum rates of change in ($F_0 − F$)/F_0 are shown. Fura-2 F values were normalized by their respective F_0 values. n = 36 regions of interest for five islets from two Tmx⁻ control mice and 43 regions of interest for eight islets from two βMek1/2DKO mice. All data are represented as means ± SEM. D: Alteration of cytosolic Ca²⁺ concentrations provoked by photolysis of a caged-Ca²⁺ compound in the islets of 15-week-old βMek1/2DKO and Tmx⁻ control mice fed NCD. The average of six regions of interest from one Tmx⁻ control islet and the average of six regions of interest from one βMek1/2DKO islet are shown. E: Total number of exocytotic events occurring in the islets on caged Ca²⁺ stimulation, as normalized to an arbitrary area (800 μm²) of islets. **$P <$ 0.01, n = 10 islets from two Tmx⁻ control mice and 10 islets from two βMek1/2DKO mice. All data are represented as mean ± SEM. F and G: The profiles of βMek1/2DKO and Tmx⁻ control mice fed NCD; body weight (F) and blood glucose levels (G). n = 7–8. All data are represented as mean ± SEM. H: Plasma insulin concentrations at indicated weeks (w) of age in βMek1/2DKO and Tmx⁻ control mice fed NCD. n = 7–9. All data are represented as means ± SEM. I and J: Blood glucose levels after intraperitoneal injection of glucose (2.0 g/kg body wt) in βMek1/2DKO and Tmx⁻ control mice fed NCD. n = 7–9. All data are represented as mean ± SEM. K: Plasma insulin concentrations after intraperitoneal injection of glucose (3.0 g/kg body wt) in 12-week-old βMek1/2DKO and Tmx⁻ control mice fed NCD. *$P <$ 0.05, n = 12. All data are represented as mean ± SEM. See also Supplementary Figs. 6 and 7. ipGTT, intraperitoneal GTT.

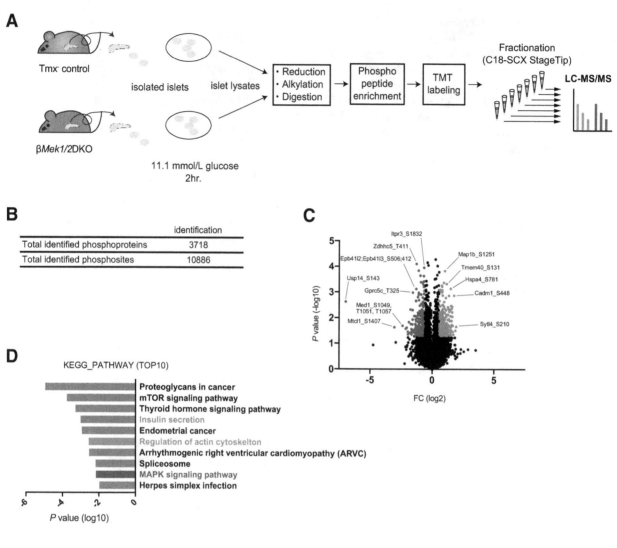

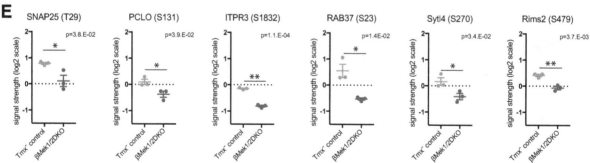

Figure 6—Phosphoproteomics analyses of pooled islets from β*Mek1/2*DKO and Tmx⁻ control mice. *A*: The workflow of phosphoproteomics with isolated islets. *B*: Summary of the phosphoproteomics data. *C*: Volcano plot displaying the distribution of significantly changed phosphosites between the β*Mek1/2*DKO and Tmx⁻ control islets. Phosphosites with significantly changed values between β*Mek1/2*DKO and Tmx⁻ control islets are highlighted in red (*P* value <0.05, fold change > 1.5) and blue (*P* value <0.05, fold change < −1.5). Several proteins with low *P* values and high absolute fold change values are shown with their gene names and changed phosphosites. *n* = 3. *D*: The results of GO analyses of the 190 molecules harboring the 241 sites that were phosphorylated at significantly lower levels in β*Mek1/2*DKO mouse islets than in the Tmx⁻ control mouse islets (*P* value <0.05, fold change < −1.5). Top 10 GO terms in the KEGG_-PATHWAY category are shown with raw *P* values. *E*: The signal strengths of phosphosites of interest, i.e., SNAP25, PCLO, ITPR3, RAB37, SYTL4, and RIMS2, in islets from β*Mek1/2*DKO and Tmx⁻ control mice fed NCD. **P* < 0.05, ***P* < 0.01, *n* = 3. All data are represented as mean ± SEM. See also Supplementary Fig. 8. LC-MS/MS, liquid chromatography–tandem mass spectrometry.

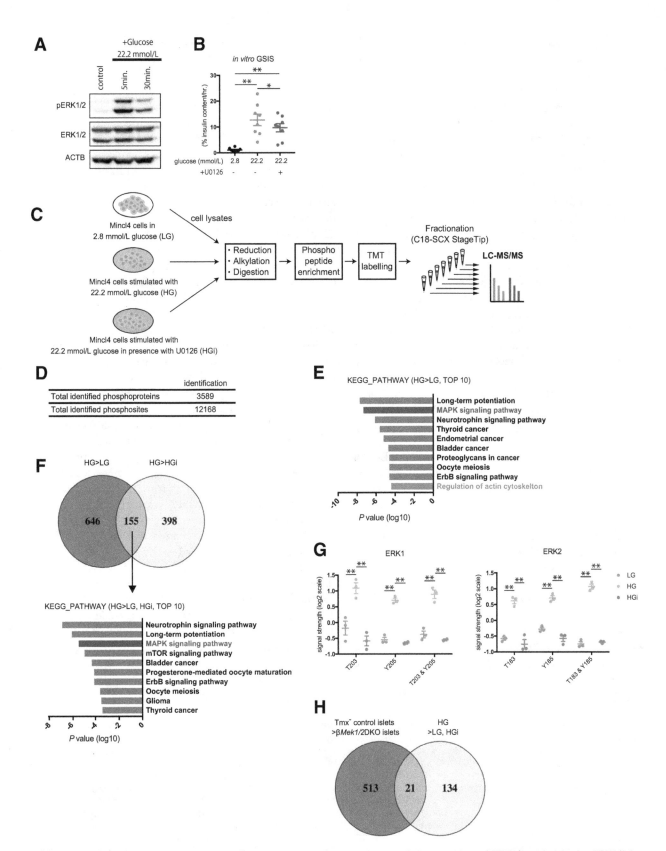

Figure 7—Phosphoproteomics analyses of MINcl4 cells stimulated with glucose. *A*: Immunoblots of ERK1/2 and phospho-ERK1/2 in MINcl4 cells. MINcl4 cells were maintained in KRBB with 0.2% BSA supplemented with 2.8 mmol/L glucose for 2 h at 37°C. Subsequently, the cells were incubated for indicated times in KRBB with 0.2% BSA containing either 2.8 mmol/L glucose or 22.2 mmol/L glucose. *B*: In vitro GSIS test performed with MINcl4 cells. MINcl4 cells were maintained in KRBB with 0.2% BSA supplemented with 2.8 mmol/L glucose for 2 h at 37°C. At 30 min before glucose stimulation, U0126 (10 μmol/L) or vehicle (0.1% DMSO) was added to the buffer. The cells

We began by investigating the islets of murine type 2 diabetic models and found reductions in the levels of ERK1/2 phosphorylation in the islets of *db/db* mice, which were associated with a progressive decline in their plasma insulin levels as they grew. In contrast, the levels of ERK1/2 phosphorylation were not reduced, or remained even higher, in the islets of DIO mice, where only mild hyperglycemia was observed with relatively maintained plasma insulin levels. Of note, the mechanism causing the observed differences in phosphorylation levels of ERK1/2 and MEK1/2 in the islets of different mouse models is unclear, while there could be composite mechanisms reflected in the differences in the levels of responsible humoral factors, potentially including insulin, or in the cellular sensitivity to these stimuli, leading to the altered activation status of the signaling cascade.

While we found that MEK/ERK signaling is necessary for adaptive hyperplasia of β-cells in obesity, it is reported that obesity in humans only leads to a mild increase in β-cell mass compared with mouse models (1). Interestingly, however, a cohort of nonobese patients with type 2 diabetes showed lower proportion of phospho-ERK1/2$^+$ cells in insulin$^+$ cells with lower V_β compared with subjects without diabetes. As β*Mek1/2*DKO mice on NCD showed significantly lower islet area at 23 weeks of age, it is plausible that MEK/ERK signaling is required not only for adaptive β-cell hyperplasia in obesity but also for maintenance of β-cell mass under lean conditions, where the defects of MEK/ERK signaling could lead to hyperglycemia due to insulin insufficiency. In support of the MEK/ERK involvements in human diabetes pathogenesis, several genome-wide association studies showed an association between type 2 diabetes and a single nucleotide polymorphism (SNP) (rs5945326) near dual-specificity phosphatase 9 (*DUSP9*), an ERK-selective cytoplasmic phosphatase, in different ancestries (38–40). Other SNPs, SNP rs1894299 on *DUSP9* and SNP rs9648716 on *BRAF*, a kinase upstream for MEK1/2, are also reported to be associated with type 2 diabetes (41,42).

To determine the functional significance of MEK/ERK signaling in β-cells, we created a murine model with *Mek1/2* abrogation and investigated its metabolic phenotypes. Our analyses collectively underscored the importance of MEK/ERK signaling–mediated cell proliferation in compensatory β-cell expansion under insulin-resistant conditions, which is plausible in light of the well-established roles that MEK/ERK signaling plays in cell proliferation (3). On the other hand, our data also indicate a significant role that MEK/ERK signaling plays in GSIS response, as revealed by the lower plasma insulin levels on a glucose challenge with comparable insulin sensitivity and the lower numbers of exocytotic events in two-photon excitation microscopy analyses in the islets of β*Mek1/*2DKO mice. Of note, our analyses indicated impairment in the regulation of exocytosis machinery downstream of the Ca^{2+} influx in the β-cells of β*Mek1/*2DKO mice. It has been suggested that reorganization of the actin cytoskeletal network is required for insulin granules to properly access cellular membrane in both the first and second phases of GSIS response (43,44). Our phosphoproteomics analyses of the isolated islets from β*Mek1/*2DKO mice showed that the levels of phosphorylation in the proteins related to exocytosis and cytoskeleton were altered on *Mek1/2* abrogation, suggesting that MEK/ERK signaling regulates these molecules by altering their phosphorylation levels and thus is involved in proper GSIS response. Additionally, as dramatic changes in cytoskeletal organization are also known to occur during mitotic processes (45), the MEK/ERK signaling–mediated cytoskeletal modifications could also be a part of mechanisms for cell proliferation regulated by MEK/ERK signaling.

We noticed that 21 sites with significantly higher phosphorylation levels in HG condition than in LG and HGi conditions were also identified in the less phosphorylated phosphosites in β*Mek1/2*DKO islets, whereas the overlap between the phosphosites identified in these two models was not large. These data could be interpreted to indicate that upstream inputs other than glucose could have been involved in the regulation of altered phosphosites detected in the islets, including those derived from the non–β-cell components producing humoral factors in a paracrine manner. Further analyses are needed to fully

---

were then incubated for 1 h in KRBB with 0.2% BSA containing 2.8 mmol/L glucose or 22.2 mmol/L glucose and U0126 (10 μmol/L) or vehicle (0.1% DMSO). The media were collected after 1 h incubation with glucose. For the insulin content measurement, the insulin was extracted from the islets by overnight incubation with acid ethanol at −20°C. *$P < 0.05$, **$P < 0.01$, $n = 8$. All data are represented as mean ± SEM. *C*: The workflow of phosphoproteomics with MIN6l4 cells. *D*: Summary of the phosphoproteomics data. *E*: The results of GO analyses of the 282 molecules harboring the 373 sites that were phosphorylated at significantly higher levels in HG condition than in LG condition (P value <0.05, fold change > 1.5). Top 10 GO terms in the KEGG_PATHWAY category are shown with raw P values. *F*: The overlap between the phosphosites with significantly higher phosphorylation levels in HG condition than in LG condition (P value <0.05) and the phosphosites with significantly higher phosphorylation levels in HG condition than in HGi condition (P value <0.05) (upper) and the results of GO analyses of the 112 molecules harboring the 155 phosphosites with significantly higher phosphorylation levels in HG condition than in both LG and HGi conditions (P value <0.05). Top 10 GO terms in the KEGG_PATHWAY category were shown with raw P values (lower). *G*: The signal strength of ERK1^{T203}, ERK1^{Y205}, ERK1$^{T203, Y205}$, ERK2^{T183}, ERK2^{Y185}, and ERK2$^{T183, Y185}$. **$P < 0.01$, $n = 3$. All data are represented as means ± SEM. *H*: The overlap between the 534 phosphosites that were phosphorylated at significantly lower levels in β*Mek1/2*DKO mouse islets than in the Tmx$^-$ control mouse islets (P value <0.05) and the 155 phosphosites with significantly higher phosphorylation levels in HG condition compared with both LG and HGi conditions (P value <0.05). See also Supplementary Fig. 9 and Supplementary Table 2. hr., hour; LC-MS/MS, liquid chromatography–tandem mass spectrometry; p, phosphorylated.

elucidate the roles that MEK/ERK signaling plays in exocytosis regulation, which will include determining the upstream stimulants as well as the exact substrates of MEK/ERK signaling in β-cells during GSIS response and the significance of such posttranscriptional modifications for the functions of the exocytosis machineries.

Of note, while our experimental design properly controlled the effects of hGH expression from the *MIP-Cre/ERT* construct (12,13), we could not strictly rule out the possibility that the transient nuclear translocation of Cre/ERT protein could have modified the phenotypes of β*Mek1/2*DKO mice, which is one of the limitations in our study.

Finally, from a therapeutic perspective, our results suggest that activation of the MEK/ERK pathway in pancreatic β-cells may have therapeutic potential for diabetes, in that it is expected to increase β-cell mass and enhance GSIS response at the same time. However, it has been reported that pharmacological inhibition, rather than activation, of MEKs improves glucose homeostasis in diabetic mouse models through control of peroxisome proliferator–activated receptor γ (PPARγ) in adipose tissues, thereby ameliorating insulin resistance (46). Besides, the RAS/RAF/MEK/ERK signaling is one of the major pathways known to be activated through mutations in cancer (47,48). Thus, simply activating MEK/ERK signaling in a systemic manner may have deleterious consequences. Instead, identifying and targeting the responsible mechanisms whereby ERK becomes less phosphorylated in the islets under diabetic conditions may represent a more promising strategy for the development of antidiabetes therapeutics.

Taken together, our data provide evidence that MEK/ERK signaling has bifunctional roles in β-cells in maintaining glucose homeostasis, suggesting that defects in MEK/ERK signaling could contribute to β-cell maladaptation in the pathogenesis of diabetes. Further research targeting the MEK/ERK pathway is required to formulate optimal therapeutic strategies for diabetes.

Acknowledgments. The authors thank Dr. H. Ishihara (Nihon University School of Medicine) for providing MIN6 clone 4 cell lines. The authors also greatly appreciate the technical support of Dr. W. Nishimura (International University of Health and Welfare Graduate School) in delivering embryonic pancreases. The authors' thanks are also due to M. Nakano and T. Oyama for assistance in immunohistochemistry as well as F. Takahashi, Y. Masaki, and R. Honma for technical assistance.

Funding. This work was supported by Japan Society for the Promotion of Science KAKENHI grants JP16K19067 (to Y.M.I.) and JP19K16547 (to Y.M.I.) and National Center for Global Health and Medicine grants 29-1021 (to Y.M.I.) and 20A1011 (to Y.M.I.).

Duality of Interest. M.M. is supported by LSI Medience Corporation through the cross-appointment system of University of Tsukuba. No other potential conflicts of interest relevant to this article were reported.

Author Contributions. Y.M.I. organized and performed the experiments, wrote the manuscript, and secured funding. K.U. conceptualized, organized, and wrote the manuscript and secured funding. M.A. organized and wrote the manuscript. N.K., S.O., S.T., H.S., and K.S. performed the experiments. H.K. provided expertise and analyzed the study data. J.A. performed phosphoproteomics analyses. M.M. performed transcriptomic analyses. H.M. provided human data. Y.M. and N.T. performed two-photon excitation imaging analyses. J.C. provided mouse strains. All authors reviewed, edited, and approved the manuscript. K.U. is the guarantor of this work and, as such, had full access to all the data in the study and takes responsibility for the integrity of the data and the accuracy of the data analysis.

References

1. Weir GC, Bonner-Weir S. Islet β cell mass in diabetes and how it relates to function, birth, and death. Ann N Y Acad Sci 2013;1281:92–105
2. Kahn SE, Hull RL, Utzschneider KM. Mechanisms linking obesity to insulin resistance and type 2 diabetes. Nature 2006;444:840–846
3. Wortzel I, Seger R. The ERK cascade: distinct functions within various subcellular organelles. Genes Cancer 2011;2:195–209
4. Sidarala V, Kowluru A. The regulatory roles of mitogen-activated protein kinase (MAPK) pathways in health and diabetes: lessons learned from the pancreatic β-cell. Recent Pat Endocr Metab Immune Drug Discov 2017;10:76–84
5. Aoidi R, Maltais A, Charron J. Functional redundancy of the kinases MEK1 and MEK2: rescue of the Mek1 mutant phenotype by Mek2 knock-in reveals a protein threshold effect. Sci Signal 2016;9:ra9
6. Gehart H, Kumpf S, Ittner A, Ricci R. MAPK signalling in cellular metabolism: stress or wellness? EMBO Rep 2010;11:834–840
7. Ueki K, Okada T, Hu J, et al. Total insulin and IGF-I resistance in pancreatic beta cells causes overt diabetes. Nat Genet 2006;38:583–588
8. Lawrence M, Shao C, Duan L, McGlynn K, Cobb MH. The protein kinases ERK1/2 and their roles in pancreatic beta cells. Acta Physiol (Oxf) 2008;192:11–17
9. Chen H, Gu X, Liu Y, et al. PDGF signalling controls age-dependent proliferation in pancreatic β-cells. Nature 2011;478:349–355
10. Assmann A, Ueki K, Winnay JN, Kadowaki T, Kulkarni RN. Glucose effects on beta-cell growth and survival require activation of insulin receptors and insulin receptor substrate 2. Mol Cell Biol 2009;29:3219–3228
11. Burns CJ, Squires PE, Persaud SJ. Signaling through the p38 and p42/44 mitogen-activated families of protein kinases in pancreatic beta-cell proliferation. Biochem Biophys Res Commun 2000;268:541–546
12. Oropeza D, Jouvet N, Budry L, et al. Phenotypic characterization of MIP-CreERT1Lphi mice with transgene-driven islet expression of human growth hormone. Diabetes 2015;64:3798–3807
13. Brouwers B, de Faudeur G, Osipovich AB, et al. Impaired islet function in commonly used transgenic mouse lines due to human growth hormone minigene expression. Cell Metab 2014;20:979–990
14. Yamato E, Tashiro F, Miyazaki J. Microarray analysis of novel candidate genes responsible for glucose-stimulated insulin secretion in mouse pancreatic β cell line MIN6. PLoS One 2013;8:e61211
15. Kaneko K, Ueki K, Takahashi N, et al. Class IA phosphatidylinositol 3-kinase in pancreatic β cells controls insulin secretion by multiple mechanisms. Cell Metab 2010;12:619–632
16. Mitok KA, Freiberger EC, Schueler KL, et al. Islet proteomics reveals genetic variation in dopamine production resulting in altered insulin secretion. J Biol Chem 2018;293:5860–5877
17. Ueki K, Yamauchi T, Tamemoto H, et al. Restored insulin-sensitivity in IRS-1-deficient mice treated by adenovirus-mediated gene therapy. J Clin Invest 2000;105:1437–1445
18. Sakuraba H, Mizukami H, Yagihashi N, Wada R, Hanyu C, Yagihashi S. Reduced beta-cell mass and expression of oxidative stress-related DNA damage in the islet of Japanese type II diabetic patients. Diabetologia 2002;45:85–96
19. Mizukami H, Takahashi K, Inaba W, et al. Involvement of oxidative stress-induced DNA damage, endoplasmic reticulum stress, and autophagy deficits in the decline of β-cell mass in Japanese type 2 diabetic patients. Diabetes Care 2014;37:1966–1974
20. Morito N, Yoh K, Usui T, et al. Transcription factor MafB may play an important role in secondary hyperparathyroidism. Kidney Int 2018;93:54–68

21. Takahashi N, Kishimoto T, Nemoto T, Kadowaki T, Kasai H. Fusion pore dynamics and insulin granule exocytosis in the pancreatic islet. Science 2002;297:1349–1352

22. Takahashi N, Hatakeyama H, Okado H, et al. Sequential exocytosis of insulin granules is associated with redistribution of SNAP25. J Cell Biol 2004;165:255–262

23. Abe Y, Hirano H, Shoji H, et al. Comprehensive characterization of the phosphoproteome of gastric cancer from endoscopic biopsy specimens. Theranostics 2020;10:2115–2129

24. Adachi J, Hashiguchi K, Nagano M, et al. Improved proteome and phosphoproteome analysis on a cation exchanger by a combined acid and salt gradient. Anal Chem 2016;88:7899–7903

25. Lee GH, Proenca R, Montez JM, et al. Abnormal splicing of the leptin receptor in diabetic mice. Nature 1996;379:632–635

26. Hull RL, Kodama K, Utzschneider KM, Carr DB, Prigeon RL, Kahn SE. Dietary-fat-induced obesity in mice results in beta cell hyperplasia but not increased insulin release: evidence for specificity of impaired beta cell adaptation. Diabetologia 2005;48:1350–1358

27. Dalbøge LS, Almholt DL, Neerup TS, et al. Characterisation of age-dependent beta cell dynamics in the male db/db mice. PLoS One 2013;8:e82813

28. Boucherat O, Nadeau V, Bérubé-Simard FA, Charron J, Jeannotte L. Crucial requirement of ERK/MAPK signaling in respiratory tract development. Development 2014;141:3197–3211

29. Talchai C, Xuan S, Lin HV, Sussel L, Accili D. Pancreatic β cell dedifferentiation as a mechanism of diabetic β cell failure. Cell 2012;150:1223–1234

30. Takahashi N, Sawada W, Noguchi J, et al. Two-photon fluorescence lifetime imaging of primed SNARE complexes in presynaptic terminals and β cells. Nat Commun 2015;6:8531

31. Huang W, Sherman BT, Lempicki RA. Systematic and integrative analysis of large gene lists using DAVID bioinformatics resources. Nat Protoc 2009;4:44–57

32. Rorsman P, Ashcroft FM. Pancreatic β-cell electrical activity and insulin secretion: of mice and men. Physiol Rev 2018;98:117–214

33. Trexler AJ, Taraska JW. Regulation of insulin exocytosis by calcium-dependent protein kinase C in beta cells. Cell Calcium 2017;67:1–10

34. Maj M, Hoermann G, Rasul S, Base W, Wagner L, Attems J. The microtubule-associated protein tau and its relevance for pancreatic beta cells. J Diabetes Res 2016;2016:1964634

35. Anhê GF, Torrão AS, Nogueira TC, et al. ERK3 associates with MAP2 and is involved in glucose-induced insulin secretion. Mol Cell Endocrinol 2006;251:33–41

36. Khoo S, Cobb MH. Activation of mitogen-activating protein kinase by glucose is not required for insulin secretion. Proc Natl Acad Sci U S A 1997;94:5599–5604

37. Dioum EM, Osborne JK, Goetsch S, Russell J, Schneider JW, Cobb MH. A small molecule differentiation inducer increases insulin production by pancreatic β cells. Proc Natl Acad Sci U S A 2011;108:20713–20718

38. Li H, Gan W, Lu L, et al.; DIAGRAM Consortium; AGEN-T2D Consortium. A genome-wide association study identifies GRK5 and RASGRP1 as type 2 diabetes loci in Chinese Hans. Diabetes 2013;62:291–298

39. Hara K, Fujita H, Johnson TA, et al.; DIAGRAM Consortium. Genome-wide association study identifies three novel loci for type 2 diabetes. Hum Mol Genet 2014;23:239–246

40. Voight BF, Scott LJ, Steinthorsdottir V, et al.; MAGIC investigators; GIANT Consortium. Twelve type 2 diabetes susceptibility loci identified through large-scale association analysis. Nat Genet 2010;42:579–589

41. Suzuki K, Akiyama M, Ishigaki K, et al. Identification of 28 new susceptibility loci for type 2 diabetes in the Japanese population. Nat Genet 2019;51:379–386

42. Zhao W, Rasheed A, Tikkanen E, et al.; CHD Exome+ Consortium; EPIC-CVD Consortium; EPIC-Interact Consortium; Michigan Biobank. Identification of new susceptibility loci for type 2 diabetes and shared etiological pathways with coronary heart disease. Nat Genet 2017;49:1450–1457

43. Arous C, Halban PA. The skeleton in the closet: actin cytoskeletal remodeling in β-cell function. Am J Physiol Endocrinol Metab 2015;309:E611–E620

44. Hoboth P, Müller A, Ivanova A, et al. Aged insulin granules display reduced microtubule-dependent mobility and are disposed within actin-positive multigranular bodies. Proc Natl Acad Sci U S A 2015;112:E667–E676

45. Kunda P, Baum B. The actin cytoskeleton in spindle assembly and positioning. Trends Cell Biol 2009;19:174–179

46. Banks AS, McAllister FE, Camporez JP, et al. An ERK/Cdk5 axis controls the diabetogenic actions of PPAR-γ. Nature 2015;517:391–395

47. Roberts PJ, Der CJ. Targeting the Raf-MEK-ERK mitogen-activated protein kinase cascade for the treatment of cancer. Oncogene 2007;26:3291–3310

48. Iezzi A, Caiola E, Scagliotti A, Broggini M. Generation and characterization of MEK and ERK inhibitors- resistant non-small-cells-lung-cancer (NSCLC) cells. BMC Cancer 2018;18:1028

49. Tamarina NA, Roe MW, Philipson L. Characterization of mice expressing Ins1 gene promoter driven CreERT recombinase for conditional gene deletion in pancreatic β-cells. Islets 2014;6:e27685

50. Bélanger LF, Roy S, Tremblay M, et al. Mek2 is dispensable for mouse growth and development. Mol Cell Biol 2003;23:4778–4787

51. Bissonauth V, Roy S, Gravel M, Guillemette S, Charron J. Requirement for Map2k1 (Mek1) in extra-embryonic ectoderm during placentogenesis. Development 2006;133:3429–3440

Altered β-Cell Prohormone Processing and Secretion in Type 1 Diabetes

Teresa Rodriguez-Calvo,[1] Yi-Chun Chen,[2] C. Bruce Verchere,[3] Leena Haataja,[4] Peter Arvan,[4] Pia Leete,[5] Sarah J. Richardson,[5] Noel G. Morgan,[5] Wei-Jun Qian,[6] Alberto Pugliese,[7] Mark Atkinson,[8] Carmella Evans-Molina,[9,10,11] and Emily K. Sims[9]

Diabetes 2021;70:1038–1050 | https://doi.org/10.2337/dbi20-0034

Analysis of data from clinical cohorts, and more recently from human pancreatic tissue, indicates that reduced prohormone processing is an early and persistent finding in type 1 diabetes. In this article, we review the current state of knowledge regarding alterations in islet prohormone expression and processing in type 1 diabetes and consider the clinical impact of these findings. Lingering questions, including pathologic etiologies and consequences of altered prohormone expression and secretion in type 1 diabetes, and the natural history of circulating prohormone production in health and disease, are considered. Finally, key next steps required to move forward in this area are outlined, including longitudinal testing of relevant clinical populations, studies that probe the genetics of altered prohormone processing, the need for combined functional and histologic testing of human pancreatic tissues, continued interrogation of the intersection between prohormone processing and autoimmunity, and optimal approaches for analysis. Successful resolution of these questions may offer the potential to use altered prohormone processing as a biomarker to inform therapeutic strategies aimed at personalized intervention during the natural history of type 1 diabetes and as a pathogenic anchor for identification of potential disease-specific endotypes.

The pancreatic β-cell integrates humoral, metabolic, neural, and paracrine inputs to regulate the production, release, and processing of the hormones insulin and islet amyloid polypeptide (IAPP) (1). In type 1 diabetes, immune-mediated death and dysfunction of pancreatic β-cells lead to reduced circulating levels of insulin and IAPP. The physiological role of insulin as a critical regulator of carbohydrate metabolism is well established. Whereas the biological function of IAPP is not fully understood, studies suggest that it may act centrally to suppress food intake and gastric emptying; and within the islet, IAPP may suppress glucagon secretion (2). Both insulin and IAPP are synthesized as prohormones that undergo sequential processing in the secretory pathway within the β-cell (1,3) (Fig. 1). Multiple studies have identified evidence of increased proinsulin or proIAPP relative to mature insulin or IAPP expression, either in circulation or in the islet, at various stages in the natural history of type 1 diabetes (4–8). For years, conventional dogma suggested that by the time of clinical onset, a large majority of β-cell mass (i.e., 85–90%) has been destroyed, with ultimate progression to complete loss of insulin and IAPP. However, large cohort studies have shown that many individuals continue to secrete low levels of C-peptide for years after type 1 diabetes diagnosis (9). Recent studies have also highlighted persistent secretion of incompletely processed

[1]Institute of Diabetes Research, Helmholtz Zentrum Muenchen - German Research Center for Environmental Health, Munich-Neuherberg, Germany

[2]Department of Surgery, University of British Columbia and BC Children's Hospital Research Institute, Vancouver, Canada

[3]Departments of Surgery and Pathology and Laboratory Medicine, University of British Columbia, Centre for Molecular Medicine and Therapeutics, and BC Children's Hospital Research Institute, Vancouver, Canada

[4]Division of Metabolism, Endocrinology & Diabetes, University of Michigan Medical Center, Ann Arbor, MI

[5]Exeter Centre of Excellence for Diabetes, Institute of Biomedical & Clinical Science, University of Exeter Medical School, Exeter, U.K.

[6]Biological Sciences Division, Pacific Northwest National Laboratory, Richland, WA

[7]Diabetes Research Institute, Leonard M. Miller School of Medicine, University of Miami, Miami, FL

[8]Departments of Pathology and Pediatrics, Diabetes Institute, University of Florida, Gainesville, FL

[9]Center for Diabetes and Metabolic Diseases, Wells Center for Pediatric Research, Department of Pediatrics, Indiana University School of Medicine, Indianapolis, IN

[10]Departments of Cellular and Integrative Physiology, Medicine, and Molecular Biology, Indiana University School of Medicine, Indianapolis, IN

[11]Richard L. Roudebush VA Medical Center, Indianapolis, IN

Corresponding author: Emily K. Sims, eksims@iu.edu

Received 22 November 2020 and accepted 26 February 2021

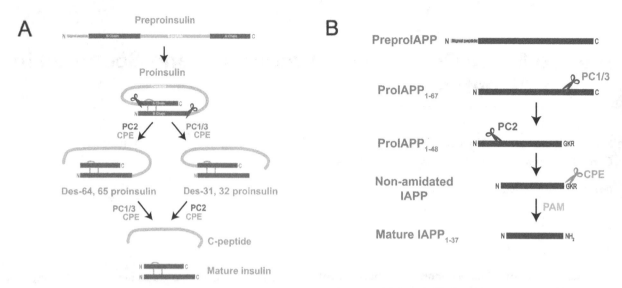

Figure 1—Processing of proinsulin and processing of proIAPP follow similar steps. Insulin and IAPP follow similar pathways of biogenesis, and processing occurs through a mostly common repertoire of enzymes located within the secretory pathway of the β-cell (1,3). *A*: Insulin production begins with translation of preproinsulin mRNA to form preproinsulin, which is a polypeptide that contains an N-terminal signal peptide, A and B chains, and a connecting C-peptide and is 100 amino acids in length. Preproinsulin is subsequently translocated into the lumen of the ER, where the N-terminal signal peptide is cleaved and three disulfide bonds are formed between the B and A chains to yield proinsulin. Proinsulin is transported to the Golgi complex and is sorted into immature secretory granules. Within the secretory granules, proinsulin is proteolytically processed to form C-peptide and the mature insulin molecule. Proteolytic processing of proinsulin is the result of sequential cleavage steps by prohormone convertase 1/3 (PC1/3), prohormone convertase 2 (PC2), and carboxypeptidase E (CPE). The classically described pathway of proinsulin processing involves an initial cleavage by PC1/3 at the junction of the B chain and C-peptide (on the C-terminal side of two basic amino acids, Arg^{31} and Arg^{32}), forming split 32,33 proinsulin. CPE trims dibasic residues at the C-terminal end of the split forms to yield des-31,32 proinsulin, followed by cleavage at the junction of the A chain and C-peptide by PC2 and trimming by CPE to yield insulin and C-peptide. Processing may also begin with PC2 cleavage (C-terminal to Lys^{64}–Arg^{65}) to form split 65,66 proinsulin. CPE trimming yields des-64,65 proinsulin, which is cleaved further by PC1/3 to form insulin and C-peptide. Ex vivo studies as well as analysis of circulating forms of proinsulin in humans, revealing higher levels of the des-31,32 proinsulin intermediate in comparison with des-64,65 proinsulin, support a model where initial cleavage by PC1/3 is strongly favored. *B*: Similar to preproinsulin, the signal peptide of pre-proIAPP is removed, creating the 67-residue IAPP precursor proIAPP. The C-terminal end of proIAPP is first cleaved by PC1/3 and CPE to produce the proIAPP$_{1-48}$ intermediate, which is then cleaved at its N-terminal end by PC2. The C-terminus of IAPP is amidated by peptidyl α-amidating monooxygenase (PAM). Alternative processing of proIAPP may occur in states of β-cell dysfunction, and the plasma proIAPP$_{1-48}$–to–total IAPP ratio is elevated in subjects with type 1 diabetes (6). Recent analyses have suggested that among human β-cells, PC1/3 may be more critical than PC2 for β-cell proinsulin processing, although impacts on human proIAPP processing remain to be tested (62).

forms of proinsulin and proIAPP in patients with long-duration type 1 diabetes, even in cohorts characterized by the absence of detectable serum C-peptide, suggesting the continued presence of proinsulin-producing cells that do not effectively process prohormones (6,8,10). Analyses of pancreata from organ donors with type 1 diabetes have extended these findings to the tissue level (4,8).

Mechanistic studies have begun to link β-cell stress, occurring either from extrinsic sources or due to activation of intrinsic molecular pathways within the β-cell, with disruptions in normal prohormone processing (1,11) (Fig. 2). Moreover, T cell autoreactivity has been demonstrated against regions of the incompletely processed forms of proinsulin and proIAPP, suggesting a role for altered prohormone processing in immune activation (12,13). In response to these emerging findings, levels of circulating prohormones relative to mature hormones are actively being studied for their potential as noninvasive indicators of type 1 diabetes risk, as well as biomarkers of therapeutic efficacy, in efforts designed for disease prevention or intervention (14).

Prohormones in the Circulation

A substantial body of work suggests that elevations in relative levels of circulating prohormones can provide insights into β-cell stress at different stages during the evolution of type 1 diabetes. Most studies in individuals at risk for or with a diagnosis of type 1 diabetes have shown elevations in ratios of proinsulin or proIAPP relative to mature insulin/C-peptide or IAPP rather than absolute elevations in circulating prohormones in comparison with control samples (6–8,15,16).

Circulating Proinsulin–to–C-peptide Ratios Predict Disease Progression in Individuals at Risk for Type 1 Diabetes

Analyses from natural history cohorts of islet autoantibody-positive (Aab$^+$) individuals without diabetes who ultimately develop type 1 diabetes have shown that these individuals exhibit elevated proinsulin–to–C-peptide (PI/C) ratios in comparison with Aab$^−$ control subjects. These efforts also suggest that fasting PI/C ratios are inversely associated with first-phase insulin responses during intravenous glucose tolerance tests or hyperglycemic clamps

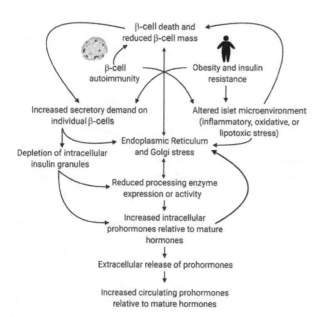

Figure 2—Potential pathologic etiologies of increased circulating immature islet prohormones relative to mature hormones. Potential etiologies arising from sources extrinsic and intrinsic to the β-cell, as well as interactions, are displayed.

(15,16). Among Aab⁺ relatives, elevated PI/C ratios are also associated with increased risk of progression to type 1 diabetes and can complement the use of Aab for risk prediction, with longitudinal ratios inversely related to time to diagnosis (7,15,17,18). PI/C ratios appear to be most elevated in younger at-risk children (i.e., age <10 years) who progress to type 1 diabetes, suggesting that this subgroup of individuals may exhibit more severe β-cell stress during disease progression (7).

PI/C Ratio Is Elevated in Many Individuals With New or Recent-Onset Type 1 Diabetes

Not surprisingly, comparisons with Aab⁻ nonrelative control subjects show elevations of PI/C in individuals with new or recent-onset type 1 diabetes, especially younger children, consistent with high levels of β-cell stress at diagnosis (19,20). However, other efforts have shown differing results regarding whether improvements versus maintained elevations in PI/C occur after exogenous insulin therapy is started, during the clinical remission often referred to as the honeymoon period (19–21). This could be related to varied participant age at the time of diagnosis (youth vs. adult), as well as the degree and/or duration of improved β-cell function over this period (19–21). A recent study testing treatment of children and young adults with recent-onset type 1 diabetes with an IgG1-κ monoclonal antibody specific for human TNF-α showed stable PI/C ratios in drug-treated participants compared with progressive increases over time in placebo (22). Intriguingly, higher PI/C ratio at the time of type 1 diabetes diagnosis was noted in studies decades ago showing an

improved response to cyclosporin treatment, suggesting that high PI/C ratios, as a proxy or readout of β-cell stress, could be leveraged to identify individuals who might benefit from a disease-modifying intervention (19). Such findings are consistent with data from other immunomodulatory interventions identifying individuals with active disease and β-cell dysfunction as robust treatment responders (23). Ideally, such biomarkers could also be leveraged to help in selection and optimization of specific interventions.

Elevations in Circulating PI/C and ProIAPP-to-IAPP Ratios Persist in Established Type 1 Diabetes

Very elevated PI/C ratios, suggestive of severe β-cell stress, are consistently present in individuals with long-standing type 1 diabetes and residual detectable C-peptide decades after diagnosis (8,10). Ratios tend to be higher in those diagnosed at very young ages (i.e., <7 years), again suggesting a more severe disease phenotype in younger children (8). Even in those individuals with long-standing type 1 diabetes and undetectable stimulated C-peptide, circulating proinsulin can be identified. The reported percentage of individuals with undetectable C-peptide but persistent proinsulin secretion has varied from 16% to up to 90%, depending on the characteristics of the assays used and cohorts studied (8,10,24,25). In addition, many individuals with undetectable or minimal residual C-peptide, but detectable proinsulin, do not exhibit the expected increase in stimulated circulating proinsulin that is observed in control subjects or those with type 1 diabetes exhibiting higher residual C-peptide (10). While measurements of the levels of the IAPP precursor, proIAPP, relative to mature IAPP have not been performed across the entire natural history of type 1 diabetes, children with long-standing type 1 diabetes and islet transplant recipients with type 1 diabetes exhibit elevated ratios of a proIAPP processing intermediate (proIAPP$_{1-48}$) relative to total IAPP (6). Interestingly, unlike PI/C, ratios of proIAPP$_{1-48}$ to mature IAPP do not appear to be elevated in individuals with type 2 diabetes (6,26).

Elevated PI/C Ratios May Be Present in Some Aab⁻ Relatives of Individuals With Type 1 Diabetes and in Aab⁺ Nonprogressors

Several older studies in relatives of individuals with type 1 diabetes testing negative for islet autoimmunity have described elevations in circulating absolute and normalized proinsulin in comparison with unrelated control subjects, suggesting that some individuals may inherit a predisposition to abnormal prohormone processing that predates detectable autoimmunity. Islet cell cytoplasmic antibody (ICA)⁺ and ICA⁻ individuals without diabetes with an identical twin affected by type 1 diabetes showed an absolute increase in fasting proinsulin in comparison with unrelated control subjects (27). Despite normal insulin and glucose values, testing in groups of Swedish and Swiss first-degree relatives of patients with type 1 diabetes who were ICA[+] and ICA[−] also showed HLA-independent increases in fasting absolute proinsulin values in comparison with control subjects, although ICA[−] relatives showed less pronounced elevations (28,29). An important caveat to these results is the use of older, less sensitive assays for assessment of islet autoimmunity. In contrast, more recent testing in first-degree relatives from the Belgian Diabetes Registry demonstrated similar random PI/C ratio values among Aab[+] relatives that did not progress to diabetes during follow-up, Aab[−] relatives, and a small group of nonrelative Aab[−] control subjects (17).

Prohormones in Islets

Increased PI/C ratios in the circulation months to years before clinical diagnosis (7,15,17,18) point to a potential functional β-cell defect appearing very early in the type 1 diabetes disease process. However, until recently, whether this relative increase in circulating proinsulin could be linked to abnormal proinsulin expression in the pancreas remained largely unknown. Recent access to human pancreas samples through the Network for Pancreatic Organ donors with Diabetes (nPOD) and the Exeter Archival Diabetes Biobank (EADB) coupled with improvements in image analysis methodologies has provided a unique opportunity to study these phenomena in samples from control subjects without diabetes (Fig. 3) as well as across multiple phases of type 1 diabetes (4,5,8) (Figs. 4 and 5). Here, analysis has shown that islets from Aab[+] individuals exhibit an increase in absolute pancreatic proinsulin area and in the proinsulin-to-insulin ratio without a significant reduction in insulin area or β-cell mass (5) (Fig. 4A). Moreover, islets from Aab[+] donors show changes in the subcellular localization of proinsulin, which was predominantly localized in secretory vesicles in Aab[+] individuals with multiple Aab, as opposed to the normal juxtanuclear localization. Taken together, these findings suggest that proinsulin maturation might already be defective in the prediabetic pancreas, independently of the loss of β-cell mass. The same analysis reported elevations in the proinsulin-to-insulin ratio in pancreatic samples from living individuals with recent-onset type 1 diabetes collected through the Diabetes Virus Detection Study (DiViD) (5). Continued elevation of ratios despite exogenous insulin therapy suggests that β-cells remain dysfunctional at the time of diagnosis, even when their workload is diminished.

Further studies demonstrated that residual β-cells containing insulin and proinsulin could be found in individuals with short and long duration of type 1 diabetes (4). Islets from donors with type 1 diabetes exhibit overall reductions in insulin, proinsulin, and C-peptide in pancreatic protein extracts in comparison with nondiabetic control subjects. However, the levels of proinsulin were higher than expected and comparable with those of Aab[+] individuals. Both the proinsulin-to-insulin and PI/C ratios were significantly elevated in individuals with type 1 diabetes.

Furthermore, insulin mRNA was low but detectable in almost all subjects with type 1 diabetes (4). In agreement with these studies, populations of proinsulin-enriched, insulin-depleted cells have been described in a subset of individuals with long-standing type 1 diabetes (30) (Fig. 5A). This depletion of insulin-positive granules might suggest β-cell exhaustion (degranulation) with (or perhaps even without) a dramatic reduction in β-cell mass.

Abnormal Proinsulin and Insulin Colocalization May Be Associated With Specific Endotypes of Type 1 Diabetes

Recent work has focused on the influence of age at diagnosis on the expression and distribution of insulin and proinsulin in the pancreas (8). Analysis of samples from the EADB and the nPOD collections showed that in children diagnosed early in life (before 7 years), most β-cells exhibited a high degree of insulin and proinsulin colocalization (8) (example in Fig. 4B). This population also displayed a hyperimmune profile characterized by abundant islet-infiltrating CD20[+] and CD8[+] cells. The authors proposed that these features represent one particular "endotype" coined as type 1 diabetes endotype 1 (T1DE1) (6). By contrast, in samples from individuals diagnosed at or after the age of 13 years, >70% of islets displayed little colocalization and had a lower proportion of CD20[+] cells in inflamed islets. It was also noted that, irrespective of age at diagnosis, for the islets of people in whom β-cells persisted for >5 years after diagnosis there were low rates of proinsulin-to-insulin colocalization. Such islets were most prevalent in subjects diagnosed at age ≥13 years. Taken together with work described above, these findings suggest that there is a strong interplay among abnormal proinsulin processing, β-cell function, and immune activity in children diagnosed very early in life. Continued study of pancreata from children and adults at multiple stages of disease should help to confirm whether disease endotypes exist (rather than a continuously variable set of pancreatic phenotypes) and may suggest routes to personalized therapeutic intervention.

Prohormone Processing Is Altered in Type 1 Diabetes

The studies described above demonstrate that proinsulin is elevated in islets before and after onset of type 1 diabetes and that relative circulating levels of proinsulin remain increased in individuals with long-standing disease. From these findings, it seems very likely that the efficiency of prohormone processing is unable to keep up with prohormone production during the course of type 1 diabetes. Potential etiologies of these findings are further discussed in Table 1. A likely contributing etiology is increased insulin secretory demand or rapid insulin release in association with reduced β-cell mass (31), resulting in mature secretory granule depletion and resultant depletion of processing enzymes. It is also possible that an intrinsic prohormone processing defect may arise during the course of the disease. Expression patterns of proinsulin and proIAPP processing enzymes (prohormone convertase

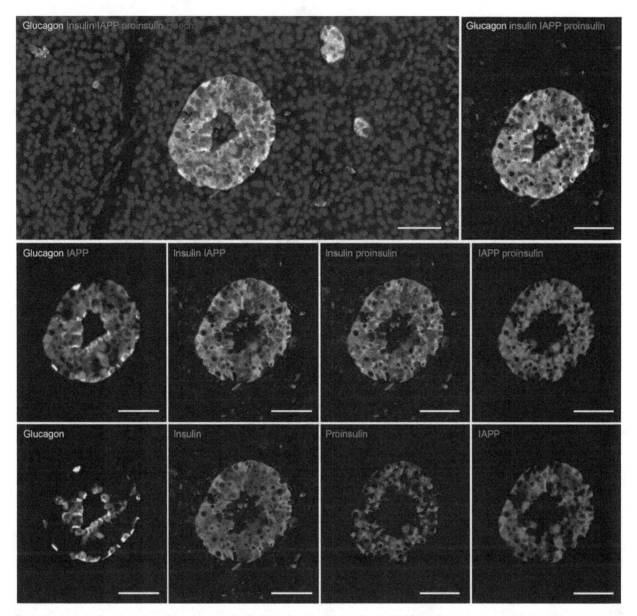

Figure 3—Immunofluorescent staining showing distribution of proinsulin, insulin, and IAPP in islets from a control donor without diabetes. Scale bars = 50 μm in the low-magnification image and 25 μm in the rest. Anti-proinsulin antibody (GS-9A8; Developmental Studies Hybridoma Bank) (detects the B-C junction and so cross-reactive with intact proinsulin, 65,66 split proinsulin, and des-64,65 proinsulin [validated in 63]) and anti-IAPP antibody (HPA053194; Atlas) were used.

1/3 [PC1/3], prohormone convertase 2 [PC2], and carboxypeptidase E [CPE]) have been investigated in islets from individuals with short and long disease duration. One study found significant reductions in PC1/3 mRNA but not in PC2 or CPE (4). Similarly, in another study, with use of laser-capture microdissection and mass spectrometry (MS), significant reductions were reported in PC1/3 and a tendency to lower CPE but no difference in PC2 (30).

Mechanistic studies testing human islet prohormone processing in the context of type 1 diabetes are fairly limited in number. Cytokine treatment for 24 h of isolated islets from donors without diabetes was associated with a significant reduction in mRNA expression levels of PC1/3, CPE, and PC2 (30). Longer (48–72 h) in vitro exposure of human islets to cytokine combinations resulted in reduced protein concentrations of PC1/3 and PC2 in association with an increase in medium proinsulin-to-insulin ratio, supporting the idea that islet inflammatory stress might be associated with intrinsic reductions in prohormone processing (32). Accumulation of misprocessed proteins can have dramatic effects on β-cell survival and mRNA translation through activation of cell-intrinsic stress pathways. Indeed, β-cells exposed to proinflammatory cytokines are

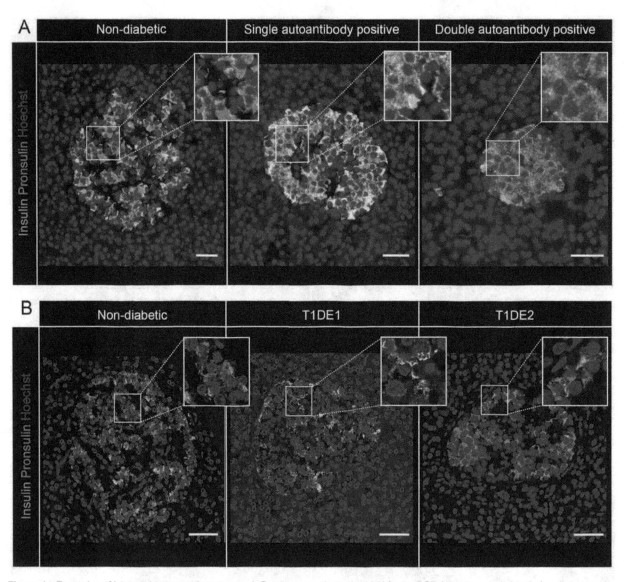

Figure 4—Examples of islet prohormone phenotypes. *A*: Pancreas sections obtained from nPOD from three individuals (no diabetes, single islet Aab positive, and double islet Aab positive) showing representative examples of increases in proinsulin-positive area (staining further described and quantified in multiple donor samples in 5). Anti-proinsulin antibody was used (GS-9A8; Developmental Studies Hybridoma Bank) (detects the B-C junction and so cross-reactive with intact proinsulin, 65,66 split proinsulin, and des-64,65 proinsulin [validated in 63]). Sections were imaged with a Zeiss Axio Scan.Z1 slide scanner. Scale bars = 25 μm. *B*: Representative pancreas sections from three individuals obtained from the EADB and nPOD (no diabetes and donors with T1DE1 and T1DE2) showing increased colocalization of insulin and proinsulin in T1DE1 in comparison with no diabetes and T1DE2 (staining further described and quantified in multiple sections in 8). Anti-proinsulin primary antibody was used (ab8301; Abcam) (detects the B-C junction and so cross-reactive with intact proinsulin, 65,66 split proinsulin, and des-64,65 proinsulin). Sections were imaged with use of high-resolution confocal (Leica DMi8, SP8) microscopy. Scale bars = 50 μm.

prone to endoplasmic reticulum (ER) stress and apoptosis (33), while islets from individuals with type 1 diabetes have increased levels of the ER stress markers BIP and CHOP, the latter of which has been associated with β-cell death (34). Defects in protein processing could theoretically contribute to β-cell death in type 1 diabetes, perhaps through exacerbation of increased secretory demands or in ways that are analogous to some monogenic forms of diabetes that occur due to proinsulin misfolding and ER stress

(35,36). Misfolded proinsulin has not been identified in secretory granules; however, β-cells under conditions of ER stress independent of cytokines could also potentially contribute unprocessed proinsulin and/or proIAPP to the circulation via "leakage" or cell death. Aberrant processing of proIAPP to mature IAPP has been hypothesized to contribute to IAPP aggregation and amyloid formation (37), which has recently been detected in pancreata of some donors with long-standing type 1 diabetes (38) (Fig. 5*B*). As IAPP

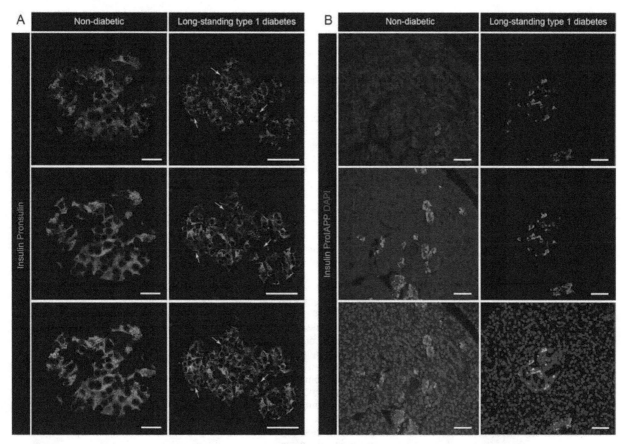

Figure 5—Examples of islet prohormone phenotypes. *A* and *B*: Immunostaining of pancreas sections, obtained from individuals through nPOD, showing islets. *A*: From a donor without diabetes (scale bars = 20 μm) and a donor with type 1 diabetes with islets showing increased numbers of proinsulin-enriched, insulin-poor cells, indicated with yellow arrows (scale bars = 50 μm). *B*: From a donor without diabetes and a donor with type 1 diabetes with islets exhibiting staining for C-terminally extended proIAPP. Sections were imaged with a ZEISS LSM 700 confocal microscope (*A*) and a Leica SP5 confocal microscope (*B*). Scale bars = 50 μm. Staining in *A* is further described and quantified in 30. Anti-proinsulin antibody (GS-9A8; Developmental Studies Hybridoma Bank) (detects the B-C junction and so cross-reactive with intact proinsulin, 65,66 split proinsulin, and des-64,65 proinsulin [validated in 63]) and anti-proIAPP antibody (F063; gift from Medimmune) (raised to an epitope in the C-terminal flanking of peptide of human proIAPP and predicted to detect intact proIAPP) were used.

aggregates are a trigger for inflammation and β-cell stress (6,37), it is plausible that impaired handling of proIAPP or IAPP could contribute to β-cell dysfunction and loss in type 1 diabetes, as is suggested in the case of type 2 diabetes (38).

In addition, accumulating evidence indicates a link between prohormone processing and T cell–mediated autoreactivity (12). T cell repertoire studies have identified autoreactivity against multiple epitopes of preproinsulin, proinsulin, and proIAPP, while analysis of the β-cell HLA-I peptidome has confirmed that many of these epitopes can be presented by the β-cell (12,39,40). Specifically, in the case of insulin, subcellular targeting and protein modifications impact processing pathways, as well as efficiency and regulation of antigen presentation (41). Errors in processing can lead to posttranslational modifications of the native protein; posttranslationally modified insulin-derived epitopes have improved HLA-I binding capacity and induce T cell activation (42). Moreover, the physiologic release of granule contents directly into the

bloodstream may allow for an opportunity to interact with distant antigen-presenting cells outside of the pancreas (12). Importantly, islet autoantibodies are absent at diagnosis of inherited forms of diabetes related to protein misfolding and ER stress, pointing away from widespread activation of islet autoimmunity under conditions of β-cell stress (35,36). However, it is possible that β-cell stress is linked to increased antigen presentation and T cell–mediated autoreactivity in individuals with a genetic predisposition to autoimmunity.

Lingering Questions Regarding Prohormones in Type 1 Diabetes

The existing body of work quantifying circulating and tissue levels of proinsulin and proIAPP has provided convincing data that during the natural history of type 1 diabetes, prohormone processing cannot keep pace with prohormone production. PI/C ratios are increased in many at-risk individuals before, at, and after diagnosis and are associated with disease progression, particularly in young

Table 1—Key exploratory questions regarding the pathophysiology of disproportionate β-cell prohormone levels and secretion

Key question	Important points to consider or test
What are the specific pathologic etiologies leading to elevations in circulating and β-cell expression of prohormones relative to mature hormones in type 1 diabetes?	• Are relative elevations in circulating prohormones compared with mature hormones due to a defect in proinsulin processing or a simple reflection of β-cell exhaustion, resulting in release of immature granules with more unprocessed prohormone? 　○ Elevated levels of prohormones relative to mature hormones observed in at-risk populations and after clinical diagnosis, rather than elevations in absolute prohormone levels, may point more toward a β-cell exhaustion phenotype with mature granule depletion over primary defects in proinsulin processing (4–8). 　○ Absolute increases in islet proinsulin area along with findings of reduced expression of islet prohormone processing enzymes in islets from donors with type 1 diabetes support the idea of defective prohormone processing, but processing enzyme levels could also theoretically be impacted by reduced β-cell counts per islet or granule depletion (4,5,30). 　○ Proinflammatory cytokine–induced increases in media proinsulin-to-insulin ratio in association with reduced islet processing enzyme expression support the idea of an intrinsic defect associated with β-cell proinflammatory stress (30,32). • Similar to increased PI/C ratios after partial pancreatectomy (31), could altered prohormone processing in type 1 diabetes result in part from the impact of reduced β-cell mass on insulin secretory demand on individual β-cells? • Could increases in β-cell death due to ER stress result in leakage of prohormone contents from cells leading to increased levels in circulation? • Do changes in the human islet microenvironment impact prohormone processing and relative secretion in concert? • Systematic comparisons of circulating prohormones as well as tissue prohormone and processing enzyme expression performed with the same reagents in samples from individuals with or at risk for type 1 and type 2 diabetes could help with identification of distinct pathological contributors to β-cell stress resulting in differing timing or phenotypes of altered prohormone processing and secretion. • Do some individuals with a high genetic risk inherit β-cells with an intrinsic functional defect, either at baseline or in response to environmental stressors? 　○ The rs2611215 single nucleotide polymorphism that has been linked to increased type 1 diabetes risk could theoretically affect CPE expression, and, thus, prohormone processing may be impacted in this subset of individuals (57). 　○ Answers to this question could be informed by genetic studies in type 2 diabetes cohorts, where clustering analysis has identified single nucleotide polymorphisms potentially leading to impaired proinsulin processing (58). • Could reduced prohormone processing serve as a readout of other particular immune phenotypes or disease endotypes beyond the constellation of features suggested as the T1DE1 endotype (8)?
How do differences in the immune system's interactions with β-cells under conditions of abnormal prohormone expression contribute to the pathophysiology of type 1 diabetes?	• Do altered interactions with the immune system occur early in the disease process due to formation of neoantigens, via misfolding, alternative translation, or posttranslational modifications (reviewed in 12)? If so, does this occur in predisposed individuals at baseline or in response to an environmental exposure, such as a viral infection (59)? • What mechanisms link CD20⁺ B cells to impaired prohormone processing? Do insulitis profiles associated with large numbers of CD20⁺ B cells yield increased β-cell stress? Or do stressed β-cells somehow attract more severe insulitis with a higher proportion of CD20⁺ cells (8)? • Does increased susceptibility to β-cell stress exacerbate β-cell failure and death once autoimmunity is established? • Is reduced expression of processing enzymes and subsequent reduced prohormone processing part of a dedifferentiated β-cell phenotype that is able to evade autoimmunity (45,46)?
Which prohormone forms (i.e., intact/unprocessed prohormones vs. partially processed forms) are relevant to β-cell stress in type 1 diabetes?	• Although both intact/unprocessed proinsulin and partially processed des-31,32 proinsulin forms are elevated in type 2 diabetes, specific quantification of relative proportions of intact vs. partially processed prohormone forms of either proinsulin or proIAPP has not been reported in type 1 diabetes (47). • What are the relationships between increased relative proportions of proinsulin and proIAPP in circulation and pancreas tissue?

Continued on p. 1046

Table 1—Continued

Key question	Important points to consider or test
	• Do different pathophysiologic etiologies of β-cell stress result in differing elevations in relative levels of prohormone forms?
	• Why are PI/C and proIAPP$_{1-48}$–to–total IAPP ratios similarly elevated in type 1 but not type 2 diabetes (6)?
	• How do differences in clearance of prohormone species in comparison with mature hormones impact circulating prohormone–to–mature hormone ratios in type 1 diabetes?

children. Even many years after diagnosis, persistent secretion of proinsulin and proIAPP has been documented, reflecting the existence of severely dysfunctional β-cells in long-standing disease. However, several lingering questions regarding the natural history and physiology of circulating prohormones remain. These will be important to answer moving forward in order to implement use of circulating prohormones as biomarkers to guide type 1 diabetes prediction, progression, and treatment. Similarly, despite the increasing number of studies in islet tissue on absolute or relative prohormone accumulation and processing, there are still conceptual gaps in our understanding of prohormone conversion dynamics and storage, both in "normal" β-cells of humans without diabetes and in cells influenced by different types of stressors.

Natural History of Circulating Prohormones in Health and Disease

Studies often show significant elevations in PI/C ratios in comparisons with control subjects, but in many cases, values overlap with those of control subjects. This might be related to several factors, including heterogenous phenotypes or endotypes of type 1 diabetes, which do not uniformly involve high levels of intrinsic β-cell stress (43). Overlap with values of control subjects could also reflect disease heterogeneity due to physiologic differences in "normal" PI/C ratios during different life stages, especially for pediatric age-groups advancing through puberty, or groups of adults compared with children. Both adults and pubertal children can exhibit increases in insulin resistance relative to prepubertal children, and knowing the expected "normal" range for PI/C ratios and proIAPP-to-IAPP ratios more definitively during growth and aging will be important for understanding what constitutes an "abnormal" value (44).

Pragmatically, another important hurdle in the implementation of prohormone measurements as biomarkers for use in prediction and intervention efforts will be development of a better definition of the expected natural history of increasing prohormones/mature hormones as type 1 diabetes develops. Longitudinal data are needed in adequately powered studies of diverse at-risk populations that allow for improved characterization of patterns of change over time. While proIAPP has been measured in established type 1 diabetes, it is not clear how patterns of secretion change during earlier disease

stages or whether there is concordance between proIAPP and proinsulin secretion at different disease stages. Such analyses will allow for a better understanding of whether certain groups of individuals are at risk for abnormal values, either at baseline or in association with environmental stressors. Along these lines, older data in ICA$^-$ first-degree relatives are intriguing but must be followed up using newer biochemical Aab assays. Additionally, ratios may increase progressively over time or could change in a relapsing-remitting pattern, in association with periods of active autoimmune disease or intermittent environmental stressors. Such factors have important implications for the timing of screening and prediction approaches—but will also be informative in tracking of the disease course in individuals. In addition, samples from successful intervention studies should be tested to identify whether circulating prohormones can be used as an early marker of successful treatment response. Such analyses would also serve to identify whether circulating prohormones could be used to identify reversible β-cell stress and predict treatment "responders" to immunomodulation.

Pathologic Etiologies and Consequences of Altered Prohormone Processing

Several important unanswered questions revolve around the pathophysiologic relevance of increases in circulating prohormones in type 1 diabetes (outlined in Table 1). First, given that multiple pathways could theoretically increase the relative proportion of β-cell prohormone expression and secretion, what are the specific pathologic etiologies leading to these outcomes in type 1 diabetes? Exploration of this question will lead to a better understanding of whether defects in prohormone processing can serve as a readout of particular immune phenotypes and/or disease endotypes (8).

Work from several investigators suggests that the immune system could react differently to β-cells under situations in which abnormal prohormone expression occurs (reviewed in 12). Alternatively, increased susceptibility to β-cell stress could exacerbate β-cell failure and death once autoimmunity is established. In contrast, recent preclinical work suggests a model wherein partially dedifferentiated β-cells may be selected for their ability to evade autoimmunity. Along these lines, loss of processing enzyme

Table 2—Optimizing measurements of proportional elevations of prohormones in type 1 diabetes

Factor	Important considerations
Timing of sampling	• Samples from all participants should be optimally obtained at consistent timing relative to fasting vs. glucose or mixed-meal stimulation. • For normalization, prohormones and mature hormones should be measured in samples obtained from the same time point. • Fasting PI/C ratios reportedly elevated in individuals at risk for or diagnosed with type 1 diabetes. • Stimulated PI/C ratios may be less impacted relative to fasting values in longer-duration type 1 diabetes, but definitive understanding of timing of peak PI/C ratios in these populations requires more robust study that includes multiple stimulated time points.
Prohormone measurements • Proinsulin assay	• Commercially available assays include radioimmunoassays and ELISA. • Does assay of interest test intact (unprocessed) proinsulin or total proinsulin (unprocessed + different combinations of partially processed split products depending on assay)? Cross-reactivity with partially processed proinsulin species is common in most commercial proinsulin and insulin assays. No commercial assays are currently available that quantify des-64,65 proinsulin or des-31,32 proinsulin individually. • Antibody-based assays are well established but often not well characterized. Because standards for partially processed forms of proinsulin are not widely available for external validation, there is uncertainty regarding which proinsulin products commercially available antibodies recognize. • Has assay of interest been externally validated to show reproducible results? • Is assay of interest calibrated based on 84/611 (older) or 09/296 (newer) intact proinsulin standard (60)? Due to diminishing supply, in 2014 the original World Health Organization intact proinsulin standard was switched to the 09/296 standard (60). Because of this, although newer intact and total proinsulin assays are calibrated based on the 09/296 standard, several older assays are calibrated against the prior 84/611 standard, thereby limiting direct comparison of results, given that values obtained with assays based on different standards are not quantitatively equivalent. • While partially processed split products do not add discriminatory capability above that of intact proinsulin for samples from control subjects and patients with type 2 diabetes, this has not been tested in type 1 diabetes (47). • Targeted MS-based techniques may allow for antibody-independent measurements and validation of antibody-based assays. But such assays are still in the developmental stage at research laboratories.
• ProIAPP assay	• Externally validated proIAPP$_{1-48}$ ELISA is available through research laboratories only (6). • Assays for intact proIAPP$_{1-67}$ and other intermediate forms are currently under development. • Targeted MS-based techniques are currently under development.
Mature hormone measurements	• Understanding of proportional elevations in prohormones requires careful quantification of levels relative to mature hormones. Thus, optimizing mature hormone measurement is also a key goal.
• C-peptide or insulin assay	• Elevations in both PI/C and proinsulin-to-insulin ratios have been described in circulation for certain populations relevant to type 1 diabetes (7,28,29,61). • PI/C ratio outperforms proinsulin-to-insulin ratio to predict incident diabetes in insulin-resistant populations, as circulating insulin values can reflect altered hepatic insulin clearance (26). • Measurement of endogenous insulin levels may be confounded by use of insulin analogs. • International standards are available for both C-peptide and insulin. • Certain immunoassays for C-peptide and insulin may cross-react with proinsulin species. • MS-based based assays for C-peptide and intact insulin are available through commercial laboratories (e.g., Quest Diagnostics).
• IAPP assay	• Commercially available assays include radioimmunoassays and ELISA. • Commercial assays have not been externally validated. • Externally validated immunoassay for mature, C-terminally amidated IAPP is available through research laboratories (5). • No international standard exists for cross calibration of assays. • MS-based techniques are currently under development.

expression and the reduced ability to complete prohormone processing could be viewed as part of a dedifferentiated β-cell phenotype (45,46). How these potentially conflicting paradigms contribute to type 1 pathophysiology is not clear and should be a focus of future studies.

Although both intact/unprocessed proinsulin and partially processed des-31,32 proinsulin forms are elevated in type 2 diabetes (47), the relative proportion of intermediate and intact forms of proinsulin and proIAPP is still unclear in type 1 diabetes. Separate quantification of both intact and partially processed prohormone forms in the

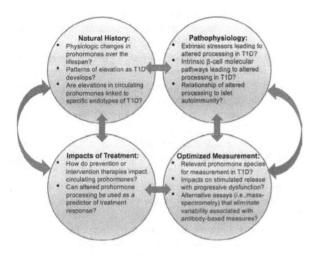

Figure 6—Key next steps in the field moving forward. Key next steps involve determining the natural history of abnormal relative prohormone expression in the islet and circulation during the progression of type 1 diabetes (T1D), better understanding the pathophysiology leading to these findings, defining the impact of disease treatment, and optimizing prohormone measurement.

circulation and pancreas from individuals with type 1 and type 2 diabetes, and of relationships between increased relative proportions of proinsulin and proIAPP, may clarify the pathophysiologic etiologies of altered ratios.

Studies testing both pancreas tissue and serum from the same individual would be optimal to address these questions, but such samples are challenging to obtain from living individuals. However, recent advances have provided the opportunity to study live pancreatic tissue from organ donors and therefore correlate anatomical and physiological data. Slices of whole pancreas tissue with preserved endocrine, exocrine, and immune tissue compartments can be obtained from donors with or without type 1 diabetes (48). With use of these, it may be feasible to measure basal and stimulated prohormone secretion as well as to evaluate enzymatic prohormone processing in both nondiabetic and diabetic tissue environments. A preliminary study in pancreas slices from a donor with type 1 diabetes has confirmed that, in some cases, significant β-cell mass is preserved at disease onset and that insulin deficiency can result from β-cell dysfunction (5,48). These findings corroborate data generated from islets, isolated from living donors with recent-onset type 1 diabetes in DiViD, that were dysfunctional initially but recovered glucose responsiveness during culture. Expanding these studies will be key to defining the role of β-cell dysfunction in type 1 diabetes.

Optimizing Prohormone Measurement

Strategies and challenges in optimizing prohormone measurement are outlined in Table 2. Of note, the use of highly specific and reliable assays for multiple forms of prohormone (e.g., intact, des-64,65, and des-31,32 proinsulins) will be critical to gaining a more detailed

understanding of prohormone processing in type 1 diabetes. Immunoassays have been developed for detecting intact proinsulin (49), total proinsulin (which includes intact + partially processed proinsulin forms) (50,51), C-peptide, insulin, and proIAPP$_{1-48}$ (6). Unfortunately, the performance characteristics of prohormone immunoassays, which are limited by the inherent exclusive dependence on reproducible antibody reagents, are often not well documented (52). For proinsulin, obtaining optimal specificity can be particularly challenging due to the structural similarities among proinsulin, its partially processed forms, insulin, and C-peptide and the low concentration of proinsulin in comparison with insulin/C-peptide (52). Specifically, proinsulin and mature insulin or C-peptide immunoassays often cross-react with intact proinsulin as well as a combination of proinsulin split products, resulting in a degree of inaccuracy in quantification of proinsulin or insulin levels from clinical data. Although to date there are no widely accepted guidelines or standardized approaches, careful independent validation is needed in confirming consistency of findings (53,54).

A promising alternative means to develop highly specific assays for prohormone products is the use of targeted MS. These techniques (55,56) provide direct measurements of surrogate peptides from any given protein with well-characterizable specificity and multiplexing capacity but without the need for affinity reagents. In principle, it is highly feasible to develop targeted MS assays for specific forms of prohormone processing products in serum, tissue, and secretome (10); however, the current limitations of targeted MS assays lie in the achievable sensitivity and analytical throughput. Further developments are needed to achieve the sensitivity required for such detection. The rigor and reproducibility of immunoassays could be substantially improved if the specificities and performance are validated and standardized with use of antibody-free targeted MS-based assays along with improved calibration standards.

Conclusions: Key Next Steps in the Field Moving Forward

In summary, analysis of pancreatic tissue and data from clinical cohorts indicate that prohormone processing insufficiency is an early and persistent component of type 1 diabetes pathogenesis. The body of work outlined herein has identified a number of exploratory questions for the type 1 diabetes research community and suggests several key next steps that should be taken to clarify the role of altered prohormone expression and secretion in type 1 diabetes (Fig. 6). These questions largely focus around continued and longitudinal testing of relevant clinical populations, studies that probe the genetics of impaired prohormone processing in type 1 diabetes, combined functional and histologic testing of human pancreas tissues, and continued interrogation of how prohormone processing intersects with immune activation and autoreactivity. A key tenet of this work is the need for reliable and well-validated assays that can detect and distinguish intact prohormones and processing intermediates. Successful resolution of these questions may offer the potential to use altered prohormone processing as an anchor that can subsequently be used to cluster different endotypes of disease enveloping a large set of variables (e.g., age, genetic background, severity of insulitis and its composition, and rate of progression). Ultimately, such an approach could inform clinical therapeutic strategies aimed at intervening in the natural history of type 1 diabetes.

Acknowledgments. Schematic figures were created with BioRender (BioRender.com). The authors apologize to investigators whose work they were unable to include in this article due to space limitations. The authors also acknowledge the support of the nPOD Slice Prohormone Processing Interest Group, which includes the coauthors as well as Clive Wasserfall, Irina Petrache, Mingder Yang, Harry Nick, Gladys Teitelman, Adam Swenson, and Sirlene Cechin.

Funding. This effort was supported by nPOD (Research Resource Identifier: SCR_014641), a collaborative type 1 diabetes research project sponsored by JDRF (grant 5-SRA-2018-557-Q-R) and The Leona M. & Harry B. Helmsley Charitable Trust (2018PG-T1D053). T.R.-C. receives funding from JDRF (5-CDA-2020-949-A-N), E.K.S. receives funding from the National Institute of Diabetes and Digestive and Kidney Diseases (NIDDK) (R03 DK117253 01A1S1 and R01DK121929) and JDRF (grant 2-SRA-2017-498-M-B), P.A. receives funding from NIDDK (R01DK48280), and C.B.V. receives funding from JDRF (1-INO-2019-794-S-B) and Canadian Institutes of Health Research (PJT-153156).

Duality of Interest. No potential conflicts of interest relevant to this article were reported.

References

1. Vasiljević J, Torkko JM, Knoch KP, Solimena M. The making of insulin in health and disease. Diabetologia 2020;63:1981–1989

2. Westermark P, Andersson A, Westermark GT. Islet amyloid polypeptide, islet amyloid, and diabetes mellitus. Physiol Rev 2011;91:795–826

3. Weiss M, Steiner DF, Philipson LH. Insulin biosynthesis, secretion, structure, and structure-activity relationships. In *Endotext*. Feingold KR, Anawalt B, Boyce A, et al., Eds. South Dartmouth, MA, 2000

4. Wasserfall C, Nick HS, Campbell-Thompson M, et al. Persistence of pancreatic insulin mRNA expression and proinsulin protein in type 1 diabetes pancreata. Cell Metab 2017;26:568–575.e3

5. Rodriguez-Calvo T, Zapardiel-Gonzalo J, Amirian N, et al. Increase in pancreatic proinsulin and preservation of β-cell mass in autoantibody-positive donors prior to type 1 diabetes onset. Diabetes 2017;66:1334–1345

6. Courtade JA, Klimek-Abercrombie AM, Chen YC, et al. Measurement of pro-islet amyloid polypeptide (1-48) in diabetes and islet transplants. J Clin Endocrinol Metab 2017;102:2595–2603

7. Sims EK, Chaudhry Z, Watkins R, et al. Elevations in the fasting serum proinsulin–to–C-peptide ratio precede the onset of type 1 diabetes. Diabetes Care 2016;39:1519–1526

8. Leete P, Oram RA, McDonald TJ, et al.; TIGI Study Team. Studies of insulin and proinsulin in pancreas and serum support the existence of aetiopathological endotypes of type 1 diabetes associated with age at diagnosis. Diabetologia 2020;63:1258–1267

9. Davis AK, DuBose SN, Haller MJ, et al.; T1D Exchange Clinic Network. Prevalence of detectable C-peptide according to age at diagnosis and duration of type 1 diabetes. Diabetes Care 2015;38:476–481

10. Sims EK, Bahnson HT, Nyalwidhe J, et al.; T1D Exchange Residual C-peptide Study Group. Proinsulin secretion is a persistent feature of type 1 diabetes. Diabetes Care 2019;42:258–264

11. Tersey SA, Nishiki Y, Templin AT, et al. Islet β-cell endoplasmic reticulum stress precedes the onset of type 1 diabetes in the nonobese diabetic mouse model. Diabetes 2012;61:818–827

12. Mallone R, Eizirik DL. Presumption of innocence for beta cells: why are they vulnerable autoimmune targets in type 1 diabetes? Diabetologia 2020;63: 1999–2006

13. Atkinson MA, Bluestone JA, Eisenbarth GS, et al. How does type 1 diabetes develop? The notion of homicide or β-cell suicide revisited. Diabetes 2011;60:1370–1379

14. Sims EK, Evans-Molina C, Tersey SA, Eizirik DL, Mirmira RG. Biomarkers of islet beta cell stress and death in type 1 diabetes. Diabetologia 2018;61: 2259–2265

15. Van Dalem A, Demeester S, Balti EV, et al.; Belgian Diabetes Registry. Prediction of impending type 1 diabetes through automated dual-label measurement of proinsulin:C-peptide ratio. PLoS One 2016;11:e0166702

16. Røder ME, Knip M, Hartling SG, Karjalainen J, Akerblom HK; The Childhood Diabetes in Finland Study Group. Disproportionately elevated proinsulin levels precede the onset of insulin-dependent diabetes mellitus in siblings with low first phase insulin responses. J Clin Endocrinol Metab 1994; 79:1570–1575

17. Truyen I, De Pauw P, Jørgensen PN, et al.; Belgian Diabetes Registry. Proinsulin levels and the proinsulin:c-peptide ratio complement autoantibody measurement for predicting type 1 diabetes. Diabetologia 2005;48:2322–2329

18. Truyen I, De Grijse J, Weets I, et al.; Belgian Diabetes Registry. Identification of prediabetes in first-degree relatives at intermediate risk of type 1 diabetes. Clin Exp Immunol 2007;149:243–250

19. Snorgaard O, Hartling SG, Binder C. Proinsulin and C-peptide at onset and during 12 months cyclosporin treatment of type 1 (insulin-dependent) diabetes mellitus. Diabetologia 1990;33:36–42

20. Watkins RA, Evans-Molina C, Terrell JK, et al. Proinsulin and heat shock protein 90 as biomarkers of beta-cell stress in the early period after onset of type 1 diabetes. Transl Res 2016;168:96–106.e1

21. Schölin A, Nyström L, Arnqvist H, et al.; Diabetes Incidence Study Group in Sweden (DISS). Proinsulin/C-peptide ratio, glucagon and remission in new-onset type 1 diabetes mellitus in young adults. Diabet Med 2011;28:156–161

22. Quattrin T, Haller MJ, Steck AK, et al.; T1GER Study Investigators. Golimumab and beta-cell function in youth with new-onset type 1 diabetes. N Engl J Med 2020;383:2007–2017

23. Herold KC, Bundy BN, Long SA, et al.; Type 1 Diabetes TrialNet Study Group. An anti-CD3 antibody, teplizumab, in relatives at risk for type 1 diabetes. N Engl J Med 2019;381:603–613

24. Heding LG, Ludvigsson J. Human proinsulin in insulin-treated juvenile diabetics. Acta Paediatr Scand Suppl 1977;270:48–52

25. Steenkamp DW, Cacicedo JM, Sahin-Efe A, Sullivan C, Sternthal E. Preserved proinsulin secretion in long-standing type 1 diabetes. Endocr Pract 2017;23:1387–1393

26. Loopstra-Masters RC, Haffner SM, Lorenzo C, Wagenknecht LE, Hanley AJ. Proinsulin-to-C-peptide ratio versus proinsulin-to-insulin ratio in the prediction of incident diabetes: the Insulin Resistance Atherosclerosis Study (IRAS). Diabetologia 2011;54:3047–3054

27. Heaton DA, Millward BA, Gray IP, et al. Increased proinsulin levels as an early indicator of B-cell dysfunction in non-diabetic twins of type 1 (insulin-dependent) diabetic patients. Diabetologia 1988;31:182–184

28. Spinas GA, Snorgaard O, Hartling SG, Oberholzer M, Berger W. Elevated proinsulin levels related to islet cell antibodies in first-degree relatives of IDDM patients. Diabetes Care 1992;15:632–637

29. Lindgren FA, Hartling SG, Dahlquist GG, Binder C, Efendić S, Persson BE. Glucose-induced insulin response is reduced and proinsulin response

increased in healthy siblings of type 1 diabetic patients. Diabet Med 1991;8: 638–643

30. Sims EK, Syed F, Nyalwidhe J, et al. Abnormalities in proinsulin processing in islets from individuals with longstanding T1D. Transl Res 2019; 213:90–99

31. Mezza T, Ferraro PM, Sun VA, et al. Increased β-cell workload modulates proinsulin-to-insulin ratio in humans. Diabetes 2018;67:2389–2396

32. Hostens K, Pavlovic D, Zambre Y, et al. Exposure of human islets to cytokines can result in disproportionately elevated proinsulin release. J Clin Invest 1999;104:67–72

33. Eizirik DL, Pasquali L, Cnop M. Pancreatic β-cells in type 1 and type 2 diabetes mellitus: different pathways to failure. Nat Rev Endocrinol 2020;16: 349–362

34. Marhfour I, Lopez XM, Lefkaditis D, et al. Expression of endoplasmic reticulum stress markers in the islets of patients with type 1 diabetes. Diabetologia 2012;55:2417–2420

35. Fonseca SG, Ishigaki S, Oslowski CM, et al. Wolfram syndrome 1 gene negatively regulates ER stress signaling in rodent and human cells. J Clin Invest 2010;120:744–755

36. Liu M, Hodish I, Haataja L, et al. Proinsulin misfolding and diabetes: mutant INS gene-induced diabetes of youth. Trends Endocrinol Metab 2010; 21:652–659

37. Denroche HC, Verchere CB. IAPP and type 1 diabetes: implications for immunity, metabolism and islet transplants. J Mol Endocrinol 2018;60:R57–R75

38. Kahn SE, Templin AT, Hull RL, Verchere CB. Probing the meaning of persistent propeptide release in type 1 diabetes. Diabetes Care 2019;42:183–185

39. Gonzalez-Duque S, Azoury ME, Colli ML, et al. Conventional and neo-antigenic peptides presented by β cells are targeted by circulating naïve CD8+ T cells in type 1 diabetic and healthy donors. Cell Metab 2018;28:946–960.e6

40. James EA, Pietropaolo M, Mamula MJ. Immune recognition of β-cells: neoepitopes as key players in the loss of tolerance. Diabetes 2018;67:1035–1042

41. Hsu HT, Janßen L, Lawand M, et al. Endoplasmic reticulum targeting alters regulation of expression and antigen presentation of proinsulin. J Immunol 2014;192:4957–4966

42. Sidney J, Vela JL, Friedrich D, et al. Low HLA binding of diabetes-associated CD8+ T-cell epitopes is increased by post translational modifications. BMC Immunol 2018;19:12

43. Battaglia M, Ahmed S, Anderson MS, et al. Introducing the endotype concept to address the challenge of disease heterogeneity in type 1 diabetes. Diabetes Care 2020;43:5–12

44. Ball GD, Huang TT-K, Gower BA, et al. Longitudinal changes in insulin sensitivity, insulin secretion, and β-cell function during puberty. J Pediatr 2006;148:16–22

45. Talchai C, Xuan S, Lin HV, Sussel L, Accili D. Pancreatic β cell dedifferentiation as a mechanism of diabetic β cell failure. Cell 2012;150: 1223–1234

46. Lee H, Lee YS, Harenda Q, et al. Beta cell dedifferentiation induced by IRE1α deletion prevents type 1 diabetes. Cell Metab 2020;31:822–836.e5

47. Kahn SE, Halban PA. Release of incompletely processed proinsulin is the cause of the disproportionate proinsulinemia of NIDDM. Diabetes 1997;46: 1725–1732

48. Panzer JK, Hiller H, Cohrs CM, et al. Pancreas tissue slices from organ donors enable in situ analysis of type 1 diabetes pathogenesis. JCI Insight 2020;5:e134525

49. Houssa P, Dinesen B, Deberg M, et al. First direct assay for intact human proinsulin. Clin Chem 1998;44:1514–1519

50. Sobey WJ, Beer SF, Carrington CA, et al. Sensitive and specific two-site immunoradiometric assays for human insulin, proinsulin, 65-66 split and 32-33 split proinsulins. Biochem J 1989;260:535–541

51. Clark PM, Levy JC, Cox L, Burnett M, Turner RC, Hales CN. Immunoradiometric assay of insulin, intact proinsulin and 32-33 split proinsulin and radioimmunoassay of insulin in diet-treated type 2 (non-insulin-dependent) diabetic subjects. Diabetologia 1992;35:469–474

52. Clark PM. Assays for insulin, proinsulin(s) and C-peptide. Ann Clin Biochem 1999;36:541–564

53. Rodland KD. As if biomarker discovery isn't hard enough: the consequences of poorly characterized reagents. Clin Chem 2014;60:290–291

54. Hoofnagle AN, Wener MH. The fundamental flaws of immunoassays and potential solutions using tandem mass spectrometry. J Immunol Methods 2009;347:3–11

55. Lange V, Picotti P, Domon B, Aebersold R. Selected reaction monitoring for quantitative proteomics: a tutorial. Mol Syst Biol 2008;4:222

56. Addona TA, Abbatiello SE, Schilling B, et al. Multi-site assessment of the precision and reproducibility of multiple reaction monitoring-based measurements of proteins in plasma. Nat Biotechnol 2009;27:633–641

57. Onengut-Gumuscu S, Chen WM, Burren O, et al.; Type 1 Diabetes Genetics Consortium. Fine mapping of type 1 diabetes susceptibility loci and evidence for colocalization of causal variants with lymphoid gene enhancers. Nat Genet 2015;47:381–386

58. Udler MS, Kim J, von Grotthuss M, et al.; Type 2 diabetes genetic loci informed by multi-trait associations point to disease mechanisms and subtypes: a soft clustering analysis. PLoS Med 2018;15:e1002654

59. Colli ML, Paula FM, Marselli L, et al. Coxsackievirus B tailors the unfolded protein response to favour viral amplification in pancreatic β cells. J Innate Immun 2019;11:375–390

60. Moore M, Ferguson J, Rigsby P, Hockley J, Burns C. WHO International Collaborative Study of the Proposed 1st International Standard for Human Proinsulin. World Health Org., 2014. Accessed 30 January 2019. Available from https://www.who.int/biologicals/bs_2237is_for_human_proinsulin_updated.pdf

61. Hartling SG, Lindgren F, Dahlqvist G, Persson B, Binder C. Elevated proinsulin in healthy siblings of IDDM patients independent of HLA identity. Diabetes 1989;38:1271–1274

62. Ramzy A, Asadi A, Kieffer TJ. Revisiting proinsulin processing: evidence that human β-cells process proinsulin with prohormone convertase (PC) 1/3 but not PC2. Diabetes 2020;69:1451–1462

63. Asadi A, Bruin JE, Kieffer TJ. Characterization of antibodies to products of proinsulin processing using immunofluorescence staining of pancreas in multiple species. J Histochem Cytochem 2015;63:646–662

A High-Fat Diet Attenuates AMPK α1 in Adipocytes to Induce Exosome Shedding and Nonalcoholic Fatty Liver Development In Vivo

Chenghui Yan,[1,2] Xiaoxiang Tian,[2] Jiayin Li,[2,3] Dan Liu,[2] Ding Ye,[1] Zhonglin Xie,[1] Yaling Han,[2] and Ming-Hui Zou[1]

Diabetes 2021;70:577–588 | https://doi.org/10.2337/db20-0146

Exosomes are important for intercellular communication, but the role of exosomes in the communication between adipose tissue (AT) and the liver remains unknown. The aim of this study is to determine the contribution of AT-derived exosomes in nonalcoholic fatty liver disease (NAFLD). Exosome components, liver fat content, and liver function were monitored in AT in mice fed a high-fat diet (HFD) or treated with metformin or GW4869 and with AMPKα1-floxed (Prkaα1[fl/fl]/wild-type [WT]), Prkaα1[−/−], liver tissue-specific Prkaα1[−/−], or AT-specific Prkaα1[−/−] modification. In cultured adipocytes and white AT, the absence of AMPKα1 increased exosome release and exosomal proteins by elevating tumor susceptibility gene 101 (TSG101)–mediated exosome biogenesis. In adipocytes treated with palmitic acid, TSG101 facilitated scavenger receptor class B (CD36) sorting into exosomes. CD36-containing exosomes were then endocytosed by hepatocytes to induce lipid accumulation and inflammation. Consistently, an HFD induced more severe lipid accumulation and cell death in Prkaα1[−/−] and AT-specific Prkaα1[−/−] mice than in WT and liver-specific Prkaα1[−/−] mice. AMPK activation by metformin reduced adipocyte-mediated exosome release and mitigated fatty liver development in WT and liver-specific Prkaα1[−/−] mice. Moreover, administration of the exosome inhibitor GW4869 blocked exosome secretion and alleviated HFD-induced fatty livers in Prkaα1[−/−] and adipocyte-specific Prkaα1[−/−] mice. We conclude that HFD-mediated AMPKα1 inhibition promotes NAFLD by increasing numbers of AT CD36-containing exosomes.

Exosomes are nanosized biovesicles (30–100 nm) secreted by cells, and they contain miRNAs, mRNAs, and proteins from parent cells (1). When internalized by recipient cells, exosomes exert regulatory effects by delivering their internal bioactive components (2). Increasing evidence indicates that exosomes play important roles in intercellular communications, including the immune response (3), tumor progression (4), and cell metabolism (5). Understanding the molecular mechanisms by which exosome biogenesis and heterogeneity are regulated by cells, including the cargo components and secretion, is a major challenge.

Adipose tissue (AT) is an important endocrine organ that has a central role regulating energy metabolism (6,7). Obesity-induced AT damage and ectopic deposition are the primary pathological factors that lead to insulin resistance, diabetes, and a nonalcoholic fatty liver (NAFL) (8–10). Notably, AT is a major source of exosomes. For example, exosome secretion is observed in cultured AT (11,12) and adipocytes (13). In addition, obesity significantly increases exosome secretion from AT in vivo (14). In contrast, specific stimuli that are associated with a reduction in body weight, such as starvation and rapamycin, significantly reduce exosome secretion (15,16). These results strongly suggest that AT is a major source of circulating exosomes and that body weight dynamics modulate circulating exosome levels. Because obesity is closely associated with the development of metabolic disorders, including NAFL disease (NAFLD), it is imperative that the role of AT-derived exosomes in the development of a NAFL is identified.

[1]Center for Molecular and Translational Medicine, Georgia State University, Atlanta, GA

[2]Cardiovascular Research Institute and Department of Cardiology, General Hospital of Northern Theater Command, Shenyang, China

[3]College of Life and Health Sciences, Northeastern University, Shenyang, China

Corresponding author: Chenghui Yan, yanch1029@163.com, or Yaling Han, hanyaling@263.net

Received 12 February 2020 and accepted 19 November 2020

This article contains supplementary material online at https://doi.org/10.2337/figshare.13259768.

AMPK is a ubiquitous energy-sensing enzyme within cells (17–19) that is critical to maintaining metabolic homeostasis. AMPK activation is thought to mediate the beneficial effects of metformin, the most widely used antidiabetic drug worldwide (20,21). Intriguingly, reduced AMPK activity in white AT (WAT) occurs in obese animals and humans (22). The effect of attenuated AMPK activity on exosome biogenesis, cargo contents, and shedding in WAT remains unknown. In this study, we report that AMPKα1 activation in WAT mitigates high-fat diet (HFD)–induced NAFL by ablating exosome biogenesis and secretion.

RESEARCH DESIGN AND METHODS

Cell Culture and Induction of Adipocyte Differentiation

The mouse preadipocyte cell line 3T3L1 and HepG2 cells were cultured in high-glucose Dulbecco's minimal essential medium with 10% exosome-depleted FBS (System Biosciences, Palo Alto, CA), 1% Glutamax (Invitrogen, Carlsbad, CA), 1% nonessential amino acids (Invitrogen), 1% sodium pyruvate (Invitrogen), and 1% penicillin/streptomycin (Gibco, Grand Island, NY). Cultured cells were incubated at 37°C in a humidified atmosphere of 5% CO_2 and 95% air. 3T3L1 cell differentiation was carried out as described previously (23). Briefly, 3T3L1 cells were cultured in preadipocyte differentiation medium (ScienCell Research Laboratories, Carlsbad, CA) for 7–10 days to induce their differentiation into mature adipocytes.

Palmitic Acid Preparation and Treatments

Differentiated 3T3L1 adipocytes were treated with palmitic acid (PA) (0.3 mmol/L) dissolved in 0.5% albumin (Sigma-Aldrich, St. Louis, MO) for 12 or 24 h. To induce endocytosis or lipid accumulation, HepG2 cells were treated with exosomes with or without PA.

Exosome Isolation and Counting

Media were collected after culturing of cells or AT under the designated conditions. Exosomes were extracted with Total Exosome Isolation Kits (Thermo Fisher Scientific, Waltham, MA) according to the manufacturer's instructions. Exosome pellets were suspended in PBS. To quantify isolated exosomes, acetylcholinesterase activity assays were performed using the EXOCET system (System Biosciences). To characterize exosomes, the isolated preparations were analyzed with a dynamic light-scattering system (Zetasizer Nano; Malvern Panalytical, Malvern, U.K.) and transmission electron microscopy (TEM).

Western Blotting and Immunoprecipitation

Cell or AT exosome protein were extracted using radioimmunoprecipitation assay buffer (sc-24948; Santa Cruz Biotechnology, Dallas, TX) and quantified using the BCA protein assay (#23225; Pierce Biotechnology, Rockford, IL). Immunoprecipitates and cell or exosome lysates were subjected to Western blotting with specific primary antibodies (Supplementary Table 1) followed by detection with

horseradish peroxidase–conjugated secondary antibodies and enhanced chemiluminescence.

Histology and Immunohistochemistry

Liver tissue sections or HepG2 cells were stained with hematoxylin and eosin (H&E) or Oil Red O to quantify the lesion sizes. For immunostaining, HepG2 cells were incubated first with cleaved caspase-3 antibodies (Cell Signaling Technology, Danvers, MA) and subsequently with fluorochrome-conjugated secondary antibodies.

Proteomic Profiling Mass Spectrometry System

Samples were dissolved in lysis buffer composed of 7 mol/L urea (Bio-Rad Laboratories, Hercules, CA), 2 mol/L thiourea (Sigma-Aldrich), and 0.1% 3-cholamidopropyl dimethylammonio 1-propanesulfonate (Bio-Rad Laboratories). Then, the tissues were ground with three TiO_2 abrasive beads (70 Hz for 120 s) followed by centrifugation at 5,000g for 5 min at 4°C. The supernatant was collected and centrifuged at 15,000g for 30 min at 4°C. The final supernatants were collected and stored at −80°C until use. Desalted peptides were labeled with iTRAQ reagents (iTRAQ Reagent-8PLEX Multiplex Kit; Sigma-Aldrich) according to the manufacturer's instructions. Briefly, the iTRAQ-labeled peptide mix was fractionated using a C18 column (Waters BEH C18 4.6 × 250 mm, 5 μm; Waters Corporation, Milford, MA) on a Rigol L3000 HPLC system (Rigol, Beijing, China) operating at 1 mL/min with a column oven set at 50°C. Mobile phases A (2% acetonitrile [ACN], pH adjusted to 10.0 using NH_4OH) and B (98% ACN, pH adjusted to 10.0 using NH_4OH) were used to develop a gradient elution. The acquired peptide fractions were suspended with 20 μL buffer A (0.1% formic acid and 2% ACN) and centrifuged at 14,000g for 10 min. Next, 10 μL of the supernatants were injected into the nano-ultrahigh-performance liquid chromatography tandem mass spectrometry (MS) system consisting of a Nanoflow HPLC system (EASY-nLC 1000) and Orbitrap Fusion Lumos MS (Thermo Fisher Scientific). Identification parameters were set as follows: precursor ion mass tolerance, ±15 ppm; fragment ion mass tolerance, ±20 mmu; maximum missed cleavages, 2; static modification, carboxyamidomethylation (57.021 Da) of Cys residues; and dynamic modifications, oxidation modification (+15.995 Da) of Met residues. Primary data with a P value ≤0.05 and a difference ratio ≥1.2 were selected for further analysis.

Quantitative Real-time PCR

Total RNA was extracted from cells or AT with an RNeasy Mini Kit (#74106; Qiagen, Hilden, Germany) and reverse transcribed with an iScript cDNA synthesis kit (#170-8891; Bio-Rad Laboratories). Real-time PCR was performed with the CFX96 Real-Time System (Bio-Rad Laboratories). The primer sequences used for amplifying mouse genes were as follows: Gapdh forward, 5′-CTA C CCC ACG GCA AGT TCA-3′ and reverse, 5′-CCA GTA GAC TCC ACG ACA AC-3′; tumor susceptibility gene 101 (Tsg101) forward,

5'-CCA TCC CCT CTA GTG CTC GTC-3' and reverse, 5'-TGC GGA AGA GTC GGT AGT CT-3'; Cd63 forward, 5'-TCA TCC AAA CGT GTA TCC TTC TG-3' and reverse, 5'-CTT GTG CTC GGA CCC TTT TCT-3'; and Cd36 forward, 5'-TGA TTA ACG GGA CAG ACG GAG AC-3' and reverse, 5'-ACG TTC TCA AAG CTG CTG AAA GTG-3'.

Gene Silencing

siRNAs targeting mouse *Prkaα1* (sc-29647), *Prkaα2* (sc-38924), *Cd63* (sc-35792), *Tsg101* (sc-36753), and *Cd36* (sc-37245) were purchased from Santa Cruz Biotechnology. Mouse 3T3L1 cells were transfected with 10 μmol/L siRNA using Lipofectamine RNAiMAX (13778150; Life Technologies, Carlsbad, CA) according to the manufacturer's instructions.

Generation of Hepatocyte- or Adipocyte-Specific Prkaα1 Knockout Mice

$Prkaα1^{-/-}$ and $Prkaα2^{-/-}$ mice were generated as previously described (24,25). $Prkaα1^{fl/fl}$ mice were provided by Dr. Benoit Viollet. Hepatocyte- or adipocyte-specific *Prkaα1* knockout mice were generated by crossing $Prkaα1^{fl/fl}$ mice with Alb^{Cre} or $Adiponectin^{Cre}$ ($Adipo^{Cre}$) transgenic mice. The mice were fed an HFD (60% kcal fat from lard; D12492; Research Diets, New Brunswick, NJ) or a normal diet, followed by collection of WAT or liver tissue. Animal studies were approved by the Institutional Animal Care and Use Committee at Georgia State University. Serum cholesterol and triglyceride levels were measured using Infinity reagents from Thermo Fisher Scientific according to the manufacturer's instructions (26).

Statistical Analyses

Data obtained were analyzed using SPSS version 24.0 (IBM Corporation, Armonk, NY) and are presented as mean ± SEM. Statistical differences were analyzed by one-way ANOVA followed by Tukey post hoc test. Differences were considered significant at $P < 0.05$.

Data and Resource Availability

The data sets generated during and/or analyzed during the current study are available from the corresponding author upon reasonable request.

RESULTS

Inactivation of AMPK Increases Exosome Secretion in Adipocytes

To elucidate the relationship between AMPKα and exosome secretion in adipocytes, adipocytes were treated with either the AMPK activator AICAR (1 mmol/L) or the AMPK inhibitor compound C (CC; 50 μmol/L) (27) for 6–24 h. Exosomes were then isolated and purified. TEM and diameter analyses revealed approximately spherical vesicles (Supplementary Fig. 1A) that had diameters of 40–200 nm (Supplementary Fig. 1B). Consistent with an earlier report of adipocytes (27), Western blotting showed that adipocyte treatment with AICAR for 6 h significantly increased AMPK phosphorylation at Thr172. AMPK activation was associated with a significant reduction in exosome number

(Fig. 1A and Supplementary Fig. 1B). In contrast, CC dramatically reduced AMPKα phosphorylation (Supplementary Fig. 1C and D) and simultaneously increased exosomes in adipocytes (Fig. 1A and Supplementary Fig. 1B).

CD81 and CD63 are the two major exosome marker proteins, and their expression in exosomes can be used to quantify exosome secretion by cells or tissues (28,29). We next investigated the effect of altered AMPK activity on CD81 and CD63 levels in adipocyte-derived exosomes. Inhibition of AMPK by CC treatment significantly increased CD81 and CD63 levels in exosomes (Fig. 1B–D). Conversely, activation of AMPK by AICAR significantly decreased CD81 and CD63 levels in exosomes (Fig. 1B–D). These results suggest that AMPK activity negatively regulates exosome secretion in adipocytes.

Silencing of AMPKα1, But Not AMPKα2, Increases Exosome Secretion in Cultured Adipocytes

Noting that AMPK has two catalytic isoforms, AMPKα1 and α2 (25), we next identified the AMPKα isoform that regulates exosome secretion in adipocytes. Adipocytes were transfected with si*Prkaa1* (*Prkaα1* siRNA) or si*Prkaα2*-(*Prkaα2* siRNA). Silencing of *Prkaα1*, but not *Prkaα2*, dramatically increased exosome secretion in adipocytes (Fig. 1F–H). Consistent with this finding, *Prkaα1* silencing caused a robust increase in CD63 and CD81 levels in adipocyte-derived exosomes (Fig. 1F–H). *Prkaα2* silencing had no effect on CD63 and CD81 levels in the exosomes (Fig. 1E–H).

Deletion of AMPKα1 Enhances Exosome Release From Cultured WAT

We further verified that AMPKα1 inactivation increased exosome release ex vivo by collecting exosomes from the medium of cultured wild-type (WT; C57BL/6J), *Prkaα1*-knockout ($Prkaα1^{-/-}$), and *Prkaα2*-knockout ($Prkaα2^{-/-}$) mouse WATs. Similar to the findings with cultured adipocytes, $Prkaα1^{-/-}$ WAT shed more exosomes (Fig. 1I) and had higher levels of exosomal CD63 and CD81 proteins (Fig. 1J–L) when compared with WT WAT. Deletion of *Prkaα2* had no effect on exosome number or exosomal CD63 and CD81 levels (Fig. 1J–L). Taken together, our results indicate that AMPKα1, but not AMPKα2, inhibits exosome secretion in adipocytes.

AMPKα1 Deficiency Enhances Exosome Release Independently of CD63

There are two pathways that regulate exosome secretion: the endosomal sorting complexes required for transport (ESCRT)–dependent and ESCRT-independent pathways (30,31). To determine the mechanism by which AMPK regulates exosome release, we first quantified CD63 expression in adipocytes treated with AICAR (1 mmol/L) or CC (50 μmol/L). AICAR treatment significantly increased CD63 protein levels. Conversely, CC treatment decreased CD63 protein level in adipocytes (Supplementary Fig. 2A and B). However, neither AICAR nor CC altered CD63 mRNA expression in adipocytes (Supplementary Fig. 2C). Similarly, *Prkaα1* silencing reduced CD63 protein levels

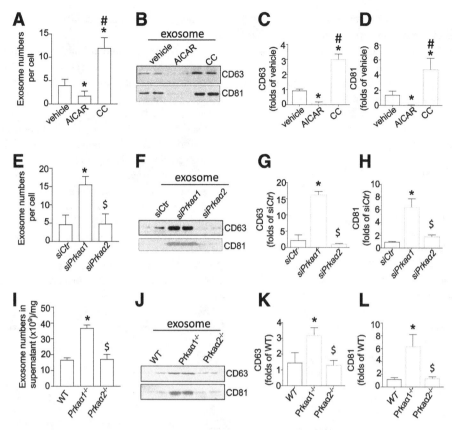

Figure 1—AMPKα1 inhibition enhances exosome release from adipocytes and WAT. *A*: The exosomes internalized by adipocytes that were treated with AICAR (1 mmol/L) or CC (50 nmol/L) were counted using the EXOCET Kit. *B*: Samples with equal amounts of exosomes were analyzed for CD63 and CD81 with Western blotting. *C* and *D*: Densitometric analysis of the Western blots from *B*. *E*: Quantification of exosomes in the medium of 3T3L1-derived adipocytes that were transfected with si*Prkaα1* or si*Prkaα2*. *F*: Samples with equal amounts of exosomes were analyzed for CD63 and CD81 by Western blotting. *G* and *H*: Densitometric analysis of the Western blots from *F*. *I*: Quantification of exosomes in WAT in WT, *Prkaα1*$^{-/-}$, and *Prkaα2*$^{-/-}$ mice (*n* = 5). *J*: Samples with equal amounts of exosomes were analyzed for CD63 and CD81 by Western blotting. *K* and *L*: Densitometric analysis of the Western blots from *J*. *P < 0.05 vs. control (*n* = 3); #P < 0.05 vs. control group treated with AICAR treatment; $P < 0.05 vs. control group treated with siPrkaα1$^{-/-}$ or Prkaα1$^{-/-}$ group (*n* = 3).

(Supplementary Fig. 2*D* and *E*), but had no effect on CD63 mRNA expression (Supplementary Fig. 2*F*). To determine whether reduced CD63 mediated AMPKα1 deficiency–enhanced exosome secretion, adipocytes were treated with the ceramide-induced exosome inhibitor GW4869 (32). GW4869 enhanced CD63 protein levels (Supplementary Fig. 2*H* and *I*) and reduced exosome secretion in a dose-dependent manner (Supplementary Fig. 2*G*).

To further investigate the effects of reduced CD63 on AMPKα1 deficiency–enhanced exosome secretion, adipocytes that underwent CD63 siRNA transfection were treated with CC to inhibit AMPK activity. *Cd63* silencing did not alter exosome numbers in cells transfected with control siRNA and did not prevent CC-enhanced exosome numbers in adipocytes (Supplementary Fig. 2*J*). These results suggest that AMPKα1 inhibition or silencing increases adipocyte exosome secretion independently of CD63.

AMPKα1 Deficiency Enhances Exosome Biogenesis by Upregulating TSG101

TSG101 is a core component of the ESCRT pathway and plays an important role in the biogenesis of multivesicular

bodies (MVBs) (33). Therefore, we investigated whether TSG101 was required for AMPKα1-regulated exosome release. To this end, we first studied the effect of TSG101 on AMPKα1 expression. AICAR significantly reduced TSG101 protein levels, and CC markedly enhanced TSG101 protein levels (Fig. 2*A* and *B*). Neither AICAR nor CC affected TSG101 mRNA expression (Supplementary Fig. 3*A*).

Next, we tested if AMPKα1 directly regulated TSG101 expression by transfecting 3T3L1-derived adipocytes with control siRNA or *Prkaα1* siRNA (si*Prkaα1*). Silencing *Prkaα1*, but not *Prkaα2*, robustly increased TSG101 protein levels (Fig. 2*C* and *D*). Neither si*Prkaα1* nor si*Prkaα2* affected TSG101 mRNA expression (Supplementary Fig. 3*B*).

To validate the results with cultured adipocytes, we measured TSG101 expression in cultured WATs from WT, *Prkaα1*$^{-/-}$, and *Prkaα2*$^{-/-}$ mice. Consistent with the prior data, TSG101 levels in *Prkaα1*$^{-/-}$ WAT were significantly higher than TSG101 levels in either WT or *Prkaα2*$^{-/-}$ WATs (Fig. 2*E* and *F*).

Next, we investigated if increased TSG101 protein was required for AMPKα1-mediated exosome release. Our data indicated that *Tsg101* silencing in adipocytes (Supplementary

Fig. 4) abolished CC-enhanced exosome secretion (Fig. 2G) and elevated levels of the exosomal proteins CD63 and CD81 (Fig. 2H–J). Furthermore, TEM revealed that the number of MVBs in si*Prkaα1*-treated adipocytes was significantly higher when compared with si*Control* (si*Ctr*)–treated cells. Silencing both *Tsg101* and *Prkaα1* dramatically reduced the biogenesis of MVBs (Fig. 2K). Taken together, TSG101 is required for AMPKα1 inhibition–induced exosome formation and exosomal protein expression in adipocytes.

PA Increases Exosome Release by Inhibiting AMPKα1

Obesity increases exosome secretion from WAT (12,13), and PA suppresses AMPK activity in WAT. We hypothesized that PA promotes exosome secretion from WAT via AMPK inhibition. To test this hypothesis, we treated adipocytes with AICAR (1 mmol/L) for 4 h, followed by treatment with PA (300 μmol/L) for 24 h. We next analyzed exosome secretion and found that PA treatment dramatically increased exosome secretion associated with low levels of phosphorylated AMPKα (Supplementary Fig. 5A–C). Further, PA-induced exosome increase

was abolished by AICAR treatment (Supplementary Fig. 5A–C).

Next, we determined if *Prkaα1* overexpression inhibited PA-enhanced exosome secretion. Overexpression of the adenovirus encoding for *Prkaα1* almost completely prevented PA-enhanced exosome secretion (Supplementary Fig. 5D). We further examined if AMPKα1 inhibition blocked the effect of AICAR on PA-enhanced exosome secretion. AICAR treatment abolished PA-increased exosome secretion in WT WATs and $Prkaα2^{-/-}$ WATs but had no effect on $Prkaα1^{-/-}$ WATs (Supplementary Fig. 5E). Moreover, the increase of exosomal proteins CD63 and CD81 induced by PA was also inhibited by AICAR treatment (Supplementary Fig. 5F and G). These results suggest that PA increases exosome release by inhibiting AMPKα1.

PA-Treated Exosomes Released From AMPKα1-Deficient Adipocytes Exacerbate Hepatocyte Damage

To understand the contribution of WAT-derived exosomes to liver damage, we investigated the response of cultured hepatocytes to exosomes derived from PA-treated adipocytes.

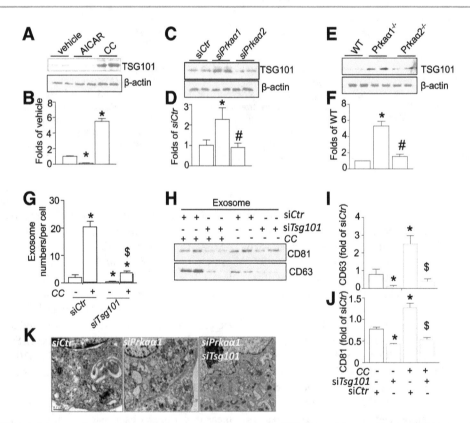

Figure 2—AMPKα1 deficiency enhances exosome biogenesis by upregulating TSG101. *A*: Western blot for TSG101 in adipocytes treated with AICAR or CC. *B*: Densitometric analysis of TSG101 Western blots from *A*. *C*: Western blot for TSG101 in adipocytes transfected with siCtr, *siPrkaα1*, and *siPrkaα2* siRNA. *D*: Densitometric analysis of TSG101 Western blots from *B*. *E*: Western blot for TSG101 in WT, *Prkaα1$^{-/-}$*, and *Prkaα2$^{-/-}$* adipocytes. *F*: Densitometric analysis of TSG101 Western blots from *E*. *G*: Quantification of exosomes in the medium from adipocytes transfected with si*Tsg101* and treated with or without *CC*. *H*: Western blot for CD63 and CD81 in exosomes derived from adipocytes transfected with si*Tsg101* and treated with or without *CC*. *I* and *J*: Densitometric analysis of CD63 and CD81 Western blots from *H*. *K*: Representative TEM images of MVBs in adipocytes that were transfected with *siPrkaa1 or siTsg101* siRNA and treated with or without CC. Red arrows indicate MVBs. Scale bar = 0.5 μm. *$P < 0.05$ vs. control; #$P < 0.05$ vs. *siPkraα1* or Prkaα1$^{-/-}$ group; $$P < 0.05$ vs. CC-treated *siCtr* group (*n* = 3).

HepG2 cells were treated with equal amounts of exosomes isolated from siCtr- or siPrkaα-transfected adipocytes that were pretreated with or without PA. Interestingly, exosome uptake by HepG2 cells was nonuniform. HepG2 cells favored exosomes that were derived from siPrkaα1-transfected adipocytes pretreated with PA (Fig. 3A and B). Oil Red O staining indicated that lipid accumulation was exacerbated in HepG2 cells that internalized these endosomes (Fig. 3C and D). There was no significant difference in endocytosis or lipid accumulation in HepG2 cells after incubation with exosomes from either siCtr- or siPrkaα1-treated adipocytes without the PA pretreatment (Fig. 3A–D). Importantly, incubating HepG2 cells with PA-pretreated siCtr exosomes increased interleukin-6 (IL-6) and MCP-1 levels, and this effect was augmented with siPrkaα1 exosomes (Fig. 3E–I). Meanwhile, cleaved caspase-3 levels also increased in HepG2 cells after incubation with PA-pretreated siCtr exosomes. Again, the effect in HepG2 cells was amplified after incubation with siPrkaα1 exosomes derived from PA pretreated adipocytes (Fig. 3G and J). These results were verified with immunostaining for cleaved caspase-3 (Fig. 3K and L). Collectively, these data indicate that exosomes derived from PA-pretreated siPrkaα1-deficient adipocytes exacerbate HepG2 cell damage.

PA Treatment Increases CD36 Sorting Into Adipocyte-Derived Exosomes

Next, we investigated whether the protein content of the exosomes derived from PA-treated adipocytes affected exosome internalization. Using a nontargeted proteomic profiling MS system, we found that CD36, a lipid transport receptor, was expressed in higher amounts in the exosomes derived from PA-treated adipocytes (Fig. 4A). To verify our results, we used Western blotting to probe CD36 expression in exosomes derived from PA-treated WT or $Prka\alpha1^{-/-}$ WATs. Interestingly, WT and $Prka\alpha1^{-/-}$ exosomes did not exhibit increased CD36 levels when quantifying WATs. However, CD36 protein levels were significantly higher in exosomes from PA-pretreated WT and $Prka\alpha1^{-/-}$ cells when compared with cells that were not treated with PA (Fig. 4B and C). The highest expression of CD36 was detected in exosomes derived from PA-pretreated $Prka\alpha1^{-/-}$ adipocytes. Increased CD63 and CD81 protein levels were detected in exosomes derived from $Prka\alpha1^{-/-}$, PA-treated WT, and PA-treated $Prka\alpha1^{-/-}$ WATs (Fig. 4B–E). These results suggest that PA treatment increases CD36 sorting into exosomes.

TSG101 Facilitates CD36 Sorting Into Exosomes

To explore the mechanism of CD36 sorting into exosomes, we measured the expression of CD36 in PA-treated WT and $Prka\alpha1^{-/-}$ WATs. Consistent with a previous report (34), PA treatment significantly increased CD36 protein and mRNA levels in WT and $Prka\alpha1^{-/-}$ WATs (Fig. 4F–H). It is important to note that AMPKα1 deficiency alone did not change CD36 mRNA and protein expression in WAT. Next, we explored how CD36 is packaged into the exosomes

derived from PA-treated adipocytes. Immunoprecipitation indicated that CD36 is associated with TSG101 in both the cytosol and exosomes (Fig. 4I). Furthermore, CD36 protein was absent from endosomes after Tsg101 silencing (Fig. 4J and K). Taken together, our results suggest that TSG101 binds to CD36 and recruits CD36 into exosomes.

CD36 Silencing Does Not Affect Exosome Secretion but Decreases Exosome Internalization and HepG2 Damage

To determine whether CD36 was involved in exosome biogenesis, Cd36 expression was knocked down in adipocytes that were transfected with siCtr or $siPrka\alpha1^{-/-}$. Cd36 silencing did not change either total exosome numbers or cytosol TSG101 protein levels in siCtr or $siPrka\alpha1^{-/-}$ adipocytes (Supplementary Fig. 6A–D). Although CD36 silencing significantly reduced exosomal CD36 protein content, it did not affect CD63 expression in exosomes (Supplementary Fig. 6E–G), indicating that Cd36 silencing does not affect exosome secretion in adipocytes.

Next, we investigated if CD36 in exosomes mediated lipid uptake and HepG2 cell damage. HepG2 cells were treated with equal numbers of exosomes isolated from adipocytes that were transfected with siCtr and siCd36. As illustrated in Fig. 5A and B, these experiments revealed a significant decrease in the endocytosis of exosomes derived from Cd36-knockdown adipocytes. Adipocyte pretreatment with PA did not have a pronounced effect on exosome uptake by HepG2 cells. In agreement with the observed endocytosis patterns, the exosomes derived from the Cd36-knockdown adipocytes were associated with decreased lipid accumulation (Fig. 5C and D) and apoptosis in HepG2 cells (Fig. 5E and F). These data suggest that the presence of CD36 augments exosome endocytosis, lipid accumulation, and apoptosis in HepG2 cells.

WAT-Specific AMPKα1 Deletion Enhances HFD-Induced Exosome Release in Serum and WAT

To determine the role of AMPKα1 in exosome secretion from WAT in vivo, we isolated exosomes from the serum and WAT of HFD-fed $Prka\alpha1^{-/-}$, $Prka\alpha1^{fl/fl}$, $Prka\alpha1^{fl/fl}$:$Adipo^{Cre+}$, and $Prka\alpha1^{fl/fl}$:Alb^{Cre+} mice. The HFD treatment significantly increased serum exosome numbers in $Prka\alpha1^{-/-}$ and $Prka\alpha1^{fl/fl}$:$Adipo^{Cre+}$ mice, but not in $Prka\alpha1^{fl/fl}$:Alb^{Cre+} and $Prka\alpha1^{fl/fl}$ mice (Fig. 6A). In addition, CD63 expression increased in the exosomes isolated from $Prka\alpha1^{-/-}$ and $Prka\alpha1^{fl/fl}$:$Adipo^{Cre+}$ mice when compared with the $Prka\alpha1^{fl/fl}$:Alb^{Cre+} and $Prka\alpha1^{fl/fl}$ mice (Fig. 6B). Similarly, PA treatment increased exosome numbers and CD63 protein levels in $Prka\alpha1^{-/-}$ and $Prka\alpha1^{fl/fl}$:$Adipo^{Cre+}$ WATs, but not in $Prka\alpha1^{fl/fl}$:Alb^{Cre+} and $Prka\alpha1^{fl/fl}$ WATs (Fig. 6C and D). These results indicate that an AMPKα1 deficiency in WAT enhances HFD-induced exosome release in serum and WAT.

Absence of AMPKα1 in WAT Exacerbates an HFD-Induced Fatty Liver

To evaluate if WAT derived-exosomes were involved in an HFD-induced fatty liver, we fed $Prka\alpha1^{fl/fl}$, $Prka\alpha1^{-/-}$,

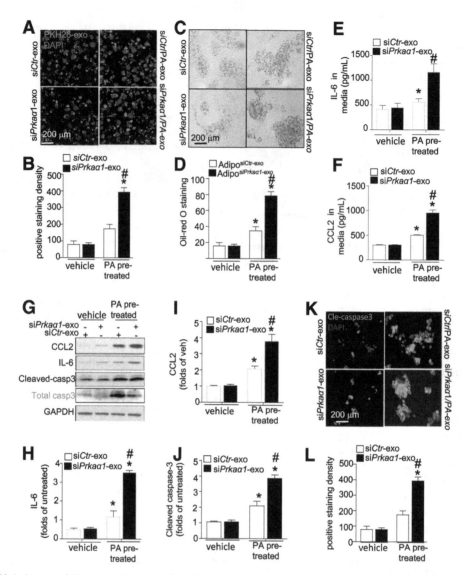

Figure 3—AMPKα1 downregulation exacerbates HepG2 cell damage induced by exosomes derived from PA-treated adipocytes. HepG2 cells were treated with exosomes (exo) derived from adipocytes (Adipo) that were pretreated with or without PA and transfected with *siCtr* or *siPrkaα1*. *A*: Immunofluorescence analysis of HepG2 cells that internalized PKH26-labeled exosomes. *B*: Quantitative analysis of exosome internalization by HepG2 cells. *C*: Representative images of Oil Red O staining. *D*: Quantification of Oil Red O staining. ELISA for IL-6 (*E*) and CCL2 (*F*) in the supernatant of HepG2 cells. *G*: Western blot for IL-6, CCL2, total caspase-3 (casp3), and cleaved caspase-3 in HepG2 cells. *H–J*: Densitometric analysis of Western blots for IL-6, CCL2, and cleaved caspase-3. *K*: Immunostaining for cleaved caspase-3 (Cle-caspase3) in HepG2 cells. *L*: Quantification of cleaved caspase-3 staining. *$P < 0.05$ vs. control; #$P < 0.05$ vs. vehicle group ($n = 3$). si*Ctr*-exo, exosome derived from adipocytes transfected with control siRNA; si*Ctr*/PA-exo, exosome derived from adipocytes transfected with control siRNA and pretreated with PA; si*Pkraα1*-exo, exosome derived from adipocytes transfected with *Pkraa1* siRNA; si*Pkraα1*/PA-exo, exosome derived from adipocytes transfected with *Pkraa1* siRNA and pretreated with PA.

Prkaα1^{fl/fl}:*Adipo*^{Cre+}, and *Prkaα1*^{fl/fl}:*Alb*^{Cre+} mice an HFD for 3 months. An HFD had a greater effect on increased overall mouse body weight (Fig. 6*E*), the amount of weight gained (Fig. 6*F*), increased liver weight (Fig. 6*G*), and the ratio of liver weight to body weight (Fig. 6*H*) in *Prkaα1*^{−/−} and *Prkaa1*^{fl/fl}:*Adipo*^{Cre+} mice when compared with *Prkaα1*^{fl/fl} and *Prkaa1*^{fl/fl}:*Alb*^{Cre+} mice. In addition, serum and hepatic triglycerides (Fig. 6*H*), cholesterol (Fig. 6*H*), AST, ALT, and inflammatory factors tumor necrosis factor-α and IL-6 levels (Supplementary Fig. 7) were higher in *Prkaa1*^{−/−} and *Prkaa1*^{fl/fl}:*Adipo*^{Cre+} mice when compared with *Prkaa1*^{fl/fl} and

Prkaa1^{fl/fl}:*Alb*^{Cre+} mice (Fig. 6*I–L*). The elevated lipid accumulation and fatty liver development in *Prkaa1*^{−/−} and *Prkaa1*^{fl/fl}:*Adipo*^{Cre+} mice were verified by Oil Red O and H&E staining (Fig. 6*M*). These results confirm that an AMPKα1 deficiency in ATs aggravates HFD-induced liver impairment.

Metformin Inhibits an HFD-Induced Fatty Liver and Exosome Secretion by Activating AMPKα1 in WAT

To address if AMPKα1 activation mitigated HFD-induced liver impairment by reducing exosome secretion in vivo,

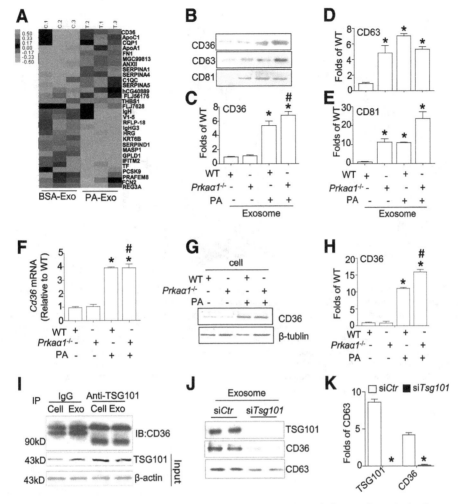

Figure 4—TSG101 facilitates CD36 sorting into exosomes in PA-treated adipocytes. *A*: Proteomic analysis of exosomes derived from adipocytes treated with or without PA. *B*: Western blot for CD36, CD63, and CD81 in exosomes from PA-treated (300 μmol/L) WT and *Prkaα1*$^{-/-}$ WAT. *C–E*: Densitometric analysis of CD36, CD63, and CD81 Western blots from *B. F*: Expression of Cd36 mRNA in PA-treated WT and *Prkaα1*$^{-/-}$ WAT. *G*: Western blot for CD36 in PA-treated WT and *Prkaα1*$^{-/-}$ WAT. *H*: Densitometric analysis of Western blots for CD36 from *G. I*: IP assay for the interaction between TSG101 and CD36 in the cytosol and exosome (Exo) lysates. *J*: Western blot for CD36 in 3T3L1 cells transfected with or without *Tsg101*. *K*: Quantitative data for TSG101. *$P < 0.05$ vs. control ($n = 3$); #$P < 0.05$ vs. PA-treated group ($n = 3$). IB, immunoblotting.

we treated *Prkaa1*$^{fl/fl}$, *Prkaa1*$^{-/-}$, *Prkaa1*$^{fl/fl}$:*Adipo*$^{Cre+}$, and *Prkaa1*$^{fl/fl}$:*Alb*$^{Cre+}$ mice with an HFD and metformin (5 mg/kg/day in drinking water) (35) for 3 months. Metformin administration significantly ameliorated lipid accumulation (Supplementary Fig. 8*A* and *B*), liver weight (Supplementary Fig. 8*C*), and the ratio of liver weight to body weight (Supplementary Fig. 8*D*) in *Prkaa1*$^{fl/fl}$ *and Prkaa1*$^{fl/fl}$:*Alb*$^{Cre+}$ mice. However, metformin treatment failed to mitigate an HFD-induced fatty liver in *Prkaa1*$^{-/-}$ and *Prkaa1*$^{fl/fl}$:*Adipo*$^{Cre+}$ mice. Notably, metformin significantly reduced HFD-induced exosome release into serum and WAT in *Prkaa1*$^{fl/fl}$:*Alb*$^{Cre+}$ and *Prkaa1*$^{fl/fl}$ mice, but not in *Prkaa1*$^{-/-}$ and *Prkaa1*$^{fl/fl}$:*Adipo*$^{Cre+}$ mice (Supplementary Fig. 8*E* and *F*). These results indicate that metformin mitigates HFD-induced liver impairment or inhibits exosome shedding by specific activation of AMPKα1 in WAT in vivo.

Blocking Exosome Shedding Ablates HFD-Induced NAFL

To validate that exosome shedding aggravated fatty liver development induced by an AMPKα1 deficiency in vivo, we inhibited exosome secretion with intraperitoneal injections of GW4869 (0.5 mg/kg/day) in HFD-fed *Prkaa1*$^{-/-}$ and *Prkaa1*$^{fl/fl}$:*Adipo*$^{Cre+}$ mice for 8 weeks. GW4869 is a ceramide-induced exosome inhibitor (32). Consistent with its known function, GW4869 administration significantly reduced exosome secretion from WAT (Fig. 7*A*) and was associated with decreased liver weights (Fig. 7*B*) and liver weight to body weight ratios (Fig. 7*C*) in all four HFD-fed strains of mice. Importantly, Oil Red O and H&E staining revealed that GW4869 treatment attenuated lipid accumulation and fatty liver development in both *Prkaa1*$^{-/-}$ and *Prkaa1*$^{fl/fl}$:*Adipo*$^{Cre+}$ mice (Fig. 7*D–F*). In summary, our results support the framework that

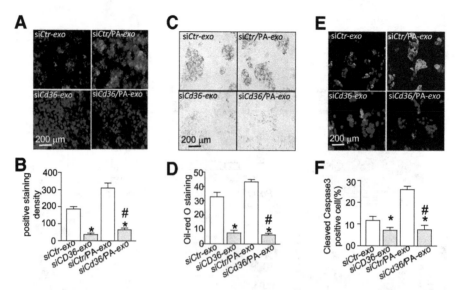

Figure 5—Silencing CD36 attenuates exosome internalization and HepG2 damage. *A*: HepG2 cells were treated with exosomes (exo) derived from adipocytes that were transfected with *siCtr or siCd36* and treated with or without PA. *B*: Quantitative analysis of exosome internalization by HepG2 cells. *C*: Representative images of Oil Red O staining in HepG2 cells treated by exosomes derived from adipocytes that were transfected with *siCtr or siCd36* and treated with or without PA. *D*: Quantification of Oil Red O staining. *E*: Immunostaining for cleaved caspase-3 in HepG2 cells treated by exosomes derived from adipocytes that were transfected with *siCtr or siCd36* and treated with or without PA. *F*: Quantification of cleaved caspase-3 staining. *siCD36-exo*, exosome derived from adipocytes transfected with si*Cd36*; *siCd36/PA-exo*, exosome derived from adipocytes transfected with si*Cd36* and pretreated with PA; *siCtr-exo*, exosome derived from adipocytes transfected with si*Control*; *siCtr/PA-exo*, exosome derived from adipocytes transfected with si*Control* and pretreated with PA. *$P < 0.05$ vs. *siCtr*-exo group ($n = 3$); #$P < 0.05$ vs. *siCtr*/PA-exo group ($n = 3$).

inhibiting exosome secretion from WAT prevents an HFD-induced fatty liver.

DISCUSSION

In this study, we have demonstrated that AMPKα1 is a critical molecule that regulates exosome synthesis, content, and shedding in WAT. Inactivation of AMPKα1 in WAT increased exosome release and mediated the development of an NAFL. Furthermore, AMPKα1 knockdown increased exosome shedding and promoted CD36 accumulation in exosomes that were derived from adipocytes treated with PA. Collectively, the effects of AMPKα1 knockdown mediated PA-induced hepatocyte damage. We also found that an HFD induced more severe liver damage in $Prkaa1^{-/-}$ and AT-specific $Prkaa1^{-/-}$ mice. Activation of AMPK by metformin reduced exosome release and contributed to a fatty liver in WT and liver-specific $Prkaa1^{-/-}$ mice. Inhibiting exosome secretion with GW4869 alleviated an HFD-induced fatty liver in $Prkaa1^{-/-}$ and adipocyte-specific $Prkaa1^{-/-}$ mice. Our study suggests that inhibition of exosome release from WAT is a novel therapeutic target for treating NAFLD (Supplementary Fig. 9).

The most important finding of our study was that AMPKα1 inhibition in WAT contributed to an NAFL caused by an HFD through increased exosome numbers and CD36 protein content. We observed exosomes derived from WT or AMPKα1-deficient adipocytes did not induce significant hepatocyte damage. However, after the addition of an adipocyte PA pretreatment, the uptake of exosomes derived from AMPKα1-deficient adipocytes was increased and damaging to hepatocytes. These data suggest that exosomes derived from PA-treated adipocytes are different and that these differences have detrimental effects on liver structure and function. Consistent with this hypothesis, we found that an AMPKα1-specific deficiency in WAT, but not in the liver, aggravated an HFD-induced NAFL. The AMPKα1-specific knockdown in WAT was accompanied by increased exosomes in both serum and WAT. Moreover, GW4869, but not metformin, dramatically mitigated fatty liver development in $Prkaa1^{fl/fl}$: $Adipo^{Cre+}$ mice.

The following evidence supports our conclusion: first, in adipocytes, activation of AMPK inhibited PA-induced exosome secretion, and conversely, repression of AMPK enhanced exosome secretion. Second, the absence of AMPKα1, but not the AMPKα2 isoform, increased exosome secretion in WAT. Third, AMPKα1 knockdown in adipocytes enhanced exosome secretion due to increased microvesicle biogenesis mediated by elevated TSG101 expression. Finally, repression of AMPKα1 led to elevated TSG101 protein levels, but had no effect on mRNA expression, which indicated that AMPKα1 may regulate TSG101 degradation. Taken together, these results strongly support the hypothesis that decreased AMPKα1 levels instigate lipid deposition in the liver through TSG101-mediated exosome biogenesis.

We have elucidated the mechanisms by which AMPKα1 downregulation affects exosomal contents and induces

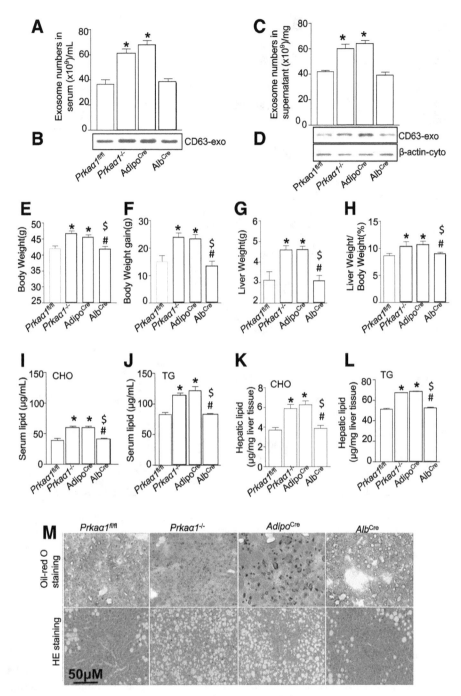

Figure 6—AMPKα1 deficiency increases HFD-enhanced exosome shedding from WAT and exacerbates lipid accumulation in the liver. *A*: Quantification of serum exosomes (exo) in *Prkaα1$^{fl/fl}$*, *Prkaα1$^{-/-}$*, *Adipo^{Cre}*, and *Alb^{Cre}* mice fed an HFD for 3 months (*n* = 4 for each group). *B*: Western blot for CD63 in the exosomes from *A*. *C*: Quantification of exosomes in the supernatant of *Prkaα1$^{fl/fl}$*, *Prkaα1$^{-/-}$*, *Adipo^{Cre}*, and *Alb^{Cre}* WAT. *D*: Western blot for CD63 in the exosomes from *C*. *E–M*: *Prkaα1$^{fl/fl}$*, *Prkaα1$^{-/-}$*, *Adipo^{Cre}*, and *Alb^{Cre}* mice were fed an HFD for 3 months. *E*: Body weight. *F*: Increase in body weight. *G*: Liver weight. *H*: Ratio of liver weight to body weight. *I*: Serum cholesterol (CHO) levels. *J*: Serum triglyceride (TG) levels. *K*: Hepatic CHO levels. *L*: Hepatic TG levels. *M*: Representative images of Oil Red O and H&E (HE) staining of the liver tissues. *P < 0.05 vs. *Prkaα1$^{fl/fl}$* mice; #P < 0.05 vs. *Prkaα1$^{-/-}$* mice (*n* = 3); $P < 0.05 vs. *Adipo^{Cre}* mice (*n* = 3). *Adipo^{Cre}*, *Prkaα1$^{fl/fl}$:Adipo^{Cre}* mice; *Alb^{Cre}*, *Prkaα1$^{fl/fl}$:Alb^{Cre}* mice.

HepG2 cell damage under PA stimulation. A nontargeted proteomic profiling MS array revealed there were 43 different proteins in the exosomes derived from PA-treated adipocytes. Among the exosomal proteins, CD36 was the most abundant. Importantly, CD36 mediates lipid uptake in vitro and in vivo. CD36 silencing has previously been found to attenuate lipid accumulation in liver tissue (36). Therefore, we explored the role of CD36 NAFL development

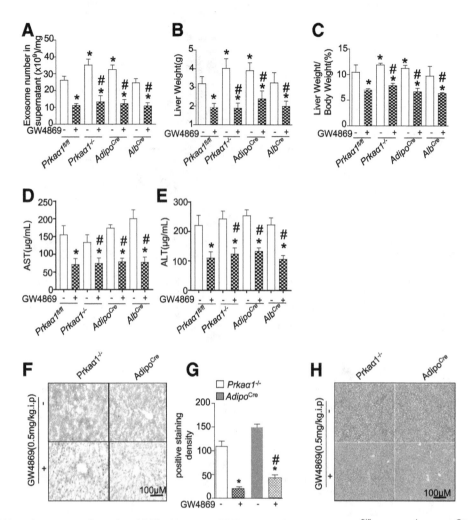

Figure 7—Inhibition of exosome release from WAT mitigates an HFD-induced fatty liver. *Prkaα1$^{fl/fl}$*, *Prkaα1$^{-/-}$*, *Adipo^{Cre}*, and *Alb^{Cre}* mice were fed an HFD and GW4869 (0.5 mg/kg/day, i.p.) for 3 months. *A*: Quantification of exosomes in the supernatant. *B*: Liver weight. *C*: Ratio of liver weight to body weight. *D*: AST. *E*: ALT. *F*: Representative images of Oil Red O staining. *G*: Quantification of Oil Red O staining (*n* = 6). *H*: Representative images of H&E staining. **P* < 0.05 vs. *Prkaα1$^{fl/fl}$* mice; *#P* < 0.05 vs. every group of mice treated with vehicle. *Adipo^{Cre}*, *Prkaα1$^{fl/fl}$:Adipo^{Cre}* mice; *Alb^{Cre}*, *Prkaα1$^{fl/fl}$:Alb^{Cre}* mice.

by investigating exosome secretion in adipocytes after CD36 silencing. Interestingly, *Cd36* silencing did not affect exosome secretion; however, exosome internalization by hepatocytes and hepatocyte damage were significantly mitigated. These data suggest that CD36 is a primary mediator of fatty liver development due to its high expression in obesity and HFD-treated adipocytes. In addition, an AMPKα1 deficiency increased TSG101 expression and promoted CD36 to sort into exosomes.

Our results indicate that AMPK activators, such as metformin, might have therapeutic effects on NAFLD. No studies have evaluated whether metformin improves long-term patient-oriented outcomes, such as progression from NAFLD to nonalcoholic steatohepatitis, cirrhosis, hepatocellular carcinoma, or death from liver failure. Rather, a considerable body of evidence on the hepatic effects of

metformin have yielded mixed results, indicating there is potentially modest benefit that has yet to be confirmed due to the small sample sizes and short terms of the studies and inconsistently reported outcomes (37–41). NAFLD is intricately linked to insulin resistance and its associated metabolic features (e.g., higher body weight, BMI, and waist circumference), so by improving metabolic features of NAFLD, metformin could also improve management of this liver disease. Indeed, a systematic review by Li et al. (42) demonstrated that metformin can improve biochemical and metabolic features in NAFLD. Larger randomized controlled trials of sufficient duration that use histological end points are needed to assess the effectiveness of this drug in modifying the progression of NAFLD.

In summary, our results demonstrate that AMPKα1 downregulation contributes to an HFD-induced NAFL.

AMPKα1 downregulation enhances the communication between WAT and the liver via increased exosome biogenesis and secretion. Inhibiting exosome release from WAT by AMPK activation is a novel therapeutic target for treating NAFL development.

Funding. This study was supported by the National Natural Science Foundation of China (grants 81670276 to Y.H. and 82070300 to C.Y.). This study was also supported in part by the National Institutes of Health grants HL079584, HL080-499, HL089920, and HL110488 (to M.-H.Z.).

Duality of Interest. No potential conflicts of interest relevant to this article were reported.

Author Contributions. M.-H.Z. conceived the project. C.Y. and M.-H.Z. designed the study and wrote the manuscript. X.T., J.L., and D.L. conducted confocal microscopy imaging, IP, and Western blotting. D.Y. conducted site-directed mutagenesis. C.Y. and Z.X. wrote the manuscript. All authors approved the manuscript. C.Y. is the guarantor of this work and, as such, had full access to all of the data in the study and takes responsibility for the integrity of the data and the accuracy of the data analysis.

References

1. Pegtel DM, Gould SJ. Exosomes. Annu Rev Biochem 2019;88:487–514

2. Nazari-Shafti TZ, Emmert MY. The link between exosomes phenotype and mode of action in the context of cardioprotection. Eur Heart J 2019;40:3361

3. LeBleu VS, Kalluri R. Exosomes exercise inhibition of anti-tumor immunity during chemotherapy. Immunity 2019;50:547–549

4. Gao L, Wang L, Dai T, et al. Tumor-derived exosomes antagonize innate antiviral immunity. Nat Immunol 2018;19:233–245

5. Ying W, Riopel M, Bandyopadhyay G, et al. Adipose tissue macrophage-derived exosomal miRNAs can modulate in vivo and in vitro insulin sensitivity. Cell 2017;171:372–384.e12

6. Chen Y, Pfeifer A. Brown fat-derived exosomes: small vesicles with big impact. Cell Metab 2017;25:759–760

7. Thomou T, Mori MA, Dreyfuss JM, et al. Adipose-derived circulating miRNAs regulate gene expression in other tissues. Nature 2017;542:450–455

8. Sciorati C, Clementi E, Manfredi AA, Rovere-Querini P. Fat deposition and accumulation in the damaged and inflamed skeletal muscle: cellular and molecular players. Cell Mol Life Sci 2015;72:2135–2156

9. Furman D, Campisi J, Verdin E, et al. Chronic inflammation in the etiology of disease across the life span. Nat Med 2019;25:1822–1832

10. Sanyal AJ. Past, present and future perspectives in nonalcoholic fatty liver disease. Nat Rev Gastroenterol Hepatol 2019;16:377–386

11. Ji C, Guo X. The clinical potential of circulating microRNAs in obesity. Nat Rev Endocrinol 2019;15:731–743

12. Crewe C, Joffin N, Rutkowski JM, et al. An endothelial-to-adipocyte extracellular vesicle axis governed by metabolic state. Cell 2018;175:695–708.e13

13. Kita S, Maeda N, Shimomura I. Interorgan communication by exosomes, adipose tissue, and adiponectin in metabolic syndrome. J Clin Invest 2019;129: 4041–4049

14. Akbar N, Azzimato V, Choudhury RP, Aouadi M. Extracellular vesicles in metabolic disease. Diabetologia 2019;62:2179–2187

15. Zou W, Lai M, Zhang Y, et al. Exosome release is regulated by mTORC1. Adv Sci (Weinh) 2018;6:1801313

16. Sato K, Meng F, Glaser S, Alpini G. Exosomes in liver pathology. J Hepatol 2016;65:213–221

17. Foretz M, Guigas B, Viollet B. Understanding the glucoregulatory mechanisms of metformin in type 2 diabetes mellitus. Nat Rev Endocrinol 2019;15: 569–589

18. Jordan S, Tung N, Casanova-Acebes M, et al. Dietary intake regulates the circulating inflammatory monocyte pool. Cell 2019;178:1102–1114.e17

19. Steinberg GR, Carling D. AMP-activated protein kinase: the current landscape for drug development. Nat Rev Drug Discov 2019;18:527–551

20. Patra KC, Weerasekara VK, Bardeesy N. AMPK-mediated lysosome biogenesis in lung cancer growth. Cell Metab 2019;29:238–240

21. Foretz M, Guigas B, Bertrand L, Pollak M, Viollet B. Metformin: from mechanisms of action to therapies. Cell Metab 2014;20:953–966

22. Hardie DG. AMPK—sensing energy while talking to other signaling pathways. Cell Metab 2014;20:939–952

23. Mizunoe Y, Sudo Y, Okita N, et al. Involvement of lysosomal dysfunction in autophagosome accumulation and early pathologies in adipose tissue of obese mice. Autophagy 2017;13:642–653

24. Wang B, Nie J, Wu L, et al. AMPKα2 protects against the development of heart failure by enhancing mitophagy via PINK1 phosphorylation. Circ Res 2018; 122:712–729

25. Wang Q, Wu S, Zhu H, et al. Deletion of PRKAA triggers mitochondrial fission by inhibiting the autophagy-dependent degradation of DNM1L. Autophagy 2017; 13:404–422

26. Liu Z, Zhu H, Dai X, et al. Macrophage liver kinase B1 inhibits foam cell formation and atherosclerosis. Circ Res 2017;121:1047–1057

27. Lorente-Cebrián S, Bustos M, Marti A, Martinez JA, Moreno-Aliaga MJ. Eicosapentaenoic acid stimulates AMP-activated protein kinase and increases visfatin secretion in cultured murine adipocytes. Clin Sci (Lond) 2009;117:243–249

28. Ban LA, Shackel NA, McLennan SV. Extracellular vesicles: a new frontier in biomarker discovery for non-alcoholic fatty liver disease. Int J Mol Sci 2016;17:376

29. Sahoo S, Losordo DW. Exosomes and cardiac repair after myocardial infarction. Circ Res 2014;114:333–344

30. Roche JV, Nesverova V, Olsson C, Deen PM, Törnroth-Horsefield S. Structural insights into AQP2 targeting to multivesicular bodies. Int J Mol Sci 2019;20:5351

31. Bänfer S, Schneider D, Dewes J, et al. Molecular mechanism to recruit galectin-3 into multivesicular bodies for polarized exosomal secretion. Proc Natl Acad Sci U S A 2018;115:E4396–E4405

32. Wang Y, Jia L, Xie Y, et al. Involvement of macrophage-derived exosomes in abdominal aortic aneurysms development. Atherosclerosis 2019;289:64–72

33. Colombo M, Moita C, van Niel G, et al. Analysis of ESCRT functions in exosome biogenesis, composition and secretion highlights the heterogeneity of extracellular vesicles. J Cell Sci 2013;126:5553–5565

34. Costantino S, Akhmedov A, Melina G, et al. Obesity-induced activation of JunD promotes myocardial lipid accumulation and metabolic cardiomyopathy. Eur Heart J 2019;40:997–1008

35. Miller RA, Chu Q, Xie J, Foretz M, Viollet B, Birnbaum MJ. Biguanides suppress hepatic glucagon signalling by decreasing production of cyclic AMP. Nature 2013;494:256–260

36. Zhao L, Zhang C, Luo X, et al. CD36 palmitoylation disrupts free fatty acid metabolism and promotes tissue inflammation in non-alcoholic steatohepatitis. J Hepatol 2018;69:705–717

37. Pan CS, Stanley TL. Effect of weight loss medications on hepatic steatosis and steatohepatitis: a systematic review. Front Endocrinol (Lausanne) 2020;11:70

38. Fan H, Pan Q, Xu Y, Yang X. Exenatide improves type 2 diabetes concomitant with non-alcoholic fatty liver disease. Arq Bras Endocrinol Metabol 2013;57:702–708

39. Feng W, Gao C, Bi Y, et al. Randomized trial comparing the effects of gliclazide, liraglutide, and metformin on diabetes with non-alcoholic fatty liver disease. J Diabetes 2017;9:800–809

40. Garinis GA, Fruci B, Mazza A, et al. Metformin versus dietary treatment in nonalcoholic hepatic steatosis: a randomized study. Int J Obes 2010;34:1255–1264

41. Handzlik G, Holecki M, Kozaczka J, et al. Evaluation of metformin therapy using controlled attenuation parameter and transient elastography in patients with non-alcoholic fatty liver disease. Pharmacol Rep 2019;71:183–188

42. Li Y, Liu L, Wang B, Wang J, Chen D. Metformin in non-alcoholic fatty liver disease: a systematic review and meta-analysis. Biomed Rep 2013;1:57–64

Deciphering the Complex Communication Networks That Orchestrate Pancreatic Islet Function

Jonathan Weitz,[1,2] Danusa Menegaz,[1] and Alejandro Caicedo[1,2,3,4]

Diabetes 2021;70:17–26 | https://doi.org/10.2337/dbi19-0033

Pancreatic islets are clusters of hormone-secreting endocrine cells that rely on intricate cell-cell communication mechanisms for proper function. The importance of multicellular cooperation in islet cell physiology was first noted nearly 30 years ago in seminal studies showing that hormone secretion from endocrine cell types is diminished when these cells are dispersed. These studies showed that reestablishing cellular contacts in so-called pseudoislets caused endocrine cells to regain hormone secretory function. This not only demonstrated that cooperation between islet cells is highly synergistic but also gave birth to the field of pancreatic islet organoids. Here we review recent advances related to the mechanisms of islet cell cross talk. We first describe new developments that revise current notions about purinergic and GABA signaling in islets. Then we comment on novel multicellular imaging studies that are revealing emergent properties of islet communication networks. We finish by highlighting and discussing recent synthetic approaches that use islet organoids of varied cellular composition to interrogate intraislet signaling mechanisms. This reverse engineering of islets not only will shed light on the mechanisms of intraislet signaling and define communication networks but also may guide efforts aimed at restoring islet function and β-cell mass in diabetes.

Cells have an innate ability to form tissues. Indeed, within the pancreas, the endocrine cells responsible for maintaining glucose homeostasis coalesce during development into small organs called islets. In the islet, the insulin-secreting β-cells make direct cellular contacts with other β-cells as well as with other endocrine cell types, including the glucagon secreting α-cells and the somatostatin-secreting δ-cells. The importance of these cellular contacts for islet cell physiology was first reported nearly 30 years ago when Halban, Meda, Wollheim, Weir, Pipeleers, and colleagues showed that hormone secretion is diminished in dispersed cells compared with intact islet clusters (1–3). Results from these creative experiments showed that β-cells in islets roughly secrete 18 times more insulin than single β-cells and that β-cell pairs secrete four to five times more insulin than expected from their sum (1,3,4). Thus, cooperation between β-cells in the islet is not additive but highly synergistic.

This arithmetical anomaly poses a significant problem to the investigator: the complexity of cellular interactions in the tissue makes it difficult to comprehend organ function. To properly perform their homeostatic functions, these specialized endocrine cells have developed intricate cell-cell communication mechanisms that rely on the recognition of the state of activity of their neighboring cells. These communication mechanisms include direct contact signaling with neighboring cells and with the extracellular matrix (gap junctions, ephrins, cadherins, and integrins) as well as noncontact signaling through secretion of paracrine factors (5). Loss of these communication mechanisms has a profound effect on the secretory function of endocrine cells in the pancreatic islet. This article discusses current developments in the field of islet endocrine cell cross talk, emphasizing novel analytical and synthetic approaches that are overcoming major roadblocks in studying communication networks in the islet.

Analytic Approaches to Dissect Out the Complexity of Islet Communication

When dispersed, islet cells have the urge to reaggregate (6), and once they have formed clusters they secrete more

[1]Department of Medicine, University of Miami Leonard M. Miller School of Medicine, Miami, FL

[2]Diabetes Research Institute, University of Miami Leonard M. Miller School of Medicine, Miami, FL

[3]Department of Physiology and Biophysics, University of Miami Leonard M. Miller School of Medicine, Miami, FL

[4]Program in Neuroscience, University of Miami Leonard M. Miller School of Medicine, Miami, FL

Corresponding author: Jonathan Weitz, jrw64@med.miami.edu, or Alejandro Caicedo, acaicedo@miami.edu

Received 27 May 2020 and accepted 1 October 2020

insulin in response to glucose (3). To understand the sociobiology that makes endocrine cells work more efficiently in clusters, islets can be examined using analytical tools, that is, by manipulating and imaging individual components and measuring the impact on the whole islet. In this section, we discuss recent developments that are helping define intraislet signaling by using analytical approaches. The research work we describe employs two different strategies to decipher the complexity of islet communication, namely, dissecting out individual components of cell-cell communication and multicellular imaging of islet networks.

Dissecting Out the Role of Purinergic and GABA Signaling in Islet Communication

There are three basic types of communication between islet cells: electrical coupling through gap junctions, direct cell-to-cell contacts, and paracrine interactions. Paracrine signaling involves release of a chemical signal, which travels through the local microcirculation or interstitial fluid to reach its target cell. The list of putative signaling molecules in the islet keeps increasing (e.g., urocortin 3 [7]). The emerging importance of paracrine signaling from α- and δ-cells in orchestrating insulin secretion was reviewed recently (7,8). Here, we focus on new findings related to the paracrine roles of purinergic signals (ATP and adenosine) and GABA because they illustrate the versatility and intricacy of cell-cell communication in the islet.

ATP is known to be stored in insulin granules and is thus cosecreted with insulin. Interestingly, ATP may leave the granule before or even without insulin in what is known as kiss-and-run exocytosis. This ATP first encounters and binds to receptors on β-cells, thus triggering signaling cascades that amplify insulin secretion from human islets (Fig. 1). Initially, these effects were reported to be mediated by ionotropic P2X$_3$ purinergic receptors (9), but newer studies revised this picture to include metabotropic P2Y1 receptors (10,11). ATP affects other endocrine cells as well (12). In its journey through the interstitium, ATP also faces the resident macrophage. Macrophages in general are endowed with purinergic receptors, and indeed two recent studies from our group show that macrophages in mouse and human islets are exquisite sensors of extracellular ATP (13,14). Of note, the results indicate that islet resident macrophages partially depend on endogenous ATP input from β-cells to produce and secrete cytokines and metalloproteinases. Furthermore, purinergic receptor expression in islet macrophages was found to be downregulated in obese and diabetic states. In these states, the loss of ATP sensing in macrophages may reduce their secretory capacity and impair their interactions with the microenvironment.

As soon as ATP starts percolating through the interstitial space it is cleaved by potent ATPases that generate other purinergic signals such as ADP (15). ADP may be further cleaved to adenosine once it approaches ectonucleotidase-coated capillaries. This adenosine likely inhibits the activity of vascular pericytes, thus dilating capillaries and increasing local blood flow, as shown recently (16). These effects are mimicked by stimulation of β-cells with high glucose concentrations and can be blocked with an A1 receptor antagonist (16). These novel findings demonstrate how purinergic signals released from β-cells accomplish multiple tasks in the islets: 1) by potentiating insulin secretion, ATP increases the speed and robustness of the β-cell's early response to a rise in glycemia; 2) by signaling to macrophages, ATP conveys information about the β-cell's secretory status, therefore allowing macrophages to properly adjust tissue homeostasis; and 3) by inhibiting pericytes, adenosine regulates islet blood flow to deliver insulin more efficiently. Thanks to their versatility, purinergic signals are thus able to recruit multiple cell types that help orchestrate hormone secretion and maintain islet integrity (Fig. 1).

GABA has been postulated as a paracrine signal since it was reported to inhibit α-cells (17). Recent studies characterized in detail native, high-affinity GABA$_A$ receptors in human β-cells (18). Because GABA also inhibits immune cells, it was further suggested that it could protect β-cells under immune attack (19). In 2017, a study appeared describing GABA as an inducer of α-to-β-cell conversion in vivo, which was presented as an unprecedented hope toward improved therapies for diabetes (20). The results were sensational and triggered a research mania. However, efforts at reproducing these results failed, as long-term treatment of mice and rhesus monkeys with GABA (or artemisinins) did not cause α-to-β-cell transdifferentiation (21,22). In brief, GABA may be famous as a paracrine signal but infamous as a transdifferentiating factor.

It was interesting to follow this debate, in particular because we were aware that it had not been established unequivocally how GABA is secreted in the islet. Like other paracrine signals, islet GABA release was described to depend on exocytosis, although researchers suspected a large tonic glucose-independent background release of GABA (23). A recent study now shows that the β-cell effluxes GABA from a cytosolic pool in a pulsatile manner (24) (Fig. 2). Moreover, knocking down expression of subunits for volume-regulated anion channels (VRACs) abolished GABA release, indicating that VRACs are critical for GABA secretion in the islet. GABA content in β-cells is depleted and secretion is disrupted in islets from patients with type 1 and patients with type 2 diabetes, suggesting that loss of GABA correlates with diabetes pathogenesis (24). It still has to be established whether this constitutive GABA secretion promotes the oscillatory activity pattern of the islet and whether its loss contributes to the erratic oscillations in insulin secretion seen in type 2 diabetes. In several ways, the notion that GABA in the islet behaves as an organic osmolyte whose extracellular levels oscillate periodically is highly unconventional. More than 30 years after the seminal work of Rorsman et al. (17), many aspects of GABA signaling in the islet remain mysterious and deserve further investigation.

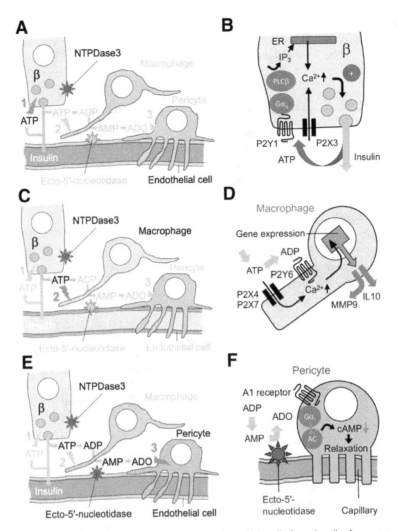

Figure 1—The fate of extracellular ATP in the islet. *A*: ATP is released together with insulin from β-cells. As soon as it leaves the granule, ATP acts on purinergic receptors on β-cells to potentiate insulin secretion, thus establishing a positive-feedback loop (1). *B*: Transduction mechanisms and effects of ATP activation of β-cells. *C*: ATP further activates macrophages (2). ATP is hydrolyzed by NTPDase3, producing ADP (and AMP), which can also activate macrophages. *D*: Transduction mechanisms and effects of purinergic activation of resident macrophages. *E*: On its way through the interstitial space, AMP encounters ectonucleotidases on endothelial cells, which produces adenosine (ADO). Adenosine inhibits vascular pericytes (3), allowing capillaries to dilate. This increases local blood flow. *F*: Transduction mechanisms and effects of purinergic inhibition of islet pericytes.

Using Functional Multicellular Imaging to Identify Complex Intraislet Networks

A different analytical approach to reveal communication networks is to study multicellular activity in intact islets. In the last decade, different groups have examined coordinated responses in islets using complex microfluidic devices (25,26), pancreas slices (27), in vivo imaging of intraocular islet grafts (28), or intravital imaging in Zebrafish (29). Mathematical modeling is then applied to the data sets for understanding of how individual events produce episodic hormone responses (e.g., multicellular islet models [30]). The new analytical approaches are showing that β-cell collectives work as broadscale complex networks and share similarities in global statistical features and structural design principles with the internet and social networks (29,30).

These studies are revealing properties of the islet network that are only apparent if the population is examined as an ensemble. A common thread appears to be β-cell heterogeneity. Physiologists have been aware for decades that the β-cell and other endocrine cell populations are heterogenous (31), a feature that was only recently confirmed at the molecular level (reviewed in 32). Heterogeneity, a natural trait of most cell collectives, introduces robustness and plasticity—for instance, different β-cell response patterns to glucose allow insulin secretion to be fine-tuned. That some β-cells recover from stress while others continue secreting reduces the islet's vulnerability to insults. Using high-speed multicellular Ca^{2+} imaging combined with correlation analyses, Hodson and colleagues (33) found rare superconnected hub cells whose activity tends to precede that of the remainder of

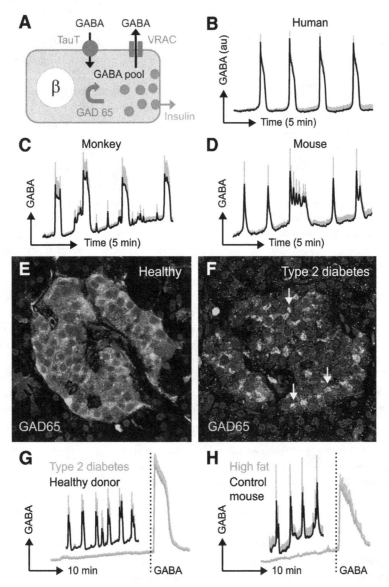

Figure 2—β-cells secrete the paracrine signal GABA constitutively and in a pulsatile manner. *A*: Cartoon depicting the mechanisms of GABA synthesis, transport across the membrane, and efflux from β-cells. The GABA-synthesizing enzyme GAD65 increases the cytoplasmic pool of GABA. This GABA leaves the cell via the VRAC. GABA is recaptured by the taurine transporter TauT. *B–D*: Detection of GABA by cytosolic Ca^{2+} flux in $GABA_B$ receptor–expressing biosensor cells shows that GABA secretion is periodic in human (*B*), monkey (*Macaca fascicularis*) (*C*), and mouse (*D*) islets. *E* and *F*: Confocal images of pancreatic sections from a donor without diabetes (*E*) and a donor with type 2 diabetes (*F*) show a redistribution of the enzyme during diabetes (arrows). *G* and *H*: GABA secretion measured as in *B–D* is impaired in human type 2 diabetes (*G*) as well as in mice fed a high-fat diet (*H*). For the original study on the mechanisms of GABA secretion, see Menegaz et al. (24). All experiments were performed at 3 mmol/L glucose concentration. au, arbitrary units.

the population. These studies provide evidence that pacemaker-like β-cells exist in the islet. Thus, some β-cells may be more equal than others.

A shortcoming is that each analytical modality seems to identify its own type of heterogeneity, and it is difficult to find biological correlates. Another caveat of these multicellular recordings is that they rely heavily on data obtained with indicators for bulk cytoplasmic Ca^{2+} concentrations. This Ca^{2+} signal represents the sum of multiple inputs, has temporal features that reflect the indicator's Ca^{2+} binding kinetics, and, unlike local Ca^{2+} influx through particular Ca^{2+} channels, is not necessarily coupled to secretory output. The imaging techniques to assess islet signaling are not fast enough to measure the primary electrical signal of the islet, the action potential. Fluorescent imaging can only predict electrical connectivity of an islet. Microelectrode array–based technologies or the use of modern optical probes for membrane voltage may provide a clearer assessment of connectivity. This is important because examining discrete pulsatile secretory events in intact human islets did not reveal leaders and followers (34) (discussion of the hub cell model in

35,36). Molecular biology data suggest that β-cell subpopulations transition through different states (stressed vs. active) multiple times over the course of their life span, suggesting that there are no fixed populations (32). Also, an exposed dominant cell would render fragile a system whose robustness is based on ensemble activity. But maybe that is how diabetes can ensue. These comments notwithstanding, it is clear that multicellular imaging studies coupled to mathematical modeling are revealing emergent properties of islet communication networks that will complete our model of islet biology and explain its fragility.

Synthetic Approaches: Reverse Engineering Strategies to Elucidate Mechanisms of Intraislet Communication

Mathematical modeling using data from multicellular imaging may be a first step in providing a synthesis, but in general the reductionist (analytical) approach identifies individual components in a biological system without characterizing the system's entirety. Synthetic approaches can be used to overcome this limitation by combining a known set of isolated components to reconstruct the system and understand its complexity. Researchers can thus recreate miniaturized or simplified versions of an organ in vitro. These so-called organoids self-organize and reassemble in ways that mimic the original tissue composition. Importantly, they recapitulate specific functions of the organ (Fig. 3).

Reverse engineering is the process by which a man-made object (in engineering) or an organ (biomedical research) is deconstructed to reveal its design or architecture or to extract knowledge from the object or organ. By deconstructing and reassembling components, an engineer can determine the contribution of each of the individual components. Engineers have used this approach for centuries to build bridges, cars, and computers. Islet biologists have applied the same approach by reconstructing the individual cellular components of islets to create islet-like organoids, also known as pseudoislets. These pseudoislets have been created from cell lines, primary cells, or stem cells. Recent advances in islet cell-cell communication based on the use of pseudoislets are discussed here. Before we delve more into the subject, it is important to note that pseudoislet formation does not always produce the architecture of the islet cells from which the pseudoislets were made. This could impact paracrine signaling, hub cell or leader cell contacts, and many other signaling events within the islet.

Pseudoislets Made of Hormone-Secreting Cell Lines

Using islet hormone-secreting cell lines for islet research is an attractive approach that has numerous advantages: they can be propagated in culture and are easily transformable and cost-effective. Cell lines such as MIN6 are generally maintained as adherent monolayers in tissue culture but, when subcultured in tissue culture flasks precoated with gelatin (1%), develop into three-dimensional pseudoislets (4). MIN6 cells also form pseudoislets when cultured in dishes without tissue culture treatment and

can be formed with suspension culture (for example, see 37). For human pseudoislet formation, innovative plates with microwells are required. Like primary islets, pseudoislets depend on cell adhesion molecules such as E-cadherin and N-cadherin to maintain their structure (4,38). Pseudoislets have been made from numerous islet hormone-secreting cell lines including the insulin-secreting MIN6 cells (4), glucagon-secreting αTC, and somatostatin-secreting TGP-52 cells (39,40).

Interestingly, reaggregation of αTC and MIN6 cells induced spontaneous organization of the rodent islet core-mantle structure (6,41,42). These findings suggest an intrinsic hardwiring in the islet endocrine cytoarchitecture. Studies suggest cell-cell contact mechanisms such as those mediated by Robo receptor signaling may control the cytoarchitectural arrangement (43). There is no doubt that studies using cell lines have revealed fundamental mechanisms of insulin secretion (44). However, immortalized cells are highly proliferative. Proliferating β-cells lose the phenotype typical of β-cells and secrete less insulin than their differentiated counterparts. Most primary β-cells, by contrast, are fully differentiated and can be as old as the animal in which they reside (45). Nonimmortalized cells such as primary islets or terminally differentiated stem cells thus seem more suitable for studying islet physiology.

Pseudoislets Made of Cells Derived From Primary Islets

Primary islets have been the workhorse for diabetes research since 1967, when the islet isolation protocol was established (46). Since then, numerous fundamental communication mechanisms have been discovered with use of intact islets. Although these findings contribute to our understanding of islet biology, using a reverse engineering approach by dismantling primary islets and reconstructing the cellular pieces back together offers researchers a unique discovery tool. One advantage of using pseudoislets derived from primary cells compared with native intact islets is that they can be readily manipulated genetically (47,48). These studies have opened the door for new functional studies in human islets using delivery of viral constructs including designer receptors exclusively activated by designer drugs (DREADDS [49]), overexpression (47), and knockdown studies using shRNA (50). A further advantage is that insulin and glucagon secretion are maintained in human pseudoislets over a longer culture period (51). In addition to traditional methods of obtaining islets, pseudoislets derived from primary cells can now be commercially obtained as well. Companies such as InSphero AG (Schlieren, Switzerland), and likely others in the future, are helping to facilitate research. The techniques described above may prove useful for engineering islets that result in a better clinical success in the context of therapeutic transplantation of islets into patients with diabetes.

Stem Cell–Derived Pseudoislets

Human embryonic stem cells and induced pluripotent stem cells (iPSCs) can now be differentiated into β-like

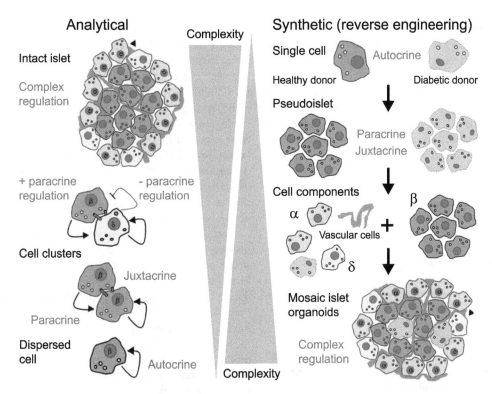

Figure 3—Illustration of analytical and synthetic strategies to decode complex cell-cell interactions in the pancreatic islet. Left: In analytical approaches the islet is broken down, either literally or using imaging tools, to dissect out individual signaling components (autocrine, paracrine, and juxtacrine). Right: In synthetic approaches, the islet is reconstructed from individual components. This reverse engineering reestablishes step-by-step the different signaling mechanisms. The advantages and limitations of these strategies are discussed in the text. Two light-green diabetic β-cells are included in the cell components in the pseudoislet below. The red squiggly line denotes vascular cells.

cells and matured into pseudoislet organoids (52,53). Because of the proliferative capacity of organoid clusters, their production from stem cells offers a unique solution to a major challenge in the field of human islet transplantation, namely the paucity of islet donors. Although these organoid clusters often contain polyhormonal cells that have defects in glucose-stimulated insulin secretion and lack expression of key β-cell–specific transcription factors (54,55), recent improved protocols of stem cell differentiation into β-like cells have shown that these cells secrete insulin in response to glucose and improve glucose tolerance after transplantation into diabetic mice (56). Of note, an important step of this protocol is to cluster and resize iPSC-derived β-cell pseudoislets (~360 μm) into pseudoislets that span 170 μm after resizing. This resizing step improved insulin secretion by nearly 25%. Interestingly, this size is close to the typical islet size in nearly all vertebrate species (100–200 μm diameter) despite the wide range of total pancreatic volume. Thus, there seems to be a limit to how beneficial cell crowding is and there may be an ideal cell number for concerted cell-cell communication. While hypoxia contributes largely to islet size limitation in vitro (57), the mechanisms that determine islet organ size in vivo still require investigation.

Perhaps the most intriguing applications for stem cell–derived pseudoislets have yet to reach their full potential. Pseudoislets derived from donor stem cells of donors with

diabetes may provide a feasible means to deliver personalized medicine to patients, allowing exploration of the mechanisms causing β-cell failure in the particular donor. A crucial step toward reaching this goal will be to develop reliable systems for modeling diabetes. Recently, several studies have reported generating β-like cells from human pluripotent stem cells from donors with type 1 diabetes (T1D) (58). In addition to endocrine cells, iPSCs from donors have been used to generate immune cells from T1D patients (59). In the future, a complete model for diabetes pathogenesis would not only include T1D donor endocrine cells derived from iPSCs but would additionally include other cell types that may play a role in diabetes pathogenesis. These studies may help overcome another major roadblock for therapeutic islet transplantation: the current need for immunosuppression. Whereas immunosuppression concerns may be addressed by encapsulating of organoids (60), it should be feasible to manipulate cell-surface signaling and the anti-inflammatory transcriptional machinery to make islet organoids less immunogenic.

Cellular Aspects Missing From Most Pseudoislet Studies

It should be noted that pseudoislets may not necessarily be less physiological than cultured primary islets. Isolation of pancreatic islets from their natural environment is a traumatic event that requires exocrine tissues to be digested and islets to be rescued from this debris. Not surprisingly, islet isolation changes gene expression patterns in the islet (61). The cytoarchitecture may be maintained in isolated islets (i.e., core/mantle structure in mouse islets), but many cellular components that are important for islet function are lost during extended culture. These cells include immune cells (62), endothelial cells (63), and nerves (64). Future protocols to produce hybrid pseudoislets consisting of several cell types may more faithfully reproduce the complex natural anatomy of the islet. This section will discuss how incorporating these critical cell types in pseudoislet organoids may improve our understanding of islet physiology and diabetes pathophysiology.

Local Immune Cells

Islet resident macrophages are emerging as important players in β-cell proliferation (65,66), sensing of β-cell activity (13,14), islet inflammation (67), and antigen presentation (68). Therefore, macrophages should be considered in future pseudoislet studies. These studies may reveal basic physiological questions that remain unanswered, such as, what are the local signals that recruit resident macrophages to the islet or how do islet immune cells respond to therapeutic intervention? Addressing these questions using pseudoislets in vitro or after transplantation may lead to therapeutic advances in diabetes through immunomodulation.

Although tissue-resident immune cells may proliferate locally (69), recruitment of immune cells also plays an important role in type 1 and type 2 diabetes (70,71). The diverse repertoire of immune cells found in the islet during diabetes includes natural killer cells, cytotoxic T cells, B cells, and macrophages (72). A large proportion of these immune cells are recruited to the islet through the islet microvasculature. Mixed lymphocyte islet culture allows studying activation of responding lymphocytes, cytokine secretion, and changes in islet cell antigen expression (73). Coculture of diabetogenic CD4 and CD8 T cells with islet showed that these immune cells secrete soluble factors promoting β-cell proliferation, suggesting that infiltrating may have surprising therapeutic effects (74). We are not aware of similar studies that evaluate the impact of immune cells using pseudoislets. While these studies highlight how soluble factors from immune cells affect islet function, a properly functioning vasculature network is needed to model the recruitment, infiltration, and extravasation of immune cells into the pseudoislet as well as the direct interactions between immune cells and β-cells.

Vascular Cells

The specialized network of capillaries in the islet allows for efficient transport of micronutrients to pancreatic endocrine cells and of islet hormones out of the islet. Building and maintaining the islet vasculature require proper coordination between vascular cells, stromal cells, and endocrine cells of the islet parenchyma. In addition to the factors that maintain the vasculature in the long-term

(e.g., VEGF), islet blood flow can be acutely modulated by local signals derived from β-cells (adenosine) and by neural input from sympathetic nerves (16). There is evidence that the islet microcirculation is dysfunctional during diabetes (75,76), as well as after islet transplantation (77). By incorporating the islet vasculature into pseudoislet organoids, studies could help improve graft revascularization after islet transplantation. Moreover, as secretion is polarized toward the vasculature (78), a "vascularized" pseudoislet would provide a more physiological model for study of hormone release. Moreover, reincorporation of vascular cells will likely contribute to build the extracellular matrix of the islet organoid.

Vascularized organoids have helped investigators gain insight into physiology and pathophysiology in other research areas including liver (79), lung (80), and brain (81). Therefore, methods to deliver endothelial cells to pseudoislets would be a powerful tool for future islet research. Indeed, mosaic pseudoislets can be generated in vitro by mixing of dispersed islets with endothelial progenitor cells (82). This approach can be extended by transplantation of mosaic pseudoislets and determination of how the graft's structure and function recapitulate the features of islets in the pancreas (83).

Innervation

The pancreatic islet is innervated by parasympathetic, sympathetic, and sensory nerves (64). While the innervation density and target cells may vary between species (64), the signaling molecules they release (e.g., acetylcholine and norepinephrine) have been shown to regulate islet blood flow (16) and promote insulin secretion in both mouse and human islets (84,85). The loss of sympathetic innervation seen in T1D may result in a substantial impairment of glucagon responses (86). Inclusion of neurons in organoid culture may enable investigating the neural defects observed in the islet in autoimmune diabetes.

How can islet innervation be engineered in vitro? Given that vascular endothelial growth factor (VEGF) coordinates islet innervation via vasculature scaffolding (87), it is likely that a pseudoislet organoid will need a functional vasculature before inclusion of neuronal cells in a pseudoislet organoid. Neurons could be added to a pseudoislet mix of endocrine and vascular cells. This would mimic the close association that neuro-insular complexes have with the peripheral vasculature of the islet. An alternative is to coculture neuronal organoids with pseudoislets. This would allow exploring the factors that attract neuronal projections to the islet and studying how innervation affects islet function. Here, the classical assay of Nobel Prize winner Rita Levi-Montalcini comes to our minds: a sensory ganglion is dissected out, cultured, and examined for nerve fiber outgrowth after exposure to different factors. This approach has been used recently to show that β-cells migrate toward explants of sympathetic ganglia, thus demonstrating that nervous input provides inductive cues for islet architecture (88). One can only imagine the myriad of possible combinations of different types of ganglia with pseudoislets of varying compositions. Of note, this approach can be extended to the in vivo situation by cotransplantation of two types of organoids into the anterior chamber of the eye, as has been done for tissues from different brain regions (89).

Conclusions

The decoding of paracrine signaling in the islet has significantly increased our understanding of the biology of this important micro-organ. The rate of new discoveries in islet research is at an all-time high. As we were writing this article, two new interesting articles on islet organoids were published (90,91). Hence, it is hard to reconcile all these findings and fit them into a cohesive physiological model. We have discussed studies using tried-and-tested methodologies as well as new analytical and synthetic approaches and mentioned the discoveries that they generated. We propose that more research with pseudoislets is needed to decipher complex interactions between endocrine, vascular, nerve, and immune cells. Generating mosaic islet organoids will be crucial for creating disease-modeling platforms aimed at revealing mechanisms of diabetes pathogenesis. While the source of tissue material in pilot studies will likely be renewable cell sources, such as cell lines, we advocate the use of human islets when possible, given their increased availability and relevance for the human disease. The studies discussed in this review have provided insight into the mechanisms of intraislet communication and how they impact insulin secretion. Knowing how interactions between different cell types change under stress conditions could inform approaches to increase or restore β-cell function in diabetes.

Funding. The authors' work was supported by the Diabetes Research Institute Foundation and National Institutes of Health grants R56DK084321 (A.C.), R01DK084321 (A.C.), R01DK111538 (A.C.), R01DK113093 (A.C.), U01DK120456 (A.C.), R33ES025673 (A.C.), and R21ES025673 (A.C.); Leona M. and Harry B. Helmsley Charitable Trust grants G-2018PG-T1D034 and G-1912-03552; and the American Heart Association 19POST34450054 (J.W.).

Duality of Interest. No potential conflicts of interest relevant to this article were reported.

References

1. Halban PA, Wollheim CB, Blondel B, Meda P, Niesor EN, Mintz DH. The possible importance of contact between pancreatic islet cells for the control of insulin release. Endocrinology 1982;111:86–94

2. Weir GC, Halban PA, Meda P, Wollheim CB, Orci L, Renold AE. Dispersed adult rat pancreatic islet cells in culture: A, B, and D cell function. Metabolism 1984;33: 447–453

3. Pipeleers D, in't Veld PI, Maes E, Van De Winkel M. Glucose-induced insulin release depends on functional cooperation between islet cells. Proc Natl Acad Sci U S A 1982;79:7322–7325

4. Hauge-Evans AC, Squires PE, Persaud SJ, Jones PM. Pancreatic beta-cell-to-beta-cell interactions are required for integrated responses to nutrient stimuli: enhanced Ca2+ and insulin secretory responses of MIN6 pseudoislets. Diabetes 1999;48:1402–1408

5. Lammert E, Thorn P. The role of the islet niche on beta cell structure and function. J Mol Biol 2020;432:1407–1418

6. Halban PA, Powers SL, George KL, Bonner-Weir S. Spontaneous reassociation of dispersed adult rat pancreatic islet cells into aggregates with three-dimensional architecture typical of native islets. Diabetes 1987;36: 783–790

7. Huising MO, van der Meulen T, Huang JL, Pourhosseinzadeh MS, Noguchi GM. The difference δ-cells make in glucose control. Physiology (Bethesda) 2018; 33:403–411

8. Rodriguez-Diaz R, Tamayo A, Hara M, Caicedo A. The local paracrine actions of the pancreatic α-cell. Diabetes 2020;69:550–558

9. Jacques-Silva MC, Correa-Medina M, Cabrera O, et al. ATP-gated P2X3 receptors constitute a positive autocrine signal for insulin release in the human pancreatic beta cell. Proc Natl Acad Sci U S A 2010;107:6465–6470

10. Khan S, Yan-Do R, Duong E, et al. Autocrine activation of P2Y1 receptors couples Ca (2+) influx to Ca (2+) release in human pancreatic beta cells. Diabetologia 2014;57:2535–2545

11. Wuttke A, Idevall-Hagren O, Tengholm A. P2Y1 receptor-dependent diacylglycerol signaling microdomains in β cells promote insulin secretion. FASEB J 2013;27:1610–1620

12. Burnstock G, Novak I. Purinergic signalling in the pancreas in health and disease. J Endocrinol 2012;213:123–141

13. Weitz JR, Makhmutova M, Almaça J, et al. Mouse pancreatic islet macrophages use locally released ATP to monitor beta cell activity. Diabetologia 2018; 61:182–192

14. Weitz JR, Jacques-Silva C, Qadir MMF, et al. Secretory functions of macrophages in the human pancreatic islet are regulated by endogenous purinergic signaling. Diabetes 2020;69:1206–1218

15. Fotino C, Dal Ben D, Adinolfi E. Emerging roles of purinergic signaling in diabetes. Med Chem 2018;14:428–438

16. Almaca J, Weitz J, Rodriguez-Diaz R, Pereira E, Caicedo A. The pericyte of the pancreatic islet regulates capillary diameter and local blood flow. Cell Metab 2018; 27:630–644.e4

17. Rorsman P, Berggren PO, Bokvist K, et al. Glucose-inhibition of glucagon secretion involves activation of GABAA-receptor chloride channels. Nature 1989; 341:233–236

18. Korol SV, Jin Z, Jin Y, et al. Functional characterization of native, high-affinity GABAA receptors in human pancreatic β cells. EBioMedicine 2018;30:273–282

19. Soltani N, Qiu H, Aleksic M, et al. GABA exerts protective and regenerative effects on islet beta cells and reverses diabetes. Proc Natl Acad Sci U S A 2011; 108:11692–11697

20. Ben-Othman N, Vieira A, Courtney M, et al. Long-term GABA administration induces alpha cell-mediated beta-like cell neogenesis. Cell 2017;168:73–85.e11

21. Ackermann AM, Moss NG, Kaestner KH. GABA and artesunate do not induce pancreatic α-to-β cell transdifferentiation in vivo. Cell Metab 2018;28:787–792.e3

22. van der Meulen T, Lee S, Noordeloos E, et al. Artemether does not turn α cells into β cells. Cell Metab 2018;27:218–225.e4

23. Braun M, Ramracheya R, Bengtsson M, et al. Gamma-aminobutyric acid (GABA) is an autocrine excitatory transmitter in human pancreatic beta-cells. Diabetes 2010;59:1694–1701

24. Menegaz D, Hagan DW, Almaça J, et al. Mechanism and effects of pulsatile GABA secretion from cytosolic pools in the human beta cell. Nat Metab 2019;1: 1110–1126

25. Benninger RK, Hofmann O, Onfelt B, et al. Fluorescence-lifetime imaging of DNA-dye interactions within continuous-flow microfluidic systems. Angew Chem Int Ed Engl 2007;46:2228–2231

26. Rocheleau JV, Walker GM, Head WS, McGuinness OP, Piston DW. Microfluidic glucose stimulation reveals limited coordination of intracellular Ca2+ activity oscillations in pancreatic islets. Proc Natl Acad Sci U S A 2004;101:12899–12903

27. Marciniak A, Cohrs CM, Tsata V, et al. Using pancreas tissue slices for in situ studies of islet of Langerhans and acinar cell biology. Nat Protoc 2014;9:2809–2822

28. Speier S, Nyqvist D, Cabrera O, et al. Noninvasive in vivo imaging of pancreatic islet cell biology. Nat Med 2008;14:574–578

29. Janjuha S, Pal Singh S, Ninov N. Analysis of beta-cell function using single-cell resolution calcium imaging in Zebrafish islets. J Vis Exp 2018:57851

30. Westacott MJ, Ludin NWF, Benninger RKP. Spatially organized β-cell subpopulations control electrical dynamics across islets of Langerhans. Biophys J 2017;113:1093–1108

31. Pipeleers D. The biosociology of pancreatic B cells. Diabetologia 1987;30:277–291

32. Dominguez-Gutierrez G, Xin Y, Gromada J. Heterogeneity of human pancreatic β-cells. Mol Metab 2019;27S:S7–S14

33. Johnston NR, Mitchell RK, Haythorne E, et al. Beta cell hubs dictate pancreatic islet responses to glucose. Cell Metab 2016;24:389–401

34. Almaça J, Liang T, Gaisano HY, Nam HG, Berggren PO, Caicedo A. Spatial and temporal coordination of insulin granule exocytosis in intact human pancreatic islets. Diabetologia 2015;58:2810–2818

35. Rutter GA, Ninov N, Salem V, Hodson DJ. Comment on Satin et al. "Take me to your leader": an electrophysiological appraisal of the role of hub cells in pancreatic islets. Diabetes 2020;69:830–836. Diabetes 2020;69:e10–e11

36. Satin LS, Zhang Q, Rorsman P. "Take me to your leader": an electrophysiological appraisal of the role of hub cells in pancreatic islets. Diabetes 2020;69:830–836

37. Lock LT, Laychock SG, Tzanakakis ES. Pseudoislets in stirred-suspension culture exhibit enhanced cell survival, propagation and insulin secretion. J Biotechnol 2011;151:278–286

38. Parnaud G, Lavallard V, Bedat B, et al. Cadherin engagement improves insulin secretion of single human β-cells. Diabetes 2015;64:887–896

39. Kelly C, Parke HG, McCluskey JT, Flatt PR, McClenaghan NH. The role of glucagon- and somatostatin-secreting cells in the regulation of insulin release and beta-cell function in heterotypic pseudoislets. Diabetes Metab Res Rev 2010;26:525–533

40. Ishihara H, Maechler P, Gjinovci A, Herrera PL, Wollheim CB. Islet beta-cell secretion determines glucagon release from neighbouring alpha-cells. Nat Cell Biol 2003;5:330–335

41. Brereton H, Carvell MJ, Persaud SJ, Jones PM. Islet alpha-cells do not influence insulin secretion from beta-cells through cell-cell contact. Endocrine 2007;31:61–65

42. Kojima N, Takeuchi S, Sakai Y. Engineering of pseudoislets: effect on insulin secretion activity by cell number, cell population, and microchannel networks. Transplant Proc 2014;46:1161–1165

43. Adams MT, Gilbert JM, Hinojosa Paiz J, Bowman FM, Blum B. Endocrine cell type sorting and mature architecture in the islets of Langerhans require expression of Roundabout receptors in β cells. Sci Rep 2018;8:10876

44. Dyachok O, Idevall-Hagren O, Sågetorp J, et al. Glucose-induced cyclic AMP oscillations regulate pulsatile insulin secretion. Cell Metab 2008;8:26–37

45. Arrojo EDR, Lev-Ram V, Tyagi S, et al. Age mosaicism across multiple scales in adult tissues. Cell Metab 2019;30:343–351.e3

46. Lacy PE, Kostianovsky M. Method for the isolation of intact islets of Langerhans from the rat pancreas. Diabetes 1967;16:35–39

47. Caton D, Calabrese A, Mas C, et al. Lentivirus-mediated transduction of connexin cDNAs shows level- and isoform-specific alterations in insulin secretion of primary pancreatic beta-cells. J Cell Sci 2003;116:2285–2294

48. Arda HE, Li L, Tsai J, et al. Age-dependent pancreatic gene regulation reveals mechanisms governing human β cell function. Cell Metab 2016;23:909–920

49. Walker JT, Haliyur R, Nelson HA, et al. Integrated human pseudoislet system and microfluidic platform demonstrate differences in GPCR signaling in islet cells. JCI Insight 2020;5:e137017

50. Harata M, Liu S, Promes JA, Burand AJ, Ankrum JA, Imai Y. Delivery of shRNA via lentivirus in human pseudoislets provides a model to test dynamic regulation of insulin secretion and gene function in human islets. Physiol Rep 2018;6:e13907

51. Misun PM, Yesildag B, Forschler F, et al. In vitro platform for studying human insulin release dynamics of single pancreatic islet microtissues at high resolution. Adv Biosyst 2020;4:e1900291

52. Tateishi K, He J, Taranova O, Liang G, D'Alessio AC, Zhang Y. Generation of insulin-secreting islet-like clusters from human skin fibroblasts. J Biol Chem 2008;283:31601–31607

53. Kim Y, Kim H, Ko UH, et al. Islet-like organoids derived from human pluripotent stem cells efficiently function in the glucose responsiveness in vitro and in vivo. Sci Rep 2016;6:35145

54. Basford CL, Prentice KJ, Hardy AB, et al. The functional and molecular characterisation of human embryonic stem cell-derived insulin-positive cells compared with adult pancreatic beta cells. Diabetologia 2012;55:358–371

55. D'Amour KA, Bang AG, Eliazer S, et al. Production of pancreatic hormone-expressing endocrine cells from human embryonic stem cells. Nat Biotechnol 2006;24:1392–1401

56. Velazco-Cruz L, Song J, Maxwell KG, et al. Acquisition of dynamic function in human stem cell-derived β cells. Stem Cell Reports 2019;12:351–365

57. Lehmann R, Zuellig RA, Kugelmeier P, et al. Superiority of small islets in human islet transplantation. Diabetes 2007;56:594–603

58. Millman JR, Xie C, Van Dervort A, Gürtler M, Pagliuca FW, Melton DA. Generation of stem cell-derived β-cells from patients with type 1 diabetes. Nat Commun 2016;7:11463

59. Joshi K, Elso C, Motazedian A, et al. Induced pluripotent stem cell macrophages present antigen to proinsulin-specific T cell receptors from donor-matched islet-infiltrating T cells in type 1 diabetes. Diabetologia 2019;62:2245–2251

60. Vegas AJ, Veiseh O, Gürtler M, et al. Long-term glycemic control using polymer-encapsulated human stem cell-derived beta cells in immune-competent mice. Nat Med 2016;22:306–311

61. Ahn YB, Xu G, Marselli L, et al. Changes in gene expression in beta cells after islet isolation and transplantation using laser-capture microdissection. Diabetologia 2007;50:334–342

62. Lacy PE, Finke EH. Activation of intraislet lymphoid cells causes destruction of islet cells. Am J Pathol 1991;138:1183–1190

63. Nyqvist D, Köhler M, Wahlstedt H, Berggren PO. Donor islet endothelial cells participate in formation of functional vessels within pancreatic islet grafts. Diabetes 2005;54:2287–2293

64. Rodriguez-Diaz R, Speier S, Molano RD, et al. Noninvasive in vivo model demonstrating the effects of autonomic innervation on pancreatic islet function. Proc Natl Acad Sci U S A 2012;109:21456–21461

65. Banaei-Bouchareb L, Gouon-Evans V, Samara-Boustani D, et al. Insulin cell mass is altered in Csf1op/Csf1op macrophage-deficient mice. J Leukoc Biol 2004;76:359–367

66. Brissova M, Aamodt K, Brahmachary P, et al. Islet microenvironment, modulated by vascular endothelial growth factor-A signaling, promotes β cell regeneration. Cell Metab 2014;19:498–511

67. Ying W, Lee YS, Dong Y, et al. Expansion of islet-resident macrophages leads to inflammation affecting β cell proliferation and function in obesity. Cell Metab 2019;29:457–474.e5

68. Vomund AN, Zinselmeyer BH, Hughes J, et al. Beta cells transfer vesicles containing insulin to phagocytes for presentation to T cells. Proc Natl Acad Sci U S A 2015;112:E5496–E5502

69. Calderon B, Carrero JA, Ferris ST, et al. The pancreas anatomy conditions the origin and properties of resident macrophages. J Exp Med 2015;212:1497–1512

70. Diana J, Simoni Y, Furio L, et al. Crosstalk between neutrophils, B-1a cells and plasmacytoid dendritic cells initiates autoimmune diabetes. Nat Med 2013;19:65–73

71. Ehses JA, Perren A, Eppler E, et al. Increased number of islet-associated macrophages in type 2 diabetes. Diabetes 2007;56:2356–2370

72. Willcox A, Richardson SJ, Bone AJ, Foulis AK, Morgan NG. Analysis of islet inflammation in human type 1 diabetes. Clin Exp Immunol 2009;155:173–181

73. Swift SM, Rose S, London NJ, James RF. Development and optimization of the human allogeneic mixed lymphocyte islet (MLIC) and acinar (MLAC) coculture system. Transpl Immunol 1996;4:169–176

74. Dirice E, Kahraman S, Jiang W, et al. Soluble factors secreted by T cells promote β-cell proliferation. Diabetes 2014;63:188–202

75. Hogan MF, Hull RL. The islet endothelial cell: a novel contributor to beta cell secretory dysfunction in diabetes. Diabetologia 2017;60:952–959

76. Carlsson PO, Jansson L. Disruption of insulin receptor signaling in endothelial cells shows the central role of an intact islet blood flow for in vivo β-cell function. Diabetes 2015;64:700–702

77. Carlsson PO, Palm F, Mattsson G. Low revascularization of experimentally transplanted human pancreatic islets. J Clin Endocrinol Metab 2002;87:5418–5423

78. Low JT, Zavortink M, Mitchell JM, et al. Insulin secretion from beta cells in intact mouse islets is targeted towards the vasculature. Diabetologia 2014;57:1655–1663

79. Takebe T, Sekine K, Enomura M, et al. Vascularized and functional human liver from an iPSC-derived organ bud transplant. Nature 2013;499:481–484

80. Nashimoto Y, Hayashi T, Kunita I, et al. Integrating perfusable vascular networks with a three-dimensional tissue in a microfluidic device. Integr Biol 2017;9:506–518

81. Cakir B, Xiang Y, Tanaka Y, et al. Engineering of human brain organoids with a functional vascular-like system. Nat Methods 2019;16:1169–1175

82. Penko D, Mohanasundaram D, Sen S, et al. Incorporation of endothelial progenitor cells into mosaic pseudoislets. Islets 2011;3:73–79

83. Beger C, Cirulli V, Vajkoczy P, Halban PA, Menger MD. Vascularization of purified pancreatic islet-like cell aggregates (pseudoislets) after syngeneic transplantation. Diabetes 1998;47:559–565

84. Duttaroy A, Zimliki CL, Gautam D, Cui Y, Mears D, Wess J. Muscarinic stimulation of pancreatic insulin and glucagon release is abolished in m3 muscarinic acetylcholine receptor-deficient mice. Diabetes 2004;53:1714–1720

85. Molina J, Rodriguez-Diaz R, Fachado A, Jacques-Silva MC, Berggren PO, Caicedo A. Control of insulin secretion by cholinergic signaling in the human pancreatic islet. Diabetes 2014;63:2714–2726

86. Mundinger TO, Mei Q, Foulis AK, Fligner CL, Hull RL, Taborsky GJ Jr. Human type 1 diabetes is characterized by an early, marked, sustained, and islet-selective loss of sympathetic nerves. Diabetes 2016;65:2322–2330

87. Reinert RB, Cai Q, Hong JY, et al. Vascular endothelial growth factor coordinates islet innervation via vascular scaffolding. Development 2014;141:1480–1491

88. Borden P, Houtz J, Leach SD, Kuruvilla R. Sympathetic innervation during development is necessary for pancreatic islet architecture and functional maturation. Cell Rep 2013;4:287–301

89. Goldowitz D, Seiger A, Olson L. Degree of hyperinnervation of area dentata by locus coeruleus in the presence of septum or entorhinal cortex as studied by sequential intraocular triple transplantation. Exp Brain Res 1984;56:351–360

90. Lebreton F, Lavallard V, Bellofatto K, et al. Insulin-producing organoids engineered from islet and amniotic epithelial cells to treat diabetes. Nat Commun 2019;10:4491

91. Wang D, Wang J, Bai L, et al. Long-term expansion of pancreatic islet organoids from resident Procr + progenitors. Cell 2020;180:1198–1211.e19

Distinct Molecular Signatures of Clinical Clusters in People With Type 2 Diabetes: An IMI-RHAPSODY Study

Roderick C. Slieker,[1,2] Louise A. Donnelly,[3] Hugo Fitipaldi,[4] Gerard A. Bouland,[1] Giuseppe N. Giordano,[4] Mikael Åkerlund,[4] Mathias J. Gerl,[5] Emma Ahlqvist,[4] Ashfaq Ali,[6] Iulian Dragan,[7] Petra Elders,[8] Andreas Festa,[9,10] Michael K. Hansen,[11] Amber A. van der Heijden,[8] Dina Mansour Aly,[4] Min Kim,[6,12] Dmitry Kuznetsov,[7] Florence Mehl,[7] Christian Klose,[5] Kai Simons,[5] Imre Pavo,[9] Timothy J. Pullen,[13,14] Tommi Suvitaival,[6] Asger Wretlind,[6] Peter Rossing,[6,15] Valeriya Lyssenko,[16,17] Cristina Legido Quigley,[6,11] Leif Groop,[4,18] Bernard Thorens,[19] Paul W. Franks,[4,20] Mark Ibberson,[7] Guy A. Rutter,[13,21] Joline W.J. Beulens,[2,22] Leen M. 't Hart,[1,2,23] and Ewan R. Pearson[3]

Diabetes 2021;70:2683–2693 | https://doi.org/10.2337/db20-1281

Type 2 diabetes is a multifactorial disease with multiple underlying aetiologies. To address this heterogeneity, investigators of a previous study clustered people with diabetes according to five diabetes subtypes. The aim of the current study is to investigate the etiology of these clusters by comparing their molecular signatures. In three independent cohorts, in total 15,940 individuals were clustered based on five clinical characteristics. In a subset, genetic ($N = 12,828$), metabolomic ($N = 2,945$), lipidomic ($N = 2,593$), and proteomic ($N = 1,170$) data were obtained in plasma. For each data type, each cluster was compared with the other four clusters as the reference. The insulin-resistant cluster showed the most distinct molecular signature, with higher branched-chain amino acid, diacylglycerol, and triacylglycerol levels and aberrant protein levels in plasma were enriched for proteins in the intracellular PI3K/Akt pathway. The obese cluster showed higher levels of cytokines. The mild diabetes cluster with high HDL showed the most beneficial molecular profile with effects opposite of those seen in the insulin-resistant cluster. This study shows that clustering people with type 2 diabetes can identify underlying molecular mechanisms related to pancreatic islets, liver, and adipose tissue metabolism. This provides novel biological insights into the diverse aetiological processes that would not be evident when type 2 diabetes is viewed as a homogeneous disease.

---

[1]Department of Cell and Chemical Biology, Leiden University Medical Center, Leiden, the Netherlands

[2]Department of Epidemiology and Data Science, Amsterdam Public Health Institute, Amsterdam UMC, location VUmc, Amsterdam, the Netherlands

[3]Population Health & Genomics, School of Medicine, University of Dundee, Dundee, U.K.

[4]Genetic and Molecular Epidemiology Unit, Lund University Diabetes Centre, Department of Clinical Sciences, Clinical Research Centre, Lund University, SUS, Malmö, Sweden

[5]Lipotype GmbH, Dresden, Germany

[6]Steno Diabetes Center Copenhagen, Gentofte, Denmark

[7]Vital-IT Group, SIB Swiss Institute of Bioinformatics, Lausanne, Switzerland

[8]Department of General Practice and Elderly Care Medicine, Amsterdam Public Health Research Institute, Amsterdam UMC, location VUmc, Amsterdam, the Netherlands

[9]Eli Lilly Regional Operations GmbH, Vienna, Austria

[10]1st Medical Department, LK Stockerau, Niederösterreich, Austria

[11]Cardiovascular and Metabolic Disease Research, Janssen Research & Development, Spring House, PA

[12]Institute of Pharmaceutical Science, Faculty of Life Sciences and Medicines, King's College London, London, U.K.

[13]Department of Diabetes, Guy's Campus, King's College London, London, U.K.

[14]Section of Cell Biology and Functional Genomics, Division of Diabetes, Endocrinology and Metabolism, Department of Metabolism, Digestion and Reproduction, Imperial College London, London, U.K.

[15]Department of Clinical Medicine, University of Copenhagen, Copenhagen, Denmark

[16]Department of Clinical Science, Center for Diabetes Research, University of Bergen, Bergen, Norway

[17]Genomics, Diabetes and Endocrinology Unit, Department of Clinical Sciences Malmö, Lund University Diabetes Centre, Skåne University Hospital, Malmö, Sweden

[18]Finnish Institute of Molecular Medicine, Helsinki University, Helsinki, Finland

[19]Center for Integrative Genomics, University of Lausanne, Lausanne, Switzerland

[20]Department of Nutrition, Harvard School of Public Health, Boston, MA

[21]Lee Kong Chian School of Medicine, Nan Yang Technological University, Singapore

[22]Julius Center for Health Sciences and Primary Care, University Medical Center Utrecht, Utrecht, the Netherlands

[23]Molecular Epidemiology, Department of Biomedical Data Sciences, Leiden University Medical Center, Leiden, the Netherlands

Type 2 diabetes is a multifactorial disease with multiple underlying aetiologies (1,2). In an attempt to address this heterogeneity, investigators of a recent study stratified people with any form of diabetes into five clusters based on six clinical variables: age, GAD antibodies, BMI, HbA^{1c}, insulin resistance (HOMA2 of insulin resistance), and β-cell function estimates (HOMA2 of β-cell function) (3). Based on this work, we clustered and cross validated individuals into five clusters in three large cohorts based on age, BMI, random or fasting C-peptide, HbA^{1c}, and HDL, largely reproducing the All New Diabetics in Scania (ANDIS) clusters and using more readily measured clinical variables (4).

The results reported in the original and subsequent articles showed that people in different clusters had different risks for a number of diabetes-related outcomes (3,5–7). The autoimmunity and insulin-deficient cluster was defined by a high HbA$_{1c}$ at diagnosis, had ketoacidosis and retinopathy (7) more often, and progressed more rapidly onto insulin compared to the other clusters (3). The insulin-resistant cluster showed a higher frequency of nonalcoholic fatty liver disease, and people in this group were at increased risk of developing chronic kidney disease (3). The differences in progression and characteristics of the different clusters suggest that these groups represent different underlying aetiologies. For example, differences in genotype frequency across clusters based on candidate loci were observed and this was further illustrated in a follow-up study where it was shown that individuals in different clusters have differences in portioned polygenic risk scores for diabetes-related outcomes (3,8).

A systematic deconvolution of the different etiological processes underlying the clusters is currently lacking. To address this, we investigate each cluster's molecular signature using metabolomics, lipidomics, proteomics, and genomics to better understand the underlying aetiological processes representative of patients with diabetes in that cluster.

RESEARCH DESIGN AND METHODS

Cohort Descriptions

Data from 15,940 individuals from three cohorts, the Hoorn Diabetes Care System (DCS) (Netherlands), Genetics of Diabetes Audit and Research in Tayside Scotland (GoDARTS) (Scotland), and ANDIS (Sweden), were used in this cross-sectional study. Inclusion criteria for IMI-RHAPSODY were age of diagnosis ≥35 years, clinical data available within 2 years after diagnosis, GAD$^-$, no missing data in one of the five clinical variables used for cluster-ing, and the presence of genome-wide association study (GWAS) data. Individuals were clustered using K-means clustering based on five clinical characteristics: age at sampling, BMI, HbA$_{1c}$, HDL, and C-peptide. Of note, C-peptide was included in the clustering as a proxy of insulin resistance, while HDL has previously been recognized as a risk factor for time to insulin requirement. Details on the cohorts and clustering have previously been published (4). Briefly, DCS is an open prospective cohort that started in 1998 comprising >14,000 individuals with type 2 diabetes from the northwest part of the Netherlands (9). The Ethical Review Committee of the VU University Medical Center, Amsterdam, approved the study. People visit DCS annually as part of routine care. GoDARTS is a study comprising individuals with diabetes from the Tayside region of Scotland (N = 391,274; January 1996) who were added to the Diabetes Audit and Research in Tayside Scotland (DARTS) register (10). The GoDARTS study was approved by the Tayside Medical Ethics Committee. Longitudinal retrospective and prospective anonymized data were collected, including data on prescribing, biochemistry, and clinical data. In ANDIS, people were recruited with incident diabetes within Scania County, Sweden, from January 2008 to November 2016.

Molecular Measures

An overview of the sample selection procedure is given in Supplementary Fig. 1A. Individuals were selected based on the shortest time between diagnosis date and sampling date without taking into account cluster assignment. Analysis of small charged molecule analytes (metabolomics, ultrahigh-performance liquid chromatography–tandem mass spectrometry [UHLPC-MS/MS]) was performed in the largest set (N = 2,945), followed by lipidomics (N = 2,593 [Lipotype lipidomics platform; Lipotype, Dresden, Germany]) and proteomics (N = 1,170 [somascan Platform; SomaLogic]). Of note, the smaller sets were selected from the larger set based on the samples being collected closest to the time of diagnosis, so in the smallest set of 1,170, GWAS, metabolomics, lipidomics, and proteomics were available (Supplementary Fig. 1A). Molecular measures were taken close to diagnosis (Supplementary Table 2). Quality control (QC) was performed in a similar way for metabolomics, lipidomics, and proteomics. A participant's data were excluded if their profile was a strong outlier based on principal components analysis and the data of the individual measurements was clearly distinct from the other samples.

Corresponding authors: Leen M. 't Hart, lmthart@lumc.nl, and Ewan R. Pearson, e.z.pearson@dundee.ac.uk

Received 22 December 2020 and accepted 1 August 2021

This article contains supplementary material online at https://doi.org/10.2337/figshare.15113193.

R.C.S., L.A.D., L.M.'t.H., and E.R.P. contributed equally.

Genetic Data

In DCS, genetic data were generated with the Illumina HumanCoreExome array. In GoDARTS genetic data were generated with the Affymetrix Genome-Wide Human SNP Array 6.0 and the Illumina HumanOmniExpress array. In ANDIS, genotyping was performed with InfiniumCoreExome-24 v1-1 BeadChip arrays (Illumina, San Diego, CA) at Lund University Diabetes Centre. Samples were excluded for ambiguous gender, call rate <95%, and any duplicate or related individuals (pi_hat $\geq$ 0.2). Single nucleotide polymorphisms (SNPs) were excluded for monomorphic SNPs, SNPs with a minor allele frequency (MAF) <0.05, and SNPs with missingness rate >0.05. Differences in diabetes-related genetic risk were based on 403 relatively independent diabetes-associated SNPs identified in a recent large GWAS meta-analysis (11). Genetic data were imputed using the Michigan Imputation Server against the reference panel Human Reference Consortium R1.1 with default settings, i.e., phasing with Eagle v2.3 and population of European descent (12). SNPs with minor allele frequency <5% were discarded from the analyses, leaving 394 SNPs across the three studies.

Metabolomics

Fifteen small charged molecules were measured in plasma with targeted UHLPC-MS/MS (Steno Diabetes Center) (13). In DCS, 1,267 individuals were included for metabolomics measurements. All passed QC, and data for 1,230 individuals overlapped with the cluster data. In GoDARTS, 898 individuals were included in the analysis; 1 failed QC, and among the 897 remaining individuals, data for 894 overlapped with the cluster data. In ANDIS, 896 individuals were included in the analysis; 4 failed QC, and of the 892 remaining samples, 821 overlapped with the cluster data.

Lipidomics

A total of 614 plasma lipids common to the three cohorts were determined with use of an Q Exactive mass spectrometer (Thermo Fisher Scientific) equipped with a TriVersa NanoMate ion source (Advion Biosciences) on the Lipotype lipidomics platform (14). Samples were divided into analytical batches of 84 samples each. Lipid identification was performed on unprocessed mass spectra files with LipotypeXplorer (15). Only lipid identifications with a signal-to-noise ratio >5, and a signal intensity fivefold higher than in corresponding blank samples, were considered for further data analysis. Batch correction was applied using eight reference samples per 96-well. Amounts were also corrected for analytical drift if the P value of the slope was <0.05 with an R^2 >0.75 and the relative drift was >5%. In DCS, 900 individuals were included for lipidomics measurements; all passed QC, and data for 877 overlapped with the cluster data. In GoDARTS, 898 individuals were included in the analysis; 1 failed QC, and of the 897 remaining samples, 894 overlapped with one of the clusters. In ANDIS, 896 individuals

were included in the analysis; 5 failed QC, and of the 891 remaining samples, 820 overlapped with one of the clusters. Lipid nomenclature is used as previously described, and SwissLipids database identifiers are provided (16) (Supplementary Table 1). After QC 162 lipid species were used in this study. The median coefficient of subspecies variation of the 162 lipids used as accessed by reference samples was 9.49% across all three cohorts.

Protein Measurements

Protein levels (1,195 proteins) in plasma were measured on the SomaLogic somascan platform (Boulder, CO) in 600 individuals each, for both DCS and GoDARTS. Individuals were removed if they were strong outliers based on a principal components analysis. In DCS, 600 individuals were included for proteomics measurements, 11 failed QC, and data for 573 overlapped with data for one of the clusters. In GoDARTS, 600 individuals were included in the analysis; 1 failed QC, and of the 599 remaining samples, 597 overlapped with one of the clusters.

Statistical Analysis

Molecular data were log transformed and z-scaled before analysis on a federated node system. Data for each of the cohorts were stored on a local node using Opal, an open-source data warehouse (Open Source Software for BioBanks [OBiBa]). A central node responsible for federated node access, user administration, and software deployment was set up at SIB Swiss Institute of Bioinformatics. Clinical and molecular data were harmonized according to the CDISC Study Data Tabulation Model (www.cdisc.org).

To identify molecular measures specific for a cluster, a generalized linear model was used to test each of the molecular measures in each cluster, where cluster i was compared against reference group j, where j was a combined group of the other clusters. Effect sizes represent change per log SD of the tested molecular measure. Genetic data were not transformed and represent change in allele frequency. For example, cluster 1 was compared with clusters 2–5 combined and cluster 2 was compared with clusters 1 and 3–5. Main results presented are based on an unadjusted model (log and z-scaled). Next, as an exploratory sensitivity analysis, models were adjusted for the extreme characteristic of a cluster to investigate whether the observed effect was independent of the extreme characteristic. This was only done for those clusters with extreme characteristics. Models were run on each of the cohorts separately and meta-analyzed with the R package meta (17). Meta-analyzed P values were adjusted with the Benjamini-Hochberg procedure, and a false discovery rate (FDR)-adjusted P value <0.05 was considered significant.

Partitioned polygenic risk scores (pPRS) were obtained from Udler et al. (18). In each individual cohort, dosages of SNPs were multiplied with the scores for each cluster, which resulted in a risk score per individual for each of the five clusters: β-cell (30 SNPs), proinsulin (7 SNPs), obesity (5 SNPs), lipodystrophy (20 SNPs), and liver (5 SNPs). Differences in pPRS were tested with a linear model for one cluster with the other clusters as the reference group. Next, results from the three cohorts were meta-analyzed with use of the metagen function from the meta package. P values were Bonferroni adjusted and considered significant at $P_{adjusted} < 0.05$.

Pathway enrichment on the proteomics was performed based on Kyoto Encyclopedia of Genes and Genomes (KEGG) pathways with the use of the R package STRINGdb (1.24.0). The entire SomaLogic set (1,195 proteins) was used as the background set. P values of enriched pathways were adjusted using the Benjamini-Hochberg procedure, and an FDR-adjusted P value <0.05 was considered significant.

Effect sizes of proteins associated with estimated glomerular filtration rate (eGFR) and incident cardiovascular disease (CVD) were obtained from Yang et al. (2020) (19). Up- and downregulated proteins in each of the clusters ($P_{FDR} < 0.05$) were selected. Effect sizes in the current study were compared to Yang et al. obtained 1) correlation coefficient of protein levels and eGFR and 2) hazard ratios (HRs) from the Cox proportional hazards models for CVD in individuals without chronic kidney disease (19).

Analyses were performed with R statistics (version 3.6.2). Figures were produced with the R packages ggplot2 (v3.3.0) and omicCircos (v1.22.0).

Data and Resource Availability

The data sets generated during and/or analyzed during the current study are not publicly available but are available from the corresponding author upon reasonable request.

RESULTS

In this cross-sectional study, 15,940 individuals from three cohorts were included as previously described (4). We reproduced the original ANDIS severe insulin-deficient (SIDD), severe insulin resistance (SIRD), and mild obesity-related diabetes (MOD) clusters and refined the mild age-related diabetes (MARD) cluster into two: a subset with high HDL (MDH) and one without any particular defining features (MD). The characteristics of the clusters and those of the individuals used for molecular characterization (genetic data, metabolites, lipids, and proteins) are given in Supplementary Table 2 and Supplementary Table 3.

SIDD

For SIDD, no differences were observed in allele frequency of known type 2 diabetes loci compared with the other clusters (Supplementary Table 4) or in the pPRS (Supplementary Fig. 2). Two metabolites, tyrosine (Fig. 1A and Fig. 1B) and asymmetric/symmetric dimethylarginine (Fig. 1C and Supplementary Table 5), were significantly lower in SIDD versus all other clusters. The effect sizes attenuated slightly after adjustment for the primary variable HbA_{1c} that defined the SIDD cluster (Supplementary Fig. 3B and Supplementary Table 5). Of the lipids, eight were downregulated and one upregulated. Out of the eight downregulated lipids, three belonged to the sphingomyelin class, four

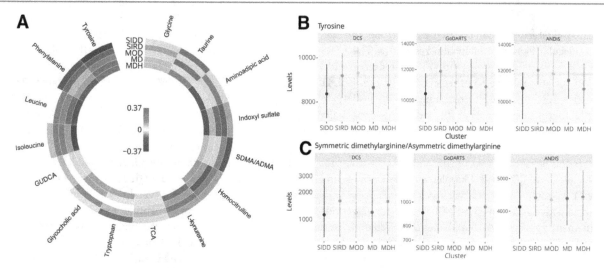

Figure 1—Metabolite levels in the five clusters. *A*: Change in metabolites levels in each of the clusters versus all others. Colors represent effect size in log SD; red, upregulation, and blue, downregulation. GUDCA, glycoursodeoxycholic acid; SDMA/ADMA, symmetric dimethylarginine/asymmetric dimethylarginine; TCA, taurocholic acid. *B*: Levels of tyrosine in DCS, GoDARTS, and ANDIS. SIDD and SIRD $P_{FDR} <$ 0.05. *C*: Levels of (a)symmetric dimethylarginine. SIDD and SIRD $P_{FDR} \leq$ 0.05. Dots represent the median, and the vertical line represents the interquartile range.

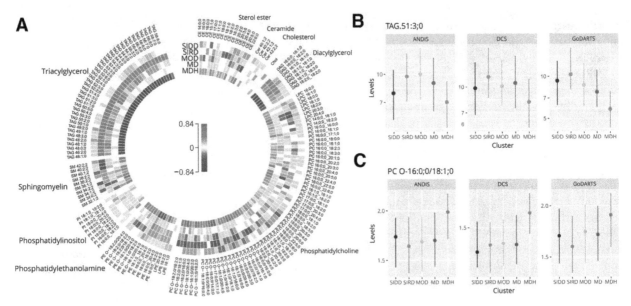

Figure 2—Lipid levels in the five clusters. *A*: Change in lipid levels in each of the clusters versus all others. Colors represent effect size in log SD: red, upregulation, and blue, downregulation. *B*: Levels of TAG 51:3;0 in DCS, GoDARTS, and ANDIS. SIRD, MOD, and MDH $P_{FDR} \leq 0.05$. *C*: Levels of PC *O*-16:0;0/18:1;0. SIRD, MOD, and MDH $P_{FDR} \leq 0.05$. Dots represent the median, and the vertical line represents the interquartile range.

belonged to the phosphatidylcholine (PC) class, and one was a cholesterol ester (Fig. 2*A* and Supplementary Table 6). The sole upregulated lipid was a cholesterol ester (CE 20:2;0). Seven of nine lipids remained significant after adjustment (Supplementary Fig. 3*C* and Supplementary Table 6). Finally, eight proteins were differentially expressed, with four up- and four downregulated (Supplementary Fig. 4*A*–*D*), where the effect sizes remained similar after adjustment (Supplementary Fig. 3*D* and Supplementary Table 7).

SIRD

The SIRD cluster was characterized by a strong and distinct molecular signature of insulin resistance. The pPRS for β-cell function and proinsulin (18) were decreased in the SIRD cluster relative to other clusters (β-cell, β 1.41 [95% CI −2.21 to −0.62]; proinsulin, −0.28 [−0.41 to −0.15]) (Supplementary Fig. 2), indicating genetically higher β-cell function in the SIRD group. Five diabetes-associated SNPs all showed a lower risk allele frequency. The top SNP (rs3802177-A) of SIRD mapped to the protective allele in *SLC30A8* (Supplementary Table 4 and Table 1). In a sensitivity analysis, only the *SLC30A8* variant remained significant after adjustment for C-peptide (Supplementary Fig. 3*A*, Supplementary Table 4, and Table 1). The SIRD cluster showed eight upregulated metabolites, including four amino acids, i.e., tyrosine, leucine, isoleucine, and phenylalanine (Fig. 1*A* and Supplementary Fig. 5*A* and *B*). Two were metabolites of the amino acid L-tryptophan, i.e., L-kynurenine and indoxyl sulfate. Adjustment for C-peptide attenuated the effect (Supplementary Fig. 3*B* and Supplementary Table 5).

Eighty-nine lipids were changed in SIRD, with 45 (50.6%) upregulated and 44 downregulated (49.4%) (Fig. 2*A*). Of the 45 upregulated lipids, 43 were in the diacylglycerol (DAG) and triacylglycerol (TAG) class, with TAG 51:3;0 as the strongest associating lipid (Fig. 2*B* and Supplementary Table 6), while the remaining two upregulated lipids were PCs containing the n-3 fatty acid docosahexaenoic acid (22:6;0, PC 18:0;0_22:6;0, PC 16:0;0_22:6;0). Of the 44 downregulated lipids, the most represented were the PC class (27 lipids [61.4%]), especially with the ether PCs (38.6%), with PC *O*-16:0;0/18:1;0 being the strongest downregulated lipid (Fig. 2*A* and *C* and Supplementary Table 6). Also, most ether phosphatidylethanolamines (four lipids [9.1%]) and sphingomyelin species (seven lipids [15.9%]) were downregulated. The changes in lipids seemed to be dependent on the high C-peptide levels, with effect sizes of DAGs and TAGs close to zero after adjustment for the latter (Supplementary Fig. 3*C* and Supplementary Table 6).

Of the 1,195 plasma proteins investigated, 367 proteins were differentially expressed, with 158 proteins downregulated and 209 upregulated. Several top proteins were upregulated independent of C-peptide levels, including two metalloproteinases, matrix metalloproteinase-7 (MMP-7) and MMP-12, and MIC-1 (Supplementary Table 7). Metalloproteinases are associated with multiple physiological processes but also with atherosclerosis and diabetes-related nephropathy (20,21). MIC-1 (GDF-15) is known to be associated with insulin resistance (22). The identified proteins showed a strong enrichment in pathways, including cytokine–cytokine receptor interaction (50 proteins, P_{FDR}

Table 1—Significant SNPs in each of the clusters

Variant	Cluster	Chr	Position	Gene	Risk allele	REF	ALT	Risk AF in cluster	Effect	Lower	Upper	P	I^2	Heterogeneity	FDR
rs3802177	SIRD	8	118185025	SLC30A8	G	G	A	↓	0.07	0.04	0.10	$2.19 \cdot 10^{-5}$	0.09	0.14	$8.64 \cdot 10^{-3}$
rs10811660	SIRD	9	22134068	CDKN2A/B	G	G	A	↓	0.05	0.02	0.07	$8.72 \cdot 10^{-5}$	0.00	0.59	$1.72 \cdot 10^{-2}$
rs7903146	SIRD	10	114758349	TCF7L2	T	C	T	↑	−0.10	−0.15	−0.05	$1.59 \cdot 10^{-4}$	0.62	0.02	$2.08 \cdot 10^{-2}$
rs11708067	SIRD	3	123065778	ADCY5	A	A	G	↓	0.05	0.02	0.08	$3.76 \cdot 10^{-4}$	0.00	0.31	0.04
rs243024	SIRD	2	60583665	BCL11A	A	G	A	↑	−0.06	−0.10	−0.03	$6.12 \cdot 10^{-4}$	0.10	0.14	0.05
rs1421085	MOD	16	53800954	FTO	C	T	C	↑	0.06	0.03	0.09	$3.99 \cdot 10^{-5}$	0.00	0.53	0.01
rs10893829	MOD	11	128042575	ETS1	T	T	C	↓	0.04	0.02	0.06	$6.62 \cdot 10^{-5}$	0.00	0.35	0.01
rs523288	MOD	18	57848369	MC4R	T	A	T	↑	0.05	0.02	0.08	$1.54 \cdot 10^{-4}$	0.00	0.23	0.02
rs8107974	MOD	19	19388500	TM6SF2	T	A	T	↓	−0.04	−0.06	−0.02	$2.60 \cdot 10^{-4}$	0.32	0.09	0.03
rs10096633	MD	8	19830921	LPL	C	C	T	↑	−0.04	−0.05	−0.02	$7.60 \cdot 10^{-5}$	0.00	0.57	0.03
rs10096633	MDH	8	19830921	LPL	C	C	T	↓	0.07	0.05	0.09	$1.04 \cdot 10^{-11}$	0.00	0.25	$4.08 \cdot 10^{-9}$

AF, allele frequency; ALT, alternative allele; Chr, chromosome; REF, reference allele.

$= 8.69 \cdot 10^{-56}$), chemokine signaling pathway (26 proteins, $P_{FDR} = 1.81 \cdot 10^{-34}$), Axon guidance (26 proteins, $P_{FDR} = 3.55 \cdot 10^{-34}$) and PI3K-Akt signaling pathway (29 proteins, $P_{FDR} = 1.05 \cdot 10^{-29}$). There was a significant reduction in 3-phosphoinositide–dependent protein kinase 1 (PDPK1) (Fig. 3A and C), which, when activated by insulin, activates Akt/PKB and increases glucose uptake via GLUT4 (23). Plasma Akt itself was also decreased in SIRD (Fig. 3A). Insulin tended to be higher in SIRD, although this was not significant (Fig. 3B), while the insulin receptor was significantly upregulated (Fig. 3A). In the downstream signaling cascade of the PI3K-Akt pathway, PDPK1 (Fig. 3C), RAC1, AMPK, HSP90, 14-3-3, and p53 were differentially expressed (Supplementary Fig. 5C–I). Of note, the proteins associated with SIRD were only modestly driven by C-peptide levels (Supplementary Fig. 3D).

Next, we overlapped identified proteins with those previously associated with eGFR and incident CVD (19). Proteins upregulated in SIRD were previously associated with lower eGFR levels, including cystatin C ($\rho = -0.74$, $P = 1.12 \cdot 10^{-163}$), tumor necrosis factor receptor superfamily member 1A (TNF sR-I) ($\rho = -0.65$, $P = 2.51 \cdot 10^{-114}$), and neuroblastoma suppressor of tumorigenicity 1 (DAN) ($\rho = -0.64$, $P = 2.29 \cdot 10^{-109}$) (Supplementary Fig. 7A). Conversely, proteins positively associated with eGFR were downregulated including epidermal growth factor receptor (ERBB1) ($\rho = 0.44$, $P = 1.96 \cdot 10^{-46}$) and α-2-antiplasmin ($\rho = 0.41$, $P = 1.42 \cdot 10^{-38}$). For incident CVD, angiopoietin-2 (HR 1.66, $P = 2.20 \cdot 10^{-16}$) and MMP-12 (HR 1.65, $P = 2.20 \cdot 10^{-16}$) were upregulated risk factors in SIRD, while ERBB1 (HR 0.59, $P = 2.20 \cdot 10^{-16}$) was protective for CVD and downregulated in SIRD (Supplementary Fig. 7B).

MOD

In MOD, the pPRS for obesity was significantly higher (β 0.51 [95% CI 0.34–0.68]) (Supplementary Fig. 2) compared with other clusters. Individual diabetes-associated risk alleles associated with high BMI were also more frequent in MOD, i.e., FTO (rs1421085-C) and the MC4R locus (rs523288-T) (Supplementary Table 4 and Table 1). Of note, both loci are also in the pPRS, although different SNPs in linkage disequilibrium. Naturally, adjustment for BMI attenuated the effect size for both SNPs (Supplementary Fig. 3A and Supplementary Table 4).

Isoleucine was the sole metabolite that was differentially upregulated in MOD (Fig. 1A, Supplementary Fig. 4A, and Supplementary Table 5), and this difference was completely eliminated after adjustment for BMI. The lipid profile of the MOD cluster was largely similar to the SIRD cluster (Fig. 2A and Supplementary Table 6); i.e., in MOD, acyl phosphatidylethanolamine species were upregulated, but not the ether phosphatidylethanolamines. Cholesterol esters and PC species containing the n-3 fatty acids eicosapentaenoic acid (20:5;0) and docosahexaenoic acid (22:6;0) were downregulated, while these were upregulated or not significantly changed in the SIRD cluster. However,

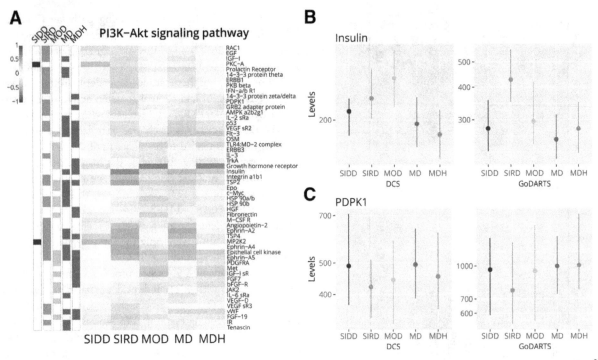

Figure 3—Proteins in the PI3K/Akt pathway in the five clusters. *A*: Effect sizes of proteins in the PI3K/Akt pathway ($P_{FDR} = 1.05 \cdot 10^{-29}$) with upregulation (red) in the cluster vs. all others and downregulation (blue). Bars on the left indicate whether proteins are statistically significant in a specific cluster. Dots represent the median, and the vertical line represents the interquartile range. *B*: Levels of insulin in DCS, GoDARTS, and ANDIS. MDH $P_{FDR} \leq 0.05$. *C*: Levels of PDPK1. Dots represent the median, and the vertical line represents the interquartile range. SIRD $P_{FDR} \leq 0.05$.

cholesterol esters and PC species containing 20:3;0 fatty acids are upregulated in MOD while downregulated or not significantly changed in the SIRD cluster. In total, 61 lipids were affected, of which 40 were upregulated. Among these, the DAGs (15%) and TAGs (57.5%) were strongly enriched. Of the 21 downregulated lipids, the majority were PCs (61.9%). The effect size for DAG and TAG changes were strongly reduced after adjustment for BMI (Supplementary Fig. 3C and Supplementary Table 6). Interestingly, the largest effect size was seen in the TAGs with the lowest number of acyl chain carbons and double bonds (Supplementary Fig. 6A and B), while the TAGs with more acyl chain carbons and double bonds were not significantly altered in MOD. In a previous study, saturated or monounsaturated TAGs were associated with increased diabetes risk, including TAG 46:1, TAG 48:0, and TAG 48:1, which were also significantly upregulated in the MOD cluster (24).

Of the 1,195 proteins, 261 were differentially expressed in MOD with the majority downregulated (158 proteins [60.5%]) (Supplementary Table 7). After adjustment for BMI, several remained significant, although their effect sizes were attenuated, including NCAM-120, DKK3, and CRDL1 (Supplementary Fig. 3D and Supplementary Table 7). DKK3 has been associated with increased adipogenesis in fat cells (25). CRDL1 has been shown to be predictive of β-cell function (26). The role of NCAM-120 is largely

unclear. The strongest enrichment was found for cytokine–cytokine receptor interaction, with 38 proteins (42.7%, $P_{FDR} = 2.08 \cdot 10^{-43}$) overlapping (Supplementary Fig. 8). The strongest upregulated proteins in this pathway were leptin (Supplementary Fig. 4B), growth hormone receptor, and interleukin-1 receptor antagonist protein, while interleukin-1 receptor type 1 (IL-1 sRi) was downregulated. Adjustment for BMI influenced the effect size of several proteins, including leptin, FABP, and CRP (Supplementary Fig. 3D and Supplementary Table 7). Finally, upregulated proteins identified in MOD were generally positively associated with eGFR and protective for CVD, including the growth hormone receptor (HR 0.62, $P = 2.20 \cdot 10^{-16}$) (Supplementary Fig. 7).

MDH

The MDH cluster showed a higher pPRS relative to the other clusters for β-cell function (β 0.61 [95% CI 0.33–0.38]) (Supplementary Fig. 2). Among the diabetes-associated SNPs, a lower risk allele frequency was observed for a SNP near *LPL* (rs10096633-T) (Supplementary Table 4 and Supplementary Table 1). With respect to metabolite, lipid, and peptide levels the MDH cluster showed opposite effects compared with the SIRD and MOD cluster. The amino acids that were upregulated in SIRD were generally downregulated in MDH (Fig. 1A and Supplementary Table 5). Only the difference in isoleucine level was significant and phenylalanine borderline insignificant. In addition, taurine was significantly upregulated in MDH. After adjustment for HDL the effect sizes strongly attenuated (Supplementary Fig. 3B and Supplementary Table 5).

Of the 162 lipids, 135 lipids were affected in MDH, with 52 downregulated and 83 upregulated (Supplementary Table 6). Opposite SIRD and MOD, DAGs (13.5%), TAGs (73.1%), and acyl phosphatidyletnanolamines (9.6%) were downregulated in MDH, while PCs (65.1%) were upregulated, especially the ether PCs (PC O-, 25.6%) (Supplementary Table 6). The TAGs with a smaller number of acyl chain carbons and double bonds showed the lowest protein levels versus the other clusters, while the differences attenuated with increasing number of acyl chain carbons and double bonds (Supplementary Fig. 6A and B). In addition, upregulation was seen for cholesterol esters (13.3%), sphingomyelins (10.8%), and all ether phosphatidylethanolamines (9.6%), which point in the opposite direction in the SIRD cluster (Supplementary Table 6). Adjustment for HDL strongly decreased the effect size for DAGs and TAGs (Supplementary Fig. 3C and Supplementary Table 6).

Of the 1,195 proteins, 270 were differentially expressed in the MDH cluster (119 down- and 151 upregulated). The effect size of the proteins changed very modestly after adjustment for HDL (Supplementary Fig. 3D). The peptide profile of the MDH cluster was opposite that of MOD (Supplementary Fig. 9 [$r = -0.82$]). As such, among the top proteins similar proteins were identified, such as CRDL1, that remained significant after adjustment for HDL. The pathway enrichment resembled that of SIRD and MOD, with enrichment for cytokine–cytokine receptor interaction (31 proteins, $P_{FDR} = 7.04 \cdot 10^{-32}$), pathways in cancer (22 proteins, $P_{FDR} = 2.35 \cdot 10^{-24}$), and the PI3K-Akt signaling pathway (22 proteins, $P_{FDR} = 5.56 \cdot 10^{-23}$). In the PI3K-Akt signaling pathway, growth hormone receptor was downregulated, as well as insulin (Fig. 3B and Supplementary Table 7). Effect sizes were generally not solely driven by increased HDL levels (Supplementary Fig. 3D and Supplementary Table 7). MDH-associated proteins in relation to eGFR showed a pattern similar to that of SIRD (Supplementary Fig. 7A and B), with proteins associated with lower eGFR being upregulated as well as proteins associated with higher risk for CVD, the latter including Follistatin-related protein 3 (HR 1.55, $P = 2.20 \cdot 10^{-16}$) and HCC-1 (HR 1.54, $P = 2.20 \cdot 10^{-16}$).

MD

The MD cluster was generally less well-defined, with only one significant SNP and no significant pPRSs, lipids, or metabolites. There was a higher risk allele frequency (C allele) in MD—opposite that of MDH—compared with the other clusters near the *LPL* gene (rs10096633-T) (Supplementary Table 4). In contrast to the few signals for lipids or metabolites, 354 proteins were differentially expressed in the MD cluster, with the majority downregulated (209 proteins [59.0%]). Enrichment was found for

Axon guidance (20 proteins, $P_{FDR} = 1.12 \cdot 10^{-30}$), cytokine–cytokine receptor interaction (25 proteins, $P_{FDR} = 3.48 \cdot 10^{-25}$), and PI3K-Akt signaling pathway (21 proteins, $P_{FDR} = 4.28 \cdot 10^{-23}$). While similar pathways were found to be enriched in comparison with the SIRD cluster, the effect sizes were correlated but reversed ($r = -0.88$) (Supplementary Fig. 9). In line with this, insulin and its receptor were significantly downregulated in MD. Finally, in MD upregulated proteins were generally associated with better eGFR levels and lower risk for CVD (Supplementary Fig. 7A and B).

DISCUSSION

Based on five clinical variables, people with type 2 diabetes from three large European cohorts were assigned to five separate clusters. The molecular phenotyping of the clusters revealed that, in addition to differences in clinical characteristics, there were also profound differences in underlying molecular profiles, which related to pancreatic islet biology (in SIDD), liver (in SIRD), and adipose tissue metabolism (in MOD and MDH).

The SIRD cluster was characterized by a molecular profile that fits with insulin resistance, i.e., upregulation of DAGs, branched-chain amino acids (BCAAs), and insulin and downregulation of PI3K-Akt pathway–related proteins and PCs. The MOD cluster showed overlap with the SIRD cluster, but with a more pronounced molecular profile of obesity. Individuals in the MDH cluster showed the opposite effect of SIRD and MOD, with, relative to the other clusters, low levels of TAG, DAG, and BCAAs but higher levels of ether PCs and phosphatidylethanolamines, sphingomyelins, and cholesterol esters. The results were in part, but not fully, driven by the identifying characteristic of the cluster, except for SIDD, which showed consistent results after adjustment for HbA$_{1c}$. For example, effect sizes of TAGs and DAGs in SIRD and MDH were influenced by adjustment for C-peptide and HDL, respectively. The lower frequency of diabetes-associated risk alleles could be explained by the fact that most diabetes SNPs are associated with reduced insulin secretion. People in the SIRD cluster have diabetes not because of lower insulin secretion but, rather, because of high insulin resistance (and consequent greater β-cell function).

The SIDD cluster was characterized by greater insulin sensitivity and lower β-cell function than the other clusters based on the clinical characteristics. SIDD was characterized by low tyrosine levels and (a)symmetric dimethylargine, CE 16:1;0, PC O-34;1, and PC O-34;2 compared with the other clusters; higher levels of these metabolites and lipids have been associated with higher type 2 diabetes risk (27–30). Higher CE 16:1;0 has also been associated with higher fasting plasma glucose and 2-h postloading glucose (31). Moreover, in SIDD, CRP was downregulated, and this is in line with a previous report that CRP levels are generally higher in those with insulin resistance and not low secretion (32).

The SIRD—and to some extent the MOD—cluster showed opposing metabolite, lipid, and protein profiles compared with the MDH cluster (Fig. 4). The SIRD cluster was characterized by a molecular signature compatible with insulin resistance inside cells. In SIRD, the frequency of protective alleles was higher for HOMA2 of β-cell function–associated variants. Evidence was found for downregulation of insulin-mediated glucose uptake across the different omics levels, where, for example, higher levels of BCAA and DAG/TAG were observed. BCAAs have been shown to be risk factors for developing incident type 2 diabetes in observational studies; their causal role has also been suggested (33). Both BCAAs and DAG inhibit insulin receptor substrate 1 (IRS1) (34). DAGs activate PKC isoforms, which inhibit PI3K activation by phosphorylating the inhibitory serine 307 of IRS1 instead of tyrosine (34,35). BCAAs target the intramuscular mammalian target of rapamycin/ribosomal protein S6 kinase β-1 (mTOR/p70S6K) signaling pathway, as shown in in vitro and rodent in vivo studies, which also inhibits the PI3K/Akt pathway via IRS1 and IRS2, depending on the cell type (34). Inhibition of PI3K/Akt reduces the GLUT4 translocation. In SIRD, multiple proteins were downregulated in PI3K/Akt and the GLUT4 translocation pathway, including Akt, PDPK1, and RAC1, while insulin was strongly upregulated (36,37). Furthermore, upregulation was seen in three ephrin family members (ephrin A2, A2, A5). Inhibition of the ephrin receptors has been shown to enhance glucose-stimulated insulin secretion in mice (38). Although these results might suggest changes in the insulin or glucose responsiveness of relevant metabolic tissues (e.g., muscle, liver, or adipose), proteins were measured in plasma in the current study and, as such, are unlikely to reflect changes in intracellular signaling. Future studies will be needed to determine the tissue(s) of origin of these biomarkers and the mechanisms through which

they are released. For example, tissue-specific knockout of proteins identified in plasma in cell lines or model organisms might provide insight into both the role and tissue of origin. The higher BMI in individuals in the MOD cluster was in line with the higher allele frequency of variants associated with a higher BMI, i.e., variants near *FTO* and *MC4R*. Interestingly, variants near *TM6SF2* were also associated with this cluster. *TM6SF2* is known to be associated with nonalcoholic steatohepatitis (39). The metabolic and lipid profile of MOD resembled that of SIRD. An interesting observation was that the number of acyl chain carbons and double bonds was associated with the effect size in some clusters, in particular MOD and MDH. In MOD lipids with a higher number of acyl chain carbons and double bonds the effect size was much lower compared with those with lower numbers. These findings are in line with those of a previous publication, which showed that TAGs with a lower number of acyl chain carbons and double bonds were elevated in T2D case versus control subjects (24). In addition, lipids that were associated with increased diabetes risk were generally saturated or monounsaturated fatty acids (24). MOD was further characterized by upregulation of leptin, growth hormone receptor, and multiple interleukins and IL-1Ra. People with a high BMI have high levels of leptin, which may be a marker of leptin resistance (40). IL-1Ra is negatively correlated with QUICKI, where higher levels associate with higher insulin resistance (32).

The MDH cluster was the cluster with the most beneficial profile and had a molecular signature of insulin sensitivity. This cluster had high HDL levels, low BCAA levels, low DAGs, and high levels of ether PCs relative to the other clusters (Fig. 4). Regarding the peptide level, the effects were opposite those of the MOD cluster. The MDH cluster displayed high levels of anti-inflammatory fatty acids, which have been associated with improved insulin sensitivity in animal studies (41–43).

In the study by Ahlqvist et al. (3), the SIRD cluster was associated with poorer renal function. In the current study we compare the identified proteins with proteins previously associated with eGFR levels and CVD risk (19). We show that proteins identified in the current study upregulated in the SIRD and MDH cluster are generally associated with lower eGFR levels and higher risk for CVD and, conversely, those downregulated in these two clusters are associated with higher eGFR levels and lower CVD risk. An explanation may be that individuals in the SIRD and MDH cluster are generally older compared with those in the other three clusters. These results also further confirm the added value of adding HDL to the clustering, as the MOD and MD cluster were much more alike than MD and MDH. The proteins upregulated in the MD and MOD cluster were associated with higher eGFR levels and lower CVD risk.

The strengths of the current study include the large number of individuals, the use of multiple cohorts, and

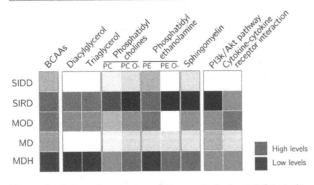

Figure 4—Schematic overview of the results in the current study. BCAAs, DAGs, TAGs, and phosphatidylethanolamine (PE) were upregulated in SIRD and to a lesser extend MOD, while being downregulated in MDH. PE O-, sphingomyelins, and proteins associated with the PI3K/Akt pathway were downregulated in SIRD. In MOD, proteins were found upregulated that have been associated with cytokine-cytokine interaction.

the use of multiple molecular layers to characterize the clusters. A limitation is that the identified markers are measured in plasma and, as such, they cannot be directly linked to specific metabolic tissues. Second, while we adjusted models for the characteristic of that cluster to identify markers that were not simply proxies of the clinical features that defined the cluster, we cannot estimate whether we were able to fully adjust for that characteristic. Third, in the current study we compared the levels of molecular measures between individuals with type 2 diabetes and not relative to those of healthy control subjects. We therefore cannot infer which cluster would be closest to the general population. Fourth, we use a validated quantitative method to measure metabolites that have previously been linked to diabetes, but the limitation of this targeted method is that other metabolites are not measured. As such, we may have missed metabolites with differential levels across clusters. Finally, the cohorts used are mainly comprised of people of European descent and these results may not be generalizable to other populations.

Conclusion

In the current study, clusters were identified in three cohorts, based on five different clinical characteristics. The underlying molecular signatures of each cluster were markedly different (Fig. 4), suggesting different underlying etiopathological processes. As expected, the identified molecular signatures reflected the underlying phenotype to some extent but often remained associated after adjustment. Our study provides important new granularity on the likely molecular processes involved in diabetes pathology in each of the diabetes subgroups.

Acknowledgments. The authors acknowledge the support of the Health Informatics Centre, University of Dundee, for managing and supplying the anonymized data.

Funding. This project has received funding from the Innovative Medicines Initiative 2 Joint Undertaking under grant agreement no. 115881 (IMI-RHAPSODY). This Joint Undertaking receives support from the European Union's Horizon 2020 research and innovation program and EFPIA. This work is supported by the Swiss State Secretariat for Education, Research and Innovation (SERI) under contract number 16.0097-2. E.R.P. was supported by a Wellcome Trust investigator award (102820/Z/13/Z). G.A.R. was supported by a Wellcome Trust Senior Investigator Award (WT098424AIA) and Investigator Award (212625/Z/18/Z), MRC program grants (MR/R022259/1, MR/J0003042/1, MR/L020149/1), and Diabetes UK project grants (BDA/11/0004210, BDA/15/0005275, BDA 16/0005485). This DCS study was in part supported by a grant from the Foundation for the National Institutes of Health through the Accelerating Medicines Partnership (no. HART17AMP).

The opinions expressed and arguments employed herein do not necessarily reflect the official views of these funding bodies.

Duality of Interest. K.S. is CEO of Lipotype. K.S. and C.K. are shareholders of Lipotype. M.J.G. is an employee of Lipotype. G.A.R. has received grant funding and consultancy fees from Sun Pharmaceuticals and Les Laboratoires Servier. M.K.H. is an employee of Janssen Research & Development, LLC. A.F. and I.P. are employees of Eli Lilly Regional Operations. No other potential conflicts of interest relevant to this article were reported.

Author Contributions. R.C.S., L.A.D., J.W.J.B., L.M.'t.H., and E.R.P. designed the study and drafted the manuscript. R.C.S., L.A.D., H.F., G.A.B., and M.Å. performed the analyses. I.D., D.K., and M.I. set up a federated node system for data analysis. R.C.S., L.A.D., H.F., M.J.G., E.A., A.A., D.M.A., M.K., F.M., T.S., A.W., C.L.Q., and M.I. were involved in the data preprocessing and QC. G.N.G., A.F., M.K.H., D.M.A., I.P., T.J.P., V.L., L.G., B.T., P.W.F., and G.A.R. contributed to the data acquisition and project logistics. M.J.G., C.K., and K.S. generated the Lipotype data. A.A., T.S. A.W., P.R., and C.L.Q. generated the metabolomics data. All authors contributed to data interpretation. All authors critically revised the manuscript and approved the final version. R.C.S. and L.A.D. are the guarantors of this work and, as such, had full access to all the data in the study and take responsibility for the integrity of the data and the accuracy of the data analysis.

References

1. McCarthy MI. Painting a new picture of personalised medicine for diabetes. Diabetologia 2017;60:793–799

2. Pearson ER. Type 2 diabetes: a multifaceted disease. Diabetologia 2019;62:1107–1112

3. Ahlqvist E, Storm P, Käräjämäki A, et al. Novel subgroups of adult-onset diabetes and their association with outcomes: a data-driven cluster analysis of six variables. Lancet Diabetes Endocrinol 2018;6:361–369

4. Slieker RC, Donnelly LA, Fitipaldi H, et al. Replication and cross-validation of T2D subtypes based on clinical variables: an IMI-RHAPSODY study. medRxiv 2020

5. Dennis JM, Shields BM, Henley WE, Jones AG, Hattersley ATH. Disease progression and treatment response in data-driven subgroups of type 2 diabetes compared with models based on simple clinical features: an analysis using clinical trial data. Lancet Diabetes Endocrinol 2019;7:442–451

6. Zaharia OP, Strassburger K, Strom A, et al.; German Diabetes Study Group. Risk of diabetes-associated diseases in subgroups of patients with recent-onset diabetes: a 5-year follow-up study. Lancet Diabetes Endocrinol 2019;7:684–694

7. Safai N, Ali A, Rossing P, Ridderstråle M. Stratification of type 2 diabetes based on routine clinical markers. Diabetes Res Clin Pract 2018;141:275–283

8. Aly DM, Dwivedi OP, Prasad RB, et al. Aetiological differences between novel subtypes of diabetes derived from genetic associations. 30 September 2020 [preprint]. medRxiv:2020.09.29.20203935

9. van der Heijden AA, Rauh SP, Dekker JM, et al. The Hoorn Diabetes Care System (DCS) cohort. A prospective cohort of persons with type 2 diabetes treated in primary care in the Netherlands. BMJ Open 2017;7:e015599

10. Hébert HL, Shepherd B, Milburn K, et al. Cohort profile: Genetics of Diabetes Audit and Research in Tayside Scotland (GoDARTS). Int J Epidemiol 2018;47:380–381j

11. Mahajan A, Taliun D, Thurner M, et al. Fine-mapping type 2 diabetes loci to single-variant resolution using high-density imputation and islet-specific epigenome maps. Nat Genet 2018;50:1505–1513

12. Das S, Forer L, Schönherr S, et al. Next-generation genotype imputation service and methods. Nat Genet 2016;48:1284–1287

13. Ahonen L, Jäntti S, Suvitaival T, et al. Targeted clinical metabolite profiling platform for the stratification of diabetic patients. Metabolites 2019;9:184

14. Surma MA, Herzog R, Vasilj A, et al. An automated shotgun lipidomics platform for high throughput, comprehensive, and quantitative analysis of blood plasma intact lipids. Eur J Lipid Sci Technol 2015;117:1540–1549

15. Herzog R, Schwudke D, Schuhmann K, et al. A novel informatics concept for high-throughput shotgun lipidomics based on the molecular fragmentation query language. Genome Biol 2011;12:R8

16. Aimo L, Liechti R, Hyka-Nouspikel N, et al. The SwissLipids knowledgebase for lipid biology. Bioinformatics 2015;31:2860–2866

17. Schwarzer G. meta: an R package for meta-analysis. R News 2007;7:40–45

18. Udler MS, Kim J, von Grotthuss M, et al. Clustering of type 2 diabetes genetic loci by multi-trait associations identifies disease mechanisms and subtypes: a soft clustering analysis. 2018;15:e1002654

19. Yang J, Brody EN, Murthy AC, et al. Impact of kidney function on the blood proteome and on protein cardiovascular risk biomarkers in patients with stable coronary heart disease. J Am Heart Assoc 2020;9:e016463

20. Hu W, Wei R, Wang L, Lu J, Liu H, Zhang W. Correlations of MMP-1, MMP-3, and MMP-12 with the degree of atherosclerosis, plaque stability and cardiovascular and cerebrovascular events. Exp Ther Med 2018;15:1994–1998

21. McLennan SV, Kelly DJ, Schache M, et al. Advanced glycation end products decrease mesangial cell MMP-7: a role in matrix accumulation in diabetic nephropathy? Kidney Int 2007;72:481–488

22. Carstensen M, Herder C, Brunner EJ, et al. Macrophage inhibitory cytokine-1 is increased in individuals before type 2 diabetes diagnosis but is not an independent predictor of type 2 diabetes: the Whitehall II study. Eur J Endocrinol 2010;162:913–917

23. Beg M, Abdullah N, Thowfeik FS, Altorki NK, McGraw TE. Distinct Akt phosphorylation states are required for insulin regulated Glut4 and Glut1-mediated glucose uptake. eLife 2017;6:e26896

24. Rhee EP, Cheng S, Larson MG, et al. Lipid profiling identifies a triacylglycerol signature of insulin resistance and improves diabetes prediction in humans. J Clin Invest 2011;121:1402–1411

25. Huang X, Fu C, Liu W, et al. Chemerin-induced angiogenesis and adipogenesis in 3 T3-L1 preadipocytes is mediated by lncRNA Meg3 through regulating Dickkopf-3 by sponging miR-217. Toxicol Appl Pharmacol 2019;385:114815

26. Belongie KJ, Ferrannini E, Johnson K, Andrade-Gordon P, Hansen MK, Petrie JR. Identification of novel biomarkers to monitor β-cell function and enable early detection of type 2 diabetes risk. PLoS One 2017;12:e0182932

27. Fiodorenko-Dumas Z, Dumas I, Mastej K, Adamiec R. Physical activity - related changes in ADMA and vWF levels in patients with type 2 diabetes: a preliminary study. Adv Clin Exp Med 2017;26:601–608

28. Yu E, Ruiz-Canela M, Razquin C, et al. Changes in arginine are inversely associated with type 2 diabetes: a case-cohort study in the PREDIMED trial. Diabetes Obes Metab 2019;21:397–401

29. Ruiz-Canela M, Guasch-Ferré M, Toledo E, et al. Plasma branched chain/aromatic amino acids, enriched Mediterranean diet and risk of type 2 diabetes: case-cohort study within the PREDIMED Trial. 2018;61:1560–1571

30. Zheng Y, Ceglarek U, Huang T, et al. Weight-loss diets and 2-y changes in circulating amino acids in 2 randomized intervention trials. Am J Clin Nutr 2016;103:505–511

31. Meikle PJ, Wong G, Barlow CK, et al. Plasma lipid profiling shows similar associations with prediabetes and type 2 diabetes. PLoS One 2013;8:e74341

32. Saltevo J, Laakso M, Jokelainen J, Keinänen-Kiukaanniemi S, Kumpusalo E, Vanhala M. Levels of adiponectin, C-reactive protein and interleukin-1 receptor antagonist are associated with insulin sensitivity: a population-based study. Diabetes Metab Res Rev 2008;24:378–383

33. Lotta LA, Scott RA, Sharp SJ, et al. Genetic predisposition to an impaired metabolism of the branched-chain amino acids and risk of type 2 diabetes: a Mendelian randomisation analysis. PLoS Med 2016;13:e1002179

34. Gancheva S, Jelenik T, Álvarez-Hernández E, Roden M. Interorgan metabolic crosstalk in human insulin resistance. Physiol Rev 2018;98:1371–1415

35. Li Y, Soos TJ, Li X, et al. Protein kinase C Theta inhibits insulin signaling by phosphorylating IRS1 at Ser(1101). J Biol Chem 2004;279:45304–45307

36. Sylow L, Nielsen IL, Kleinert M, et al. Rac1 governs exercise-stimulated glucose uptake in skeletal muscle through regulation of GLUT4 translocation in mice. J Physiol 2016;594:4997–5008

37. Ueda S, Kitazawa S, Ishida K, et al. Crucial role of the small GTPase Rac1 in insulin-stimulated translocation of glucose transporter 4 to the mouse skeletal muscle sarcolemma. FASEB J 2010;24:2254–2261

38. Jain R, Jain D, Liu Q, et al. Pharmacological inhibition of Eph receptors enhances glucose-stimulated insulin secretion from mouse and human pancreatic islets. Diabetologia 2013;56:1350–1355

39. Koo BK, Joo SK, Kim D, et al. Additive effects of PNPLA3 and TM6SF2 on the histological severity of non-alcoholic fatty liver disease. J Gastroenterol Hepatol 2018;33:1277–1285

40. Gruzdeva O, Borodkina D, Uchasova E, Dyleva Y, Barbarash O. Leptin resistance: underlying mechanisms and diagnosis. Diabetes Metab Syndr Obes 2019;12:191–198

41. Lalia AZ, Lanza IR. Insulin-sensitizing effects of omega-3 fatty acids: lost in translation? Nutrients 2016;8:329

42. Oh DY, Talukdar S, Bae EJ, et al. GPR120 is an omega-3 fatty acid receptor mediating potent anti-inflammatory and insulin-sensitizing effects. Cell 2010;142:687–698

43. Storlien LH, Kraegen EW, Chisholm DJ, Ford GL, Bruce DG, Pascoe WS. Fish oil prevents insulin resistance induced by high-fat feeding in rats. Science 1987;237:885–888

Effects of Gastric Bypass Surgery on the Brain: Simultaneous Assessment of Glucose Uptake, Blood Flow, Neural Activity, and Cognitive Function During Normo- and Hypoglycemia

Kristina E. Almby,[1] Martin H. Lundqvist,[1] Niclas Abrahamsson,[1] Sofia Kvernby,[2] Markus Fahlström,[2] Maria J. Pereira,[1] Malin Gingnell,[3] F. Anders Karlsson,[1] Giovanni Fanni,[1] Magnus Sundbom,[2] Urban Wiklund,[4] Sven Haller,[2,5] Mark Lubberink,[2] Johan Wikström,[2] and Jan W. Eriksson[1]

Diabetes 2021;70:1265–1277 | https://doi.org/10.2337/db20-1172

While Roux-en-Y gastric bypass (RYGB) surgery in obese individuals typically improves glycemic control and prevents diabetes, it also frequently causes asymptomatic hypoglycemia. Previous work showed attenuated counterregulatory responses following RYGB. The underlying mechanisms as well as the clinical consequences are unclear. In this study, 11 subjects without diabetes with severe obesity were investigated pre- and post-RYGB during hyperinsulinemic normo-hypoglycemic clamps. Assessments were made of hormones, cognitive function, cerebral blood flow by arterial spin labeling, brain glucose metabolism by ^{18}F-fluorodeoxyglucose (FDG) positron emission tomography, and activation of brain networks by functional MRI. Post- versus presurgery, we found a general increase of cerebral blood flow but a decrease of total brain FDG uptake during normoglycemia. During hypoglycemia, there was a marked increase in total brain FDG uptake, and this was similar for post- and presurgery, whereas hypothalamic FDG uptake was reduced during hypoglycemia. During hypoglycemia, attenuated responses of counterregulatory hormones and improvements in cognitive function were seen postsurgery. In early hypoglycemia, there was increased activation post- versus presurgery of neural networks in brain regions implicated in glucose regulation, such as the thalamus and hypothalamus.

The results suggest adaptive responses of the brain that contribute to lowering of glycemia following RYGB, and the underlying mechanisms should be further elucidated.

The global rise in obesity and type 2 diabetes is one of the great challenges to public health in the 21st century. Results of bariatric surgery have shed light on several new and crucial mechanisms by which hunger, satiety, and body weight regulation, as well as glucose homeostasis, can be modified. Roux-en-Y gastric bypass (RYGB) is highly effective to prevent and reverse type 2 diabetes (1–3), with multiple pathways involved (e.g., hepatic glucose production, postprandial glucagon-like peptide 1 secretion, adipose factors) (4). Less is known about the role of neuroendocrine mechanisms and the central nervous system (CNS) in achieving favorable metabolic effects.

Besides these beneficial effects, RYGB surgery commonly leads to episodes of postprandial hypoglycemia (5), which are usually asymptomatic, pointing to an adaptive lowering of the glycemic "set point." To some extent, this resembles the clinical phenomenon known as impaired awareness of hypoglycemia (IAH), which is observed in some patients with type 1 diabetes. These patients display

[1]Department of Medical Sciences, Clinical Diabetes and Metabolism, Uppsala University, Uppsala, Sweden
[2]Department of Surgical Sciences, Uppsala University, Uppsala, Sweden
[3]Department of Neurosciences and Department of Psychology, Uppsala University, Uppsala, Sweden
[4]Department of Radiation Sciences, Umeå University, Umeå, Sweden
[5]Faculty of Medicine, University of Geneva, Geneva, Switzerland

Corresponding author: Jan W. Eriksson, jan.eriksson@medsci.uu.se

Received 19 November 2020 and accepted 25 February 2021

This article contains supplementary material online at https://doi.org/10.2337/figshare.14114159.

K.E.A. and M.H.L. contributed equally.

See accompanying article, p. 1244.

attenuation of symptoms and some counterregulatory hormonal responses during hypoglycemia compared with patients with normal hypoglycemic awareness (6). Moreover, a blunting of responses to hypoglycemia have been found in IAH in brain regions involved in hypoglycemic counterregulation, including the thalamus, hypothalamus, and brain stem and regions involved in behavioral responses, such as the striatum, amygdala, and various cortical regions (7–10).

Interestingly, attenuation of hormonal and symptomatic responses to hypoglycemia has also been observed after RYGB (11,12). In obesity and type 2 diabetes, positron emission tomography (PET) investigations performed during euglycemic-hyperinsulinemic clamp showed elevated brain glucose uptake (13,14), and this can be normalized after RYGB (15). While IAH can impair both short- and long-term cognitive performance (16,17), less is known about cognition in relation to hypoglycemia after bariatric surgery (12). In the current study, we combined hormonal, cognitive, and neuroimaging assessments during normoglycemic and hypoglycemic clamps in subjects before and after RYGB surgery.

RESEARCH DESIGN AND METHODS

This study was conducted at Uppsala University and Uppsala University Hospital. Subjects aged 18–60 years with a BMI of 35–45 kg/m^2 were recruited after a regular visit at the obesity outpatient clinic before planned bariatric surgery. Main exclusion criteria were diagnosis of diabetes, history of cardiovascular events, contraindication to PET/MRI investigation, treatment with β-blockers or CNS-active drugs, and serious psychiatric or substance abuse disorders.

The subjects came for two study visits: before RYGB (median 41 days, range 20–76 days) and then ~4 months (median 130 days, range 106–155 days) after RYGB. In accordance with local clinical guidelines, subjects received a 4-week low-caloric diet of 800–1,100 kcal/day before the RYGB, which was performed laparoscopically at the Department of Surgery, Uppsala University Hospital. On both study visits, subjects came to the PET/MR facility at 8:00 A.M. after an overnight fast. Medical history, anthropometric measures, and blood samples were obtained. Total body fat was assessed with bioimpedance (Body Composition Analyzer BC-418; Tanita).

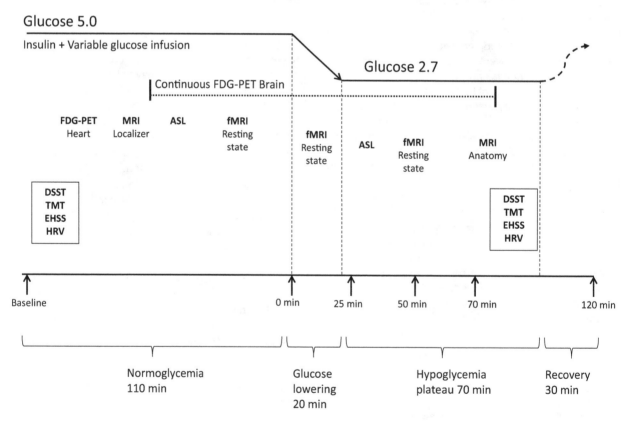

Figure 1—Schematic overview of the clamp and imaging investigations performed pre- and post-RYGB. Arrows at the bottom indicate time points for hormone blood samples. ASL, arterial spin labeling; DSST, Digital Symbol Substitution Test; EHSS, Edinburg Hypoglycemia Symptom Scale; HRV, heart rate variability; TMT, Trail Making Test.

Glucose Clamp Procedure

A schematic overview is given in Fig. 1. After blood sampling and physical examinations, the hyperinsulinemic glucose clamp started with simultaneous infusion of insulin and 20% glucose. Potassium was infused with a target rate of 8 mmol/h in order to avoid insulin-induced hypokalemia. After priming, insulin (Actrapid; Novo Nordisk, Copenhagen, Denmark) was infused at a steady-state rate of 80 mU/m^2 body surface area/min, and the rate of 20% glucose infusion was adjusted on the basis of plasma glucose readings every 5 min. During the normoglycemic phase, the target glucose level was 5.0 mmol/L, and assessments of heart rate variability (HRV), cognitive function, and hypoglycemic symptoms (Edinburgh Hypoglycemia Symptom Score [EHSS]) were performed. Approximately 30 min into the clamp, the subject was positioned in the PET/MR scanner. After an additional 30 min, ^{18}F-fluorodeoxyglucose (FDG) was rapidly infused, and PET scanning was initiated followed by arterial spin labeling (ASL) and functional MRI (fMRI), as depicted in Fig. 1. After another 50 min, plasma glucose was lowered by temporarily stopping the glucose infusion. The target was 2.7 mmol/L, which was typically reached at ~20 min, and this was then maintained for 70 min. FDG-PET, ASL, and fMRI were performed again. After ~50 min, subjects exited the scanner, and HRV, cognitive function, and EHSS assessments were again performed. The recovery phase was initiated by stopping the insulin infusion while the glucose infusion continued for 30 min at a fixed rate of 100 mg/kg body weight/h. Because of the complex technical procedures, sometimes there were slight delays in experimental periods (Table 1) and sampling times.

Cardiovascular Function

To assess autonomic nervous system activity, HRV was assessed for 6 min during normoglycemia and during late hypoglycemia in the supine position, using a single-channel electrocardiogram system (Actiwave Cardio; CamNtech Ltd., Fenstanton, U.K.), and a power spectrum analysis of HRV was performed (18). Blood pressure was measured at rest before clamps. Heart rate was measured during the normoglycemic and hypoglycemic clamps.

Cognitive Tests and Hypoglycemic Symptoms Scores

The Trail Making Test (TMT) (19) and Digit Symbol Substitution Test (DSST) (20) were performed during both the normoglycemic and the hypoglycemic phase of the clamp (19,20). To avoid bias as a result of learning effects, both the TMT and the DSST were sent by mail to the subjects before each investigation day with instructions to practice taking the tests. The TMT examines visual search, scanning, speed of processing, mental flexibility, and executive functions (21), while the DSST aims to measure cognitive operations, such as motor speed, attention, visuoperceptual functions, and associative learning

(20). Hypoglycemic symptoms were assessed with the EHSS questionnaire (22) both in the normo- and hypoglycemic clamp phases.

Biochemical Measurements

Blood samples were repeatedly drawn from an antecubital vein (Fig. 1) following arterialization using a heating pad. Analyses were performed at the Department of Clinical Chemistry and the Clinical Diabetes Research Laboratory of Uppsala University Hospital. Glucose during clamps was assessed with a Contour hand-held glucometer (Bayer). Insulin, C-peptide, and cortisol were determined with a cobas e analyzer (Roche), growth hormone (GH) and ACTH with IMMULITE 2000 XPi (Siemens Healthineers), and glucagon with ELISA (#10-1271-01; Mercodia, Uppsala, Sweden).

Brain Imaging Using PET, ASL, and fMRI

All examinations were performed using integrated PET/MR (SIGNA; GE Healthcare, Waukesha, WI), which combines a 3T MRI with a time-of-flight–capable silicone photomultiplier-based PET scanner (23). All subjects were scanned in supine position using an eight-channel head coil (MR Instruments, Inc., Minneapolis, MN). First, the subject was positioned with the field of view of the PET/MR centered over the heart. Simultaneously with a bolus injection of 2–3 MBq/kg FDG, a 10-min dynamic PET scan was started. Then, the subject was moved so that the brain was in the center of the field of view, and PET scanning was resumed at ~20 min postinjection and continued for ~120 min during normo- and hypoglycemia (Fig. 1). Arterialized venous blood samples were taken for measurement of radioactivity after the cardiac scan, prior to start of the brain scan, and repeatedly at set times during the remainder of the scan. PET image processing is described in the Supplementary Material.

A 3D fast-spin echo pseudo-continuous ASL with spiral readout and background suppression was acquired at a postlabel delay of 2,000 ms. In addition, the protocol included a high-resolution 3D T1-weighted image and a 3D T2-weighted fluid attenuated inversion recovery as anatomical references and a two-point Dixon sequence in combination with a zero echo time sequence for attenuation correction of PET data. ASL-derived cerebral blood flow (CBF) images were calculated according to the model defined by Buxton et al. (24) and recommended by Alsop et al. (25), including a correction term for full proton density reference (26–29).

fMRI during resting state implemented a standard echo-planar imaging sequence with the following fundamental parameters: whole-brain coverage, voxel size $3.4 \times 3.4 \times 3.0$ mm^3, 45 slices, 200 repetitions, repetition time 3.0 s, and echo time 3.0 ms. Analysis was carried out using tensorial independent component (IC) analysis (TICA) (30) and region of interest (ROI)-to-ROI analysis. TICA was implemented as in MELODIC

Table 1—Anthropometric and biochemical measures at the presurgery visit and after gastric bypass (postsurgery)

	Presurgery ($n = 11$)	Postsurgery ($n = 11$)	P value
Anthropometry			
Sex (male/female), n	3/8	—	—
Age (years)	35 (± 8)	—	—
Time from surgery to postsurgery visit 2 (days)	—	130 (122; 148)	—
Weight (kg)	113.8 (109.7; 132.5)	83.3 (77.2; 98.5)	**0.003**
BMI (kg/m^2)	40.2 (± 3.6)	29.9 (± 4.0)	**<0.001**
Waist (cm)	119 (± 10)	95 (± 10)	**<0.001**
Waist/hip ratio	0.90 (0.86; 0.96)	0.88 (0.83; 0.90)	0.328
Total body fat (%)	44.4 (± 7.3)	34.0 (± 10.2)	**<0.001**
SBP (mmHg)	125 (± 13)	118 (± 12)	0.138
DBP (mmHg)	80 (± 10)	73 (± 11)	0.076
Heart rate normo (bpm)*	74 (73; 78)	61 (59; 74)	**0.004**
Heart rate hypo (bpm)†	78 (70; 87)	65 (60; 80)	**0.021**
Duration of normoglycemic clamp (min)	118 (113; 129)	111 (109; 114)	0.373
Duration of hypoglycemic clamp (min)	85 (80; 93)	80 (79; 90)	0.765
Test scores			
EHSS normo	14.3 (2.3)	15.1 (3.9)	0.57
EHSS hypo	31.5 (8.4)	28.3 (7.5)	0.28
DSST normo	31.5 (13.4)	27.5 (7.1)	0.19
DSST hypo	24.3 (6.3)	27.5 (9.3)	**0.046**
TMT‡ normo	43.7 (11.9)	42.6 (14.3)	0.33
TMT‡ hypo	52.0 (19.7)	34.4 (10.5)	**0.009**
Biochemistry			
HbA$_{1c}$ (mmol/mol)	34 (34; 36)	33 (30; 34)	**0.011**
HbA$_{1c}$ (NGSP %)	5.3 (5.3; 5.4)	5.2 (4.9; 5.3)	**0.011**
P-glucose (mmol/L)	6.0 (± 0.5)	5.3 (± 0.5)	**<0.001**
S-insulin (mU/L)	10.5 (5.7; 15.8)	7.2 (4.5; 13.8)	0.113
S-C-peptide (nmol/L)	1.20 (± 0.29)	0.79 (± 0.22)	**<0.001**
HOMA-IR	2.7 (1.6; 4.3)	1.4 (1.0; 3.5)	**0.047**
P-HDL cholesterol (mmol/L)	0.99 (± 0.14)	0.97 (± 0.21)	0.651
P-LDL cholesterol (mmol/L)	3.11 (± 0.75)	2.15 (± 0.58)	**<0.001**
P-triglycerides (mmol/L)	0.99 (0.92; 2.07)	0.79 (0.71; 1.14)	**0.016**
P-glucagon (pmol/L)	9.8 (5.9; 13.8)	6.2 (4.8; 9.4)	0.131
S-cortisol (nmol/L)	182 (165; 252)	214 (166; 271)	1.000
P-ACTH (nmol/L)	2.7 (2.3; 5.5)	1.8 (1.6; 2.2)	**0.005**
S-GH (μg/L)	0.16 (0.05; 1.18)	1.80 (0.10; 7.00)	**0.008**
M-value (mg/kg LBM/min)	7.55 (± 3.90)	8.63 (± 2.53)	0.352

Data are mean (± SD) if normally distributed or median (IQR) unless otherwise indicated. P values represent comparison with paired t tests (if normally distributed) or Wilcoxon signed rank tests between pre- and postsurgery. Boldface indicates significance at $P < 0.05$. bpm, beats/min; DBP, diastolic blood pressure; HOMA-IR, HOMA of insulin resistance; hypo, hypoglycemic phase of clamp; NGSP, National Glycohemoglobin Standardization Program; normo, normoglycemic phase of clamp; P, plasma; S, serum; SBP, systolic blood pressure. *Incomplete data for four subjects. †Incomplete data for one subject. ‡TMT low value = better.

(Multivariate Exploratory Linear Decomposition into Independent Components) version 3.15, part of FSL (FMRIB Software Library, https://www.fmrib.ox.ac.uk/fsl), using standard parameters. All six runs (three presurgery, three postsurgery [see Fig. 1]) of each subject were included in one analysis. This data set of all runs in all subjects identified 20 ICs in a data-driven manner without a priori assumptions. Those 20 ICs were then default ordered by the amount of data variance explained by the ICs. The IC analysis provides a so-called S-mode (measure of activation of each component) in each run. For ROI-to-ROI analysis in the CONN toolbox (31) (https://web.conn-toolbox.org), standard parameters were used except for the additional definition of ROIs of the medial hypothalamus and lateral hypothalamus (LH) (32). The subject S-modes of the 20 ICs were used as input data for the post hoc statistical analysis between groups using Graph-Pad Prism 5 software. Neuroimaging postprocessing details and software and the full set of acquisition parameters for MRI scans are provided in the Supplementary Material.

Statistical Analysis

Data are presented as mean (± SD) or as median (interquartile range [IQR]) as indicated. For biochemical measurements, the area under the curve (AUC) and the ΔAUC from hypoglycemia 0–70 min was calculated using the trapezoid method. If sampling time was delayed because of practical reasons, the concentration at the intended time was interpolated from the adjacent measured values.

Differences in clinical and biochemical variables were analyzed using paired t tests or Wilcoxon signed rank tests as appropriate and specified. FDG-PET and ASL data were analyzed using paired t tests. Spearman correlations were performed between selected clinical and imaging measures. $P < 0.05$ was considered statistically significant. Details regarding statistical software are provided in the Supplementary Material.

Ethics

The study was approved by the Regional Research Ethics Committee of Uppsala (Dnr 2017/210). All subjects received written and verbal information prior to signing an informed consent form. The study was conducted in accordance with the Declaration of Helsinki.

Data Availability

The data and study protocol are available upon request to the corresponding author.

RESULTS

Eighteen subjects were recruited, seven of whom did not complete both visits for various reasons, including personal circumstances, difficulties gaining venous access, back pain, anxiety, or other discomfort during the imaging procedure and one patient's cancellation of surgery. Thus, 11 subjects (3 males and 8 females) completed both visits. Clinical characteristics pre- and postsurgery are summarized in Table 1. RYGB led to the expected metabolic improvements: weight loss of 30.3 kg, BMI reduction of 10.3 kg/m², and significant lowering of fasting glucose and HbA₁c.

Cardiovascular Function

There was a significant decrease in heart rate after RYGB. This was found during both normo- and hypoglycemic clamp periods ($P < 0.01$ and $P < 0.05$, respectively) (Table 1). There were no significant changes in blood pressure or HRV spectral components.

Cognitive Tests and Hypoglycemic Symptoms

These results are shown in Table 1. The DSST and TMT results showed significant improvements during hypoglycemia for the postsurgery versus presurgery comparison ($P < 0.05$ and $P < 0.01$, respectively). There were no differences during the normoglycemic phase. The EHSS symptom scores were similar postsurgery versus presurgery.

Biochemical Measurements

Glucose and hormone levels are displayed in Table 1 and Fig. 2. Clamp glucose levels tended to be slightly lower post- versus presurgery ($P = 0.137$ and $P = 0.070$ for normo- and hypoglycemia, respectively). During the recovery phase, glucose levels rose less post- versus presurgery ($P < 0.01$). Fasting C-peptide levels were lower

postsurgery but were suppressed similarly to presurgery during the clamp. Clamp insulin levels, mainly reflecting exogenous insulin, were slightly and significantly lower postsurgery. Glucagon, ACTH, cortisol, and GH all increased during the hypoglycemic clamp. Postsurgery, this increase was attenuated for glucagon ($P < 0.01$) and numerically for ACTH and cortisol response ($P = 0.08$ and $P = 0.16$, respectively, for ΔAUC; $P < 0.01$ and $P = 0.08$, respectively, for total AUC). Fasting ACTH in the morning was also lower after surgery ($P < 0.01$). The GH response was augmented post- versus presurgery ($P < 0.01$).

FDG-PET

Results from the FDG-PET investigations are shown in Figs. 3 and 4. Both the global brain FDG net influx rate (Ki) and the estimated total uptake of glucose (MRglu) were somewhat lower post- versus presurgery during normoglycemia ($P < 0.05$ for both) (Fig. 3A and B). Hypoglycemia led to an approximately fourfold increase in Ki ($P < 0.001$) (Fig. 3A) both pre- and postsurgery. The magnitude of this increase did not differ significantly pre- versus postsurgery. The whole-brain PET images of a typical subject are depicted in Fig. 3C. This increase of Ki during hypoglycemia was evident in most parts of the brain both pre- and postsurgery (Figs. 3C and 4A and C). However, this was not seen in the hypothalamic area, where Ki instead decreased during hypoglycemia, and this response was less evident post- versus presurgery (Fig. 4B and D). In hypoglycemia, the lumped constant for FDG uptake in the brain is not defined, and, therefore, MRglu estimates are not reported.

CBF

Regional CBF was assessed with ASL, and data are summarized in Fig. 5. Postsurgery, CBF during the normoglycemic phase increased significantly in all brain regions. No significant changes were found between the normo- and hypoglycemic states pre- or postsurgery.

To assess whether the increased blood flow postsurgery was specific for the brain, we also used FDG-PET scanning of the heart to calculate whole-body arterial blood-flow, i.e., cardiac output (33). In absolute terms, cardiac output (in L/min) was clearly reduced after gastric bypass surgery, whereas the cardiac index (adjusted to body surface area) was not significantly altered (mean 3.06 vs. 3.23 L/m²/min for pre- vs. postsurgery, respectively).

fMRI

Resting state fMRI was performed in three sequential periods during the clamp investigation: normoglycemia, early hypoglycemia and steady-state hypoglycemia (Fig. 1), and this was done before as well as after RYGB. TICA of MRI using the FSL software package (30) revealed one independent component (IC), which represents a functional connectivity resting-state network, explaining most variability of the data across all fMRI runs. This IC notably

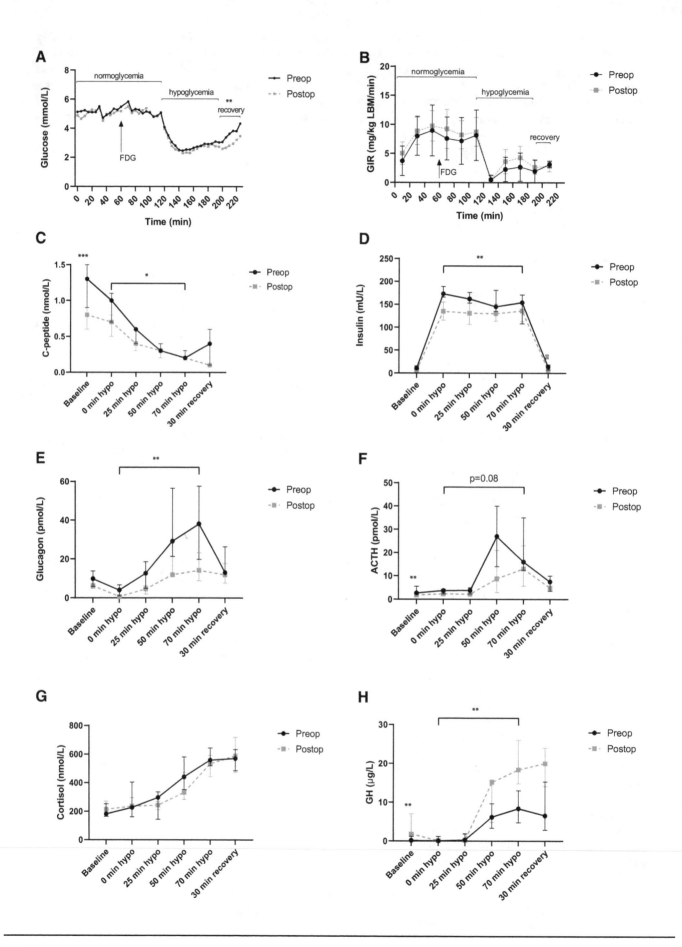

includes bilateral thalamus and hypothalamus and, to a lesser degree, right dominant frontal regions (Fig. 6A). The activity of this IC (S-mode) was significantly higher post- versus presurgery during those runs in which blood glucose was rapidly lowered, i.e., during the early hypoglycemic clamp phase ($P < 0.05$) (Fig. 6A and B).

The additional connectivity analysis was based on ROI-to-ROI analysis in the CONN toolbox using the right lateral hypothalamus (LH) (31) as the seed region. During early hypoglycemia, we observed a significantly decreased functional connectivity to left hippocampus and significantly increased functional connectivity to the cerebellar vermis regions 4 and 5 for the post- versus presurgery condition (Fig. 6C).

Correlation Analyses

There were significant correlations between EHSS score and whole-brain CBF during hypoglycemia, particularly at the postsurgery investigation ($\rho = 0.706$, $P = 0.015$). Likewise, there were positive associations between cognitive function and CBF during hypoglycemia, both pre- and post-RYGB ($P = 0.010$ and $P = 0.079$, respectively, for TMT; $P = 0.017$ and $P = 0.040$, respectively, for DSST). These latter associations were seen for CBF in several separate regions but were significant only for the basal ganglia and hippocampus (data not shown). Whole-brain FDG uptake did not correlate with any of these scores. There were no significant correlations between postsurgery changes in anthropometric measures and changes in EHSS and cognitive scores or hormonal and fMRI responses to hypoglycemia. Furthermore, time since surgery did not correlate with changes in any of the above measures.

DISCUSSION

This study demonstrates the feasibility of simultaneous metabolic and multimodal neuroimaging assessments. The findings indicate that changes in the brain's neuronal network activity, cognitive functions, as well as blood flow and energy metabolism occur after RYGB surgery in patients with severe obesity. Some RYGB effects were also found during experimental hypoglycemia, mainly on cognitive, hormonal, and fMRI readouts, and they may be of relevance for the asymptomatic hypoglycemic episodes that frequently occur in patients after RYGB (5). A nearly global attenuation of neurohormonal responses to hypoglycemia was found after RYGB, and this is likely largely due to adaptive changes within the brain. Conversely, such an adaptation is also likely to contribute to an overall lowering of glycemia and, hence, to the prevention, or

reversal, of type 2 diabetes in patients undergoing RYGB. The mechanisms behind this adaptation to low glucose levels remain elusive but may include upregulation of glucose transport into some brain regions, utilization of alternative fuels, and alterations of hypothalamic signaling and opioid-dependent pathways (34).

Cognitive Function

Both cognitive tests, TMT and DSST, showed congruent results, with scores during hypoglycemia improving post-compared with presurgery. This is compatible with an adaptation of the brain to low glucose, leading to less vulnerability of cognition during hypoglycemia. Previous studies have also reported modulation of other aspects of cognitive function following RYGB, including problem solving and pattern comparison (12,35).

Hormonal and Cardiovascular Responses

RYGB led to attenuated responses of counterregulatory hormones as well as heart rate during hypoglycemia. The blunted hormonal responses included glucagon, ACTH, and cortisol but, as reported previously (11,12), GH had a greater response following weight loss. After RYGB, glucose levels rose more slowly during the recovery phase directly after the hypoglycemic clamp, and this is most likely a consequence of the attenuated counterregulation. The finding following RYGB of a suppressed ACTH response to hypoglycemia provides additional support for a brain-mediated neuroendocrine adaptation, including the hypothalamic-pituitary-adrenal axis. Interestingly, in a recent study, we reported that enhanced counterregulatory responses are a feature of subjects with obesity and insulin resistance that might promote relative hyperglycemia and development of type 2 diabetes (36). In contrast, RYGB instead leads to an attenuated counterregulation, probably even below normal, which can contribute to the prevention or reversal of diabetes (11,12).

In our limited cohort, we did not see a significant improvement of whole-body insulin resistance, pointing to other mechanisms for the rapid glycemic effects of RYGB, such as reduced endogenous glucose production (37). Local insulin resistance in the brain has been implicated in obesity and type 2 diabetes (38). Some of the effects on brain functions and counterregulation found after RYGB in our study may be linked to improved brain insulin resistance, but this was not directly addressed and warrants further work.

In this study, we did not see any clear post-RYGB effect on autonomic nervous system reactivity during hypoglycemia, which is different from our previous report, indicating a blunted response of the sympathetic

---

Figure 2—A–H: Glucose levels, glucose infusion rates, and hormone levels during normoglycemic and hypoglycemic clamp. Data are median ± IQR (all but panel A) or mean ± SD (A). *$P < 0.05$, **$P < 0.01$, ***$P < 0.001$. P values refer to differences between pre- and postsurgery, during the hypoglycemic period (brackets, AUCs) or fasting levels (baseline). P values within brackets refer to Wilcoxon signed rank tests of ΔAUC (for all panels except D, where total AUC is shown). GIR, glucose infusion rate; hypo, hypoglycemic phase of clamp; LBM, lean body mass; Preop, preoperative; Postop, postoperative.

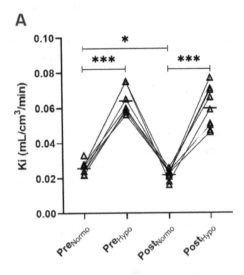

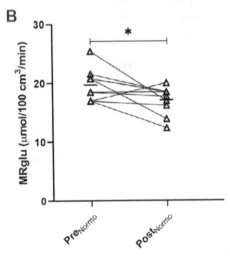

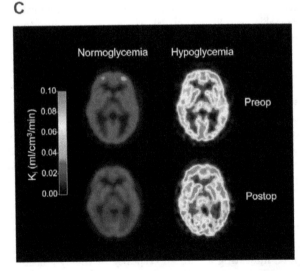

Figure 3—FDG PET of the brain. *A*: Whole-brain Ki values during normo- and hypoglycemia. *B*: MRglu during normoglycemia. *C*: Ki PET images for a typical patient pre- and postsurgery during normo- and hypoglycemia. Data in panels *A* and *B* presented as spaghetti plot of individual values with individual connecting lines and mean of all subjects at that time point (horizontal solid lines). *n* = 11.

nervous system (11). This is probably explained by HRV assessments now being done only in the very last part of the hypoglycemic period as opposed to continuous registration.

CBF, fMRI, and FDG-PET

The counterregulatory response to hypoglycemia is largely coordinated by the basal regions of the brain, in particular the hypothalamus (34). It is therefore intriguing that we found an increased activity on resting-state fMRI assessments in these regions as well as some others during hypoglycemia post- versus presurgery. Although the functional consequences of increased neural activity in these brain regions are unclear, it may be hypothesized that this network exerts an inhibitory effect on hypoglycemic counterregulation. A causal connection between such findings and the attenuated neurohormonal counterregulation reported in this and a few previous studies (11,12) is therefore plausible and intuitively appealing. However, it is beyond the reach of our current results to allow firm conclusions about this connection.

A major finding of the ASL investigations was a general increase in blood flow in all brain regions occurring after RYGB, and this was largely seen during both normoglycemia and hypoglycemia. Interestingly, we found a link between increased brain blood flow during hypoglycemia and better results on cognitive tests, compatible with a potential impact of blood flow vis-à-vis cognitive improvement following RYGB. Since there was no significant postsurgery effect on whole-body blood flow (cardiac index), we propose that the increase in CBF is secondary to effects on regional vasoregulation. Of note, impaired vasoreactivity has been reported in obese versus lean subjects, but it was rapidly normalized after RYGB (39).

In contrast to blood flow, glucose metabolic rate, as reflected by FDG uptake, in the brain dropped after RYGB when measured during normoglycemia. This is compatible with previous findings by other investigators (13,15,37) showing elevated brain glucose uptake in obese subjects during hyperinsulinemic-normoglycemic clamps and a normalization following bariatric surgery. As expected, we found an increased plasma clearance of FDG by the brain (Ki), and thus extraction fraction, during hypo- versus normoglycemia. However, Ki during hypoglycemia did not change after RYGB, and the MRglu could not be calculated because the assigned lumped constant for FDG of 0.65 during normoglycemia (14,40) is probably not applicable for hypoglycemia. This was shown in rats, where the deoxyglucose lumped constant of the brain was more

*P < 0.05, ***P < 0.001 for post- vs. presurgery (paired *t* tests). PreNormo and PostNormo: missing data for one subject; PreHypo: missing data for four subjects; PostHypo: missing data for two subjects.

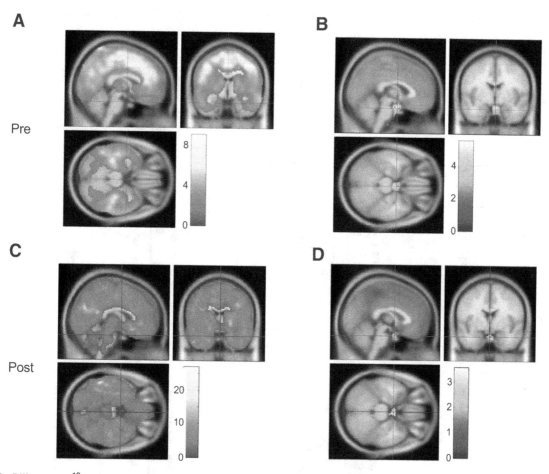

Figure 4—Difference in ^{18}F-FDG net influx rates between hypo- and normoglycemic clamp periods. PET statistical parametric mapping (SPM) T-maps show comparisons from the presurgery (*A* and *B*) and postsurgery (*C* and *D*) investigations, respectively. *A* and *C* show clusters with significantly increased ^{18}F-FDG net influx rate for hypo- vs. normoglycemia (red), whereas *B* and *D* show clusters with significant reduction (blue). The color maps represent T-values, indicating the number of pooled standard deviations between net influx rate values during hypo- vs. normoglycemia, where T > 1.96 corresponds to $P < 0.05$. Minimum cluster size for significance was 50 voxels (0.4 cm^3). The crosshairs are centered on the hypothalamic cluster in panel B and the peak coordinates (MNI) are 0, −8, −22.

than twofold higher at plasma glucose 1.9 compared with 7 mmol/L (41). It might be assumed that the overall brain glucose uptake during modest hypoglycemia in our subjects was in a similar range as in normoglycemia and, most importantly, it did not change following RYGB.

In contrast to the whole brain, there was a decrease in the hypothalamic FDG uptake rate during hypoglycemia, and this decrease appeared to be less evident post- versus presurgery. These findings may point to an involvement of glucose uptake and, potentially, sensing in the hypothalamus coordination of counterregulatory neuroendocrine responses.

The somewhat lower Ki for FDG in normoglycemia post- versus presurgery may suggest an adaptation of the postsurgery brain to become less dependent on glucose uptake per se, possibly by metabolizing glucose more efficiently or utilizing alternative energy sources, including lactate and ketones. Indeed, intravenous administration of both lactate and β-hydroxybutyrate during hypoglycemia has been shown to decrease symptoms, cognitive dysfunction, and hormonal counterregulation in healthy subjects (42).

Overall, further studies are needed to directly assess nutrient uptake and metabolism in the brain during hypoglycemia in normal subjects as well as in subjects with diabetes or obesity, also after bariatric surgery. In our present study, RYGB was followed by an altered neuronal network response to hypoglycemia in brain regions that are considered to be involved in the regulation of glucose turnover. This may contribute to the overall glucose-lowering effects of RYGB. A reduction of whole-brain glucose uptake was seen under normoglycemic conditions, and a rise in CBF was demonstrated in both normo- and hypoglycemia. Thus, it cannot be established whether the attenuation of counterregulation to hypoglycemia following RYGB is dependent on changes in brain glucose uptake and/or blood flow, and additional targeted and dynamic assessments of specific brain regions may be needed.

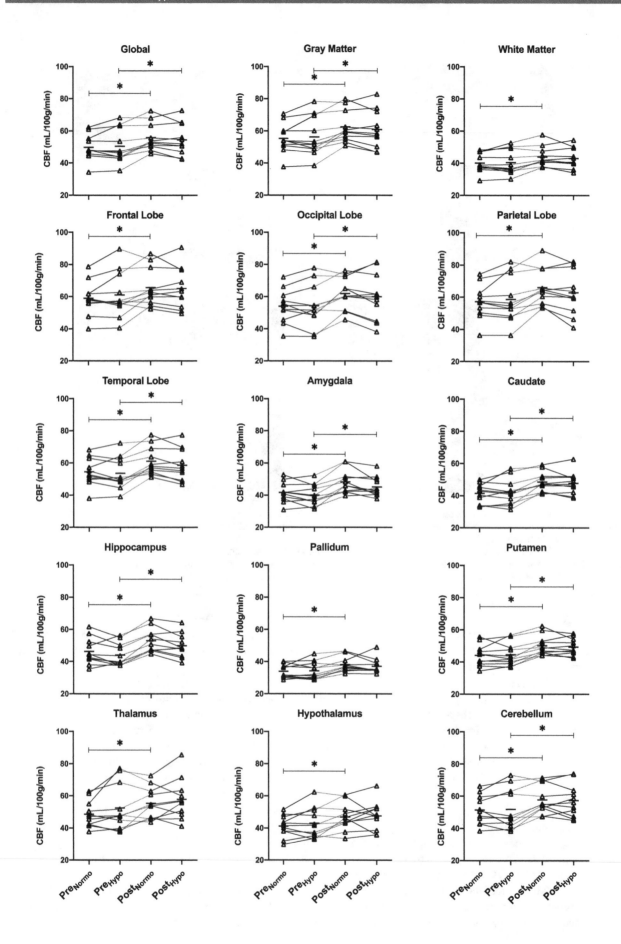

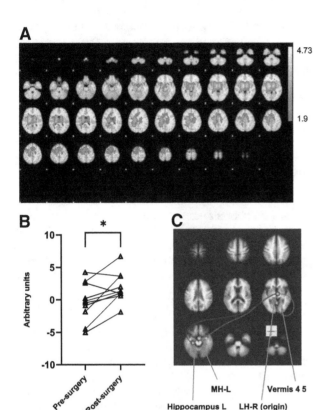

Figure 6—fMRI. *A*: TICA across all six resting fMRI runs revealed one IC, which represents a functional connectivity resting-state network, explaining most variability. This resting-state network was defined purely on the provided data without prior assumption and includes, notably, bilateral thalamus and hypothalamus. The activity of this IC was significantly higher after vs. before surgery (red color; S-mode) during the first 20 min of the hypoglycemic clamp (i.e., rapid glucose lowering) ($P < 0.05$). The color code represents T-values. *B*: Individual data of the above IC activity (S-mode) during the initial phase of hypoglycemia. *$P < 0.05$. *C*: The ROI functional connectivity analysis using the right LH as seed region as defined on the basis of previous literature (31). During initial hypoglycemia, there was a significantly decreased functional connectivity to left hippocampus and a significantly increased functional connectivity to vermis regions 4 and 5 for the post- vs. presurgery condition. Similar increases in connectivity to corresponding regions were obtained using the left LH as seed region (data not shown). $n = 10$. L, left; LH, lateral hypothalamus; MH, medial hypothalamus; R, right.

Limitations

This study protocol was laborious and challenging for patients as well as staff, and there was an ~30% dropout rate among the included subjects. Therefore, the number of subjects completing the protocol was small ($n = 11$). There were also some technical issues that led to fewer subjects for some assessments. The spatial resolution of our MR and PET exams did not allow for very detailed regional analysis, for example, at the subnucleus level of the

hypothalamus. Individual subnuclei can exert different and sometimes opposing effects on whole-body glucose turnover and energy balance (43), making the functional consequences of changes detected in hypothalamic glucose uptake or network activity uncertain. Furthermore, we have no results at present on anatomical assessments, and there may be structural effects in specific brain regions in addition to the functional changes. Previous work has suggested an increase in gray as well as white matter density in specific brain areas after RYGB, which may be related to the brain's regulation of energy balance (15,44,45). Importantly, there is yet limited understanding of the functional impact of changes in the brain's glucose uptake and blood flow rates that were found in our study.

Conclusions

The current results suggest adaptation of the brain to lower glycemic levels following RYGB. This is supported by the attenuation of several insulin-antagonistic responses to hypoglycemia. In the brain, there were changes after RYGB in neural activation by hypoglycemia in central regions and the hypothalamus that are considered important for the coordination of glucose regulation. There were also global changes in brain glucose uptake rate and blood flow, and the latter may be related to improved cognitive function. Taken together, our findings point toward a role of the brain to orchestrate maintenance of normoglycemia and thereby reverse, or prevent, type 2 diabetes following gastric bypass surgery. Although critical hormonal and metabolic effects are finally exerted in the peripheral "end organs," the glycemic set point may largely be determined and governed by the CNS.

Acknowledgments. The authors thank all study participants for their invaluable support. The authors are very grateful to research nurses Anna Åhlander, Sofia Löfving, Caroline Woxberg, and Carola Almström (all Department of Medical Sciences, Uppsala University) and Anders Lundberg, Marie Åhlman, and Gunilla Arvidsson (all Department of Surgical Sciences, Uppsala University). The authors also thank Prof. Elna-Marie Larsson (Department of Surgical Sciences, Uppsala University) for expert advice and support in the early phase of this study.

Funding. The study was funded by grants from the Swedish Diabetes Foundation (DIA2019-490), EXODIAB–Excellence of Diabetes Research in Sweden, the Ernfors Foundation, TREATMENT (EC H2020-MSCA-ITN-721236), Novo Nordisk Fonden (NNF20OC0063864), and ALF–Swedish Government Research Grants to Uppsala University Hospital.

Duality of Interest. No potential conflicts of interest relevant to this article were reported.

Author Contributions. K.E.A. contributed to the study design, supervised the experiments, performed statistical analyses on clinical characteristics, collated results from co-authors, and wrote the manuscript. M.H.L. supervised experiments, performed statistical analyses on clinical

Figure 5—Regional CBF (by ASL) for normo- and hypoglycemia states in subjects pre- and postsurgery. Data are presented as spaghetti plots of individual values with individual connecting lines and mean of all subjects at that time point (horizontal solid lines). *$P < 0.05$ (paired *t* tests, $n = 11$). hypo, hypoglycemic phase of clamp; normo, normoglycemic phase of clamp; Pre, preoperative; Post, postoperative.

characteristics and cardiovascular function, collated results from co-authors, and wrote the manuscript. N.A. contributed to the study design and performed data preparation, statistical analyses, presentation, and interpretation of cognitive tests and symptoms. S.K. examined FDG-PET imaging, performed statistical analyses, and presented and interpreted the FDG-PET results. M.F. examined ASL images, performed statistical analyses, and presented and interpreted the ASL results. M.J.P. gave statistical advice, performed the statistical analyses on metabolism and hormones, and presented these results. M.G. contributed to the study design and aided in interpreting the cognitive tests and fMRI findings. F.A.K. contributed to the study design and interpretation of major findings. G.F. performed and interpreted statistical analyses. M.S. contributed to the study design and the interpretation of major findings. U.W. performed and interpreted the HRV analyses. S.H. examined the fMRI imaging, performed the statistical analyses, and interpreted and presented the results. M.L. contributed to the study design, examined the FDG-PET imaging, and interpreted and presented the results. J.W. contributed to the study design, examined the fMRI and ASL imaging, and interpreted the results. J.W.E. was the principal investigator and, as such, designed and coordinated the study, interpreted the findings, and wrote the manuscript. All authors critically revised and approved the final manuscript. J.W.E. is the guarantor of this work and, as such, had full access to the all the data in the study and takes responsibility for the integrity of the data and the accuracy of the data analysis.

References

1. Buchwald H, Estok R, Fahrbach K, et al. Weight and type 2 diabetes after bariatric surgery: systematic review and meta-analysis. Am J Med 2009;122:248–256.e5

2. Katsogiannos P, Kamble PG, Wiklund U, et al. Rapid changes in neuroendocrine regulation may contribute to reversal of type 2 diabetes after gastric bypass surgery. Endocrine 2020;67:344–353

3. Sjöström L, Lindroos A-K, Peltonen M, et al.; Swedish Obese Subjects Study Scientific Group. Lifestyle, diabetes, and cardiovascular risk factors 10 years after bariatric surgery. N Engl J Med 2004;351:2683–2693

4. Morínigo R, Moizé V, Musri M, et al. Glucagon-like peptide-1, peptide YY, hunger, and satiety after gastric bypass surgery in morbidly obese subjects. J Clin Endocrinol Metab 2006;91:1735–1740

5. Abrahamsson N, Edén Engström B, Sundbom M, Karlsson FA. Hypoglycemia in everyday life after gastric bypass and duodenal switch. Eur J Endocrinol 2015;173:91–100

6. Cryer PE. Hypoglycemia-associated autonomic failure in diabetes. Am J Physiol Endocrinol Metab 2001;281:E1115–E1121

7. Mangia S, Tesfaye N, De Martino F, et al. Hypoglycemia-induced increases in thalamic cerebral blood flow are blunted in subjects with type 1 diabetes and hypoglycemia unawareness. J Cereb Blood Flow Metab 2012;32:2084–2090

8. Dunn JT, Cranston I, Marsden PK, Amiel SA, Reed LJ. Attenuation of amygdala and frontal cortical responses to low blood glucose concentration in asymptomatic hypoglycemia in type 1 diabetes: a new player in hypoglycemia unawareness? Diabetes 2007;56:2766–2773

9. Cranston I, Reed LJ, Marsden PK, Amiel SA. Changes in regional brain (18)F-fluorodeoxyglucose uptake at hypoglycemia in type 1 diabetic men associated with hypoglycemia unawareness and counter-regulatory failure. Diabetes 2001;50:2329–2336

10. Hwang JJ, Parikh L, Lacadie C, et al. Hypoglycemia unawareness in type 1 diabetes suppresses brain responses to hypoglycemia. J Clin Invest 2018;128:1485–1495

11. Abrahamsson N, Börjesson JL, Sundbom M, Wiklund U, Karlsson FA, Eriksson JW. Gastric bypass reduces symptoms and hormonal responses in hypoglycemia. Diabetes 2016;65:2667–2675

12. Guldstrand M, Ahrén B, Wredling R, Backman L, Lins PE, Adamson U. Alteration of the counterregulatory responses to insulin-induced hypoglycemia and of cognitive function after massive weight reduction in severely obese subjects. Metabolism 2003;52:900–907

13. Hirvonen J, Virtanen KA, Nummenmaa L, et al. Effects of insulin on brain glucose metabolism in impaired glucose tolerance. Diabetes 2011;60:443–447

14. Boersma GJ, Johansson E, Pereira MJ, et al. Altered glucose uptake in muscle, visceral adipose tissue, and brain predict whole-body insulin resistance and may contribute to the development of type 2 diabetes: a combined PET/MR study. Horm Metab Res 2018;50:e10

15. Tuulari JJ, Karlsson HK, Hirvonen J, et al. Weight loss after bariatric surgery reverses insulin-induced increases in brain glucose metabolism of the morbidly obese. Diabetes 2013;62:2747–2751

16. Chaytor NS, Barbosa-Leiker C, Ryan CM, Germine LT, Hirsch IB, Weinstock RS. Clinically significant cognitive impairment in older adults with type 1 diabetes. J Diabetes Complications 2019;33:91–97

17. Howorka K, Heger G, Schabmann A, Anderer P, Tribl G, Zeitlhofer J. Severe hypoglycaemia unawareness is associated with an early decrease in vigilance during hypoglycaemia. Psychoneuroendocrinology 1996;21:295–312

18. Almby KE, Abrahamsson N, Lundqvist MH, et al. Effects of GLP-1 on counter-regulatory responses during hypoglycemia after GBP surgery. Eur J Endocrinol 2019;181:161–171

19. Bowie CR, Harvey PD. Administration and interpretation of the Trail Making Test. Nat Protoc 2006;1:2277–2281

20. Jaeger J. Digit symbol substitution test: the case for sensitivity over specificity in neuropsychological testing. J Clin Psychopharmacol 2018;38:513–519

21. Tombaugh TN. Trail Making Test A and B: normative data stratified by age and education. Arch Clin Neuropsychol 2004;19:203–214

22. Deary IJ, Hepburn DA, MacLeod KM, Frier BM. Partitioning the symptoms of hypoglycaemia using multi-sample confirmatory factor analysis. Diabetologia 1993;36:771–777

23. Grant AM, Deller TW, Khalighi MM, Maramraju SH, Delso G, Levin CS. NEMA NU 2-2012 performance studies for the SiPM-based ToF-PET component of the GE SIGNA PET/MR system. Med Phys 2016;43:2334–2343

24. Buxton RB, Frank LR, Wong EC, Siewert B, Warach S, Edelman RR. A general kinetic model for quantitative perfusion imaging with arterial spin labeling. Magn Reson Med 1998;40:383–396

25. Alsop DC, Detre JA, Golay X, et al. Recommended implementation of arterial spin-labeled perfusion MRI for clinical applications: a consensus of the ISMRM perfusion study group and the European consortium for ASL in dementia. Magn Reson Med 2015;73:102–116

26. Dai W, Robson PM, Shankaranarayanan A, Alsop DC. Reduced resolution transit delay prescan for quantitative continuous arterial spin labeling perfusion imaging. Magn Reson Med 2012;67:1252–1265

27. Dai W, Shankaranarayanan A, Alsop DC. Volumetric measurement of perfusion and arterial transit delay using hadamard encoded continuous arterial spin labeling. Magn Reson Med 2013;69:1014–1022

28. Maleki N, Dai W, Alsop DC. Optimization of background suppression for arterial spin labeling perfusion imaging. MAGMA 2012;25:127–133

29. Dai W, Garcia D, de Bazelaire C, Alsop DC. Continuous flow-driven inversion for arterial spin labeling using pulsed radio frequency and gradient fields. Magn Reson Med 2008;60:1488–1497

30. Beckmann CF, Smith SM. Tensorial extensions of independent component analysis for multisubject FMRI analysis. Neuroimage 2005;25:294–311

31. Whitfield-Gabrieli S, Nieto-Castanon A. Conn: a functional connectivity toolbox for correlated and anticorrelated brain networks. Brain Connect 2012;2:125–141

32. Li P, Shan H, Nie B, et al. Sleeve gastrectomy rescuing the altered functional connectivity of lateral but not medial hypothalamus in subjects with obesity. Obes Surg 2019;29:2191–2199

33. Sorensen J, Stahle E, Langstrom B, Frostfeldt G, Wikstrom G, Hedenstierna G: Simple and accurate assessment of forward cardiac output by use of 1- (11) C-acetate PET verified in a pig model. J Nucl Med 2003;44:1176–1183

34. Stanley S, Moheet A, Seaquist ER. Central mechanisms of glucose sensing and counterregulation in defense of hypoglycemia. Endocr Rev 2019;40:768–788

35. Saindane AM, Drane DL, Singh A, Wu J, Qiu D. Neuroimaging correlates of cognitive changes after bariatric surgery. Surg Obes Relat Dis 2020;16: 119–127

36. Lundqvist MH, Almby K, Wiklund U, et al. Altered hormonal and autonomic nerve responses to hypo- and hyperglycaemia are found in overweight and insulin-resistant individuals and may contribute to the development of type 2 diabetes. Diabetologia 2021;64:641–655

37. Rebelos E, Immonen H, Bucci M, et al. Brain glucose uptake is associated with endogenous glucose production in obese patients before and after bariatric surgery and predicts metabolic outcome at follow-up. Diabetes Obes Metab 2019;21:218–226

38. Kullmann S, Valenta V, Wagner R, et al. Brain insulin sensitivity is linked to adiposity and body fat distribution. Nat Commun 2020;11:1841

39. Lind L, Zethelius B, Sundbom M, Edén Engström B, Karlsson FA. Vasoreactivity is rapidly improved in obese subjects after gastric bypass surgery. Int J Obes 2009;33:1390–1395

40. Wu HM, Bergsneider M, Glenn TC, et al. Measurement of the global lumped constant for 2-deoxy-2-[^{18}F]fluoro-D-glucose in normal human brain using [^{15}O]water and 2-deoxy-2-[^{18}F]fluoro-D-glucose positron emission tomography imaging. A method with validation based on multiple methodologies. Mol Imaging Biol 2003;5:32–41

41. Suda S, Shinohara M, Miyaoka M, Lucignani G, Kennedy C, Sokoloff L. The lumped constant of the deoxyglucose method in hypoglycemia: effects of moderate hypoglycemia on local cerebral glucose utilization in the rat. J Cereb Blood Flow Metab 1990;10:499–509

42. Veneman T, Mitrakou A, Mokan M, Cryer P, Gerich J. Effect of hyperketonemia and hyperlacticacidemia on symptoms, cognitive dysfunction, and counterregulatory hormone responses during hypoglycemia in normal humans. Diabetes 1994;43:1311–1317

43. Lundqvist MH, Almby K, Abrahamsson N, Eriksson JW. Is the brain a key player in glucose regulation and development of type 2 diabetes? Front Physiol 2019;10:457

44. Rullmann M, Preusser S, Poppitz S, et al. Gastric-bypass surgery induced widespread neural plasticity of the obese human brain. Neuroimage 2018;172: 853–863

45. Rullmann M, Preusser S, Poppitz S, et al. Adiposity related brain plasticity induced by bariatric surgery. Front Hum Neurosci 2019;13:290

Genetic Composition and Autoantibody Titers Model the Probability of Detecting C-Peptide Following Type 1 Diabetes Diagnosis

MacKenzie D. Williams,[1] Rhonda Bacher,[2] Daniel J. Perry,[1] C. Ramsey Grace,[1] Kieran M. McGrail,[1] Amanda L. Posgai,[1] Andrew Muir,[3] Srikar Chamala,[1] Michael J. Haller,[4] Desmond A. Schatz,[4] Todd M. Brusko,[1,4] Mark A. Atkinson,[1,4] and Clive H. Wasserfall[1]

Diabetes 2021;70:932–943 | https://doi.org/10.2337/db20-0937

We and others previously demonstrated that a type 1 diabetes genetic risk score (GRS) improves the ability to predict disease progression and onset in at-risk subjects with islet autoantibodies. Here, we hypothesized that GRS and islet autoantibodies, combined with age at onset and disease duration, could serve as markers of residual β-cell function following type 1 diabetes diagnosis. Generalized estimating equations were used to investigate whether GRS along with insulinoma-associated protein-2 autoantibody (IA–2A), zinc transporter 8 autoantibody (ZnT8A), and GAD autoantibody (GADA) titers were predictive of C-peptide detection in a largely cross-sectional cohort of 401 subjects with type 1 diabetes (median duration 4.5 years [range 0–60]). Indeed, a combined model with incorporation of disease duration, age at onset, GRS, and titers of IA–2A, ZnT8A, and GADA provided superior capacity to predict C-peptide detection (quasi-likelihood information criterion [QIC] = 334.6) compared with the capacity of disease duration, age at onset, and GRS as the sole parameters (QIC = 359.2). These findings support the need for longitudinal validation of our combinatorial model. The ability to project the rate and extent of decline in residual C-peptide production for individuals with type 1 diabetes could critically inform enrollment and benchmarking for clinical trials where investigators are seeking to preserve or restore endogenous β-cell function.

A 2015 Consensus Statement defined the preclinical staging of type 1 diabetes based on the number of islet autoantibodies and presence of dysglycemia (1). Extensive genotyping and the development of type 1 diabetes genetic risk scores (GRS), which consolidate the complex heritable components of the disease (2–4), have further improved our ability to predict disease progression and onset among islet autoantibody–positive individuals (5). Despite this substantial progress in characterizing metabolic and immunologic events during pre–type 1 diabetes, these factors are rarely monitored beyond the recent-onset phase of the disease.

Preservation of endogenous insulin production, as measured by C-peptide in serum, is the most common benchmark for type 1 diabetes interventional trials (6), and it is well known that the production of even low levels of endogenous insulin is associated with reduced severity of long-term complications (7). Though the disease was originally thought to result in complete loss of functional β-cell mass, the development of ultrasensitive C-peptide assays has largely overturned that notion (8). Indeed, C-peptide loss after type 1 diabetes diagnosis is now known to occur in a biphasic pattern with a window of exponential fall followed by a stable period (9), and many individuals with long-standing type 1 diabetes (i.e., up to 50 years' duration) continue to secrete small amounts of endogenous insulin (10). Accordingly, we observed small insulin-positive islets and insulin-positive single cells scattered throughout the exocrine pancreas tissue of organ donors with established disease (11,12); however, there is marked heterogeneity in the duration and degree of maintenance of β-cell function (13).

[1]Department of Pathology, Immunology and Laboratory Medicine, Diabetes Institute, College of Medicine, University of Florida, Gainesville, FL

[2]Department of Biostatistics, College of Public Health and Health Professions, and College of Medicine, University of Florida, Gainesville, FL

[3]Department of Pediatrics, Emory University, Atlanta, GA

[4]Department of Pediatrics, Diabetes Institute, College of Medicine, University of Florida, Gainesville, FL

Corresponding author: Clive H. Wasserfall, clive@ufl.edu

Received 15 September 2020 and accepted 1 January 2021

This article contains supplementary material online at https://doi.org/10.2337/figshare.13516808.

Early studies linked islet autoantibody positivity with more precipitous loss of residual β-cell function, particularly during the first year following type 1 diabetes diagnosis (14–16). After disease onset, islet autoantibody titers are known to decline with variable kinetics and often to undetectable levels, though autoantibodies against GAD (GADA) and insulinoma-associated protein-2 (IA–2A) are more persistent than zinc transporter 8 autoantibodies (ZnT8A) (17). Declining ZnT8A and IA–2A titers have been shown to generally parallel C-peptide production in the 2.5 years immediately following diagnosis (17), but to our knowledge, long-term associations have not been explored. Separately, C-peptide persistence has been associated with genetic risk at a number of individual loci (18–20) as well as in a combined GRS model (21). These studies prompted us to explore the complex relationships linking genetic composition, islet autoantibody titers, and residual β-cell function in both recent-onset and long-standing disease.

We hypothesized that islet autoantibody titers might serve as potential biomarkers for prediction and monitoring of the rate of decline in functional β-cell mass following the onset of type 1 diabetes and that this relationship may be governed by overall genetic load for the disease. Reported herein, we assessed the utility of a type 1 diabetes GRS (22), in combination with disease duration and age at onset, as well as GADA, IA–2A, and ZnT8A titers, for prediction of the probability of C-peptide detection in individuals with type 1 diabetes. We envision that our prediction model could be applied to stratify newly diagnosed subjects according to their anticipated C-peptide trajectories to inform enrollment or establish benchmarks that define therapeutic response in intervention studies.

RESEARCH DESIGN AND METHODS

Sample Collection

Study subjects were enrolled from outpatient clinics at the University of Florida, Nemours Children's Hospital (Orlando, FL), and Emory University under institutional review board approval at each institution. Peripheral blood was collected into vacutainer tubes for serum and genomic DNA isolation. Serum samples were separated by centrifugation. Genomic DNA was extracted with QIAGEN kits on a QIAcube (QIAGEN, Hilden, Germany) according to the manufacturer's instructions. Serum and DNA were stored at −20°C in the University of Florida Diabetes Institute (UDFI) biorepository. Samples were selected from 401 individuals with type 1 diabetes of any duration at the time of blood collection (Table 1). Because the GRS model was found to be less robust for assessment of risk in non-European populations (22), only subjects with genetically imputed European ancestry who self-reported as Caucasian were considered for study inclusion.

Autoantibody and C-Peptide Measurement

IA–2A, ZnT8A, and GADA were measured from serum with use of Islet Autoantibody Standardization Program (IASP)-validated ELISA kits (KRONUS Inc., Star, ID) according to

Table 1—Summary of demographic and genetic data for cross-sectional and longitudinal study subjects

	All	Cross-sectional	Longitudinal
Total N	401	382	19
Age at sample collection, years	19.5 ± 11.9	19.5 ± 11.9	20.4 ± 12.0
Age at onset, years	12.0 ± 9.1	11.9 ± 9.2	13.1 ± 5.4
T1D duration, years	7.5 ± 9.1	7.5 ± 9.0	7.2 ± 11.1
Ethnicity, n (%)			
Hispanic	41 (10.2)	41 (10.7)	0 (0)
Non-Hispanic	329 (82)	311 (81.4)	18 (94.7)
Not reported	31 (7.7)	30 (7.9)	1 (5.3)
Sex, n (%)			
Female	208 (51.9)	198 (51.8)	10 (52.6)
Male	193 (48.1)	184 (48.2)	9 (47.4)
HLA status, n (%)			
DR3/3	38 (9.5)	35 (9.2)	3 (15.8)
DR3/4	102 (25.4)	97 (25.4)	5 (26.3)
DR3/X	65 (16.2)	63 (16.5)	2 (10.5)
DR4/4	27 (6.7)	26 (6.8)	1 (5.3)
DR4/X	112 (27.9)	106 (27.7)	6 (31.6)
DRX/X	57 (14.2)	55 (14.4)	2 (10.5)
GRS	0.278 ± 0.027	0.278 ± 0.027	0.280 ± 0.023

Data are means ± SD unless otherwise indicated. All subjects were Caucasian (self-reported race) and of European descent (genetically imputed race). Of 401 subjects, 382 had one blood draw, 18 had two blood draws, and 1 had four blood draws. Notably, because all samples in this study were collected from subjects diagnosed with type 1 diabetes, GRS values are high compared with those in the general population without diabetes (3,4,22); hence, both the 80th and 20th GRS percentiles examined herein reflect "high genetic risk" for type 1 diabetes. T1D, type 1 diabetes.

modified protocols as previously described (23). When necessary, sera were titrated to fall within the assay's dynamic range. C-peptide was measured from serum by ultrasensitive ELISA (lower detection limit 2.5 pmol/L; Mercodia, Uppsala, Sweden), according to the manufacturer's instructions.

GRS Calculation

Genotyping of 975,000 genetic markers was performed on an Affymetrix GeneTitan with a custom Axiom genotyping array based on the Precision Medicine Research Array (~790,000 single nucleotide polymorphisms [SNPs]) modified to contain the ImmunoChip (24) complement SNP set (version 2.0), as well as additional known type 1 diabetes–associated loci (25), termed the UFDIchip (Thermo Fisher Scientific, Waltham, MA). The UFDIchip included 26 of the 30 SNPs required to compute GRS (22). The remaining four were obtained from imputation (rs2069762 [R^2 = 0.9962], rs1264813 [R^2 = 0.9962], rs689 [R^2 = 0.9486], rs3788013 [R^2 = 0.9967]) to the Human Reference Consortium (version r1.1) with use of the Michigan Imputation Server (26). GRS was calculated as previously described (3,22).

Table 2—Summary of GEE logistic regression results for prediction of C-peptide detection

Coefficient	OR	95% CI	P
Duration	0.697	(0.59, 0.82)	<0.0001
Onset age	1.070	(1.01, 1.14)	0.033
GRS	1.180	(0.87, 1.62)	0.294
Duration * GRS	0.895	(0.84, 0.96)	<0.001

The effects of type 1 diabetes duration, age at onset, GRS, and their interactions on detectable C-peptide were modeled using GEE with assumption of binomial variance and logit link. GEE models were used to account for the mixed cohort of both cross-sectional and longitudinal samples. Type 1 diabetes duration and onset age were found to be significantly predictive of C-peptide detection at the mean GRS (OR 0.697, $P < 0.0001$, and OR 1.070, $P < 0.033$, respectively). GRS was not found to be a direct significant predictor of C-peptide detection with duration = 0 ($P = 0.294$). An interaction effect between disease duration and GRS (Duration * GRS) was found to be significantly predictive of C-peptide detection (OR 0.895, $P < 0.001$). OR with 95% CI and corresponding P values are reported for disease duration, GRS, and the interaction effect between duration and GRS. Sex was not a significant predictor of C-peptide detection ($P = 0.443$) and was not included in the model.

Statistical Analysis

Generalized estimating equations (GEE) assuming binomial variance and logit link were used to model the effect of type 1 diabetes duration, age at onset, and GRS on the probability of C-peptide detection. GEE models were used to accommodate our mixed cohort of both cross-sectional ($N = 382$ subjects) and longitudinal ($N = 19$ subjects) samples. For significant predictors, the odds of C-peptide detection were compared for the 20th (GRS = 0.260) versus the 80th (GRS = 0.301) GRS quantiles within our cohort to compare lower versus higher genetic load. For comparison of younger versus older disease onset age, odds of C-peptide detection were compared for the 20th (6.0 years) versus the 80th (15.7 years) onset age quantiles. For these analyses, subjects were not binned into separate groups according to variable percentiles. Instead, the models were fit with use of GEE, and the values of different percentiles for age at onset, GRS, and autoantibody titers were then substituted into the models to calculate predicted probabilities of C-peptide detection. Therefore, percentiles represent not an interval but a single value. Table 2 reports unadjusted odds ratios (ORs) and 95% CI of population-average parameter estimates from the GEE model.

Associations of C-peptide detection with disease duration, age at onset, GRS, titers of each autoantibody, and all two-way interactions were assessed simultaneously by logistic regression with lasso penalty. Briefly, the data set was repeatedly partitioned in half for training and testing, and the probability of model inclusion for each predictor (including all two-way interaction effects) was calculated over 1,000 iterations. No variables were weighted in the analysis, and all coefficients with at least 50% inclusion frequency and their main effects are reported in Table 3. A GEE with binomial variance and logit link including these predictors

was then used to model the log odds of C-peptide detection as follows:

$$\log\left(\frac{p}{1-p}\right) = \beta_0 + (\beta_1 * age) + (\beta_2 * T) + (\beta_3 * GRS)$$

$$+ (\beta_4 * T * IA\text{-}2A) + (\beta_5 * GRS * ZnT8A)$$

$$+ (\beta_6 * GADA) + (\beta_7 * age * ZnT8A)$$

$$+ (\beta_8 * T * ZnT8A) + (\beta_9 * IA\text{-}2A)$$

$$+ (\beta_{10} * ZnT8A)$$

where p is the probability of detecting C-peptide, T is disease duration in years, and the intercept (β_0) is -0.251. The remaining β-coefficients are given in exponentiated form (as ORs) (Table 3).

Because the GEE method is based on quasi-likelihood theory, Akaike information criterion was not directly applicable for model selection. Instead we used quasi-likelihood information criterion (QIC), a modification of Akaike information criterion (27), to compare the two models (QIC results summarized in Supplementary Table 1). The calculation of QIC considers how well the model fits the data while favoring simpler models via a penalization term for the number of variables included (27). Statistical analyses were performed with R 3.6.1. Models were fit with use of the geeglm function in the geepack version 1.2 R package (28–30). When comparing the odds of detecting C-peptide between percentiles, a difference in estimated detection probability < 0.01 was considered to represent similar odds. All tests were two sided, with $P < 0.05$ considered significant. All CIs were estimated with the bootstrap method by sampling of subjects with replacement (sampling was performed 1,000 times).

Data and Resource Availability

The data sets generated during and/or analyzed during the current study are available from the corresponding author upon reasonable request. No applicable resources were generated or analyzed during the current study.

RESULTS

Disease Duration, Age at Onset, GRS, and Their Interactions Affect Probability of Detection of C-Peptide in Individuals With Type 1 Diabetes

As expected, C-peptide detection decreased with increasing disease duration (Fig. 1A). We modeled the effect of type 1 diabetes duration, age at onset, and GRS on C-peptide detection using GEE (model 1). As expected, disease duration was negatively associated with odds of detecting C-peptide: at the mean GRS (0.278), each additional duration year decreased the odds of C-peptide detection (OR 0.697 [95% CI 0.59, 0.82], $P < 0.0001$) (Table 2). Older onset age was associated with increased odds of C-peptide detection (OR 1.070 [95% CI 1.01, 1.14], $P =$

Table 3—Summary of repeated train-test split results for selection of the most significant predictors of C-peptide detection

	Probability of inclusion	Coefficient from model	OR†	P
Onset age	1.00	β_1	1.110	<0.0001
Duration	1.00	β_2	0.701	<0.001
GRS	0.80	β_3	0.748	0.061
Duration * IA–2A	0.72	β_4	0.896	0.175
GRS * ZnT8A	0.65	β_5	1.380	0.057
GADA	0.58	β_6	1.230	0.128
Onset age * ZnT8A	0.52	β_7	1.080	<0.001
Duration * ZnT8A	0.51	β_8	0.908	0.190
IA–2A	0.47	β_9	1.680	0.041
ZnT8A	0.39	β_{10}	0.625	0.198

Disease duration; onset age; GRS; titers for IA–2A, ZnT8A, and GADA; and all two-way interaction effects of predictor variables were tested for inclusion in the C-peptide model simultaneously with penalized logistic regression with repeated 10-fold cross validation for feature selection. The data set was repeatedly partitioned in half for training and testing, and the probability of each predictor (including all two-way interaction effects) being in the model was calculated over 1,000 iterations. All coefficients with at least 50% probability of inclusion and their main effects are reported. Interaction effects are denoted as two variables separated by an asterisk. The glmnet, version 3.0, package in R was used for penalized logistic regression and feature selection. †Regression coefficients (β_i) are reported in exponentiated form as ORs, such that $OR = e^{\beta}$. The coefficient values correspond to the β values from the overall model formula.

0.033). We found a significant interaction effect between disease duration and GRS on C-peptide detection odds (OR 0.895 [95% CI 0.84, 0.96], $P < 0.001$). At increasing disease durations and fixed onset age, subjects at the 80th GRS quantile had substantially lower odds of C-peptide detection compared with subjects at the 20th GRS quantile (Fig. 1B). Although younger age at onset (Fig. 1B, red curves) was generally associated with lower odds of C-peptide detection compared with older age at onset (Fig. 1B, blue curves), onset age did not affect the rate of decline in the odds of C-peptide detection over time. In contrast, higher GRS (Fig. 1B, dashed curves) was associated with a more rapid decline in the odds of C-peptide detection compared with lower GRS (Fig. 1B, solid curves). Sex was not a significant predictor of C-peptide detection ($P = 0.443$) and was therefore not included in the model.

At the median onset age (10.2 years), GRS had the greatest effect on the odds of C-peptide detection at 6.3 years' disease duration (95% CI 1.14, 8.14), while longer disease durations ($\geq$19.1 years [95% CI 10.99, 25.16]) yielded similar odds of C-peptide detection regardless of GRS. For comparison of the effect of low versus high GRS on C-peptide detection, the difference in predicted probability of detectable C-peptide between the 20th and 80th GRS percentiles was plotted according to disease duration with onset age set to either the 20th or the 80th percentile (Fig. 1C). When age at onset was at the 20th percentile (6.0 years), GRS had the greatest effect on C-peptide detection odds at 6.0 years' disease duration (95% CI 0.33, 7.54), with lower GRS corresponding to higher odds of C-peptide detection (Fig. 1C, red curve). When age at onset was set to the 80th percentile (15.7 years), GRS had the greatest effect on C-peptide detection odds at 6.9 years' duration (95% CI 1.98, 9.09) (Fig. 1C, blue curve).

At the median GRS (0.280), onset age had the largest effect on odds of C-peptide detection at 3.0 years' disease duration (95% CI 2.42, 3.57), while longer disease durations ($\geq$14.4 years [95% CI 10.39, 20.22]) yielded similar odds of C-peptide detection regardless of onset age. For comparison of the effect of older versus younger age at onset on C-peptide detection, the difference in predicted probability of detectable C-peptide between the 20th and 80th age at onset percentiles was plotted according to disease duration with GRS set to either the 20th or 80th percentile (Fig. 1D). When GRS was at the 20th percentile (0.260), age at onset had the greatest effect on C-peptide detection odds at 3.4 years' duration (95% CI 2.72, 4.32), with younger age at onset corresponding to lower odds of C-peptide detection (Fig. 1D, red curve). When GRS was set to the 80th percentile (0.301), age at onset had the greatest effect on C-peptide detection odds at 2.7 years' duration (95% CI 1.80, 3.22), with younger age at onset corresponding to lower odds of C-peptide detection (Fig. 1D, blue curve).

Incorporating GADA, IA–2A, and ZnT8A Titers Improves Model Fit

We next examined whether autoantibody titers and their interactions with disease duration, onset age, or GRS had an effect on C-peptide detection odds using logistic regression with a lasso penalty (model 2 [results summarized in Table 3]). For model 2, the most significant predictors of C-peptide detection were onset age and disease duration (each with 100% probability of model inclusion). As with model 1, older age at onset was associated with greater odds of C-peptide detection (OR 1.110, $P < 0.0001$) and longer duration was associated with decreased odds of C-peptide detection (OR 0.701, $P < 0.001$). GRS was the third most informative predictor in model 2, with 80% probability of inclusion. Higher GRS was associated with

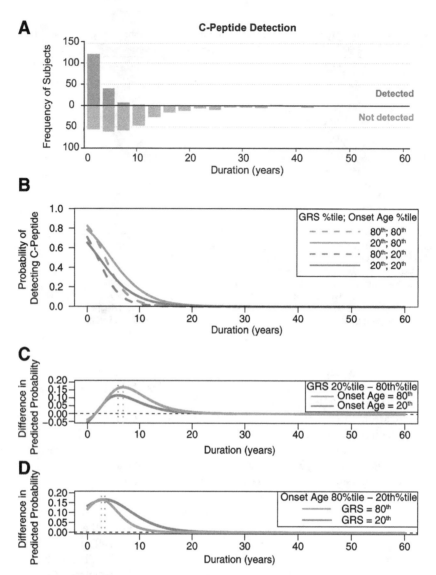

Figure 1—*A*: The *y*-axis indicates the number of individuals with (upper histogram, purple bars) and without (lower histogram, gray bars) detectable C-peptide in the cohort. *B–D*: The odds of C-peptide detection were compared for the 20th (GRS = 0.260) and the 80th (GRS = 0.301) GRS quantiles within our cohort for comparison of lower versus higher genetic load. For comparison of younger versus older onset age, odds of C-peptide detection were compared for the 20th (6.0 years) and the 80th (15.7 years) onset age quantiles. *B*: Solid curves show the predicted probability of C-peptide detection according to disease duration when GRS is at the 20th percentile and onset age is set to either the 20th percentile (red solid curve) or the 80th percentile (blue solid curve). Dashed curves show the predicted probability of C-peptide detection according to disease duration when GRS is at the 80th percentile and onset age is set to either the 20th percentile (red dashed curve) or the 80th percentile (blue dashed curve). *C*: The difference in predicted probability of detectable C-peptide between the 20th and 80th GRS percentiles was plotted according to disease duration when onset age is at either the 20th percentile (red curve) or the 80th percentile (blue curve). The vertical dotted lines mark the duration at which the difference in predicted probability between the 20th and 80th GRS percentiles is the greatest (6.0 years when onset age is at the 20th percentile [red dotted vertical line] and 6.9 years when onset age is at the 80th percentile [blue dotted vertical line]). *D*: The difference in predicted probability of detectable C-peptide between the 20th and 80th onset age percentiles was plotted according to disease duration when GRS is at either the 20th percentile (red curve) or the 80th percentile (blue curve). The vertical dotted lines mark the duration at which the difference in predicted probability between the 20th and 80th onset age percentiles is the greatest (3.4 years when GRS is at the 20th percentile [red dotted vertical line] and 2.7 years when GRS is at the 80th percentile [blue dotted vertical line]). %tile, percentile.

reduced odds of C-peptide detection (OR 0.748, *P* = 0.061). The predictive capacity of IA–2A and ZnT8A for C-peptide detection was dependent on their interactions with other variables (summarized in Table 3). In contrast, GADA titer was individually predictive of C-peptide detection, with higher titers associating with increased odds for C-peptide detection (OR 1.230, *P* = 0.128) (Fig. 2*A*), and had 58% probability of model inclusion. Although, overall, autoantibodies were less informative for C-peptide detection compared with onset age, duration, and GRS, their incorporation improved model fit compared with model 1 (Supplementary Table 1).

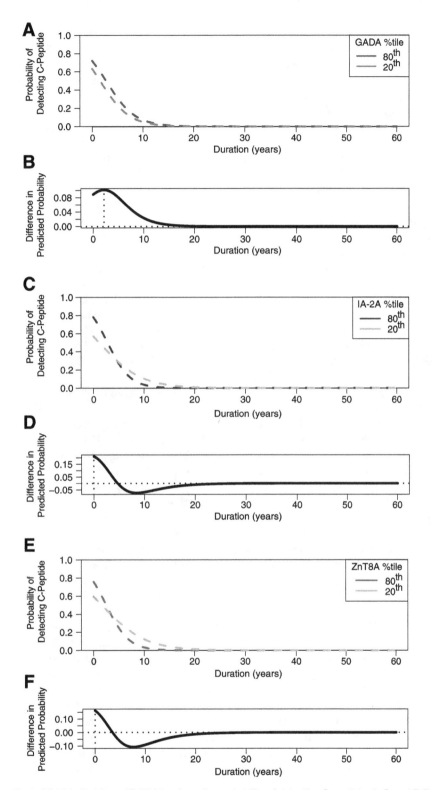

Figure 2—Significant effect of GADA, IA–2A, and ZnT8A levels on the probability of detecting C-peptide. *A*, *C*, and *E*: Dashed lines show the fitted predicted probability of C-peptide detection (*y*-axis) according to type 1 diabetes duration. GRS is set to the median. *B*, *D*, and *F*: Difference in predicted probability between the 80th and 20th autoantibody titer percentiles was plotted according to disease duration. The vertical dotted line marks the duration at which the difference in predicted probability between the 80th and 20th autoantibody percentiles was the greatest. *A*: Fitted predicted probability of C-peptide detection for subjects at the 80th GADA titer percentile (dark-red dashed line) and at the 20th GADA titer percentile (light-red dashed line). *B*: Difference in predicted probability between the 80th and 20th GADA titer percentiles according to disease duration. The vertical dotted line marks the duration at which the difference in predicted probability between the 80th and 20th GADA percentiles is the greatest (2.1 years' duration). *C*: Fitted predicted probability of C-peptide detection for subjects at the 80th IA–2A titer percentile (dark-blue dashed line) and at the 20th IA–2A titer percentile (light-blue dashed line). *D*: Difference in predicted

GADA titer had the largest effect on odds of C-peptide detection at disease duration of 2.1 years (95% CI 1.27, 2.97), while longer disease durations (≥12.6 years [95% CI 6.22, 17.87]) yielded similar odds of C-peptide detection regardless of GADA titer (Fig. 2B). While IA–2A and ZnT8A titers were not individually predictive of C-peptide detection, both interacted significantly with type 1 diabetes duration to predict C-peptide detection odds. At disease durations <4 years, higher IA–2A titers were associated with a higher probability of C-peptide presence followed by a more rapid decline in the probability of C-peptide detection compared with lower levels of IA–2A (Fig. 2C). This effect was most pronounced at disease onset (duration 0 years [95% CI 0, 6.55]) (Fig. 2D). Similarly, higher ZnT8A titers were associated with a higher probability of C-peptide detection close to disease onset (i.e., <2 years' duration) followed by a more rapid decline in the probability of C-peptide detection compared with lower ZnT8A titers (Fig. 2E). As with IA–2A, the effect of ZnT8A titer on the probability of C-peptide detection was most pronounced at disease onset (duration 0 years [95% CI 0, 7.67]) (Fig. 2F).

ZnT8A was the only autoantibody that had an interactive effect with GRS: at lower GRS values, the probability of C-peptide detection declined more rapidly when ZnT8A titer was high compared with when ZnT8A titer was low (Fig. 3A). At the 20th GRS percentile, ZnT8A titer had the greatest effect on the odds of C-peptide detection at 6.6 years' duration (95% CI 0, 7.99) (Fig. 3B). In contrast, when GRS was high, the probability of detecting C-peptide declined with increased disease duration independent of ZnT8A titer (Fig. 3C). At the 80th GRS percentile, ZnT8A titer had the greatest effect on the odds of C-peptide detection at disease onset (duration 0 years [95% CI 0, 5.07]) (Fig. 3D).

The effects of GRS and age at onset on the probability of C-peptide detection varied as a function of ZnT8A titer (Fig. 4). The effect of GRS on C-peptide detection probability was more pronounced when ZnT8A titer was low, whereas GRS had almost no effect on C-peptide detection when ZnT8A titer was high (Fig. 4A). Specifically, when ZnT8A titer was at the 20th percentile, the maximum difference in C-peptide detection probability between high and low GRS was 0.26 (at 1.6 years' duration, 95% CI 0, 3.49). However, when ZnT8A titer was at the 80th percentile, the greatest difference in C-peptide detection probability between high and low GRS was only 0.014 (at 2.5 years' duration, 95% CI 1.69, 3.27). In contrast with that of GRS, the effect of age at onset on C-peptide detection probability was more pronounced when

ZnT8A titer was high and was diminished when ZnT8A titer was low (Fig. 4B). Specifically, when ZnT8A titer was at the 80th percentile, the maximum difference in C-peptide detection probability between younger (6.0 years) and older (15.7 years) onset age was 0.41 at 2.8 years' duration (95% CI 2.02, 3.64). However, when ZnT8A titer was at the 20th percentile, the greatest difference in C-peptide detection probability between younger and older onset age was only 0.022 (at 1.7 years' duration [95% CI 0, 3.57]). Overall, high ZnT8A titer was associated with a more rapid decline in the probability of C-peptide detection compared with low ZnT8A titer, and this association was modulated by age at type 1 diabetes onset (Fig. 4B and C, dashed curves). Low ZnT8A titer was associated with a more gradual decline in probability of C-peptide detection, and this association was modulated by GRS (Fig. 4A and C, solid curves).

QIC was then used for comparisons between model 1 (initial model without autoantibody titers) (Table 2) and model 2 (prediction model based on variable inclusion frequencies) (Table 3). Despite a penalty for the higher number of variables, model 2 (QIC = 334.6) was found to have a better fit versus model 1 (QIC = 359.2) (Supplementary Table 1).

Overall, the most informative factors for C-peptide detection odds in our final model were onset age, duration, and GRS. However, inclusion of GADA, IA–2A, and ZnT8A titers improved model fit compared with model 1, which only included onset age, duration, and GRS (Supplementary Table 1). Both age at diagnosis and GRS influenced the duration at which each autoantibody was most informative (i.e., the duration at which the autoantibody effect on C-peptide was >95th percentile across all duration times) for C-peptide detection odds (Fig. 5). Specifically, when onset age was at the 20th percentile (6.0 years), both GADA and IA–2A levels were most informative for C-peptide detection from disease onset to 3 years' duration, regardless of GRS (Fig. 5A). When GRS was high, ZnT8A titer was also most informative for C-peptide detection from 0 to 3 years' duration, although the magnitude of this effect was small. In contrast, when GRS was low, ZnT8A titer was most informative for C-peptide detection at 3.2–6.2 years' duration (Fig. 5A). When onset age was at the 80th percentile (15.7 years), both IA–2A and ZnT8A levels were most informative for C-peptide detection from disease onset to 3 years' duration, regardless of GRS (Fig. 5B). GRS affected the duration at which GADA had the greatest effect on C-peptide detection odds: when GRS was high, GADA was most informative at 1.5–4.5 years' duration. When GRS was low, GADA was most

probability between the 80th and 20th IA–2A titer percentiles according to disease duration. The vertical dotted line marks the duration at which the difference in predicted probability between the 80th and 20th IA–2A titer percentiles is the greatest (0 years' duration). E: Fitted predicted probability of C-peptide detection for subjects at the 80th ZnT8A titer percentile (dark-green dashed line) and at the 20th ZnT8A titer percentile (light-green dashed line). F: Difference in predicted probability between the 80th and 20th ZnT8A titer percentiles according to disease duration. The vertical dotted line marks the duration at which the difference in predicted probability between the 80th and 20th ZnT8A titer percentiles is the greatest (0 years' duration). %tile, percentile.

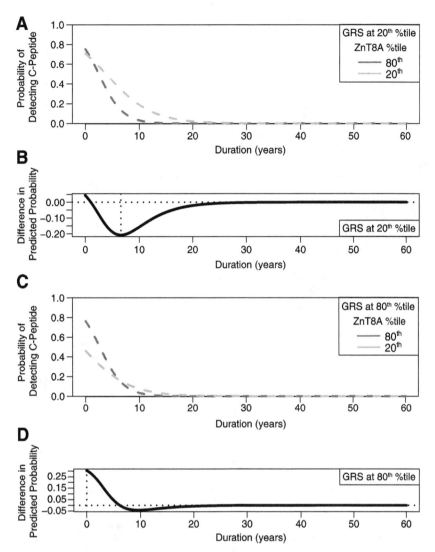

Figure 3—Interaction effect of ZnT8A titer, GRS, and type 1 diabetes duration on the probability of detecting C-peptide. For illustration of the effect of GRS on the association between ZnT8A titer and detectable C-peptide, the predicted probability of C-peptide detection was plotted with GRS set to the 20th percentile (A and B) and the 80th percentile (C and D) according to disease duration. A and C: Dashed lines show the fitted predicted probability of C-peptide detection (y-axis) at the 80th ZnT8A titer percentile (dark-green dashed line) and at the 20th ZnT8A titer percentile (light-green dashed line). B and D: Difference in predicted probability of C-peptide detection between the 80th and 20th ZnT8A titer percentiles according to disease duration. The vertical dotted line marks the duration at which the difference in predicted probability between the 80th and 20th ZnT8A titer percentiles is the greatest. A: Interaction effect between ZnT8A and type 1 diabetes duration when GRS is set to the 20th percentile. At the 20th GRS percentile, the probability of C-peptide detection declined more rapidly when ZnT8A titer was high (dark-green dashed line) compared with when ZnT8A titer was low (light-green dashed line). B: At the 20th GRS percentile, the difference in predicted probability between the 80th and 20th ZnT8A titer percentiles was the greatest at 6.6 years' duration. C: Interaction effect between ZnT8A and type 1 diabetes duration when GRS is set to the 80th percentile. At the 80th GRS percentile, the probability of C-peptide detection declined with increased disease duration, regardless of ZnT8A titer. D: At the 80th GRS percentile, the difference in predicted probability between the 80th and 20th ZnT8A titer percentiles was the greatest at disease onset (i.e., 0 years). %tile, percentile.

informative for C-peptide detection at 2.8–5.8 years' duration (Fig. 5B).

DISCUSSION

Within our cohort, the odds of detecting C-peptide following type 1 diabetes onset was best predicted by a combined model with incorporation of disease duration, age at disease onset, GRS, and titers for GADA, IA–2A, and ZnT8A. In accordance with previous studies, we found

longer disease duration and younger age at onset to be associated with lower odds of C-peptide detection in subjects with type 1 diabetes (16,31,32).

An interaction effect between GRS and disease duration was found such that higher overall genetic load for type 1 diabetes was associated with a more rapid decline in the odds of C-peptide detection. High-risk alleles from the HLA class I (A*24) and class II (DR3 and DR4) loci have been associated with younger age at onset (33), and risk

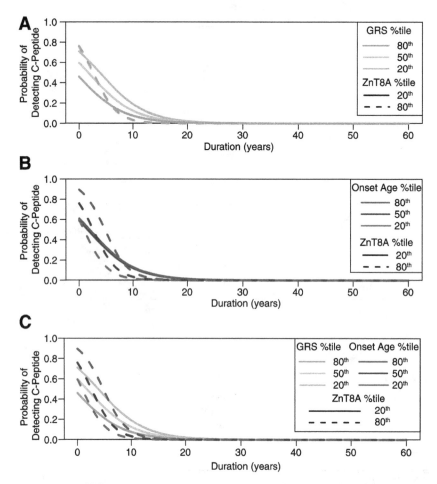

Figure 4—ZnT8A titer interacts with GRS and type 1 diabetes onset age to predict odds of C-peptide detection. *A*: The probability of C-peptide detection is plotted according to disease duration when GRS is set to the 80th (orange curves), 50th (blue curves), or 20th (green curves) percentile. Solid and dashed curves represent the probability of C-peptide detection when ZnT8A titer is at the 20th and 80th percentiles, respectively. The probability of C-peptide detection was sensitive to changes in GRS when ZnT8A titer was low (solid lines) but not when ZnT8A titer was high (dashed lines, which appear superimposed). *B*: The probability of C-peptide detection is plotted according to disease duration when onset age is set to the 80th (red curves), 50th (blue curves), or 20th (green curves) percentile. Solid and dashed curves represent the probability of C-peptide detection when ZnT8A titer is at the 20th and 80th percentiles, respectively. The probability of C-peptide detection was sensitive to changes in onset age when ZnT8A titer was high (dashed lines) but not when ZnT8A titer was low (solid lines, which appear superimposed). *C*: The probability of C-peptide detection is plotted according to disease duration with respect to ZnT8A titer, GRS, and age at disease onset. Dark dashed curves represent the probability of C-peptide detection when ZnT8A titer is high and age at onset is high (dashed dark-red curve), medium (dashed dark-blue curve), and low (dashed dark-green curve). Light solid curves represent the probability of C-peptide detection when ZnT8A titer is low and GRS is high (light-red/orange curve), medium (light-blue curve), and low (light-green curve). %tile, percentile.

conferred by these alleles comprises a large component of GRS (22). Because younger age at onset has been associated with more rapid decline in residual β-cell function (13), higher GRS was expected to also result in reduced odds of C-peptide detection through its intrinsic link with onset age. Yet, in the current study, GRS and age at onset had different effects on C-peptide detection: younger onset age resulted in a downward shift of the predicted probability curve of C-peptide detection compared with older onset age, whereas higher GRS resulted in a steeper decline in C-peptide detection odds compared with lower GRS (Fig. 1*B*). Thus, although related through high-risk HLA associations, GRS and onset age exert differing effects on the odds of C-peptide detection over time.

GADA titer was directly related to the odds of C-peptide detection, and because GADA did not have any interaction effects with other variables, it may offer unfettered utility as a biomarker. In accordance with our findings, Ziegler and Bonifacio recently addressed the observation that GAD65 autoimmunity is associated with slower progression to clinical type 1 diabetes, speculating that GADA may be reflective of β-cell–protective mechanisms (34). Longitudinal studies are required to explore whether these purported mechanisms (or the enduring effects thereof) could extend beyond clinical onset to prolong the preservation of β-cell function.

The effects of IA–2A and ZnT8A titers on C-peptide detection were dependent on their interactions with either

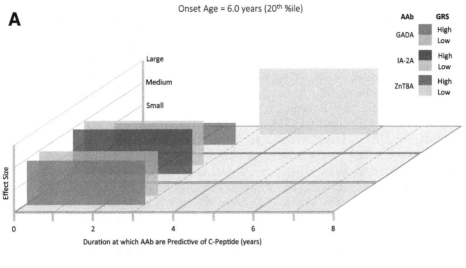

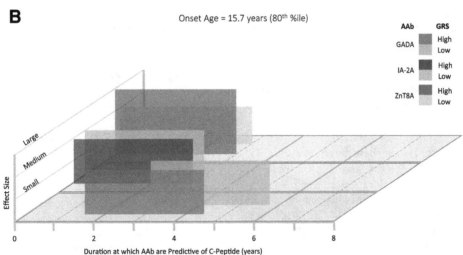

Figure 5—Duration at which autoantibodies (AAb) are most informative for C-peptide detection. Model representation illustrating the duration at which each autoantibody is most informative for C-peptide detection odds when age at disease onset is set to either the 20th percentile (6.0 years [A]) or the 80th percentile (15.7 years [B]). Boxes span the disease duration (x-axis) at which the autoantibody effect on C-peptide is >95th percentile across all duration times. The y-axis represents the effect size of each autoantibody on C-peptide detection odds. For illustration of how GRS modulates the duration at which autoantibodies are most informative in the model, each autoantibody is shown for when GRS is set to the 80th percentile and the 20th percentile. A: Duration at which GADA, IA–2A, and ZnT8A levels are informative for C-peptide detection odds when age at disease onset is set to the 20th percentile (6.0 years). At this younger onset age, GRS did not affect the duration interval at which GADA (dark- and light-red boxes) or IA–2A (dark- and light-blue boxes) were informative for C-peptide detection odds. GRS did affect the duration interval at which ZnT8A were informative for C-peptide detection odds: when GRS was high, ZnT8A titer was most informative for C-peptide detection odds from 0 to 3 years' duration (dark-green box). When GRS was low, ZnT8A titer was most informative for C-peptide detection odds at 3.2–6.2 years' duration (light-green box). B: Duration at which GADA, IA–2A, and ZnT8A levels are informative for C-peptide detection odds when age at disease onset is set to the 80th percentile (15.7 years). At this older onset age, GRS did not affect the duration interval at which IA–2A (dark- and light-blue boxes) or ZnT8A (dark- and light-green boxes) are informative for C-peptide detection odds. GRS did affect the duration interval at which GADA titer was most informative for C-peptide detection odds: when GRS was high, GADA titer was most informative at 1.5–4.5 years' duration (dark-red box). When GRS was low, GADA titer was most informative for C-peptide detection odds at 2.8–5.8 years' duration (light-red box). %tile, percentile.

disease duration (IA–2A) or disease duration, GRS, and onset age (ZnT8A). Our results suggest that, following diagnosis, subjects with low or undetectable titers of IA–2A and ZnT8A may experience a slower decline in functional β-cell mass compared with subjects with high titers and, thus, a longer period during which they could benefit from clinical interventions aimed at preserving β-cell function.

This is in agreement with previously reported findings that IA–2A and ZnT8A tend to emerge and peak closer to type 1 diabetes onset, typically following insulin autoantibodies and/or GADA seroconversion (35). Therefore, the presence of IA–2A and ZnT8A is thought to reflect a more advanced stage of disease and/or β-cell destruction. In support of this notion, Juusola et al. (36) found that among children and adolescents, ZnT8A presence at the time of diagnosis was associated with reduced C-peptide levels at 12, 18, and 24 months postonset compared with levels in ZnT8A-negative subjects.

ZnT8A was unique in that its relationship to C-peptide detection odds depended on its interaction with not only disease duration but also GRS and onset age. When ZnT8A titer was low, its effect on C-peptide detection odds was more sensitive to change in GRS and less sensitive to change in age at onset. When ZnT8A titer was high, its effect was more sensitive to change in age at onset versus GRS. Because ZnT8 was more recently identified as a type 1 diabetes autoantigen (37), fewer studies have longitudinal data on ZnT8A's association with residual β-cell function as compared with GADA and IA–2A (38,39). Notwithstanding, associations have been uncovered of ZnT8A levels, HLA alleles, and age at disease onset (36,40,41). Although these associations are supported by our model, more studies are needed to untangle the complexities of these interaction effects on residual β-cell function.

In our model, age at diagnosis and GRS influenced the effect size and duration at which the autoantibodies were most indicative of C-peptide detection, and these factors had differing effects depending on autoantibody specificity, as summarized in Fig. 5. The duration at which GADA exerted its peak effect was sensitive to changes in GRS when onset age was older (~16 years) (Fig. 5B, red). In contrast, GRS modulated the duration at which ZnT8A were most effective in the model but only when onset age was younger (~6 years) (Fig. 5A, green). IA–2A's effect was uniquely resilient to changes in onset age and GRS (Fig. 5A and B, blue). Notably, onset age and GRS influenced the magnitude of the effect of ZnT8A but not GADA or IA–2A. Hence, in terms of a clinical application, our model suggests that for individuals diagnosed with type 1 diabetes at a young age, GADA and IA–2A levels are most informative for C-peptide detection odds during the first 3 years following diagnosis, but thereafter, ZnT8A become the predominant marker, specifically among subjects with lower GRS. In older-onset subjects, IA–2A and ZnT8A levels are most informative within 3 years of diagnosis, while GADA are most informative slightly later, particularly among subjects with low GRS.

One limitation of our study is that our cohort is largely cross-sectional, and autoantibodies are known to fluctuate temporally (42). Since exogenous insulin therapy may increase autoantibody titers, insulin autoantibodies were excluded from this study. We aim to investigate the contribution of insulin autoantibodies to C-peptide detection odds in a longitudinal study that includes samples collected at diagnosis. Another caveat is the use of random serum C-peptide. Stimulated C-peptide tests, although more accurate in assessing β-cell function, are invasive, costly, and time-consuming. On the other hand, implementing fasting restrictions on patients would be difficult, and assuring compliance would not be feasible. Random C-peptide has

been shown to correlate with mixed-meal tolerance test outcomes (43) and, hence, was our most practical option. Additionally, the GRS applied here was found to be less robust for assessment of risk in non-Caucasian populations (22); thus, our analysis was restricted to subjects with genetically imputed European ancestry. Efforts to generate population-specific GRS models are underway (44), and incorporation of such GRS into our C-peptide model would theoretically allow for modeling among ethnically diverse cohorts.

Collectively, our data support a model wherein age at onset, GRS, and islet autoantibody titers can be used to project the loss of C-peptide over the course of type 1 diabetes duration. Although it requires validation in an independent longitudinal cohort, we envisage that this model, based on underlying genetic composition and minimally invasive serological markers, may be used to project C-peptide trajectory and thereby inform clinical trial inclusion criteria for a precision medicine approach.

Acknowledgments. The authors thank Ezio Bonifacio (Dresden University of Technology) for valuable feedback and constructive comments.

Funding. These studies were supported by funding from the National Institutes of Health (P01 AI042288) and JDRF (1-SRA-2019-764-A-N and 2-PDF-2016-207-A-N) and endowments from the American Diabetes Association, the McJunkin Family Charitable Foundation, and the Jeffrey Keene Family Professorship.

Duality of Interest. No potential conflicts of interest relevant to this article were reported.

Author Contributions. M.D.W. researched the data and wrote the manuscript. R.B. analyzed the data and wrote the manuscript. D.J.P., C.R.G., and K.M.M. researched the data and reviewed and edited the manuscript. A.L.P., A.M., and M.J.H. contributed to discussion and reviewed and edited the manuscript. S.C. analyzed the data and reviewed and edited the manuscript. D.A.S., T.M.B., and M.A.A. contributed to discussion and reviewed and edited the manuscript. C.H.W. conceived of the study and wrote the manuscript. C.H.W. is the guarantor of this work and, as such, had full access to all the data in the study and takes responsibility for the integrity of the data and the accuracy of the data analysis.

References

1. Insel RA, Dunne JL, Atkinson MA, et al. Staging presymptomatic type 1 diabetes: a scientific statement of JDRF, the Endocrine Society, and the American Diabetes Association. Diabetes Care 2015;38:1964–1974

2. Winkler C, Krumsiek J, Buettner F, et al. Feature ranking of type 1 diabetes susceptibility genes improves prediction of type 1 diabetes. Diabetologia 2014;57:2521–2529

3. Oram RA, Patel K, Hill A, et al. A type 1 diabetes genetic risk score can aid discrimination between type 1 and type 2 diabetes in young adults. Diabetes Care 2016;39:337–344

4. Patel KA, Oram RA, Flanagan SE, et al. Type 1 diabetes genetic risk score: a novel tool to discriminate monogenic and type 1 diabetes. Diabetes 2016;65:2094–2099

5. Redondo MJ, Geyer S, Steck AK, et al.; Type 1 Diabetes TrialNet Study Group. A type 1 diabetes genetic risk score predicts progression of islet autoimmunity and development of type 1 diabetes in individuals at risk. Diabetes Care 2018;41:1887–1894

6. Palmer JP, Fleming GA, Greenbaum CJ, et al. C-peptide is the appropriate outcome measure for type 1 diabetes clinical trials to preserve β-cell function: report of an ADA workshop, 21–22 October 2001. Diabetes 2004;53:250–264

7. Steffes MW, Sibley S, Jackson M, Thomas W. β-Cell function and the development of diabetes-related complications in the diabetes control and complications trial. Diabetes Care 2003;26:832–836

8. Oram RA, Jones AG, Besser REJ, et al. The majority of patients with long-duration type 1 diabetes are insulin microsecretors and have functioning beta cells. Diabetologia 2014;57:187–191

9. Shields BM, McDonald TJ, Oram R, et al.; TIGI Consortium. C-peptide decline in type 1 diabetes has two phases: an initial exponential fall and a subsequent stable phase. Diabetes Care 2018;41:1486–1492

10. Yu MG, Keenan HA, Shah HS, et al. Residual β cell function and monogenic variants in long-duration type 1 diabetes patients. J Clin Invest 2019;129:3252–3263

11. Wasserfall C, Nick HS, Campbell-Thompson M, et al. Persistence of pancreatic insulin mRNA expression and proinsulin protein in type 1 diabetes pancreata. Cell Metab 2017;26:568–575.e3

12. Damond N, Engler S, Zanotelli VRT, et al. A map of human type 1 diabetes progression by imaging mass cytometry. Cell Metab 2019;29:755–768.e5

13. Palmer JP. C-peptide in the natural history of type 1 diabetes. Diabetes Metab Res Rev 2009;25:325–328

14. Komulainen J, Knip M, Lounamaa R, et al.; The Childhood Diabetes in Finland Study Group. Poor beta-cell function after the clinical manifestation of type 1 diabetes in children initially positive for islet cell specific autoantibodies. Diabet Med 1997;14:532–537

15. Decochez K, Keymeulen B, Somers G, et al.; Belgian Diabetes Registry. Use of an islet cell antibody assay to identify type 1 diabetic patients with rapid decrease in C-peptide levels after clinical onset: Belgian Diabetes Registry. Diabetes Care 2000;23:1072–1078

16. Mortensen HB, Swift PGF, Holl RW, et al.; Hvidoere Study Group on Childhood Diabetes. Multinational study in children and adolescents with newly diagnosed type 1 diabetes: association of age, ketoacidosis, HLA status, and autoantibodies on residual beta-cell function and glycemic control 12 months after diagnosis. Pediatr Diabetes 2010;11:218–226

17. Wenzlau JM, Walter M, Gardner TJ, et al. Kinetics of the post-onset decline in zinc transporter 8 autoantibodies in type 1 diabetic human subjects. J Clin Endocrinol Metab 2010;95:4712–4719

18. Petrone A, Spoletini M, Zampetti S, et al.; Immunotherapy Diabetes (IMDIAB) Group. The *PTPN22* 1858T gene variant in type 1 diabetes is associated with reduced residual β-cell function and worse metabolic control. Diabetes Care 2008; 31:1214–1218

19. Fløyel T, Brorsson C, Nielsen LB, et al. CTSH regulates β-cell function and disease progression in newly diagnosed type 1 diabetes patients. Proc Natl Acad Sci U S A 2014;111:10305–10310

20. Roshandel D, Gubitosi-Klug R, Bull SB, et al.; DCCT/EDIC Research Group. Meta-genome-wide association studies identify a locus on chromosome 1 and multiple variants in the MHC region for serum C-peptide in type 1 diabetes. Diabetologia 2018;61:1098–1111

21. McKeigue PM, Spiliopoulou A, McGurnaghan S, et al. Persistent C-peptide secretion in type 1 diabetes and its relationship to the genetic architecture of diabetes. BMC Med 2019;17:165

22. Perry DJ, Wasserfall CH, Oram RA, et al. Application of a genetic risk score to racially diverse type 1 diabetes populations demonstrates the need for diversity in risk-modeling. Sci Rep 2018;8:4529

23. Wasserfall C, Montgomery E, Yu L, et al. Validation of a rapid type 1 diabetes autoantibody screening assay for community-based screening of organ donors to identify subjects at increased risk for the disease. Clin Exp Immunol 2016;185: 33–41

24. Cortes A, Brown MA. Promise and pitfalls of the ImmunoChip. Arthritis Res Ther 2011;13:101

25. Onengut-Gumuscu S, Chen WM, Burren O, et al.; Type 1 Diabetes Genetics Consortium. Fine mapping of type 1 diabetes susceptibility loci and evidence for colocalization of causal variants with lymphoid gene enhancers. Nat Genet 2015; 47:381–386

26. Das S, Forer L, Schönherr S, et al. Next-generation genotype imputation service and methods. Nat Genet 2016;48:1284–1287

27. Pan W. Akaike's information criterion in generalized estimating equations. Biometrics 2001;57:120–125

28. Yan J. geepack: yet another package for generalized estimating equations. R News 2002;2/3:12–14

29. Yan J, Fine J. Estimating equations for association structures. Stat Med 2004;23:859–874; discussion 875–877, 879–880

30. Halekoh U, Højsgaard S, Yan J. The R package geepack for generalized estimating equations. J Stat Softw 2006;15:1–11

31. Greenbaum CJ, Beam CA, Boulware D, et al.; Type 1 Diabetes TrialNet Study Group. Fall in C-peptide during first 2 years from diagnosis: evidence of at least two distinct phases from composite Type 1 Diabetes TrialNet data. Diabetes 2012; 61:2066–2073

32. Barker A, Lauria A, Schloot N, et al. Age-dependent decline of β-cell function in type 1 diabetes after diagnosis: a multi-centre longitudinal study. Diabetes Obes Metab 2014;16:262–267

33. Noble JA, Valdes AM. Genetics of the HLA region in the prediction of type 1 diabetes. Curr Diab Rep 2011;11:533–542

34. Ziegler A-G, Bonifacio E. Why is the presence of autoantibodies against GAD associated with a relatively slow progression to clinical diabetes? Diabetologia 2020;63:1665–1666

35. Ziegler A-G, Nepom GT. Prediction and pathogenesis in type 1 diabetes. Immunity 2010;32:468–478

36. Juusola M, Parkkola A, Härkönen T, et al.; Childhood Diabetes in Finland Study Group. Positivity for zinc transporter 8 autoantibodies at diagnosis is subsequently associated with reduced β-cell function and higher exogenous insulin requirement in children and adolescents with type 1 diabetes. Diabetes Care 2016;39:118–121

37. Wenzlau JM, Juhl K, Yu L, et al. The cation efflux transporter ZnT8 (Slc30A8) is a major autoantigen in human type 1 diabetes. Proc Natl Acad Sci U S A 2007; 104:17040–17045

38. Petersen JS, Dyrberg T, Karlsen AE, et al.; The Canadian-European Randomized Control Trial Group. Glutamic acid decarboxylase (GAD65) autoantibodies in prediction of beta-cell function and remission in recent-onset IDDM after cyclosporin treatment. Diabetes 1994;43:1291–1296

39. Lan MS, Wasserfall C, Maclaren NK, Notkins AL. IA-2, a transmembrane protein of the protein tyrosine phosphatase family, is a major autoantigen in insulin-dependent diabetes mellitus. Proc Natl Acad Sci U S A 1996;93:6367–6370

40. Wenzlau JM, Frisch LM, Hutton JC, Fain PR, Davidson HW. Changes in zinc transporter 8 autoantibodies following type 1 diabetes onset: the Type 1 Diabetes Genetics Consortium Autoantibody Workshop. *Diabetes Care* 2015;38(Suppl. 2): S14–S20

41. Salonen KM, Ryhänen S, Härkönen T, Ilonen J, Knip M; Finnish Pediatric Diabetes Register. Autoantibodies against zinc transporter 8 are related to age, metabolic state and HLA DR genotype in children with newly diagnosed type 1 diabetes. Diabetes Metab Res Rev 2013;29:646–654

42. Decochez K, Tits J, Coolens JL, et al. High frequency of persisting or increasing islet-specific autoantibody levels after diagnosis of type 1 diabetes presenting before 40 years of age: the Belgian Diabetes Registry. Diabetes Care 2000;23:838–844

43. Hope SV, Knight BA, Shields BM, Hattersley AT, McDonald TJ, Jones AG. Random non-fasting C-peptide: bringing robust assessment of endogenous insulin secretion to the clinic. Diabet Med 2016;33:1554–1558

44. Onengut-Gumuscu S, Chen W-M, Robertson CC, et al.; SEARCH for Diabetes in Youth; Type 1 Diabetes Genetics Consortium. Type 1 diabetes risk in African-ancestry participants and utility of an ancestry-specific genetic risk score. Diabetes Care 2019;42:406–415

The Management of Type 1 Diabetes in Adults. A Consensus Report by the American Diabetes Association (ADA) and the European Association for the Study of Diabetes (EASD)

Richard I.G. Holt,[1,2] J. Hans DeVries,[3,4] Amy Hess-Fischl,[5] Irl B. Hirsch,[6] M. Sue Kirkman,[7] Tomasz Klupa,[8] Barbara Ludwig,[9] Kirsten Nørgaard,[10,11] Jeremy Pettus,[12] Eric Renard,[13,14] Jay S. Skyler,[15] Frank J. Snoek,[16] Ruth S. Weinstock,[17] and Anne L. Peters[18]

Diabetes Care 2021;44:2589–2625 | https://doi.org/10.2337/dci21-0043

The American Diabetes Association (ADA) and the European Association for the Study of Diabetes (EASD) convened a writing group to develop a consensus statement on the management of type 1 diabetes in adults. The writing group has considered the rapid development of new treatments and technologies and addressed the following topics: diagnosis, aims of management, schedule of care, diabetes self-management education and support, glucose monitoring, insulin therapy, hypoglycemia, behavioral considerations, psychosocial care, diabetic ketoacidosis, pancreas and islet transplantation, adjunctive therapies, special populations, inpatient management, and future perspectives. Although we discuss the schedule for follow-up examinations and testing, we have not included the evaluation and treatment of the chronic microvascular and macrovascular complications of diabetes as these are well-reviewed and discussed elsewhere. The writing group was aware of both national and international guidance on type 1 diabetes and did not seek to replicate this but rather aimed to highlight the major areas that health care professionals should consider when managing adults with type 1 diabetes. Though evidence-based where possible, the recommendations in the report represent the consensus opinion of the authors.

SECTION 1: INTRODUCTION AND RATIONALE FOR THE CONSENSUS REPORT

Type 1 diabetes is a condition caused by autoimmune damage of the insulin-producing β-cells of the pancreatic islets, usually leading to severe endogenous insulin deficiency. Type 1 diabetes accounts for approximately 5–10% of all cases of diabetes. Although the incidence peaks in puberty and early adulthood, new-onset type 1 diabetes occurs in all age-groups and people with type 1 diabetes live for many decades after onset of the disease, such that the overall prevalence of type 1 diabetes is higher in adults than in children, justifying our focus on type 1 diabetes in adults (1). The global prevalence of type 1 diabetes is 5.9 per 10,000 people, while the incidence has risen rapidly over the last 50 years and is currently estimated to be 15 per 100,000 people per year (2).

[1]Human Development and Health, Faculty of Medicine, University of Southampton, Southampton, U.K.
[2]Southampton National Institute for Health Research Biomedical Research Centre, University Hospital Southampton NHS Foundation Trust, Southampton, U.K.
[3]Amsterdam UMC, Internal Medicine, University of Amsterdam, Amsterdam, the Netherlands
[4]Profil Institute for Metabolic Research, Neuss, Germany
[5]Kovler Diabetes Center, University of Chicago, Chicago, IL
[6]UW Medicine Diabetes Institute, Seattle, WA
[7]University of North Carolina School of Medicine, Chapel Hill, NC
[8]Department of Metabolic Diseases, Center for Advanced Technologies in Diabetes, Jagiellonian University Medical College, Kraków, Poland
[9]University Hospital Carl Gustav Carus, Technische Universität Dresden, Dresden, Germany
[10]Steno Diabetes Center Copenhagen, Gentofte, Denmark
[11]University of Copenhagen, Copenhagen, Denmark
[12]University of California, San Diego, CA
[13]Montpellier University Hospital, Montpellier, France
[14]Institute of Functional Genomics, University of Montpellier, CNRS, Inserm, Montpellier, France
[15]University of Miami Miller School of Medicine, Miami, FL
[16]Amsterdam UMC, Medical Psychology, Vrije Universiteit, Amsterdam, the Netherlands
[17]SUNY Upstate Medical University, Syracuse, NY
[18]Keck School of Medicine of USC, Los Angeles, CA

Corresponding author: Richard I.G. Holt, righ@soton.ac.uk

Received 25 August 2021 and accepted 25 August 2021.

Prior to the discovery of insulin a century ago, type 1 diabetes was associated with a life expectancy as short as a few months. Beginning in 1922, relatively crude extracts of exogenous insulin, derived from animal pancreases, were used to treat people with type 1 diabetes. Over the ensuing decades, insulin concentrations were standardized, insulin solutions became more pure, resulting in reduced immunogenicity, and additives, such as zinc and protamine, were incorporated into insulin solutions to increase the duration of action. In the 1980s, semisynthetic and recombinant human insulins were developed, and in the mid 1990s, insulin analogs became available. Basal insulin analogs were designed with prolonged duration of action and reduced pharmacodynamic variability compared with protamine-based (NPH) human insulin, while rapid-acting analogs were introduced with quicker onset and shorter duration than short-acting ("regular") human insulin, resulting in reduced early postprandial hyperglycemia and less later hypoglycemia several hours after the meal (3).

The discovery of insulin transformed the lives of many people, but it soon became apparent that type 1 diabetes is associated with the development of long-term complications and shortened life expectancy. Over the last 100 years, developments in insulin, its delivery, and technologies to measure glycemic indices have markedly changed the management of type 1 diabetes. Despite these advances, many people with type 1 diabetes do not reach the glycemic targets necessary to prevent or slow the progression of diabetes complications, which continue to exert a high clinical and emotional burden.

Recognizing the ongoing challenge of type 1 diabetes and the rapid development of new treatments and technologies, the European Association for the Study of Diabetes (EASD) and the American Diabetes Association (ADA) convened a writing group to develop a consensus report on the management of type 1 diabetes in adults, aged 18 years and over. The writing group was aware of both national and international guidance on type 1 diabetes and did not seek to replicate this, but rather aimed to highlight the major areas of care that health care professionals should consider when managing adults with type 1 diabetes. The consensus report has focused predominantly on current and future glycemic management strategies and metabolic emergencies. Recent advances in the diagnosis of type 1 diabetes have been considered. Unlike many other chronic conditions, type 1 diabetes places a unique burden of management on the individual with the condition. In addition to complex medication regimens, other behavioral modification is also needed; all of this requires considerable knowledge and skill to navigate between hyper- and hypoglycemia. The importance of diabetes self-management education and support (DSMES) and psychosocial care are rightly documented in the report. While acknowledging the major significance and cost of screening, diagnosing, and managing the chronic microvascular and macrovascular complications of diabetes, a detailed description of the management of these complications is beyond the scope of this report.

Two members of the writing group, one from the ADA and one from the EASD, were assigned to be the primary authors of each section. The chosen individuals had specific knowledge of the area and were tasked with reviewing and summarizing the available literature. Each section, in turn, was reviewed and approved by the entire writing group. The draft consensus report was peer reviewed (see the Acknowledgments section) and suggestions were incorporated as deemed appropriate by the authors. The revised draft report was presented at the virtual ADA Scientific Sessions in 2021, after which public comments were invited. The report was further revised in light of this consultation. Large areas of clinical practice in type 1 diabetes are based on expert opinion and cohort studies rather than RCTs and so the writing group considered both observational and clinical trial findings, rather than relying solely on unbiased RCTs and meta-analyses. The report represents the consensus opinion of the authors, given that the available evidence is incomplete.

SECTION 2: DIAGNOSIS OF TYPE 1 DIABETES

Adults with new-onset type 1 diabetes can present with a short duration of illness of 1–4 weeks or a more slowly evolving process that can be mistaken for type 2 diabetes. Several other types of diabetes, for example monogenic diabetes, can be misdiagnosed as type 1 diabetes. In older adults, pancreatic cancer may present with diabetes and weight loss. A new and emerging issue is the development of profound insulin deficiency associated with the use of immune check-point inhibitors, which may present with hyperglycemia and diabetic ketoacidosis (DKA) (4).

Most of the available data discussed below are derived from White European populations and may not be representative of other ethnic groups. The clinical presentation may differ, but the classical triad of thirst and polydipsia, polyuria, and weight loss are common symptoms of type 1 diabetes. Accurate classification of the type of diabetes has implications beyond the use of insulin treatment; education, insulin regimen, use of

---

This Consensus Report is jointly published in Diabetologia, *published by Springer-Verlag, GmbH, on behalf of the European Association for the Study of Diabetes, https://doi.org/10.1007/s00125-021-05568-3; and* Diabetes Care, *published by the American Diabetes Association, https://doi.org/10.2337/dci21-0043.*

A consensus report of a particular topic contains a comprehensive examination and is authored by an expert panel (i.e., consensus panel) and represents the panel's collective analysis, evaluation, and opinion. The need for a consensus report arises when clinicians, scientists, regulators, and/or policy makers desire guidance and/or clarity on a medical or scientific issue related to diabetes for which the evidence is contradictory, emerging, or incomplete. Consensus reports may also highlight gaps in evidence and propose areas of future research to address these gaps. A consensus report is not an American Diabetes Association (ADA) position but represents expert opinion only and is produced under the auspices of the ADA by invited experts. A consensus report may be developed after an ADA Clinical Conference or Research Symposium.

adjuvant therapies, access to newer technologies, need for psychosocial support to address the profound psychological impact of the diagnosis of diabetes, and concurrent disease screening may all depend on the diagnosis an individual receives. Furthermore, accurate diagnosis allows an assessment of the risk of diabetes in first-degree relatives and appropriate counseling. Although profound insulin deficiency is the hallmark of type 1 diabetes, some adults with type 1 diabetes maintain some insulin secretion for years after diagnosis and may not require insulin treatment at diagnosis (5), leading to diagnostic uncertainty about the type of diabetes and its management.

Differentiating Type 1 Diabetes From Type 2 Diabetes

Identifying whether an adult with newly diagnosed diabetes has type 1 diabetes may be challenging where the individual has features pointing toward both type 1 diabetes and type 2 diabetes, such as an older adult with a low or normal BMI or young adult with an elevated BMI. Ketoacidosis, once considered pathognomonic of type 1 diabetes, may occur in ketosis-prone type 2 diabetes. Misclassification of type 1 diabetes in adults is common, and over 40% of those developing type 1 diabetes after age 30 years are initially treated as having type 2 diabetes (6–8). From a patient perspective, a misdiagnosis of type 2 diabetes can cause confusion and misunderstanding, especially for those with type 1 diabetes who have overweight or obesity. This can impair the acceptance of the diagnosis and future management plans. No single clinical feature confirms type 1 diabetes in isolation (9,10). The most discriminative feature is younger age at diagnosis (<35 years), with lower BMI (<25 kg/m^2), unintentional weight loss, ketoacidosis, and glucose >20 mmol/L (>360 mg/dL) at presentation also being informative. Other features classically associated with type 1 diabetes, such as ketosis without acidosis, osmotic symptoms, family history, or a history of autoimmune diseases are weak discriminators (8–10).

The very strong relationship between type 2 diabetes incidence and age means that even "classical" features of type 1 diabetes may have a limited predictive value in older adults, as type 2 diabetes in this age-group is so common (11). The majority of older adults with

low BMI will have type 2 diabetes (9,12,13), even more so when a person's ethnicity is associated with high type 2 diabetes risk (14). Rapid progression to insulin treatment (<3 years) is strongly suggestive of type 1 diabetes at any age (6,8,15). The diagnosis of type 1 diabetes can be more difficult in adults who progress to insulin therapy more slowly. Controversy remains as to whether latent autoimmune diabetes of adulthood (LADA) is a discrete subtype, a milder form of type 1 diabetes, or a mixture of some individuals with type 1 diabetes and others with type 2 diabetes (16,17).

Differentiating Type 1 Diabetes From Monogenic Diabetes

Monogenic diabetes is found in approximately 4% of those diagnosed with diabetes before the age of 30 years; the likelihood of monogenic diabetes rises to 20% where islet antibodies are negative and C-peptide secretion is maintained (18). Monogenic diabetes is commonly mistaken for type 1 diabetes because of the young age at onset. A diagnosis of monogenic diabetes allows specific treatment with discontinuation of insulin in many cases and has implications for family members and screening for concurrent conditions (19,20).

Investigation of an Adult With Suspected Type 1 Diabetes

An algorithm for the investigation of adults with suspected type 1 diabetes is shown in Fig. 1.

Islet Autoantibodies

An assessment of islet autoantibodies at diagnosis is recommended as the primary investigation of an adult with suspected type 1 diabetes. GAD should be the primary antibody measured and, if negative, should be followed by islet tyrosine phosphatase 2 (IA2) and/or zinc transporter 8 (ZNT8) where these tests are available. Islet cell antibody (ICA) measurement is no longer recommended because it is an imprecise biological assay that has been superseded by the direct measurement of single antibodies (21,22).

In people with clinical features suggesting type 1 diabetes, the presence of one or more positive islet autoantibodies is highly predictive of rapid progression and severe insulin deficiency and

these individuals should be considered to have type 1 diabetes, even if they did not require insulin at diagnosis (23,24). As positive GAD antibodies may be found at a low level in adults without autoimmune diabetes and false positive results may occur, GAD should only be measured in those suspected to have type 1 diabetes (24).

The absence of autoantibodies does not exclude type 1 diabetes, since approximately 5–10% of White European people with new-onset type 1 diabetes have negative islet antibodies (8,9,25), and further consideration of the diagnosis is necessary. Furthermore, antibodies may disappear over time (26). In those diagnosed below the age of 35 years, type 1 diabetes is still the most likely diagnosis, particularly if there are no clinical features of type 2 diabetes or monogenic diabetes. In those aged over 35 years, type 2 diabetes becomes increasingly likely with absent islet autoantibodies and older age. However, it can be hard to differentiate between type 1 diabetes and type 2 diabetes based on age and clinical features in non-White European populations.

It is important to make a clinical decision about how to treat the person with diabetes. Regardless of any features of type 2 diabetes or absence of islet antibodies, if there is a clinical suspicion of type 1 diabetes, the individual should be treated with insulin. However, in some individuals, where the clinical course is more suggestive of type 2 diabetes, a trial of noninsulin therapy may be appropriate. Those whose diabetes is treated without insulin will require careful monitoring and education so that insulin can be rapidly initiated in the event of glycemic deterioration. Type 2 diabetes and other types of diabetes should be considered in all age-groups, but in those aged under 35 years, negative islet antibodies should raise the suspicion of monogenic diabetes.

C-Peptide Measurement

Beyond 3 years after diagnosis where there is uncertainty about diabetes type, a random C-peptide measurement (with concurrent glucose) within 5 h of eating is recommended. Where a person is treated with insulin, this test should always be performed prior to insulin discontinuation to exclude severe insulin deficiency.

Flow chart for investigation of suspected type 1 diabetes in newly diagnosed adults, based on data from White European populations

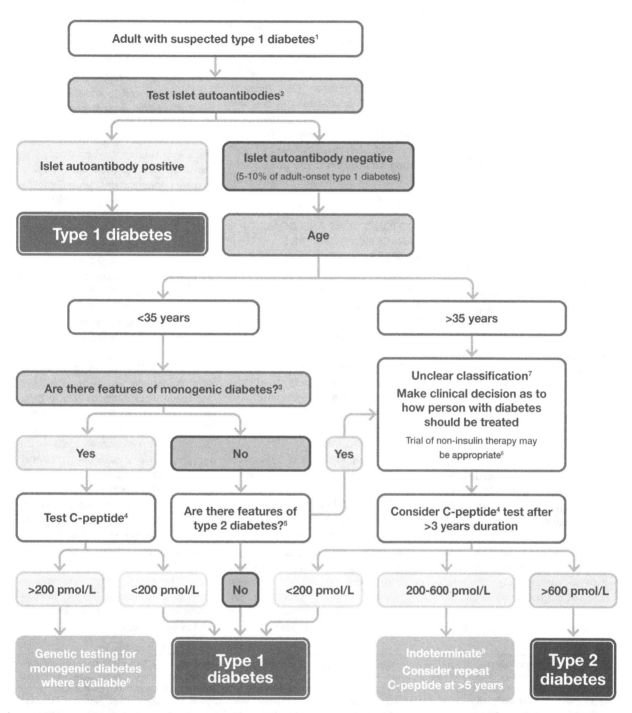

Figure 1—Flowchart for investigation of suspected type 1 diabetes in newly diagnosed adults, based on data from White European populations. [1]No single clinical feature confirms type 1 diabetes in isolation. The most discriminative feature is younger age at diagnosis (<35 years), with lower BMI (<25 kg/m^2), unintentional weight loss, ketoacidosis, and glucose >20 mmol/L (>360 mg/dL) at presentation also being informative. Other features classically associated with type 1 diabetes, such as ketosis without acidosis, osmotic symptoms, family history, or a history of autoimmune diseases are weak discriminators. [2]GAD should be the primary antibody measured and, if negative, should be followed by islet tyrosine phosphatase 2 (IA2) and/or zinc transporter 8 (ZNT8) where these tests are available. In those diagnosed below the age of 35 years who have no clinical features of type 2 diabetes or monogenic diabetes, a negative result does not change the diagnosis of type 1 diabetes since 5–10% of people with type 1 diabetes do not have antibodies. [3]Monogenic diabetes is suggested by the presence of one or more of the following features: HbA$_{1c}$ <58 mmol/mol (7.5%) at diagnosis, one parent with diabetes, features of specific monogenic cause (e.g., renal cysts, partial lipodystrophy, maternally inherited deafness, severe insulin resistance in the absence of obesity), and monogenic diabetes prediction model

Persistent C-peptide >600 pmol/L (non-fasting) is strongly suggestive of type 2 diabetes, and people with C-peptide in this range are often able to replace insulin with other agents (27–30). Routine C-peptide testing in those with clinically diagnosed type 1 diabetes of at least 3 years duration has led to reclassification in 11% of those with adult-onset diabetes (31). By contrast, low or absent C-peptide confirms the diagnosis of type 1 diabetes. Although low C-peptide concentrations may occur in some types of secondary diabetes and very long-standing type 2 diabetes, these situations are unlikely to be confused for type 1 diabetes; however, in some cases, investigation of other types of diabetes may be appropriate.

Plasma C-peptide is the recommended test where available, with modestly higher performance than urine measurement. The latter may be confounded by impaired renal function. If urinary C-peptide:creatinine ratio is used, a value <0.2 nmol/mol can be used to define severe insulin deficiency.

Genetic Testing

As monogenic diabetes was less likely to have been considered in the past, molecular genetic testing for neonatal diabetes should be considered for all people with type 1 diabetes, regardless of current age, who were diagnosed under 6 months of age as more than 80% have monogenic neonatal diabetes, and the 30–50% with ATP-sensitive potassium (K_{ATP}) channel mutations can replace insulin with sulfonylureas (32,33).

Monogenic diabetes should be considered in those with one or more of the following features: age at diagnosis of less than 35 years, HbA_{1c} <58 mmol/mol (7.5%) at diagnosis, one parent with diabetes, and features of specific monogenic cause (e.g., renal cysts, partial lipodystrophy, maternally inherited deafness, severe insulin resistance in the absence of obesity) (34). A monogenic diabetes prediction model risk calculator (www.diabetesgenes.org/mody-probability-calculator; accessed 20 August 2021) may also be used to identify which individuals diagnosed between 6 months and 35 years are at increased risk of monogenic diabetes (35). Those at increased risk should have islet autoantibody and C-peptide testing. Molecular genetic testing should only be considered if the antibodies are negative and nonfasting C-peptide is >200 pmol/L (36–38). Molecular genetic testing is not universally available.

SECTION 3: AIMS AND GOALS OF MANAGEMENT OF TYPE 1 DIABETES

The aim of diabetes care and management is to support people with type 1 diabetes to live a long and healthy life. The management strategies to achieve this aim broadly include:

- Effectively delivering exogenous insulin to maintain glucose levels as close to the individual's target range as is safely possible to prevent the development and progression of diabetes complications while:
  ○ Minimizing episodes of hypoglycemia, of all levels, including level 1 (<3.9 to ≥3.0 mmol/L [<70 to ≥54 mg/dL]) but, in particular, level 2 (<3.0 mmol/L [<54 mg/dL]) and level 3 (severe event characterized by altered mental and/or physical functioning that requires assistance from another person for recovery) hypoglycemia, and preventing episodes of DKA, while treating these appropriately should they occur.

- Effectively managing cardiovascular risk factors.
- Providing approaches, treatments, and devices that minimize the psychosocial burden of living with type 1 diabetes and, consequently, diabetes-related distress, while promoting psychological well-being.

Management strategies should adapt to new therapies and technologies as they become available, according to the wishes and desires of the person with diabetes.

The importance of glycemic management was demonstrated convincingly by the DCCT (39) and the Epidemiology of Diabetes Interventions and Complications (EDIC) follow-up study (40). With the use of intensive insulin therapy that aimed to achieve blood glucose levels close to the nondiabetes range, HbA_{1c} was lowered by ~2% (22 mmol/mol) to a mean HbA_{1c} of ~7.0% (53 mmol/mol) over a mean of 6.5 years, compared with standard care (mean HbA_{1c} ~9.0% [75 mmol/mol]) (39). The risk of primary development of retinopathy was reduced by 75%, and progression of retinopathy slowed by 54%. The development of microalbuminuria was reduced by 39% and clinical neuropathy by 60% in those assigned to intensive therapy. These benefits persisted beyond the end of the trial despite equivalent glucose levels in the two groups (HbA_{1c} ~8% [64 mmol/mol]) in the posttrial period; furthermore, reductions in incident cardiovascular disease and mortality in the intensively treated group emerged with time (40). This seminal study has been the basis for glycemic target recommendations for type 1 diabetes worldwide. The cost of intensive management was, however, a 2–3-fold increase in the rates of severe hypoglycemia, as well as weight gain.

probability >5% (www.diabetesgenes.org/exeter-diabetes-app/ModyCalculator; accessed 20 August 2021). [4]A C-peptide test is only indicated in people receiving insulin treatment. A random sample (with concurrent glucose) within 5 h of eating can replace a formal C-peptide stimulation test in the context of classification. If the result is ≥600 pmol/L, the circumstances of testing do not matter. If the result is <600 pmol/L and the concurrent glucose is <4 mmol/L (<72 mg/dL) or the person may have been fasting, consider repeating the test. Results showing very low levels (<80 pmol/L) do not need to be repeated. Where a person is insulin-treated, C-peptide must be measured prior to insulin discontinuation to exclude severe insulin deficiency. Do not test C-peptide within 2 weeks of a hyperglycemic emergency. [5]Features of type 2 diabetes include increased BMI (≥25 kg/m^2), absence of weight loss, absence of ketoacidosis, and less marked hyperglycemia. Less discriminatory features include non-White ethnicity, family history, longer duration and milder severity of symptoms prior to presentation, features of the metabolic syndrome, and absence of a family history of autoimmunity. [6]If genetic testing does not confirm monogenic diabetes, the classification is unclear and a clinical decision should be made about treatment. [7]Type 2 diabetes should be strongly considered in older individuals. In some cases, investigation for pancreatic or other types of diabetes may be appropriate. [8]A person with possible type 1 diabetes who is not treated with insulin will require careful monitoring and education so that insulin can be rapidly initiated in the event of glycemic deterioration. [9]C-peptide values 200–600 pmol/L are usually consistent with type 1 diabetes or maturity-onset diabetes of the young (MODY) but may occur in insulin-treated type 2 diabetes, particularly in people with normal or low BMI or after long duration.

The main results of the DCCT were published in 1993, before any of the current insulin analogs and diabetes technologies, except for insulin pumps, were available. Increasingly, achieving and maintaining glucose levels in the target range have become possible with fewer episodes of hypoglycemia (41–44). Although the evidence of HbA_{1c} reduction remains the most robust measure associated with chronic diabetes complications and is the only measure that is prospectively validated, more recent studies have begun to examine the relationship between time that glucose is within the target range and long-term complications and have provided the basis for glycemic targets with newer glucose monitoring technologies (45,46).

The glycemic target should be individualized considering factors that include duration of diabetes, age and life expectancy, comorbid conditions, known cardiovascular disease or advanced microvascular complications, impaired awareness of hypoglycemia (IAH), and other individual considerations, and it may change over time. Goals should be

achieved in conjunction with an understanding of the person's psychosocial needs and a reduction in diabetes distress if elevated. An HbA_{1c} goal for most adults of <53 mmol/mol (<7.0%) without significant hypoglycemia is appropriate. Following discussion between the person with diabetes and their health care team, achievement of lower HbA_{1c} levels than the goal of 53 mmol/mol (7%) may be acceptable, and even beneficial, if these can be achieved safely without adverse effects of treatment. Less-stringent HbA_{1c} goals (such as <64 mmol/mol [<8.0%]) may be appropriate for individuals with limited life expectancy or where the harms of treatment are greater than the benefits. It should be recognized that any reduction in HbA_{1c} from high initial levels has significant benefit even if the "goal" is not reached.

Capillary blood glucose monitoring (BGM) can help people with type 1 diabetes achieve these HbA_{1c} goals. A preprandial capillary plasma glucose target of 4.4–7.2 mmol/L (80–130 mg/dL) is appropriate for many people. Postprandial glucose may be targeted if HbA_{1c} goals are

not met despite reaching preprandial glucose targets. Postprandial glucose measurements should be made 1–2 h after the beginning of the meal, which generally corresponds to peak levels in people with diabetes. A peak postprandial capillary plasma glucose of <10.0 mmol/L (<180 mg/dL) is appropriate for most people with diabetes, although an ideal target for normoglycemia is <7.8 mmol/L (<140 mg/dL). Higher goals in those with limited life expectancy or where the harms of treatment are greater than the benefits are recommended (Table 1).

Further measurements that complement HbA_{1c} and BGM are assessments of the glucose management indicator (GMI) and time in range (TIR) from continuous glucose monitoring (CGM) data. GMI is calculated based on the average sensor glucose over the last 14 days and provides an approximation of a laboratory-measured HbA_{1c} in some individuals, but it may be higher or lower than actual HbA_{1c} in others (45). GMI and TIR may be more useful than HbA_{1c} for clinical management because they reflect more recent blood glucose levels and provide more detailed clinical information. A typical GMI goal is <53 mmol/mol (<7.0%). TIR is often taken as 3.9–10 mmol/L (70–180 mg/dL) for most adults and time below range (TBR) as below 3.9 mmol/L (70 mg/dL) (risk alert level), as well as less than 3.0 mmol/L (54 mg/dL) (clinically significant). Other metrics are also defined (Fig. 2). TIR is associated with microvascular complications (45,46), and a TIR of 70% roughly corresponds to an HbA_{1c} of 53 mmol/mol (7.0%). An international consensus conference reported that for most adults with type 1 diabetes, a target TIR should be above 70%, with TBR less than 4% and less than 1% for clinically significant hypoglycemia. The primary target for older people with a long duration of diabetes should be TBR less than 1% (47).

The cornerstone of type 1 diabetes therapy is insulin replacement. This is challenging because insulin demands vary widely according to meals, exercise, and many other factors. Furthermore, the insulin doses needed to prevent hyperglycemia are associated with a high risk of hypoglycemia, leaving people with type 1 diabetes walking a tightrope between high and low glucose levels. Insulin management must be supported by adequate monitoring of glucose and education and

Table 1—Glycemic targets for most adults with type 1 diabetes

Variable	Target value
HbA_{1c}	<53 mmol/mol (<7.0%)
GMI	<53 mmol/mol (<7.0%)
Preprandial glucose	4.4–7.2 mmol/L (80–130 mg/dL)
1–2 h postprandial glucose[a]	<10.0 mmol/L (<180 mg/dL)
TIR	>70%
TBR	
Readings and time <3.9 mmol/L (<70 mg/dL; level 1 and level 2 hypoglycemia)[b]	<4%
Readings and time <3.0 mmol/L (<54 mg/dL; level 2 hypoglycemia)[b]	<1%
Time above range	
Readings and time >10.0 mmol/L (>180 mg/dL; level 1 and level 2 hyperglycemia)[c]	<25%
Readings and time >13.9 mmol/L (>250 mg/dL; level 2 hyperglycemia)[c]	<5%
Glycemic variability (%CV)[d]	≤36%

All glycemic targets should be individualized and agreed with the person with diabetes. Lower or higher targets may be appropriate according to individual characteristics. [a]A postprandial glucose target of <7.8 mmol/L (<140 mg/dL) may be recommended if this can be achieved safely. Higher targets in those with limited life expectancy or where the harms of treatment are greater than the benefits are recommended. In some individuals at notably higher risk for level 3 hypoglycemia, it may be necessary to increase the glucose target range to decrease the TBR. [b]Level 1 hypoglycemia is defined as blood glucose levels <3.9 to ≥3.0 mmol/L (<70 to ≥54 mg/dL); level 2 hypoglycemia is defined as blood glucose levels <3.0 mmol/L (<54 mg/dL). [c]Level 1 hyperglycemia is defined as blood glucose levels >10.0 to ≤13.9 mmol/L (>180 to ≤250 mg/dL); level 2 hyperglycemia is defined as blood glucose levels >13.9 mmol/L (>250 mg/dL). [d]Some studies suggest that lower %CV targets (<33%) provide additional protection against hypoglycemia. GMI, glucose management indicator.

AGP Report: Continuous Glucose Monitoring

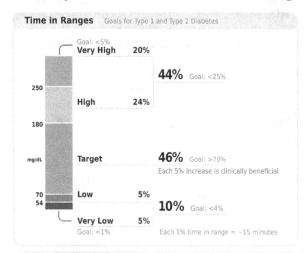

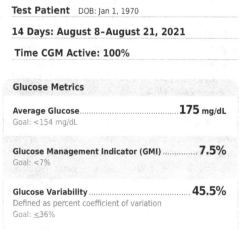

Time in Ranges Goals for Type 1 and Type 2 Diabetes

- Goal: <5% **Very High** 20%
- **44%** Goal: <25%
- **High** 24%
- **Target** **46%** Goal: >70%
  Each 5% increase is clinically beneficial
- **Low** 5%
- **10%** Goal: <4%
- **Very Low** 5%
  Goal: <1% Each 1% time in range = ~15 minutes

Test Patient DOB: Jan 1, 1970

14 Days: August 8–August 21, 2021

Time CGM Active: 100%

Glucose Metrics

Average Glucose..**175** mg/dL
Goal: <154 mg/dL

Glucose Management Indicator (GMI)..............**7.5%**
Goal: <7%

Glucose Variability...**45.5%**
Defined as percent coefficient of variation
Goal: ≤36%

Ambulatory Glucose Profile (AGP)

AGP is a summary of glucose values from the report period, with median (50%) and other percentiles shown as if they occurred in a single day.

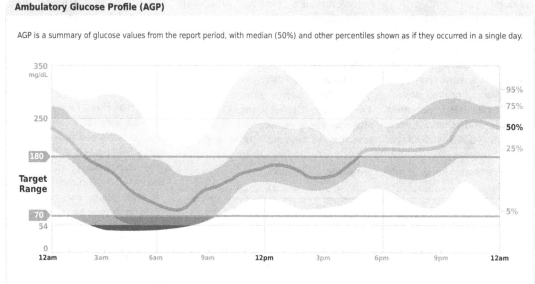

Daily Glucose Profiles

Each daily profile represents a midnight-to-midnight period.

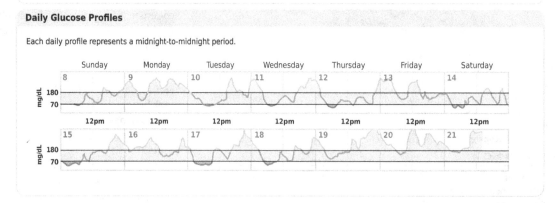

Figure 2—CGM visualization in an ambulatory glucose profile (AGP) report. Figure courtesy of R.M. Bergenstal and the International Diabetes Center, Minneapolis, MN. To convert glucose values to mmol/L, values in mg/dL should be divided by 18. DOB, date of birth.

training to allow the individual with type 1 diabetes to make the most of their treatment regimen.

The prevention of long-term complications of diabetes, particularly cardiovascular disease, extends beyond glycemic management to include the optimal management of blood pressure and use of lipid-lowering medication. There is an absence of high-quality data to guide blood pressure targets in type 1 diabetes, but RCTs in other populations have demonstrated that treatment of hypertension to a blood pressure <140/90 mmHg reduces cardiovascular events and microvascular complications. Blood pressure targets should be individualized, but a target of <140/90 mmHg is appropriate

Schematic for management of new-onset type 1 diabetes in an adult

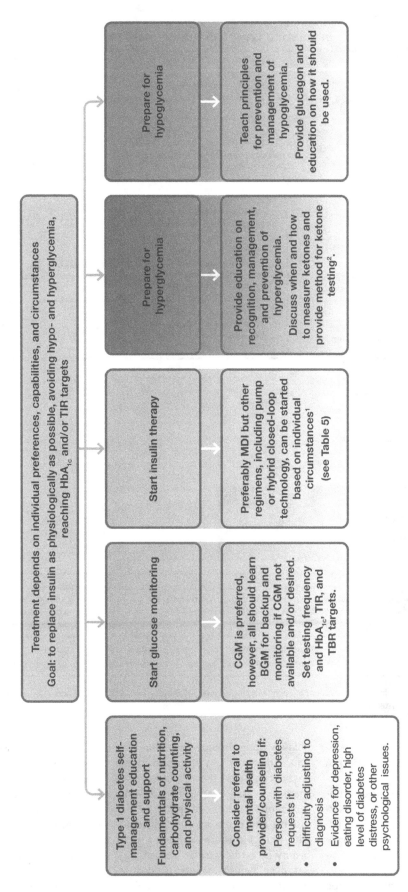

Figure 3—A framework for initial assessment and treatment of an individual with newly diagnosed type 1 diabetes. In most people, frequent follow-up until the diabetes is stabilized is needed. [1]People can switch back and forth between MDI and pump or hybrid closed-loop therapy based on preference and circumstances; however, all people must be prepared to use injected insulin therapy if pump or hybrid closed-loop systems fail or are not available. [2]The availability of blood and urine ketone measurement varies across health care systems.

General principles for management of blood glucose in existing type 1 diabetes in an adult

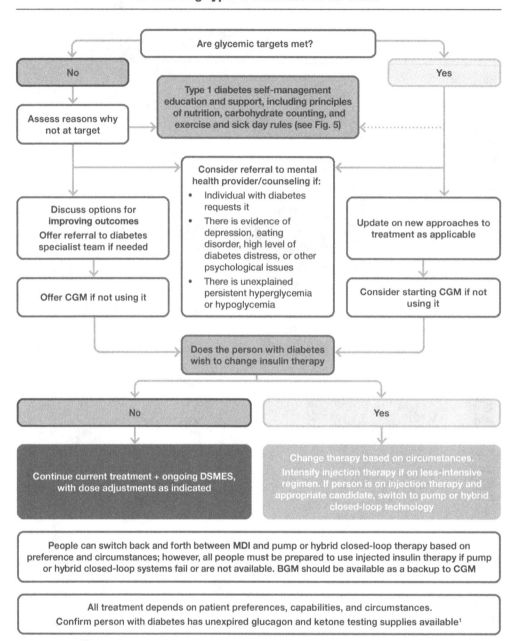

Fig. 4—A framework for the follow-up treatment of an individual with type 1 diabetes. [1]The availability of blood and urine ketone measurement varies across health care systems.

for those with a lower risk for cardiovascular disease (10-year risk of <15%). A lower target of <130/80 mmHg is recommended for those at higher cardiovascular disease risk or with evidence of microvascular complications, particularly renal disease. ACE inhibitors or angiotensin receptor blockers are recommended first-line therapies.

Similar to the situation for blood pressure, there is a paucity of trials of lipid-lowering therapy in people with type 1 diabetes, but an observational study reported that lipid-lowering therapy is associated with a 22–44% reduction in the risk of cardiovascular disease and death among individuals with type 1 diabetes without a prior history of cardiovascular disease (48). Based on type 2 diabetes guidelines, moderate-intensity statins should be considered for people aged over 40 years, and in those aged between 20–39 years with additional atherosclerotic cardiovascular disease risk factors or when the 10-year cardiovascular risk estimated by one of the risk calculators suitable for people with type 1 diabetes exceeds 10% (49–51). Additional agents, such as ezetimibe or proprotein convertase subtilisin/ kexin type 9 (PCSK9) inhibitors, may be needed.

Table 2—Schedule of care

Component of care	Details of evaluation
Medical and family history	
Diabetes history	Date of diagnosis
	Presentation at onset
	Islet autoantibodies (date)
	C-peptide (date)
	Episodes of DKA or level 3 hypoglycemia
	Hypoglycemia awareness
Family history	Type 1 diabetes or type 2 diabetes in first-degree relatives
	Other autoimmune disorders
Personal history of chronic complications	Microvascular: retinopathy, macular edema, laser/injection therapy, date of last retinal evaluation (exam or photos); peripheral neuropathy, autonomic neuropathy; nephropathy
	Macrovascular: heart, cerebrovascular and peripheral arterial disease
	Foot ulcers or amputations
Personal history of common comorbidities	Autoimmune disorders: thyroid, celiac, others[a]
	Hypertension
	Lipid disorder
	Overweight and obesity
	Eating disorders
	Hearing loss
	Sleep disorder
	Dermopathy
	Fractures
	Joint and soft tissue disorders: cheiroarthropathy, trigger finger, capsulitis, carpal tunnel syndrome
	Dental and gum health
Other	Pregnancy and contraception history
	Immunization history
Additional behavioral factors	Diet and nutrition: use of carbohydrate counting, weight history
	Physical activity
	Smoking, alcohol, substance use
	Sleep
Diabetes management	
Current insulin regimen	MDI: pens, including connected insulin pens; syringes; needles
	Insulin pump (type/model): settings; backup injection plan
BGM	Type of meter/strips
	Frequency of use
	Mean (SD), range
	Pattern
CGM	Type/model
	Data sharing; if yes, with whom
	Glucometrics
	Pattern
Other	Other diabetes medications
	Glucagon prescribed
	Ketone testing supplies prescribed (where available)
	Software/app use
Psychosocial issues	Monitor psychological well-being: diabetes-specific distress; depressive symptoms; anxiety symptoms
	Consider, also, the potential presence of fear of hypoglycemia and disordered eating
	Screen for social determinants of health and social support
	Assess cognitive status
DSMES	Assess and plan for meeting individual needs
	Consider contraception and pregnancy planning
Physical examination	Height
	Weight, BMI: every visit
	Blood pressure and pulse: at least once a year
	Skin including injection/infusion sites: every visit if skin complaints or erratic glucose readings, otherwise annual
	Cardiovascular: annual; more often if previous abnormality or symptoms
	Feet: every visit if peripheral vascular disease, neuropathy, foot complaints, or history of foot ulcer, otherwise annual

Continued on p. 2599

Table 2—Continued

Component of care	Details of evaluation
Laboratory testing	HbA_{1c} every 3–12 months Creatinine: annual; may be more often if kidney disease Urine albumin/creatinine ratio: annual Lipid panel: frequency dependent on the presence of previous lipid abnormality or treatment ALT and AST: at least once and as indicated clinically Serum potassium: if taking ACE-I, ARB, or diuretic TSH, vitamin B_{12}, vitamin D, celiac screen: at least once and as indicated clinically[a]
Goals setting	Individualized, attainable, realistic: behavioral considerations (diet and nutrition, activity, smoking cessation) Glycemic: HbA_{1c}, TIR, hypoglycemia
Treatment plan	Formulate treatment plan with shared decision-making
Referrals	As needed: podiatry, cardiology, nephrology, ophthalmology, vascular surgery, gynecology, others

[a]Individuals with type 1 diabetes are also at increased risk for the development of other autoimmune diseases, including autoimmune thyroid disorders, pernicious anemia, celiac disease, collagen vascular diseases, and Addison disease (291,292). The optimal frequency of screening for these conditions in adults has not been established. ACE-I, ACE inhibitor; ALT, alanine aminotransferase; ARB, angiotensin II receptor blocker; AST, aspartate aminotransferase; TSH, thyroid stimulating hormone.

Antiplatelet agents, such as aspirin, should be considered for all people with type 1 diabetes and existing cardiovascular disease. Antiplatelet agents may be indicated for primary prevention, but the benefit should be balanced with the increased risk of gastrointestinal bleeding.

In asymptomatic people with type 1 diabetes, routine screening for coronary artery disease is not recommended as it does not improve outcomes as long as atherosclerotic cardiovascular disease risk factors are treated. However, investigations for coronary artery disease should be considered if the person has any of the following: atypical cardiac symptoms, signs or symptoms of associated vascular disease, or electrocardiogram abnormalities.

Type 1 diabetes is a demanding condition and requires ongoing professional medical, educational, and psychosocial support. Care may differ at particular times of life, such as at the point of diagnosis, during concomitant illness or pregnancy, and later in life. Given the complexity of management, health care professionals should have the appropriate skills, training, and resources to help people with type 1 diabetes access the education, technology, knowledge, and urgent care they require. These issues are discussed in greater detail in the sections that follow. Overall approaches for people with newly diagnosed or established type 1 diabetes are shown in Figs. 3 and 4.

SECTION 4: SCHEDULE OF CARE

A detailed evaluation should be obtained at the initial consultation, and more targeted interval care at follow-up visits with a focus on person-centered care (Table 2) (52,53). A personalized approach for visit frequency is recommended, but visits should occur at least annually. More frequent contact, however, is preferred for most individuals, for example, those who have been recently diagnosed, those who are not meeting their diabetes goals, those who require cardiovascular risk management, and those who would benefit from additional self-management education and psychosocial support. The increased contact will allow additional review of glucose data and other support. Additional visits can also be useful when the therapeutic regimen changes, for example, when the insulin regimen is modified or when a new device is started.

In the past, initial and follow-up visits were primarily conducted face-to-face and telemedicine only used sporadically. With the onset of the coronavirus disease 2019 (COVID-19) pandemic, the use of telemedicine became a necessity and there was an abrupt widespread adoption of remote visits (videoconference/telephone call) to deliver diabetes care. Pre–COVID-19, results from a limited number of studies using telemedicine in different subgroups of people with type 1 diabetes suggested that remote monitoring, education, and provider visits have the potential to: improve outcomes, quality of life, and self-management; increase access to care and reduce costs; and are well-accepted with improved treatment satisfaction (54–57).

The use of telemedicine, however, should be individualized and will vary depending upon individual needs, computer literacy, and access to care (58). The health care professional and person with diabetes should be in a private space. In advance of the visit, people with diabetes should receive clear instructions on the expectations for the televisit, including how to connect to the consultation and how to upload data from their diabetes devices (glucose meters, data-collecting applications [apps], CGM devices, and insulin pumps) prior to the appointment (59). When clinically indicated and appropriate, people with diabetes should be asked to weigh themselves and perform home blood pressure measurements where possible. A list of all medications and relevant medical reports should be available. Despite the value of telemedicine,

Table 3—Key content areas of DSMES

Key content areas	Examples that focus on type 1 diabetes
Diabetes pathophysiology and treatment options	Immunology of β-cell destruction.
Healthy eating	Basic and advanced carbohydrate counting vs. intuitive dosing. Impact of composition of meals (fat, protein, glycemic index, fiber, sugar, alcohols) on glucose levels. Use of technology to enhance dosing recommendations.
Physical activity	Impact on glucose and insulin dose recommendations.
Medication usage	Types of available insulins. Methods of insulin delivery.
Monitoring and using patient-generated health data	Technology and its impact on the ability to have more frequent communication between the person with type 1 diabetes and their health care professional. Reviewing CGM, pump and connected insulin pen downloads, and apps.
Preventing, detecting and treating acute complications (including hypoglycemia, hyperglycemia, and DKA), sick day guidelines, and severe weather or situation crisis and diabetes supplies management	Euglycemic DKA. DKA prevention with pump use. Glucagon use. Ketone testing.
Preventing, detecting, and treating chronic complications, including immunizations and preventive eye, foot, dental, and renal examinations, as indicated per the individual participant's duration of diabetes and health status	Understanding the individual risk for complications in type 1 diabetes. How to prevent development and progression of complications in the future.
Healthy coping with psychosocial issues and concerns	Discussing diabetes distress and burnout.
Problem solving	Goal setting. Developing personal strategies to promote health and behavior change. Problem identification and solutions. Identifying and accessing resources. Sick day rules. Management of pump failure or pump holiday. Planning for procedures or surgery.

people should have the option to schedule an in-person visit, where possible.

SECTION 5: DIABETES SELF-MANAGEMENT EDUCATION AND SUPPORT

DSMES is an essential component of type 1 diabetes care that allows all other diabetes interventions to work optimally. The objective of DSMES is to provide those living with type 1 diabetes (and their caregivers, if applicable) with the knowledge, skills, and confidence to successfully self-manage the diabetes on a daily basis and, thereby, reduce the risks of acute and long-term complications while maintaining quality of life (60). DSMES aims to empower people with type 1 diabetes, with an emphasis on shared decision-making and active collaboration with the health care team. Where possible, DSMES programs should be evidence-based and conform to local and national standards to demonstrate effectiveness.

Levels and Content of Diabetes Self-Management Education and Support

Three levels of DSMES can be distinguished:

- Level 1 comprises provision of diabetes information and one-to-one advice.
- Level 2 refers to ongoing learning that may be informal, perhaps through a peer group.
- Level 3 DSMES refers to structured education that meets nationally agreed criteria, including an evidence-based curriculum, quality assurance of teaching standards, and regular audit. These programs are guided by learning and behavior change theories.

Several level 3 programs have been developed for adults with type 1 diabetes and have proven to be effective, both in terms of improved glycemic outcomes and improved psychosocial outcomes (61). Most programs use a group format, increasingly supplemented with digital support, including text messaging and cloud-based solutions and telemedicine (62). Structured DSMES programs most

often include multiple components and cover a broad range of topics, from pathophysiology to medical technology and healthy coping (Table 3).

Specific DSMES should not be confined to one particular moment but offered on a continuous basis and tailored to the ever-evolving individual's educational needs. People with type 1 diabetes may be diagnosed at a young age or during adulthood, and many live with type 1 diabetes throughout different life stages. Four critical times where DSMES is particularly needed can be distinguished: 1) at diagnosis; 2) when not meeting targets; 3) when transitions occur; and 4) when complications develop (Fig. 5) (63). DSMES should be revisited when a child transitions to adult diabetes services, as there may be significant knowledge gaps in someone diagnosed early in life, when education at the time was directed to the parents and caregivers. DSMES should be tailored toward an individuals' needs, taking into account cognitive function and literacy, family history and comorbidities,

Four critical times for DSMES in type 1 diabetes

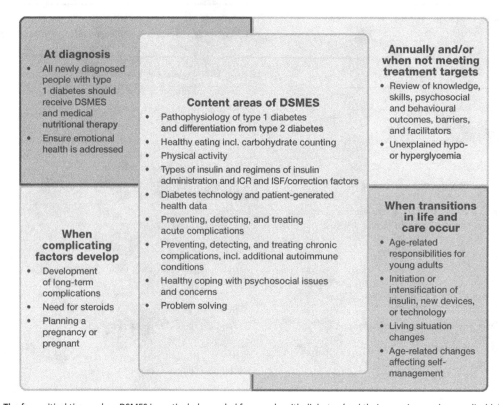

Figure 5—The four critical times when DSMES is particularly needed for people with diabetes (and their caregivers, when applicable). ICR, insulin:-carbohydrate ratio; incl., including; ISF, insulin sensitivity factor.

as well as ethnic, socio-cultural, financial, geographical, and lifestyle factors (64). A structured, periodic assessment of educational needs and barriers should be an integral part of ongoing diabetes care (see Text box: Needs Assessment for Diabetes Management, Education, and Support).

Needs Assessment for Diabetes Management, Education, and Support

Key assessment features

- Health history
- Cognition, functional health literacy and numeracy
- Diabetes distress and support systems
- Religious and cultural influences
- Health beliefs and attitudes
- Physical limitations
- Social determinants of health e.g., financial status
- Barriers

There are numerous smartphone and web-based apps that aim to help people with type 1 diabetes navigate the challenges of self-management. Although

widely used, the available evidence on the safety and effectiveness of diabetes health apps remains limited, with issues ranging from inadequate evidence on app accuracy and clinical validity to lack of training provision, poor interoperability and standardization, and insufficient data security (65).

SECTION 6: MONITORING OF GLUCOSE LEVELS

People with type 1 diabetes should have an assessment of their glucose levels with their health care professional as often as is clinically indicated, but at least annually. Glycemic status should be assessed at least every 3 months in those whose therapy has changed or who are not meeting glycemic goals.

HbA$_{1c}$

Monitoring of blood glucose has traditionally been by HbA$_{1c}$, which has been used in most studies that demonstrate the effects of lowering glucose on the development and progression of diabetes complications (39). There is a strong

correlation ($r = >0.9$) between HbA$_{1c}$ and mean blood glucose levels during the preceding 3 months when glucose levels are stable (66). In several conditions, however, HbA$_{1c}$ does not reflect mean glucose; these are mainly situations where erythrocyte turnover is altered or in the presence of hemoglobinopathies (Table 4) (67). Variability exists between individuals, but the HbA$_{1c}$ and blood glucose within an individual correlate over time (68). Although HbA$_{1c}$ is an indicator of mean glucose, it does not inform glycemic variability and hypoglycemia and, therefore, is inappropriate as the only method of glucose evaluation in type 1 diabetes (68,69).

Other biomarkers, such as fructosamine, 1,5-anhydroglucitol and glycated albumin, provide measures of mean glucose, albeit with shorter durations than HbA$_{1c}$. None of these are as well associated with diabetes complications as HbA$_{1c}$ (70).

Capillary Blood Glucose Monitoring
Capillary BGM involves the use of a hand-held meter and provides a measurement

Table 4—Nonglycemic factors that alter HbA$_{1c}$ levels (70)

Effect on HbA$_{1c}$	Factor
Apparent increase	• Age • Ethnicity: HbA$_{1c}$ is slightly higher in African Americans than in people of White Northern-European ancestry[a] • Anemias with decreased erythrocyte turnover: iron, vitamin B$_{12}$, folate • Severe hypertriglyceridemia (hypertriacylglycerolemia) • Severe hyperbilirubinemia • Chronic alcohol consumption • Chronic salicylate consumption • Chronic opioid ingestion
Apparent decrease	• Pregnancy (second and third trimester) • Anemias of chronic disease • Hemolytic anemia • Splenomegaly and splenectomy • Acute blood loss • Renal failure • Advanced liver disease drugs: dapsone; trimethoprim/sulfamethoxazole • Vitamin E ingestion • Ribavirin and interferon α • Erythrocyte transfusion
Apparent increase or decrease	• Hemoglobin variants • Vitamin C ingestion

[a]Variability within races is greater than variability between races (293).

of capillary plasma glucose. Frequent BGM measurements are important as an integrated part of diabetes management to guide insulin dosage, food intake, and prevention of hypoglycemia with exercise. Every person with type 1 diabetes should have the equipment to undertake BGM, regardless of whether they are using CGM.

BGM is needed before meals to give the user the chance to adjust the meal insulin dose if the pre-meal glucose is out of range at the time, while measurements over a few days will show whether the doses active before that meal require adjustment. Additionally, BGM is needed to prevent and detect hypoglycemia in several situations, such as: before bedtime; before driving; before, during, and after exercise; and when hypoglycemic symptoms occur. The evidence for the optimal number of daily BGM measurements is lacking and may depend on variation in the person's lifestyle. In registry studies, increased testing frequency is associated with lower HbA$_{1c}$ (71). However, even with frequent BGM, most people with type 1 diabetes will have undetected and an unacceptable high frequency of hyper- and hypoglycemia

(72). Frequent measurements are often not feasible and can be distressing. Seeing high or low glucose values can evoke feelings of frustration, anxiety, and guilt, leading many people with type 1 diabetes to measure less often than needed (73). Downloading memory-capable glucose meters can be helpful in observing patterns of hyper- or hypoglycemia and allowing the person with diabetes to reflect on insulin dose adjustment (74). Most meters meet the accuracy standards established by the International Organization for Standardization, and manufacturers need to evaluate each product's clinical performance in a broad population of users over time to ensure that their products continue to meet standards of clinical accuracy (75).

Continuous Glucose Monitoring
CGM is the standard for glucose monitoring for most adults with type 1 diabetes. CGM devices, which have been available commercially since 2006, measure interstitial glucose to provide an estimate of plasma glucose. CGM devices have evolved and improved enough in accuracy to the point where most currently available sensors are "nonadjunctive," meaning that a check with capillary BGM

before a treatment decision is taken is not required. However, BGM may still be required if there are concerns that the CGM readings do not reflect the plasma glucose.

Currently there are two types of CGM devices: one provides a continuous value of current glucose and trends to a receiver, mobile app, smartwatch, or pump (designated as real-time CGM [rt-CGM]), while the other requires the glucose level to be determined by scanning a small reader or smartphone across the transmitter (intermittently scanned CGM [is-CGM]). Historically, rt-CGM has offered a variety of alerts, both in terms of indicating when a specific glucose level is reached as well as for trends in glucose levels. Early is-CGM devices did not have these alerts but increasingly include them. In the near future, these sensors and others in development will increasingly connect to other devices, including connected insulin pens. All currently available devices can be uploaded to an internet cloud to allow people with diabetes and health care professionals to easily view the data at or between clinic visits. CGMs report a reading every 1–15 min.

rt-CGM is effective for adults with type 1 diabetes in improving HbA$_{1c}$ (particularly when high) and reducing hypoglycemia for both those using insulin pumps or multiple daily injections (MDI) (42–44,76). RCTs of the original is-CGM devices are more mixed, but observational data are supportive of their use. However, switching from is-CGM without alarms to rt-CGM improved TIR and HbA$_{1c}$ and reduced level 3 hypoglycemia (77). rt-CGM is beneficial in reducing the burden of hypoglycemia in older adults with type 1 diabetes (78) and those with IAH (44). Most people with type 1 diabetes can benefit from this technology with appropriate initial and ongoing education, including frequent observation of the glucose trends. The choice of the device should be based on individual preferences and circumstances.

Some people may not find CGM valuable as they may feel that they do not require it or find it stressful because they dislike being "attached to a device," being constantly reminded of their diabetes, or feeling exhausted by alarms (alarm fatigue). Cost considerations can also play a role.

Standardized CGM Metrics for Clinical Care

- Number of days CGM device is worn:
  - recommend 14 days
- Percentage of time CGM device is active:
  - recommend 70% of data from 14 days
- Mean glucose
- GMI
- Glycemic variability (%CV)
- Time above range
  - Percent of readings and time >13.9 mmol/L (>250 mg/dL); level 2 hyperglycemia
  - Percent of readings and time >10.0 mmol/L (>180 mg/dL); level 1 and level 2 hyperglycemia
- Time in range
  - Percent of readings and TIR 3.9–10.0 mmol/L (70–180 mg/dL)
- Time below range
  - Percent of readings and time <3.9 mmol/L (<70 mg/dL); level 1 and level 2 hypoglycemia
  - Percent of readings and time <3.0 mmol/L (<54 mg/dL); level 2 hypoglycemia

Adapted from ref. 47.

Retrospective analysis of CGM data can guide and enhance therapeutic decision-making, patient understanding, and engagement in adjusting behaviors. Standardized glucose reports with visual cues, such as the ambulatory glucose profile (AGP) and daily tracings, should be available for all CGM devices (Text box: Standardized CGM metrics for Clinical Care) (Fig. 2) (79, 80).

Although health care professionals should regularly access and review CGM data as part of clinical management, people with type 1 diabetes should be encouraged to review their own reports regularly and follow their progress over time, contacting their health care professional as needed for worsening or changing trends.

People with type 1 diabetes should be warned that contact dermatitis (both irritant and allergic) may occur with all CGM devices that attach to the skin (81–83). In some instances, the use of an implanted sensor can help avoid skin reactions in those who are sensitive to tape (84,85).

Ketone Measurement

Ketone bodies are produced when insulin concentrations are too low to prevent lipolysis. If left untreated, ketosis can lead to progressive dehydration and DKA. Measurement of ketones is important during periods of illness or hyperglycemia to facilitate the management of the hyperglycemia and prevent and/or treat DKA.

Ketone bodies may be measured in blood or urine. Urine testing, the traditional method, detects acetoacetate, but not β-hydroxybutyrate, which is measured in blood testing. This means that urine testing may give a falsely low estimate of ketosis. Furthermore, after an episode of ketoacidosis, measurement of blood ketones provides a more accurate assessment of adequate treatment as urine tests may continue to be positive for 48 h as acetone leaks from fat tissue after ketogenesis and lipolysis have stopped. Modern technology allows the rapid and accurate measurement of ketones from a finger prick blood sample using a strip and meter. Blood ketone measurement is the method of choice and so adults with type 1 diabetes should be offered blood ketone testing strips and a meter (86). Blood and urine ketone testing is not available in all countries and settings.

SECTION 7: INSULIN THERAPY

The ideal regimen of insulin replacement maintains blood glucose in the normal physiological range, as far as possible, while allowing flexibility in terms of mealtimes and activity levels. Typical insulin replacement regimens incorporate several components: basal insulin to restrain gluconeogenesis and ketogenesis in the preprandial state; mealtime insulin to cover the intake of carbohydrate and other macronutrients; and correction insulin to treat hyperglycemia.

Choice of Regimen

Most people with type 1 diabetes should use regimens that mimic physiology as closely as possible, irrespective of the presentation. This is best achieved with either MDI of subcutaneous basal insulin analogs and mealtime rapid-acting or ultra-rapid-acting insulin analogs, or with continuous subcutaneous insulin infusion of a rapid-acting insulin analog via a pump, delivered as continuous basal insulin combined with manual mealtime boluses. In the U.S., inhaled human insulin is an alternative to subcutaneous rapid-acting analogs (3). Although first-generation basal analogs and NPH insulin are frequently administered once a day, greater flexibility and better coverage of basal insulin needs may be obtained if they are administered twice daily. Trials have demonstrated that the latest basal analogs may cause less hypoglycemia than first-generation basal analogs and NPH insulin, while rapid-acting analogs achieve better mealtime coverage and less post-meal hypoglycemia than short-acting (regular) human insulin (87,88). Insulin analogs are, therefore, considered the insulins of choice.

Ultra-rapid analogs have a slightly earlier time of onset and peak action than rapid-acting analogs. These insulins reduce postprandial hyperglycemia but have otherwise not been shown to reduce HbA$_{1c}$ or hypoglycemia to a greater extent than rapid-acting analogs (3). Currently, recombinant human insulin or analogs of human insulin account for the vast majority of insulin used worldwide.

HbA$_{1c}$, TIR, and TBR are improved further when physiological MDI or pump regimens are augmented with CGM usage (89), with the greatest benefits seen with algorithm-driven automated basal (and in some systems correction) insulin delivery, which is commonly called hybrid closed-loop therapy (90, 91).

Despite these advantages, the costs of insulin analogs and CGM or pump therapy are barriers for some people,

Representative relative attributes of insulin delivery approaches in people with type 1 diabetes[1]

Injected insulin regimens	Flexibility	Lower risk of hypoglycemia	Higher costs
MDI with LAA + RAA or URAA	+++	+++	+++

Less-preferred, alternative injected insulin regimens

	Flexibility	Lower risk of hypoglycemia	Higher costs
MDI with NPH + RAA or URAA	++	++	++
MDI with NPH + short-acting (regular) insulin	++	+	+
Two daily injections with NPH + short-acting (regular) insulin or premixed	+	+	+

Continuous insulin infusion regimens	Flexibility	Lower risk of hypoglycemia	Higher costs
Hybrid closed-loop technology	+++++	+++++	++++++
Insulin pump with threshold/predictive low-glucose suspend	++++	++++	+++++
Insulin pump therapy without automation	+++	+++	++++

Figure 6—Choices of insulin regimens in people with type 1 diabetes. CGM improves outcomes with injected or infused insulin and is superior to BGM. Inhaled insulin may be used in place of injectable prandial insulin in the U.S.. [1]The number of plus signs (+) is an estimate of relative association of the regimen with increased flexibility, lower risk of hypoglycemia, and higher costs between the considered regimens. LAA, long-acting insulin analog; RAA, rapid-acting insulin analog; URAA: ultra-rapid-acting insulin analog.

while others do not wish to wear a device or inject multiple times per day. In these cases, subcutaneous regimens of human short-acting (regular) and NPH insulin or premixed insulin, with BGM as frequently as feasible, may be used at a cost of higher glucose variability with higher risk of hypoglycemia and less flexibility of lifestyle. Figure 6 shows advantages and disadvantages of more- or less-physiological insulin replacement regimens, while Table 5 provides details on various regimens that might be employed.

Mode of Delivery

There are several options for the mode of insulin delivery, and the choice of device should be individualized. Hybrid closed-loop systems are the most effective means of maintaining glucose in the normal range in people with type 1 diabetes (90,91).

MDI therapy can be administered using vials and insulin syringes or insulin pens, with the latter providing more convenience with regard to dosing, but may be at higher cost. Smaller gauge and shorter needles provide almost painless injections. Contrary to common wisdom, skin thickness is not significantly increased in individuals who have overweight or obesity. Needles as short as 4 mm, injected at a 90° angle, enter the subcutaneous space with minimal risk of intramuscular injection in most adults (92). The use of longer needles increases the risk of intramuscular injection. MDI regimens may be enhanced with emerging technology, such as bolus calculators and memory-enabled pens that keep track of insulin doses.

Different insulin pumps for subcutaneous insulin delivery are available in many countries. The primary mechanical differences between pumps are whether they utilize external tubing to connect to an infusion set or a pod directly applied to the skin and controlled via a wireless connection to a controller. Current pumps include bolus calculators programmed with personalized insulin:carbohydrate ratio and correction factors.

Hybrid closed-loop systems comprise an insulin pump, continuous glucose sensor, and a control algorithm. The algorithm controls basal insulin delivery and, in some cases, correction boluses, based on CGM data, while the user still boluses manually for meals (90,91).

Some people with type 1 diabetes are using "do-it-yourself," user-driven, open-source artificial insulin delivery systems, which use commercially available CGM systems and pumps, with software algorithms that communicate with both and can reverse-engineer the pump control of basal and corrective doses (93). Regulatory bodies do not allow health care professionals to prescribe these systems, but health care professionals should respect an individual's right to make informed choices about their care and continue to offer support to the people using these systems.

Table 5—Examples of subcutaneous insulin regimens

Regimen	Timing and distribution	Advantages	Disadvantages	Adjusting doses
Regimens that more closely mimic normal insulin secretion				
Insulin pump therapy (hybrid closed-loop, low-glucose suspend, CGM-augmented open-loop, BGM-augmented open-loop)	Basal delivery of URAA or RAA; generally 40–60% of TDD. Mealtime and correction: URAA or RAA by bolus based on ICR and/or ISF and target glucose, with pre-meal insulin ~15 min before eating.	Can adjust basal rates for varying insulin sensitivity by time of day, for exercise and for sick days. Flexibility in meal timing and content. Pump can deliver insulin in increments of fractions of units. Potential for integration with CGM for low-glucose suspend or hybrid closed-loop. TIR % highest and TBR % lowest with: hybrid closed-loop > low-glucose suspend > CGM-augmented open-loop > BGM-augmented open-loop.	Most expensive regimen. Must continuously wear one or more devices. Risk of rapid development of ketosis or DKA with interruption of insulin delivery. Potential reactions to adhesives and site infections. Most technically complex approach (harder for people with lower numeracy or literacy skills).	Mealtime insulin: if carbohydrate counting is accurate, change ICR if glucose after meal consistently out of target. Correction insulin: adjust ISF and/or target glucose if correction does not consistently bring glucose into range. Basal rates: adjust based on overnight, fasting or daytime glucose outside of activity of URAA/RAA bolus.
MDI: LAA + flexible doses of URAA or RAA at meals	LAA once daily (insulin detemir or insulin glargine may require twice-daily dosing); generally 50% of TDD. Mealtime and correction: URAA or RAA based on ICR and/or ISF and target glucose.	Can use pens for all components. Flexibility in meal timing and content. Insulin analogs cause less hypoglycemia than human insulins.	At least four daily injections. Most costly insulins. Smallest increment of insulin is 1 unit (0.5 unit with some pens). LAAs may not cover strong dawn phenomenon (rise in glucose in early morning hours) as well as pump therapy.	Mealtime insulin: if carbohydrate counting is accurate, change ICR if glucose after meal consistently out of target. Correction insulin: adjust ISF and/or target glucose if correction does not consistently bring glucose into range. LAA: based on overnight or fasting glucose or daytime glucose outside of activity time course, or URAA or RAA injections.

Continued on p. 2606

Table 5—Continued

Regimen	Timing and distribution	Advantages	Disadvantages	Adjusting doses
MDI regimens with less flexibility				
Four injections daily with fixed doses of N and RAA	Pre-breakfast: RAA ~20% of TDD. Pre-lunch: RAA ~10% of TDD. Pre-dinner: RAA ~10% of TDD. Bedtime: N ~50% of TDD.	May be feasible if unable to carbohydrate count. All meals have RAA coverage. N less expensive than LAAs.	Shorter duration RAA may lead to basal deficit during day; may need twice-daily N. Greater risk of nocturnal hypoglycemia with N. Requires relatively consistent mealtimes and carbohydrate intake.	Pre-breakfast RAA: based on BGM after breakfast or before lunch. Pre-lunch RAA: based on BGM after lunch or before dinner. Pre-dinner RAA: based on BGM after dinner or at bedtime. Evening N: based on fasting or overnight BGM.
Four injections daily with fixed doses of N and R	Pre-breakfast: R ~20% of TDD. Pre-lunch: R ~10% of TDD. Pre-dinner: R ~10% of TDD. Bedtime: N ~50% of TDD.	May be feasible if unable to carbohydrate count. R can be dosed based on ICR and correction. All meals have R coverage. Least expensive insulins.	Greater risk of nocturnal hypoglycemia with N. Greater risk of delayed post-meal hypoglycemia with R. Requires relatively consistent mealtimes and carbohydrate intake. R must be injected at least 30 min before meal for better effect.	Pre-breakfast R: based on BGM after breakfast or before lunch. Pre-lunch R: based on BGM after lunch or before dinner. Pre-dinner R: based on BGM after dinner or at bedtime. Evening N: based on fasting or overnight BGM.
Regimens with fewer daily injections				
Three injections daily: N+R or N+RAA	Pre-breakfast: ~40% N + ~15% R or RAA. Pre-dinner: ~15% R or RAA. Bedtime: 30% N.	Morning insulins can be mixed in one syringe. May be appropriate for those who cannot take injection in middle of day. Morning N covers lunch to some extent. Same advantages of RAAs over R. Least (N + R) or less expensive insulins than MDI with analogs.	Greater risk of nocturnal hypoglycemia with N than LAAs. Greater risk of delayed post-meal hypoglycemia with R than RAAs. Requires relatively consistent mealtimes and carbohydrate intake. Coverage of post-lunch glucose often suboptimal. R must be injected at least 30 min before meal for better effect.	Morning N: based on pre-dinner BGM. Morning R: based on pre-lunch BGM. Morning RAA: based on post-breakfast or pre-lunch BGM. Pre-dinner R: based on bedtime BGM. Pre-dinner RAA: based on post-dinner or bedtime BGM. Evening N: based on fasting BGM.

Continued on p. 2607

Table 5—Continued

Regimen	Timing and distribution	Advantages	Disadvantages	Adjusting doses
Twice-daily "split-mixed": N+R or N+RAA	Pre-breakfast: ~40% N + ~15% R or RAA. Pre-dinner: ~30% N + ~15% R or RAA.	Least number of injections for people with strong preference for this. Insulins can be mixed in one syringe. Least (N+R) or less (N+RAA) expensive insulins vs analogs. Eliminates need for doses during the day.	Risk of hypoglycemia in afternoon or middle of night from N. Fixed mealtimes and meal content. Coverage of post-lunch glucose often suboptimal. Difficult to reach targets for blood glucose without hypoglycemia.	Morning N: based on pre-dinner BGM. Morning R: based on pre-lunch BGM. Morning RAA: based on post-breakfast or pre-lunch BGM. Evening R: based on bedtime BGM. Evening RAA: based on post-dinner or bedtime BGM. Evening N: based on fasting BGM.

ICR, insulin:carbohydrate ratio; ISF, insulin sensitivity factor; LAA, long-acting analog; N, NPH insulin; R, short-acting (regular) insulin; RAA: rapid-acting analog; TDD, total daily insulin dose; URAA, ultra-rapid-acting analog.

Fully closed-loop automated insulin delivery systems are currently being evaluated in clinical trials being conducted by several collaborative groups in both North America and Europe (94). The expectation is that some of these will receive regulatory approval in the next few years. This should allow people with type 1 diabetes to achieve better glucose management with minimal risk of hypoglycemia. Bi-hormonal (insulin and glucagon) automated insulin delivery systems are under investigation and could also contribute to the optimization of glucose management. This is a rapidly evolving area, and readers may wish to keep abreast by referring to the "Technology" section of the ADA Standards of Care, which is a living document that is updated frequently (53).

Adverse Effects
The main adverse effect associated with insulin therapy is hypoglycemia, which is discussed in the next section. The safety and efficacy of insulin therapy is closely related to glucose monitoring and insulin dose adjustments made by the individual with diabetes or, more recently, made automatically through control algorithms. Therefore, education in the management of insulin doses is a crucial component of this therapy, both at initiation and during follow-up. This education includes rescue strategies in case of hyperglycemic or hypoglycemic deviations, including the measurement of urine or blood ketone bodies or the prescription of carbohydrate intake and glucagon, respectively.

Insulin causes body weight gain and can lead to some people with type 1 diabetes reducing their insulin doses. Clinicians should review such weight concerns related to insulin and discuss strategies to avoid undesirable weight gain.

Skin reactions to subcutaneous insulin therapy include local inflammation (often due to the pH of or additives to the insulin), insulin-induced lipoatrophy, and insulin-induced lipohypertrophy. Lipoatrophy has become rare as the purity of manufacture of human and analog insulin has improved. Lipohypertrophy is common and typically occurs when the same sites are repeatedly used for injections or pump sites; it leads to use of higher insulin doses and is a cause of glycemic variability, leading to both hyper- and hypoglycemia (95,96). People with type 1 diabetes should receive instructions about proper injection technique, including regular site rotation and skin examination, at the time of insulin initiation, with periodic reminders thereafter. Clinicians should inspect and palpate injection and infusion sites at least annually.

As described above for CGM devices, individuals should be warned about possible skin reactions to pump adhesives.

Alternative Routes of Administration

Although subcutaneous insulin therapy has been the mainstay of treatment for almost a century, this mode does not mimic physiological insulin secretion well. Healthy β-cells secrete a burst of insulin into the portal circulation at the onset of glucose intake, with approximately 70% of the insulin cleared by the liver and not entering the systemic circulation, whereas subcutaneous insulin enters the systemic circulation with some delay and is removed relatively slowly. Inhaled human insulin, available only in the U.S., has a very rapid onset of action and short duration compared with subcutaneous rapid-acting analogs (3). Inhaled insulin ameliorates early postprandial hyperglycemia well, but its short duration of action results in less control of later postprandial hyperglycemia. Additionally, inhaled insulin can cause cough or sore throat, and therapy must be monitored with periodic spirometry because of possible effects on lung function (97).

Peritoneal delivery of human short-acting (regular) insulin, with rapid transit to the portal system, can be accomplished with implantable insulin pumps or through a port connected to an intraperitoneal catheter (available only in some countries in Europe at considerable cost). Compared with subcutaneous insulin regimens, intraperitoneal insulin infusion reduces HbA_{1c}, glycemic variability, and hypoglycemia (98,99). Insulin aggregation, local infections, and catheter occlusions are reported complications of the devices used for this route of insulin delivery. In some individuals, an increased production of anti-insulin antibodies has been observed while using this route of insulin delivery. The effect on glucose levels is variable, ranging from no effect to marked glucose swings according to the binding affinity of the antibodies to insulin.

SECTION 8: HYPOGLYCEMIA

Hypoglycemia is the main limiting factor in the glycemic management of type 1 diabetes. Hypoglycemia is classified into three levels:

- Level 1 corresponds to a glucose value below 3.9 mmol/L (70 mg/dL) and greater than or equal to 3.0 mmol/L (54 mg/dL) and is named as an alert value.
- Level 2 is for glucose values below 3.0 mmol/L (54 mg/dL) and considered clinically important hypoglycemia.
- Level 3 designates any hypoglycemia characterized by altered mental state and/or physical status needing the intervention of a third party for recovery (100).

Although these were originally developed for clinical trials reporting, they are useful clinical constructs. Particular attention should be made to prevent level 2 and 3 hypoglycemia.

Level 1 hypoglycemia is common, with most people with type 1 diabetes experiencing several episodes per week. Hypoglycemia with glucose levels below 3.0 mmol/L (54 mg/dL) occurs much more often than previously appreciated (46,101). Level 3 hypoglycemia is less common but occurred in 12% of adults with type 1 diabetes over a 6-month period in a recent global observational analysis (102). Several studies have shown that rates of hypoglycemia have not declined, even with more widespread use of insulin analogs and CGM, while other studies have shown benefit with these therapeutic advances (41).

Risks for hypoglycemia, particularly level 3 hypoglycemia, include longer duration of diabetes, older age, history of recent level 3 hypoglycemia, alcohol ingestion, exercise, lower education levels, lower household incomes (41), chronic kidney disease, and IAH (103–105). Endocrine conditions, such as hypothyroidism, adrenal and growth hormone deficiency, and celiac disease may precipitate hypoglycemia. Older diabetes databases consistently documented that people with lower HbA_{1c} levels had 2–3-fold higher rates of level 3 hypoglycemia. However, in the Type 1 Diabetes Exchange Clinic Registry, the risk of level 3 hypoglycemia was increased not only in those whose HbA_{1c} was below 7.0% (53 mmol/mol), but also in people with an HbA_{1c} above 7.5% (58 mmol/mol) (41).

It is possible that the absence of a relationship between HbA_{1c} and level 3 hypoglycemia in real-world settings is explained by relaxation of glycemic targets by those with a history of hypoglycemia, or confounders, such as inadequate self-management behaviors that contribute to both hyper- and hypoglycemia. A secondary analysis of the IN CONTROL trial, where the primary analysis showed a reduction in level 3 hypoglycemia in people using CGM, demonstrated an increase in the rate of level 3 hypoglycemia with lower HbA_{1c}, similar to what was reported in the DCCT (106). This implies that lowering HbA_{1c} may still come with a higher risk of level 3 hypoglycemia.

Mortality from hypoglycemia in type 1 diabetes is not trivial. One recent trial noted more than 8% of deaths for those younger than 56 years were from hypoglycemia (107). The mechanism for this is complex, including cardiac arrhythmias, activation of both the coagulation system and inflammation, and endothelial dysfunction (108). What may not be as well recognized is that level 3 hypoglycemia is also associated with major microvascular events, noncardiovascular disease, and death from any cause, although much of this evidence is obtained from people with type 2 diabetes (108). With regard to cognitive function, in the DCCT and EDIC study, after 18 years of follow-up, severe hypoglycemia in middle-aged adults did not appear to affect neurocognitive function (109). However, independent of other risk factors and comorbidities, more episodes of severe hypoglycemia were associated with greater decrements in psychomotor and mental efficiency that were most notable after 32 years of follow-up (110). It appears that older adults with type 1 diabetes are more prone to mild cognitive impairment associated with hypoglycemia (110,111), while hypoglycemia occurs more frequently in those with cognitive impairment. CGM data were not available in the DCCT era and so the true extent of serious hypoglycemia over time is not known.

Impaired Awareness of Hypoglycemia

IAH is the reduced ability to recognize low blood glucose levels that would otherwise prompt an appropriate corrective therapy (112). Its prevalence is estimated to be close to 25% in people with type 1 diabetes but is likely to be underestimated according to CGM data (113). IAH increases the risk of level 3 hypoglycemia by sixfold (114) and may lead to the person with diabetes omitting insulin injections intentionally or loosening tight glucose management to prevent their occurrence.

The pathophysiology of IAH is still not fully understood but includes a partial or total loss of sympathoadrenal reactions to hypoglycemia that prevent catecholaminergic stimulation of hepatic glucose output and restraint of muscle glucose uptake (104). The connections between autonomic neuropathy and IAH are complex since both the defect of sympathoadrenal reaction to hypoglycemia can be a component of autonomic neuropathy and hypoglycemia itself can promote neuropathy. Indeed, recurrent hypoglycemia is a major cause of IAH. Sleep disturbance, psychological stress, and alcohol can also induce IAH (112).

In clinical practice, physicians should be proactive in asking people with type 1 diabetes whether, and at which glucose level, they feel hypoglycemia in order to identify IAH and adjust individual glucose targets to prevent the occurrence of level 3 hypoglycemia. The reference method to assess IAH is the hyperinsulinemic–hypoglycemic clamp (115), although this is not used out of a research frame due to its invasiveness, cost, and time commitment from people with diabetes. Self-reported awareness, however, agrees well with the autonomic glucose threshold (116). The Gold questionnaire and Clarke questionnaire, showing a score equal or above 4 are indicative of IAH (114,117), and the Pedersen-Bjergaard et al. questionnaire and Hypoglycemia Awareness Questionnaire (HypoA-Q) can also identify IAH (118,119). Another good test for hypoglycemia awareness is to ask, "Do your symptoms of hypoglycemia usually occur at a blood glucose level of ≥3.0 mmol/L (≥54 mg/dL) or <3.0 mmol/L (<54 mg/dL) or do you not feel symptoms?" Those responding, "less than 3.0 mmol/L (54 mg/dL)" or not experiencing symptoms

have a >4-fold increased risk of level 3 hypoglycemia (120). The U.K. National Institute for Health and Care Excellence recommended for the first time that an assessment of hypoglycemia, including awareness, should form part of clinical consultations (86).

Prevention of Hypoglycemia

Hypoglycemia is not inevitable, and several strategies can be used to reduce the risk (121). Structured education programs, such as Dose Adjustment For Normal Eating (DAFNE) and blood glucose awareness training (BGAT), which provide informed support for active insulin dose self-adjustment, are the key to the prevention of hypoglycemia and lead to sustained falls in level 3 hypoglycemia rates in those at high risk (122,123). The use of insulin analog regimens are associated with less hypoglycemia, while hybrid closed-loop systems result in both improvement in TIR and reduction in TBR (91).

Strict avoidance of hypoglycemia can help to restore hypoglycemia awareness (124). Structured diabetes education in flexible insulin therapy, which may incorporate psychotherapeutic and behavioral therapies, progressing to diabetes technology, incorporating sensors and insulin pumps, are effective treatments in those with persisting need (125). CGM use promotes the identification of current or impending low glucose levels that people may not feel. BGAT, education to optimize insulin dosing and type, and hypoglycemia avoidance motivational programs all improve hypoglycemia awareness. In some situations, it may be necessary to increase the glucose target range (124,126). Several clinical trials have not shown a reduction of IAH by using CGM despite a reduced incidence of level 3 hypoglycemia (101,112,124,126–128).

Treatment of Hypoglycemia

The recommended correction of hypoglycemia is the oral intake of approximately 15 g of glucose or equivalent simple carbohydrate when a capillary blood glucose level is <3.9 mmol/L (<70 mg/dL) (129). This should be repeated every 15 min until any symptoms have resolved and the blood glucose level is above 3.9 mmol/L (70 mg/dL). A larger amount of glucose may be

needed if glucose levels are below 3.0 mmol/L (54 mg/dL). Lower carbohydrate intakes can be used when symptoms are associated with a capillary blood glucose level above 3.9 mmol/L (70 mg/dL). As there may be a 5–15 min lag between changes in capillary blood glucose and interstitial glucose, the restoration of normoglycemia may not be detected by CGM straight away. The use of capillary glucose measurement is recommended to prevent overtreatment of the hypoglycemia.

The specific recommendations for correction of hypoglycemia or trends for hypoglycemia according to CGM in people using automated insulin delivery systems will have to be defined as this mode of therapy expands in forthcoming years. Less carbohydrate (5–15 g) may need to be ingested to correct hypoglycemia because the automated insulin delivery system should have already reduced or stopped basal insulin delivery (130).

Where there is a reduced level of consciousness, oral glucose intake is contraindicated because of risk for aspiration. Instead, glucagon via subcutaneous or intramuscular injection or nasal delivery should be given by attending people. Intravenous glucose injection is a possible alternative for health care professionals in cases of level 3 hypoglycemia.

After the acute symptoms have resolved, a further 20 g of long-acting carbohydrate as part of a snack or meal should be given and the cause of the hypoglycemic episode sought to prevent further episodes.

SECTION 9: ADDITIONAL BEHAVIORAL CONSIDERATIONS

Nutrition therapy

Nutrition, in particular carbohydrate intake, has a major effect on blood glucose levels, and people with type 1 diabetes need to understand the effect of food on their diabetes and plan meals accordingly (see Text box: Goal of nutrition therapy for type 1 diabetes). People with type 1 diabetes should be referred for individualized medical nutrition therapy provided by a registered dietitian who is knowledgeable and skilled in providing diabetes-specific nutritional advice in conjunction with the diabetes technology being used. Medical nutrition therapy delivered by a registered dietitian is associated with a reduction in HbA_{1c} of 1.0–1.9% (11–21 mmol/mol) for people with suboptimally managed type 1 diabetes when integrated into an overall management program (131).

Goal of Nutrition Therapy for Type 1 Diabetes

- Promote healthy eating patterns, emphasizing a variety of nutrient-dense foods in appropriate sizes to improve overall health and to:
  ○ Improve HbA_{1c}, blood pressure, and cholesterol and aid in maintaining weight
- Individualize nutrition needs based on personal and cultural preferences, health literacy, and access to healthy food choices
- Provide practical tools for day-to-day meal planning
- Focus on matching insulin doses with meal composition through advanced carbohydrate counting

Information from ref. 134.

There is no one eating pattern recommended for people with type 1 diabetes. The nutrition approach should be individualized based on personal preferences, socioeconomic status, cultural backgrounds, and comorbidities. Carbohydrate counting is the most common meal planning approach in type 1 diabetes. In conjunction with promoting healthy eating patterns, carbohydrate counting and insulin:carbohydrate ratios can be a useful method for adjusting mealtime insulin dosing for optimal glycemic outcomes (132,133). While low-carbohydrate and very-low-carbohydrate eating patterns have become increasingly popular and reduce HbA_{1c} levels in the short term, it is important to incorporate these in conjunction with healthy eating guidelines. Additional components of the meal, including high fat and/or high protein, may contribute to delayed hyperglycemia and the need for insulin dose adjustments. Since this is highly variable between individuals, postprandial glucose measurements for up to 3 h or more may be needed to determine initial dose adjustments (134).

The average BMI of individuals with type 1 diabetes is rising at a faster rate than the general population, partly as a result of insulin intensification and societal factors that also affect the general population, such as physical inactivity. Weight loss and maintenance interventions involving nutritional advice and physical activity should be offered to individuals with type 1 diabetes who have overweight or obesity, in conjunction with other DSMES topics. New interactive technologies using mobile phones to provide information, insulin bolus calculations based on insulin:carbohydrate ratios, and telemedicine communications with care providers may be used to aid in reducing both weight gain and the time required for education (65). In the case of extreme low weight, unhealthy eating habits should be reviewed, including the possibility of insulin omission.

Alcohol and Recreational Drug Use

Similar to the general population, many individuals with type 1 diabetes consume alcohol, although its effects on glycemic management are not always adequately considered by those with diabetes and their health care professionals. Increased alcohol consumption is associated with a higher risk of DKA and level 3 hypoglycemia (135). Some of this increase may occur through the association with other risk-taking behavior. However, excessive alcohol consumption impairs cognitive function and symptom awareness, leading to a diminished ability to self-manage the diabetes. Alcohol promotes ketosis, which in the context of consumption of sugary alcoholic beverages, may increase the risk of DKA (136). Alcohol also inhibits hepatic gluconeogenesis, leading to an increased risk of hypoglycemia for up to 24 h after the last drink (137). Hypoglycemia is particularly hazardous because of the potential to confuse the symptoms of hypoglycemia with alcohol intoxication.

Cannabis has been legalized in multiple jurisdictions. An association between recent recreational cannabis consumption and a more than twofold increased risk of DKA has been reported from countries where cannabis has been legalized, possibly related to the emergence of higher potency formulations of cannabis and other synthetic cannabinoids (138). Use of

cocaine and other stimulant-like drugs, such as amphetamine, methamphetamine, and ecstasy (or 3,4-methylenedioxy methamfetamine [MDMA]), increase glucose production and inhibit glucose clearance, which increases the risk of DKA. Having a diagnosis of a substance use disorder confers an increased all-cause mortality in populations with diabetes across a range of substances, including cocaine, opioids, and cannabis, regardless of consumption.

As many people are unlikely to spontaneously report their alcohol or drug use to clinicians, systematic screening for excess alcohol and/or drug use is recommended (139). Health care professionals have a responsibility to inform people with type 1 diabetes about the effects of drugs and alcohol on diabetes and related risks, otherwise people with diabetes will seek information elsewhere, which is frequently incorrect and misleading (140). Brief interventions to reduce risky drinking and drug use have been well validated in a variety of populations and offer the potential to improve diabetes medication taking and outcome (141). In the case of alcohol or drug addiction, referral to a specialized clinic is warranted.

Smoking

Since smoking increases the risk of macrovascular and microvascular complications in people with diabetes, smoking cessation should be promoted and supported in all individuals with type 1 diabetes. The direct effect of smoking on blood glucose levels in people with diabetes needs more research to assess the impact (142,143).

Physical Activity

People with type 1 diabetes should be encouraged to engage in a combination of aerobic and resistance exercise on most days because exercise is associated with improved fitness, increased insulin sensitivity, leading to reduced insulin requirement, improved cardiovascular health with better lipid profile and endothelial function, and decreased mortality (144–147). Independent effects on β-cell function and HbA_{1c} have not been established beyond doubt but appear beneficial. In addition, regular physical activity is associated with reduced risk of microvascular complications, osteoporosis, and cancer in people with type 1 diabetes (148). Exercise also helps maintain a healthy BMI and promotes sleep quality and mental well-being.

It is important that physical activity is performed safely. The major risks are from the acute effects of exercise on glucose concentrations, which depend on several factors, including: the baseline fitness of the individual and type, intensity, and the duration of activity; the amount of insulin in the circulation; the blood glucose concentration before exercise; and the composition of the last meal or snack. People with type 1 diabetes should be taught about the effects of exercise on glucose levels and how to balance exogenous insulin delivery and carbohydrate intake for the different forms and intensities of exercise.

Glycemic management during exercise should be made safer with CGM systems. The updated consensus statement for management of exercise in type 1 diabetes highlights very detailed suggestions regarding the use of trend arrows and adjustment of insulin doses and carbohydrate intake (149).

When discussing the importance of exercise, consideration of cardiovascular and lower extremity comorbid conditions is critical. Advice should be given about appropriate footwear and foot inspection for those with peripheral neuropathy to avoid the risk of ulceration. However, walking does not increase the risk of ulceration in people with peripheral neuropathy (150). Weight-bearing exercise should be avoided in active foot disease. If an individual has proliferative diabetic retinopathy or severe nonproliferative diabetic retinopathy, then vigorous activity requiring straining may be contraindicated because of the risk of vitreous hemorrhage or retinal detachment (151). The individual should be advised to consult an ophthalmologist prior to engaging in an intense exercise regimen.

Additional details regarding the diabetes management during physical activity or exercise have been described elsewhere (152). When there is excessive physical exercise combined with extreme low weight, an eating disorder should be considered.

Sleep
Proper sleep hygiene is essential for all individuals. Sleep may be disrupted in people with type 1 diabetes as a result of both behavioral and physiological

aspects of diabetes and its management (153). They may include hyper- and hypoglycemic episodes, blood glucose variability, and loss of blood pressure decline. However, studies performed so far have not determined causality. On the other hand, sleep disturbances including poor sleep quality and shorter sleep duration are associated with worsening glycemic levels in type 1 diabetes (154,155).

Sick Day/Illness Management
Stressful events, including illness, may affect glucose levels and increase risk of DKA. More frequent glucose and ketone measurements are necessary to identify insulin adjustments. Individuals should devise a sick day management plan in consultation with their health care professional (156). Examples of sick day protocols are available online (157,158). All recommend ingestion of adequate amounts of fluids and carbohydrates, as well as when to monitor glucose and ketone levels, give insulin, and under what circumstances a person with diabetes should seek urgent medical care.

Driving
Unrecognized hypoglycemia and rapidly dropping glucose levels are the most relevant hazards for drivers with type 1 diabetes. These risks may be reduced by the use of CGM or BGM prior to driving and at 2 hourly intervals. Local regulations and recommendations should be followed for driving with type 1 diabetes (159,160). In some countries, glucose meter downloads are essential to support applications for heavy goods and public service vehicle driving licenses. Safe driving practices should be discussed regularly with people who drive.

Employment
People with type 1 diabetes can successfully undertake a wide range of employment, but there remains prejudice against those with diabetes that can limit employment opportunities. The main concerns are associated with the risks of acute hypoglycemia as well as certain situations in which continued supply of effective insulin is not possible, for example, working in very hot climates. Additionally, chronic diabetes complications may affect the ability to

work in certain situations. For some occupations, any risk of hypoglycemia is considered unacceptable, but efforts have been made to address these risks. For example, in some countries, people with type 1 diabetes are now working as commercial airline pilots. For this reason, any person with type 1 diabetes should be supported to undertake professional activity, job, or employment for which they are otherwise qualified and can do safely (161). Employment circumstances should allow the safe use and storage of insulin and unrestrained access to glucose monitoring and self-treatment of hyper- or hypoglycemia.

Travel
Planning ahead is the key to safe and trouble-free travel for individuals with type 1 diabetes. This includes preparing diabetes-related and emergency supplies, which should be available at hand during the travel. A plan of adjusting insulin doses, especially when traveling across time zones, is essential to reduce glucose fluctuations (162). In particular, it is important to consider the impact of change in usual schedule, hot weather, reduced stress and relaxation, and changes in exercise patterns on glucose levels while on holiday.

Depending on the locale of travel destinations, it may be advisable to research the estimated carbohydrate content of local foods to aid better insulin adjustment. Frequent glucose measurement with CGM or BGM is advisable for any travel (163). Additionally, it may be helpful to have note cards written in the local language to communicate that the person has type 1 diabetes and may need urgent glucose administration if hypoglycemic.

Additional Religious and Cultural Considerations
Fasting for religious and cultural reasons is a widespread practice globally. Health care professionals should ask if the person with type 1 diabetes wishes to partake in fasting and provide guidance and support (164).

SECTION 10: PSYCHOSOCIAL CARE
Type 1 diabetes is a psychologically challenging chronic condition, with treatment outcomes highly dependent on the person's ongoing self-

care behaviors. Cognitive, emotional, and social factors are critical determinants of self-care behaviors and, consequently, treatment success (165,166). Emotional health is an important focus and outcome of person-centered diabetes care (167).

Psychosocial Problems

Diabetes-specific emotional distress affects 20–40% of people with type 1 diabetes and can be experienced at any point in time from early adulthood to older age. Two "critical" times, however, are following the diagnosis and when complications develop (168). Feeling powerless and overwhelmed by the daily self-care demands, fear of hypoglycemia, and worries about complications are among the most cited sources of distress by people with type 1 diabetes. Prolonged significant diabetes distress is associated with depressed mood and elevated HbA$_{1c}$ levels (169).

Lack of social support or feeling "policed" by family, friends, or coworkers also evokes emotional distress in individuals with type 1 diabetes (170). Conversely, social support is a protective factor, serving as a buffer against stress. Depression and anxiety symptoms are twice as prevalent among people with type 1 diabetes relative to people without diabetes, negatively impacting quality of life (171–173). Anxiety and depression often coexist and may partly overlap with symptoms of diabetes distress (174). Psychological distress, including mild to major depression, is a risk factor for poor self-care, hyperglycemia, complications, and excess mortality (174–176). The association between generalized anxiety and suboptimal blood glucose levels is less clear (177, 178).

Given the high prevalence and impact of psychosocial problems and psychological disorders in diabetes, screening and monitoring should be integral parts of diabetes care, not least because these psychological comorbidities tend to negatively affect diabetes outcomes and vice versa. Validated screening tools that can help to "flag" psychological problems that may require follow-up or referral to a mental health specialist have been developed for most problem areas and are available in multiple languages. Clinicians engaging in screening

need to understand the psychological and social issues that may complicate diabetes management, have good communication skills, and be able to refer to specialized mental health services where appropriate. Recently, a working group from the International Consortium for Health Outcomes Measurement (ICHOM) made recommendations for a standard set of practical and validated psychosocial measures (179), including the WHO-5 Well-Being Index (WHO-5) (180), Problem Areas in Diabetes (PAID) scale (181), and Patient Health Questionnaire (PHQ-9) (182). Completion of these three questionnaires takes approximately 7 min and can be scheduled prior to the visit, either online or in the waiting room. For generalized anxiety, the Generalized Anxiety Disorder 7-item (GAD-7) is recommended (183). Brief screeners for depression (two items) (184), depression and anxiety (four items) (185) and diabetes distress (five or two items) (186,187) are also available.

Assessment and periodic monitoring of emotional health, at least on an annual basis, is recommended to promote case-finding, emotional well-being, and patient satisfaction with care (188, 189). This may require changes to current service provision, for example, inviting people with diabetes to complete standardized questionnaires prior to their consultation.

Fear of hypoglycemia affects up to 10% of adults with type 1 diabetes, particularly among those experiencing repeated episodes of level 3 hypoglycemia (190). Fear of hypoglycemia may translate into avoidance behaviors aimed at keeping blood glucose at a "safe" level, resulting in persistent hyperglycemia (191). In cases of problematic fear of hypoglycemia, administering the Hypoglycemia Fear Survey (HFS) can help to identify specific worries and level of severity (192). Both disproportional high and low fear of hypoglycemia warrant attention.

Eating disorders, including anorexia nervosa, bulimia nervosa, and binge eating, are overrepresented in type 1 diabetes populations, particularly in young women (193,194) but may also occur in men. Insulin omission as a weight-loss strategy ("diabulimia") often starting in teenage years warrants special attention (195,196). If indicated, screening for

eating disorders is advised, using a validated instrument suited for use in people with type 1 diabetes, for example, the Diabetes Eating Problems Survey-Revised (DEPS-R) or Eating Disorders Inventory-3 Risk Composite (EDI-3RC) (197).

In case of a positive screen, offering a referral to specialized mental health services is recommended.

Social Determinants of Health

Social and financial hardships can negatively impact an individual's mental health, motivation, and capacity to engage in self-management practices, increasing the risk for elevated HbA$_{1c}$ and complications. In a review of social determinants of health and diabetes (198), the importance of the following domains is discussed: 1) neighborhood and physical environment (e.g., housing stability); 2) built environment (e.g., walkability, access to green spaces); 3) environmental exposures (e.g., pollution); 4) food access, availability, and affordability; and 5) health care access, affordability, and quality.

Socioeconomic challenges, particularly the inability to pay for food, insulin, other medications, and supplies, need to be recognized and addressed. Several screening tools are available (199–204). Sample questions that have been used include: How hard is it for you to pay for the very basics like food, housing, medical care, and heating? At any time since the last interview or in the last 2 years have you ended up taking less insulin than was prescribed for you because of cost? In the past 12 months has lack of transportation kept you from attending medical appointments or from getting insulin? The diabetes team should have access to a social worker and/or links to community resources to help those with these needs.

Psychosocial Interventions

All members of the diabetes care team have a responsibility for providing psychosocial care as an integral component of diabetes care. Preferably, the diabetes care team should include a mental health professional (psychiatrist, psychologist, and/or social worker) to advise the team and consult with people with diabetes in need of psychosocial support (205). Three levels of psychosocial support can be

Simplified overview of indications for β-cell replacement therapy in people with type 1 diabetes

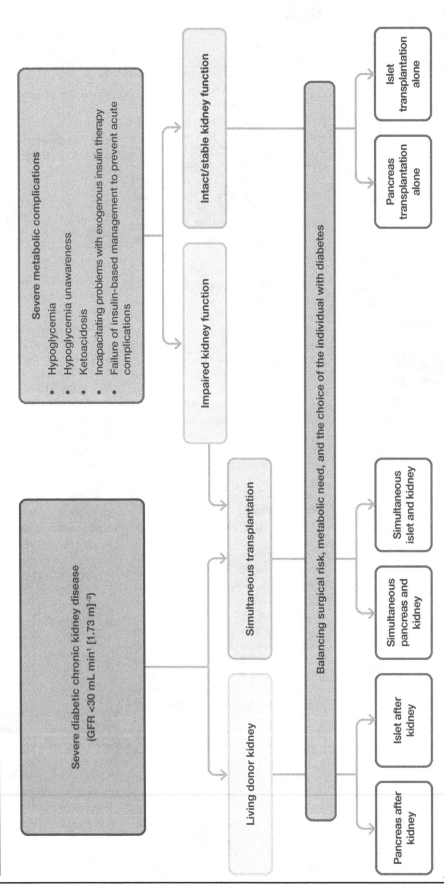

Figure 7—Simplified overview of indications for β-cell replacement therapy in people with type 1 diabetes. The two main forms of β-cell replacement therapy are whole-pancreas transplantation or islet cell transplantation. β-cell replacement therapy can be combined with kidney transplantation if the individual has end-stage renal disease, which may be performed simultaneously or after kidney transplantation. All decisions about transplantation must balance the surgical risk, metabolic need, and the choice of the individual with diabetes.

distinguished, and diabetes teams have an important role in all three levels.

At the first level, people living with type 1 diabetes do not require professional mental health care. They may engage in self-help programs and/or receive informal coaching, as well as family, peer, and community support to assist them in coping with the psychological demands of self-managing type 1 diabetes as well as socioeconomic challenges. At the second level, which concerns approximately one-quarter of individuals with type 1 diabetes, some degree of professional psychosocial support is warranted. Support for social needs can be provided by a social worker and/or community organization. It is important that therapists have a good understanding of diabetes treatments and integrate diabetes management in the psychological treatment. Psychological therapies, including time-limited (online) cognitive behavioral therapy (CBT), mindfulness, and interpersonal therapies are effective with regard to a range of psychological outcomes, including diabetes distress and depression. The effects of psychotherapy on glycemic levels are generally small but tend to increase when diabetes self-management education is incorporated in the treatment (206). Approximately 5% of the adults with type 1 diabetes are in need of psychiatric treatment, the third level, which may involve psychotropic medication that can have an impact on glycemic management. Psychiatric comorbidities, such as anorexia nervosa and schizophrenia, require close collaboration between the mental health specialist and diabetes care team (207,208).

SECTION 11: DIABETIC KETOACIDOSIS

DKA is a life-threatening but preventable acute complication of type 1 diabetes, characterized by hyperglycemia, metabolic acidosis, and ketosis. There are times when the glucose levels are normal or only minimally elevated. The underlying cause is insulin deficiency, either absolute (new diagnosis of type 1 diabetes or omission of insulin in those with diagnosed disease) or relative (increased counterregulatory hormones due to infection or other stressors without an adequate increase in insulin doses).

The prevalence of DKA and risk factors for the complication have been less-well studied in adults with type 1

diabetes than in children. In the U.S., national surveillance of emergency department visits and hospital admissions suggests a rate of 28 cases per 1,000 adults with diabetes per year, with a worrisome increase in emergency department visits and admissions for DKA seen since 2009 (209). The U.S. Type 1 Diabetes Exchange Clinic Network reported that 4.8% of participants (age 26 to 93 years) had been hospitalized for DKA in the prior year (41). In a European (predominantly Germany and Austria) registry, adults with type 1 diabetes had DKA at a rate of 2.5 per 100 patient-years (210).

As DKA occurs repeatedly in some people with diabetes, risk factors should be identified and approached in a prevention strategy. Some known risk factors are nonmodifiable, such as low socioeconomic status, younger age, female sex, and ethnicity (41,210), whereas other factors associated with increased risk of DKA are potentially modifiable. These include having had one previous episode of DKA, high HbA_{1c}, low self-management skills (including omission of insulin therapy), psychiatric disorders, infections, somatic comorbidity, alcohol and drug abuse and less interaction with the health care team (211–213). Older studies demonstrated a higher risk of DKA in those using insulin pumps, likely due to the lack of depot insulin when continuous delivery of insulin is disrupted (214). However, more recent studies have not found this to be the case (41,210, 215). Adjunctive use of sodium–glucose cotransporter (SGLT) inhibitors (see below) in adults with type 1 diabetes increases the risk of DKA by an absolute rate of about 4% per year, suggesting the need for intensive diabetes self-management education and monitoring (216,217). DKA in the setting of SGLT inhibitor use is often so-called euglycemic DKA, with initial case reports describing admission glucose levels of 5.3–12.4 mmol/L (96–224 mg/dL) (218).

Diabetes self-management education is an effective tool in reducing DKA risk. Additional medical, behavioral health interventions, including home ketone testing, and psychosocial support are often needed. Telemedicine offers the potential to reach populations with decreased access to care, and 24 h access to advice about managing hyperglycemia and ketosis/ketonemia at home can

reduce the risk of hospital admission (211).

A detailed description of the management of DKA is beyond the scope of this report but the general principles of treatment are replacement of fluid, insulin, and potassium. Different protocols for DKA treatment exist in different parts of the world (219,220). For further information regarding treatment, refer to previous reviews (221,222).

SECTION 12: PANCREAS AND ISLET TRANSPLANTATION

Whole organ pancreas and pancreatic islet transplantation are currently the only means of clinical β-cell replacement (Fig. 7). Both therapeutic options can effectively prevent hypoglycemia, restore normoglycemia, and possibly stabilize the progression of complications of type 1 diabetes (223–227). However, chronic systemic immunosuppression is needed in both forms to prevent allogeneic rejection. Therefore, the indication must thoroughly balance risk and benefit, taking into consideration psychological factors as well (228). In the U.S., islet transplantation is not yet approved for clinical use and reimbursement.

Most whole-pancreas transplants are performed simultaneously with a kidney transplant (simultaneous pancreas and kidney [SPK] transplant). This is the "gold-standard" therapy for people with type 1 diabetes and pre-final or end-stage renal disease if no contraindications (malignancies, chronic infections, insufficient self-management, and severe cardiovascular conditions) are present. SPK transplants show a 5-year pancreas graft survival of 83% and are superior to pancreas transplants alone (PTA) or pancreas after a kidney transplant (55% and 70%, respectively) (229). With an SPK transplant, most recipients can expect amelioration of problematic hypoglycemia for more than a decade (229–231).

PTA are usually performed in people who are relatively young (<50 years) and do not have obesity (<30 kg/m^2) or coronary artery disease. These selection criteria minimize operative mortality (<1%) and reduce early technical pancreas graft loss (<10%) (229,232). The main indications are a history of frequent, acute, and severe metabolic complications (hypoglycemia, hyperglycemia, ketoacidosis), clinical and emotional

Table 6—Adjunctive therapies for type 1 diabetes

Variable	Metformin	Pramlintide	GLP-1 RA	SGLT-2 or SGLT-1/2 inhibitors
HbA$_{1c}$ reduction	~1 mmol/mol (~0.1%)	3–4 mmol/mol (0.3–0.4%)	2–4 mmol/mol (0.2–0.4%)	2–4 mmol/mol (0.2–0.4%)
Fasting glucose	Minimal effect	No effect	Minimal effect	Modest decrease (0.8 mmol/L [15 mg/dL])
Postprandial glucose	Minimal effect	Significant decrease	Modest decrease	Modest decrease
TIR	No data	No data	No data	Increased (~12% at higher doses)
Insulin dose	Unchanged	Mealtime reductions	Predominantly mealtime reductions	Mealtime and basal reductions (~10% total reduction)
Body weight	Modest (~1 kg)	Modest (~1 kg)	Significant (~5 kg)	Moderate (2–3 kg)
Systolic blood pressure	No change	No change	4 mmHg decrease (with increase in heart rate)	3–4 mmHg decrease
Hypoglycemia	Low risk	Potential increase in level 3 hypoglycemia if prandial insulin doses are not decreased	Increase in hypoglycemia	Low risk
Side effects	GI side effects	GI side effects	GI side effects; increase in ketosis	Genital mycotic infections; increased risk of DKA
Approval status for type 1 diabetes in EU/U.S.	Not currently approved	U.S. approved	Not currently approved	EU approved low dose when BMI ≥27 kg/m^2
Specific groups for whom treatment may be of benefit	Women with polycystic ovary syndrome	No specific groups	Overweight and obese; high insulin dose; risk of cardiovascular and renal disease	Risk of cardiovascular and renal disease

EU, European Union; GI, gastrointestinal.

problems with exogenous insulin therapy that are incapacitating, or consistent failure of insulin-based management, including technological aids (233).

Islet transplantation, a less invasive procedure, is indicated in people with excessive glycemic lability and frequent level 3 hypoglycemia despite optimal medical therapy, and allows for inclusion of older people and those with coronary artery disease who would not be eligible for a whole-pancreas transplant (224,234, 235). Careful patient selection and protocol optimization have led to substantial clinical improvements (224). Insulin independence can be maintained for 5 years in 50% of recipients (236,237). Although achievement of insulin independence remains an important objective, several multicenter clinical trials of islet transplants in people with type 1 diabetes and problematic hypoglycemia have adopted a combination of near-normal glycemic levels (HbA$_{1c}$ <7.0% [<53 mmol/mol]) together with the elimination of level 3

hypoglycemia as the primary end point and the clinically relevant dual goal of intervention (238–240). These outcomes can translate into improved patient-reported outcomes, but research in this area is limited (241).

Regardless of the β-cell replacement approach (pancreas or islets), the majority of recipients experience reliable prevention of problematic hypoglycemia with near-normal glycemic levels. Islet and pancreas transplants are the only approaches to date that confer both sustained recovery from IAH and restoration of glucose counterregulation and, thereby, reliable protection from level 3 hypoglycemia in people with long-standing type 1 diabetes (242). However, these approaches have not been compared with the newer systems of hybrid closed-loop technology, which might render immunosuppression requiring therapies less necessary, in large long-term studies (243).

SECTION 13: ADJUNCTIVE THERAPIES

While insulin therapy is essential for people with type 1 diabetes, obtaining glycemic goals with insulin alone is difficult because of the risks of hypoglycemia. Furthermore, insulin therapy is often associated with undesirable weight gain, which may worsen insulin resistance, does not address other pathophysiological abnormalities, such as α-cell dysfunction, and does not wholly protect individuals from an increased risk of cardiovascular disease or other complications. Adjunctive therapies aim to augment insulin therapy by addressing some of these critical unmet needs.

To date, although several drugs have been licensed as adjunctive therapies, the evidence of their effectiveness on clinically relevant outcomes other than blood glucose levels, such as cardiovascular and renal disease, is limited. It is not possible to make a general recommendation about their use, but they can be considered in individual cases (Table 6). However, before these drugs are prescribed, insulin therapy should be optimized.

Metformin

Metformin has been evaluated in numerous small trials in people with type 1 diabetes with hopes that its insulin-sensitizing properties would improve glycemic management and/or reduce cardiovascular risk (244,245). The largest study to date assessed the use of metformin 1 g, twice daily, in 428 people with type 1 diabetes who were treated for 3 years, with a primary end point of changes in mean carotid intima–media thickness, a marker of cardiovascular disease risk. The study ultimately found no difference in the primary end point, minimal and nonsustained effects on HbA$_{1c}$, minimal effects on weight (~1 kg reduction), and no change in total daily insulin dose (246).

Pramlintide

Pramlintide, an amylin analog, is approved for therapeutic use as an adjunctive therapy to insulin in the U.S., but not in Europe. It remains the only U.S. Food and Drug Administration (FDA)-approved adjunctive therapy for type 1 diabetes. Injection prior to meals acts to suppress glucagon secretion, delay gastric emptying, and promote satiety (247–250). Clinical trials have shown a reduction in HbA$_{1c}$ (0.3–0.4% [3–4 mmol/mol]) and modest (~1 kg) weight loss (251–254). As a result of its adverse effects and need for additional injections, clinical uptake of pramlintide has been limited. However, co-formulations of amylin with insulin are currently in development, as is the possibility of use of pramlintide in pumps or artificial pancreas systems.

Glucagon-Like Peptide 1 Receptor Agonists

Glucagon-like peptide 1 receptor agonists (GLP-1 RA) have been explored in people with type 1 diabetes for two indications; the first aimed to ameliorate β-cell decline at the time of diagnosis and there are ongoing trials of this approach. In one study of 308 people with recently diagnosed type 1 diabetes, liraglutide, when used in combination with anti-IL-21, preserved β-cell function (255). The second

indication is as an adjunctive therapy in established type 1 diabetes by blunting glucagon secretion, decreasing gastric emptying, and promoting satiety and weight loss (256). The largest clinical trials in people with type 1 diabetes were conducted with liraglutide and showed decreases in HbA$_{1c}$ at daily doses of 1.8 mg (0.2–0.4% [2–4 mmol/mol]), decreases in weight (~5 kg), and reductions in insulin doses (257,258). However, increased rates of hypoglycemia and ketosis were shown. Subgroup analysis in people with residual C-peptide production suggests greater HbA$_{1c}$ reduction and improved safety, with lower risk of ketosis. Trials in people with type 2 diabetes have shown convincing reductions in cardiovascular events with some GLP-1 RA (259); whether these benefits would also be seen in people with type 1 diabetes is unknown. GLP-1 RA have been approved for management of obesity, but not in people with type 1 diabetes. However, given the clinical trial results in people without type 1 diabetes (260), these agents may have a role for those with type 1 diabetes who have concomitant obesity.

SGLT Inhibitors

In several phase III programs in people with type 1 diabetes, the use of SGLT-1 or SGLT-1/2 inhibitors reduced HbA$_{1c}$, improved TIR, reduced body weight, and improved blood pressure (244). However, an increased rate of DKA led to rejection of market authorization for type 1 diabetes by the FDA, whereas the European Medicines Agency has approved low-dose dapagliflozin (5 mg) and sotagliflozin (200 mg) for those with a BMI ≥27 kg/m^2 (261). While no risk mitigation strategies have been proven to lower the risk of DKA, a consensus statement on SGLT2 inhibitors and DKA suggested careful patient selection, appropriate insulin dose adjustment to avoid insulinopenia, starting with a low dose of SGLT2 inhibitors, and regular ketone measurements with prompt action to address elevated values as sensible precautions aimed at preventing DKA (216).

In people with type 2 diabetes, improved cardiovascular outcomes, mainly due to a reduction in congestive heart failure, and improved renal outcomes have been established, but there are only limited data on the applicability of these

findings to people with type 1 diabetes (262,263). However, increasingly, data on SGLT2 inhibitors have shown renal and heart failure benefits in people without diabetes, suggesting that people with type 1 diabetes and these comorbidities may also benefit.

SECTION 14: SPECIAL POPULATIONS

Pregnancy Including Preconception and Postnatal Care

Both maternal and fetal pregnancy outcomes are worse in women with type 1 diabetes compared with women without diabetes. Hyperglycemia before and during pregnancy increases the risk of complications in the pregnant woman and developing fetus and, also, affects further child development. Thus, women should be supported to achieve blood glucose ranges close to those seen in pregnant women without diabetes, with an HbA$_{1c}$ target of 48 mmol/mol (≤6.5%) (264,265). Women should aim for fasting and pre-meal glucose concentrations below 5.3 mmol/L (95 mg/dL), and postprandial values of below 7.8 mmol/L (140 mg/dL) 1 h after a meal and below 6.7 mmol/L (120 mg/dL) 2 h after a meal. Although CGM is not approved in the U.S. for use in pregnancy and no studies in pregnancy have used CGM alone, the Continuous Glucose Monitoring in Women With Type 1 Diabetes in Pregnancy Trial (CONCEPTT) showed that when CGM was used in conjunction with BGM, CGM was associated with better pregnancy outcomes (266) and is widely recommended in Europe. Many women rely on CGM during pregnancy and its use should be encouraged with the caveat that BGM should be performed if there are concerns that the CGM reading is inaccurate. When CGM is used in pregnancy, the target range is lower than outside of pregnancy (3.5–7.8 mmol/L [63–140 mg/dL]).

The major limiting step to achieving normoglycemia is hypoglycemia, which occurs more frequently in the first half of pregnancy, in part because of diminished awareness of hypoglycemia and pregnancy-associated nausea and vomiting (267). Pregnant women with type 1 diabetes are at risk for DKA at lower blood glucose levels than in the nonpregnant state and should receive education on DKA prevention and detection (268). Postpartum breastfeeding, erratic sleep and eating schedules may increase the risk of hypoglycemia and insulin dosing may require adjustment (269,270).

The management of pregnancy begins before conception as a planned pregnancy is associated with improved outcomes for both the women and offspring. Effective contraception should be used until the woman is ready for pregnancy. Choice of a safe and reliable method of contraception should be based on the preference of the woman, her individual risk factors, such as the presence of micro- or macrovascular complications, and the WHO Medical Eligibility Criteria for Contraceptive Use (271).

All women of childbearing age with type 1 diabetes should be informed about the importance of seeking professional help prior to trying to conceive; this provides an opportunity not only to improve glycemic management but to offer folic acid to prevent neural tube defects, screen for diabetes-related complications, and stop potentially teratogenic medications.

Diabetes in pregnancy is best managed by a multidisciplinary team, including a diabetologist/endocrinologist, obstetrician, dietitian, diabetes nurse/educator, and diabetes midwife. A detailed description of the management of pregnancy in women with type 1 diabetes is beyond the scope of this report but is available elsewhere (272,273).

Older People With Type 1 Diabetes

Insulin regimens in older adults should be individualized and patient safety is a key priority. Glycemic targets should be based on functional status and life expectancy, rather than chronological age. As older adults with type 1 diabetes are especially vulnerable to hypoglycemia, target glucose values should be adjusted to minimize the occurrence of hypoglycemic events. Since, in some older adults with type 1 diabetes, administration of insulin may become more difficult, simplification of insulin management may be justified in cases of individuals with complications or functional or cognitive impairment. The use of advanced technologies in older individuals is useful and should not be discontinued or a priori

excluded because of the older age (78,274).

People With Late Complications of Type 1 Diabetes

As there is no evidence that intensive glycemic management slows the progression of late microvascular complications of diabetes, glycemic targets in individuals with advanced complications should be individualized and based on the balance of risks and benefits (39,275). Diabetes management may be particularly challenging in individuals with chronic kidney disease who may be at an increased risk of hypoglycemia and in whom HbA_{1c} can be falsely low (276) and in people with gastroparesis and unpredictable rates of food absorption (277). The rate of optimizing blood glucose levels in this group of people should also be individualized as rapid improvement may be associated with transient early worsening of retinopathy or the development of acute painful neuropathy (278,279). In people with cardiovascular complications, hypoglycemia avoidance should be one of the management priorities (280).

SECTION 15: INPATIENT MANAGEMENT OF TYPE 1 DIABETES

There have been no large RCTs specifically assessing glycemic targets for inpatients with type 1 diabetes. Therefore, type 2 diabetes guidelines should be followed, which recommend target glucose ranges of 7.8–10.0 mmol/L (140–180 mg/dL) for the majority of noncritically and critically ill patients (281). However, it is important that the health care team recognizes key differences between type 1 diabetes and type 2 diabetes. People with type 1 diabetes, particularly those with concomitant chronic kidney disease, are at higher risk of hypoglycemia, which should be avoided by careful insulin and carbohydrate matching (129). Furthermore, people with type 1 diabetes are at high risk of developing ketosis if insulin is withheld (282). People with type 1 diabetes often find the inpatient care of their diabetes stressful and disempowering. A major issue for some inpatients with type 1 diabetes care is coping with fixed meal timings. Therefore, inpatients with type 1 diabetes should be clearly identified to avoid common errors, such as

omission of mealtime insulin or withholding of basal insulin for procedures or surgery.

Inpatient services should have protocols to allow people who can monitor their glucose and self-administer insulin safely to do so. Similarly, patients using diabetes devices should be allowed to use them in an inpatient setting or during outpatient procedures when proper supervision is available and the patient/caregiver is capable of managing the device(s) (283). Whenever a dedicated inpatient diabetes service is available, they should be consulted for glycemic management, DSMES, and discharge planning (284). Finally, the use of diabetes technology (CGM and insulin pumps) can be continued in selected, noncritically ill patients with clear mentation and previous training and education (285,286). Institutions should develop clear guidelines to manage inpatient type 1 diabetes safely.

SECTION 16: EMERGENT AND FUTURE PERSPECTIVES

Both xenotransplantation with porcine islets and human stem cells are under investigation to solve the problem of limited availability of donors for pancreas or islet transplantation (287). Stem cell strategies have used either patient-specific stem cells or universal allogeneic cells. In the former, the patient's own stem cells are reprogrammed or transdifferentiated to become β-cells. By contrast, generic allogeneic cells may be used for multiple patients and centrally produced from a bank of human embryonic stem cells (hESCs) or of induced pluripotent stem cells (iPSCs). One of the key issues is protecting the cells from immune attack, both rejection and recurrent autoimmunity. Three general strategies are being investigated: 1) use of immunosuppressive or immunomodulatory drugs; 2) use of a physical barrier (e.g., encapsulation) (288); and 3) gene editing for immune evasion and/or immune protection (289). Both academic and commercial groups are pursuing these approaches and some are already in clinical trials.

Immunotherapy approaches are being evaluated for their potential use in stage 1 (≥2 islet autoantibodies but normoglycemia) or stage 2 (autoantibodies and dysglycemia) type 1 diabetes to prevent stage 3 clinical type 1 diabetes, and for the preservation of β-cell function before and shortly after onset of stage 3 clinical type 1 diabetes (290). Many interventions have been tested in clinical trials but, to date, the most promising results have been from the anti-CD3 monoclonal antibody teplizumab, low-dose antithymocyte globulin (ATG), and the anti-TNF drug, golimumab. These have been shown to preserve β-cell function in recent-onset type 1 diabetes, and teplizumab also has delayed the clinical onset of type 1 diabetes. Several other trials are underway with the hope of not only preserving but even improving β-cell function and being able to interdict the type 1 diabetes disease process sufficiently to prevent the development of the disease.

SECTION 17: CONCLUSION

This report has covered many areas of the management of type 1 diabetes; however, the writing group recognizes that huge gaps exist in our knowledge in the prevention, diagnosis, and treatment of the disease. People with type 1 diabetes deserve better, higher quality research evidence on which to determine their optimal care. We are also aware of the inequalities in treatment experienced by many people with type 1 diabetes and we must advocate for better services to ensure that all individuals with type 1 diabetes have access to the care they need.

Acknowledgments. We acknowledge the support of M.I. Hill, M. Saraco, and R.A. Gabbay (all ADA, Arlington, VA), and P. Niemann, N. Buckley-Mühge, and M. Gruesser (all EASD, Dusseldorf, Germany), the Committee for Clinical Affairs of the EASD, and the Professional Practice Committee of the ADA. We acknowledge A. Jones (University of Exeter, Exeter, U.K.) for his invaluable help with the "Diagnosis of Type 1 Diabetes" section. We also acknowledge D.F. Kruger (Henry Ford Health System, Detroit, MI), G. Aleppo (Northwestern University, Chicago, IL), D. Schatz (University of Florida, Gainesville, FL), J. Speight (Australian Centre for Behavioural Research in Diabetes, Melbourne, VIC, Australia), A.-G. Ziegler (Technical University of Munich, Munich, Germany), and C. Mathieu (Katholieke Universiteit Leuven, Leuven, Belgium) for serving as internal peer reviewers for the EASD and ADA. We would like to thank C. Franklin and M. Bonar of the Leicester Diabetes Centre (Leicester, U.K.) for the graphic design of the figures and R.M. Bergenstal and the International Diabetes Center, Minneapolis (MN), for the ambulatory glucose profile (AGP) figure (Fig. 2).
Funding. The report was jointly commissioned and funded by the ADA and EASD. The authors did not receive any payment for their involvement in the writing group.

Duality of Interest. R.I.G.H. serves on the speakers' bureau for and receives research support from Novo Nordisk. He serves on the speakers' bureau for Abbott, Eli Lilly, Otsuka, and Roche. He also served as the Editor-in-Chief of *Diabetic Medicine* until December 2020. J.H.D. received research funding from Afon, Eli Lilly, and Novo Nordisk. He served on advisory boards for Adocia, Novo Nordisk, and Zealand Pharma and was on a speaker's bureau for Novo Nordisk. A.H.-F. is an auditor for the ADA's Education Recognition Program. She is a participant in a speaker's bureau for Abbott Diabetes Care and Xeris. She is also a member of Xeris' advisory board. I.B.H. receives industry research funding from Medtronic Diabetes, Insulet, and Beta Bionics. He is a consultant for Bigfoot, Roche, and Abbott Diabetes Care. M.S.K. receives research funding from Novo Nordisk and Bayer. T.K. has served on advisory boards for Abbott, Ascensia, Bioton, Boehringer Ingelheim, Dexcom, Eli Lilly, Medtronic, Roche, Sanofi, and Ypsomed. He has received research funding from Medtronic and is a participant in a speakers' bureau for Abbott, Ascensia, Bioton, Boehringer Ingelheim, Eli Lilly, Medtronic, Novo Nordisk, Roche, Sanofi, and Servier. B.L. declares that there are no relationships or activities that might bias, or be perceived to bias, their work. K.N. receives research funding from, is a member of the advisory board for, and is a stockholder in Novo Nordisk. She is an advisory board member for Medtronic and Abbott Diabetes Care and receives research funding from Dexcom, Medtronic, and Zealand Pharma. J.P. is a consultant to Sanofi, Novo Nordisk, Eli Lilly, Zealand, Mannkind, and Diasome. E.R. serves on the advisory board for Abbott, Air Liquide SI, Dexcom, Insulet, Sanofi, Roche, Novo Nordisk, and Eli Lilly, and received research support from Dexcom and Tandem. J.S.S. is a member of the board of directors for Applied Therapeutics and Dexcom. He serves on the scientific advisory board for Abvance, ActoBiotics, Adocia, Avotres, Oramed, Orgenesis, Sanofi Diabetes, Tolerion, and Viacyte. He received research support from Tolerion. He is an advisor and consultant to Boehringer Ingelheim, Dance Biopharm/Aerami Therapeutics, Enthera, Ideal Life, Imcyse, Immnomolecular Therapeutics, Novo Nordisk, Provention Bio, Sanofi Diabetes, Signos, Tolerion, and VielaBio. He is a shareholder or option holder in Abvance, Avotres, Dance Biopharm/Aerami Therapeutics, Dexcom, Ideal Life, Immnomolecular Therapeutics, Oramed, and Orgenesis. F.J.S. is consultant to Abbott, Eli Lilly, Sanofi, and Novo Nordisk, and serves on the speakers' bureau for Abbott, Eli Lilly, Sanofi, and Novo Nordisk. He has received research funding from Sanofi and Novo Nordisk. R.S.W. receives research funding from Eli Lilly, Medtronic, Insulet, Diasome, Kowa, Tolerion, Novo Nordisk, and Boehringer Ingelheim. A.L.P. serves on the advisory board for Abbott Diabetes Care, Eli Lilly, Novo Nordisk, Medscape, and Zealand Pharmaceuticals. She has received research support from Dexcom and Insulet and has received donated devices from Abbott Diabetes Care. She also has stock options from Omada Health and Livongo and is a special government employee of the FDA. No other potential conflicts of interest relevant to this article were reported.
Author Contributions. R.I.G.H. and A.L.P. were co-chairs for the consensus report

writing group. A.H.-F., I.B.H., M.S.K., J.P., J.S.S., and R.S.W. were the writing group members for the ADA. J.H.D., T.K., B.L., K.N., E.R., and F.J.S. were the writing group members for the EASD. All authors were responsible for drafting the report and revising it critically for important intellectual content. All authors approved the version to be published.

References

1. Miller RG, Secrest AM, Sharma RK, Songer TJ, Orchard TJ. Improvements in the life expectancy of type 1 diabetes: the Pittsburgh Epidemiology of Diabetes Complications study cohort. Diabetes 2012;61:2987–2992
2. Mobasseri M, Shirmohammadi M, Amiri T, Vahed N, Hosseini Fard H, Ghojazadeh M. Prevalence and incidence of type 1 diabetes in the world: a systematic review and meta-analysis. Health Promot Perspect 2020;10:98–115
3. Hirsch IB, Juneja R, Beals JM, Antalis CJ, Wright EE. The evolution of insulin and how it informs therapy and treatment choices. Endocr Rev 2020;41:733–755
4. Stamatouli AM, Quandt Z, Perdigoto AL, et al. Collateral damage: insulin-dependent diabetes induced with checkpoint inhibitors. Diabetes 2018;67:1471–1480
5. Davis AK, DuBose SN, Haller MJ, et al.; T1D Exchange Clinic Network. Prevalence of detectable C-peptide according to age at diagnosis and duration of type 1 diabetes. Diabetes Care 2015;38:476–481
6. Thomas NJ, Lynam AL, Hill AV, et al. Type 1 diabetes defined by severe insulin deficiency occurs after 30 years of age and is commonly treated as type 2 diabetes. Diabetologia 2019;62:1167–1172
7. Muñoz C, Floreen A, Garey C, et al. Misdiagnosis and diabetic ketoacidosis at diagnosis of type 1 diabetes: patient and caregiver perspectives. Clin Diabetes 2019;37:276–281
8. Hope SV, Wienand-Barnett S, Shepherd M, et al. Practical classification guidelines for diabetes in patients treated with insulin: a cross-sectional study of the accuracy of diabetes diagnosis. Br J Gen Pract 2016;66:e315–e322
9. Shields BM, Peters JL, Cooper C, et al. Can clinical features be used to differentiate type 1 from type 2 diabetes? A systematic review of the literature. BMJ Open 2015;5:e009088
10. Jones AG, Hill AV, Trippett PW, Hattersley AT, McDonald TJ, Shields BM. The utility of clinical features and glycaemia at diagnosis in classifying young adult onset diabetes (Abstract). Published 19 September 2019. Accessed 23 August 2021. Available from www.easd.org/virtualmeeting/home.html#!resources/the-utility-of-clinical-features-and-glycaemia-at-diagnosis-in-classifying-young-adult-onset-diabetes
11. Thomas NJ, Jones SE, Weedon MN, Shields BM, Oram RA, Hattersley AT. Frequency and phenotype of type 1 diabetes in the first six decades of life: a cross-sectional, genetically stratified survival analysis from UK Biobank. Lancet Diabetes Endocrinol 2018;6:122–129
12. Hillier TA, Pedula KL. Characteristics of an adult population with newly diagnosed type 2 diabetes: the relation of obesity and age of onset. Diabetes Care 2001;24:1522–1527
13. Westphal SA. The occurrence of diabetic ketoacidosis in non-insulin-dependent diabetes

and newly diagnosed diabetic adults. Am J Med 1996;101:19–24

14. Nakagami T, Qiao Q, Carstensen B, et al.; DECODE-DECODA Study Group. Age, body mass index and type 2 diabetes-associations modified by ethnicity. Diabetologia 2003;46:1063–1070

15. Prior MJ, Prout T, Miller D, Ewart R; The ETDRS Research Group. C-peptide and the classification of diabetes mellitus patients in the Early Treatment Diabetic Retinopathy Study. Report number 6. Ann Epidemiol 1993;3:9–17

16. Chung WK, Erion K, Florez JC, et al. Precision medicine in diabetes: a consensus report from the American Diabetes Association (ADA) and the European Association for the Study of Diabetes (EASD). Diabetologia 2020;63:1671–1693

17. Buzzetti R, Tuomi T, Mauricio D, et al. Management of latent autoimmune diabetes in adults: a consensus statement from an international expert panel. Diabetes 2020;69:2037–2047

18. Shields BM, Shepherd M, Hudson M, et al.; UNITED study team. Population-based assessment of a biomarker-based screening pathway to aid diagnosis of monogenic diabetes in young-onset patients. Diabetes Care 2017;40:1017–1025

19. Pearson ER, Starkey BJ, Powell RJ, Gribble FM, Clark PM, Hattersley AT. Genetic cause of hyperglycaemia and response to treatment in diabetes. Lancet 2003;362:1275–1281

20. Hattersley AT, Greeley SAW, Polak M, et al. ISPAD clinical practice consensus guidelines 2018: the diagnosis and management of monogenic diabetes in children and adolescents. Pediatr Diabetes 2018;19(Suppl. 27):47–63

21. Bingley PJ. Clinical applications of diabetes antibody testing. J Clin Endocrinol Metab 2010;95: 25–33

22. Sabbah E, Savola K, Ebeling T, et al. Genetic, autoimmune, and clinical characteristics of childhood- and adult-onset type 1 diabetes. Diabetes Care 2000;23:1326–1332

23. Littorin B, Sundkvist G, Hagopian W, et al. Islet cell and glutamic acid decarboxylase antibodies present at diagnosis of diabetes predict the need for insulin treatment. A cohort study in young adults whose disease was initially labeled as type 2 or unclassifiable diabetes. Diabetes Care 1999;22:409–412

24. Lynam A, McDonald T, Hill A, et al. Development and validation of multivariable clinical diagnostic models to identify type 1 diabetes requiring rapid insulin therapy in adults aged 18-50 years. BMJ Open 2019;9:e031586

25. Thomas NJ, Walkey HC, Kaur A, et al. The absence of islet autoantibodies in clinically diagnosed older-adult onset type 1 diabetes suggests an alternative pathology, advocating for routine testing in this age group. medRxiv. 24 March 2021 [preprint]. DOI: 10.1101/2021.03.22.21252507

26. Tridgell DM, Spiekerman C, Wang RS, Greenbaum CJ. Interaction of onset and duration of diabetes on the percent of GAD and IA-2 antibody-positive subjects in the type 1 diabetes genetics consortium database. Diabetes Care 2011;34:988–993

27. Balasubramanyam A, Garza G, Rodriguez L, et al. Accuracy and predictive value of classification schemes for ketosis-prone diabetes. Diabetes Care 2006;29:2575–2579

28. Hohberg C, Pfützner A, Forst T, et al. Successful switch from insulin therapy to

treatment with pioglitazone in type 2 diabetes patients with residual beta-cell function: results from the PioSwitch study. Diabetes Obes Metab 2009;11:464–471

29. Lee A, Morley J. Classification of type 2 diabetes by clinical response to metformin-troglitazone combination and C-peptide criteria. Endocr Pract 1999;5:305–313

30. Bell DS, Mayo MS. Improved glycemic control with use of oral hypoglycemic therapy with or without insulin. Endocr Pract 1998;4:82–85

31. Foteinopoulou E, Clarke CAL, Pattenden RJ, et al. Impact of routine clinic measurement of serum C-peptide in people with a clinician-diagnosis of type 1 diabetes. Diabet Med 2021;38:e14449

32. De Franco E, Flanagan SE, Houghton JAL, et al. The effect of early, comprehensive genomic testing on clinical care in neonatal diabetes: an international cohort study. Lancet 2015;386: 957–963

33. Pearson ER, Flechtner I, Njølstad PR, et al.; Neonatal Diabetes International Collaborative Group. Switching from insulin to oral sulfonylureas in patients with diabetes due to Kir6.2 mutations. N Engl J Med 2006;355:467–477

34. Carlsson A, Shepherd M, Ellard S, et al. Absence of islet autoantibodies and modestly raised glucose values at diabetes diagnosis should lead to testing for MODY: lessons from a 5-year pediatric Swedish national cohort study. Diabetes Care 2020;43:82–89

35. Shields BM, McDonald TJ, Ellard S, Campbell MJ, Hyde C, Hattersley AT. The development and validation of a clinical prediction model to determine the probability of MODY in patients with young-onset diabetes. Diabetologia 2012; 55:1265–1272

36. Besser REJ, Shepherd MH, McDonald TJ, et al. Urinary C-peptide creatinine ratio is a practical outpatient tool for identifying hepatocyte nuclear factor 1-α/hepatocyte nuclear factor 4-α maturity-onset diabetes of the young from long-duration type 1 diabetes. Diabetes Care 2011;34:286–291

37. McDonald TJ, Colclough K, Brown R, et al. Islet autoantibodies can discriminate maturity-onset diabetes of the young (MODY) from type 1 diabetes. Diabet Med 2011;28:1028–1033

38. Thanabalasingham G, Pal A, Selwood MP, et al. Systematic assessment of etiology in adults with a clinical diagnosis of young-onset type 2 diabetes is a successful strategy for identifying maturity-onset diabetes of the young. Diabetes Care 2012;35:1206–1212

39. Nathan DM, Genuth S, Lachin J, et al.; Diabetes Control and Complications Trial Research Group. The effect of intensive treatment of diabetes on the development and progression of long-term complications in insulin-dependent diabetes mellitus. N Engl J Med 1993;329: 977–986

40. The Diabetes Control and Complications Trial (DCCT)/Epidemiology of Diabetes Interventions and Complications (EDIC) Study Research Group. Intensive diabetes treatment and cardiovascular outcomes in type 1 diabetes: the DCCT/EDIC study 30-year follow-up. Diabetes Care 2016; 39:686–693

41. Weinstock RS, Xing D, Maahs DM, et al.; T1D Exchange Clinic Network. Severe hypoglycemia and diabetic ketoacidosis in adults with type 1 diabetes:

results from the T1D Exchange clinic registry. J Clin Endocrinol Metab 2013;98:3411–3419

42. Tamborlane WV, Beck RW, Bode BW, et al.; Juvenile Diabetes Research Foundation Continuous Glucose Monitoring Study Group. Continuous glucose monitoring and intensive treatment of type 1 diabetes. N Engl J Med 2008;359:1464–1476

43. Bolinder J, Antuna R, Geelhoed-Duijvestijn P, Kröger J, Weitgasser R. Novel glucose-sensing technology and hypoglycaemia in type 1 diabetes: a multicentre, non-masked, randomised controlled trial. Lancet 2016;388:2254–2263

44. van Beers CAJ, DeVries JH, Kleijer SJ, et al. Continuous glucose monitoring for patients with type 1 diabetes and impaired awareness of hypoglycaemia (IN CONTROL): a randomised, open-label, crossover trial. Lancet Diabetes Endocrinol 2016;4:893–902

45. Beck RW, Bergenstal RM, Riddlesworth TD, et al. Validation of time in range as an outcome measure for diabetes clinical trials. Diabetes Care 2019;42:400–405

46. Ranjan AG, Rosenlund SV, Hansen TW, Rossing P, Andersen S, Nørgaard K. Improved time in range over 1 year is associated with reduced albuminuria in individuals with sensor-augmented insulin pump-treated type 1 diabetes. Diabetes Care 2020;43:2882–2885

47. Battelino T, Danne T, Bergenstal RMA, et al. Clinical targets for continuous glucose monitoring data interpretation: recommendations from the international consensus on time in range. Diabetes Care 2019;42:1593–1603

48. Hero C, Rawshani A, Svensson A-M, et al. Association between use of lipid-lowering therapy and cardiovascular diseases and death in individuals with type 1 diabetes. Diabetes Care 2016;39:996–1003

49. Vistisen D, Andersen GS, Hansen CS, et al. Prediction of first cardiovascular disease event in type 1 diabetes mellitus: the Steno Type 1 Risk Engine. Circulation 2016;133:1058–1066

50. ClinRisk. Welcome to the QRISK3-2018 risk calculator https://qrisk.org/three. Accessed 16 July 2021. Available from https://qrisk.org/three/index.php

51. McGurnaghan SJ, McKeigue PM, Read SH, et al. (2021). CVD risk prediction T1D. Accessed 16 July 2021. Available from https://diabepi.shinyapps.io/cvdrisk/

52. American Diabetes Association. 4. Comprehensive medical evaluation and assessment of comorbidities: *Standards of Medical Care in Diabetes—2021*. Diabetes Care 2021;44(Suppl. 1):S40–S52

53. American Diabetes Association. 7. Diabetes technology: *Standards of Medical Care in Diabetes—2021*. Diabetes Care 2021;44(Suppl. 1):S85–S99

54. Borries TM, Dunbar A, Bhukhen A, et al. The impact of telemedicine on patient self-management processes and clinical outcomes for patients with Types I or II Diabetes Mellitus in the United States: a scoping review. Diabetes Metab Syndr 2019;13:1353–1357

55. Lee JY, Lee SWH. Telemedicine cost-effectiveness for diabetes management: a systematic review. Diabetes Technol Ther 2018;20:492–500

56. Tchero H, Kangambega P, Briatte C, Brunet-Houdard S, Retali G-R, Rusch E. Clinical effectiveness of telemedicine in diabetes mellitus: a

meta-analysis of 42 randomized controlled trials. Telemed J E Health 2019;25:569–583

57. Timpel P, Oswald S, Schwarz PEH, Harst L. Mapping the evidence on the effectiveness of telemedicine interventions in diabetes, dyslipidemia, and hypertension: an umbrella review of systematic reviews and meta-analyses. J Med Internet Res 2020;22:e16791

58. Duke DC, Barry S, Wagner DV, Speight J, Choudhary P, Harris MA. Distal technologies and type 1 diabetes management. Lancet Diabetes Endocrinol 2018;6:143–156

59. Crossen S, Raymond J, Neinstein A. Top 10 tips for successfully implementing a diabetes telehealth program. Diabetes Technol Ther 2020;22:920–928

60. Beck J, Greenwood DA, Blanton L, et al.; 2017 Standards Revision Task Force. 2017 National standards for diabetes self-management education and support. Diabetes Care 2017; 40:1409–1419

61. Diabetes UK. Diabetes self-management education. Accessed 11 February 2021. Available from www.diabetes.org.uk/professionals/resourc es/resources-to-improve-your-clinical-practice/ diabetes-self-management-education

62. Joubert M, Benhamou P-Y, Schaepelynck P, et al. Remote monitoring of diabetes: a cloud-connected digital system for individuals with diabetes and their health care providers. J Diabetes Sci Technol 2019;13:1161–1168

63. Powers MA, Bardsley JK, Cypress M, et al. Diabetes self-management education and support in adults with type 2 diabetes: a consensus report of the American Diabetes Association, the Association of Diabetes Care & Education Specialists, the Academy of Nutrition and Dietetics, the American Academy of Family Physicians, the American Academy of PAs, the American Association of Nurse Practitioners, and the American Pharmacists Association. Diabetes Care 2020;43:1636–1649

64. Chatterjee S, Davies MJ, Heller S, Speight J, Snoek FJ, Khunti K. Diabetes structured self-management education programmes: a narrative review and current innovations. Lancet Diabetes Endocrinol 2018;6:130–142

65. Fleming GA, Petrie JR, Bergenstal RM, Holl RW, Peters AL, Heinemann L. Diabetes digital app technology: benefits, challenges, and recommendations. A consensus report by the European Association for the Study of Diabetes (EASD) and the American Diabetes Association (ADA) Diabetes Technology Working Group. Diabetologia 2020; 63:229–241

66. Nathan DM, Kuenen J, Borg R, Zheng H, Schoenfeld D; A1c-Derived Average Glucose Study Group. Translating the A1C assay into estimated average glucose values. Diabetes Care 2008;31:1473–1478

67. Radin MS. Pitfalls in hemoglobin A1c measurement: when results may be misleading. J Gen Intern Med 2014;29:388–394

68. Beck RW, Connor CG, Mullen DM, Wesley DM, Bergenstal RM. The fallacy of average: how using hba₁c alone to assess glycemic control can be misleading. Diabetes Care 2017;40:994–999

69. Beck RW, Bergenstal RM, Cheng P, et al. The relationships between time in range, hyperglycemia metrics, and HbA1c. J Diabetes Sci Technol 2019;13:614–626

70. Krhač M, Lovrenčić MV. Update on biomarkers of glycemic control. World J Diabetes 2019;10:1–15

71. Miller KM, Beck RW, Bergenstal RM, et al.; T1D Exchange Clinic Network. Evidence of a strong association between frequency of self-monitoring of blood glucose and hemoglobin A1c levels in T1D exchange clinic registry participants. Diabetes Care 2013;36:2009–2014

72. Bode BW, Schwartz S, Stubbs HA, Block JE. Glycemic characteristics in continuously monitored patients with type 1 and type 2 diabetes: normative values. Diabetes Care 2005;28: 2361–2366

73. Moreland EC, Volkening LK, Lawlor MT, Chalmers KA, Anderson BJ, Laffel LMB. Use of a blood glucose monitoring manual to enhance monitoring adherence in adults with diabetes: a randomized controlled trial. Arch Intern Med 2006;166:689–695

74. Draznin B. Diabetes Technology: Science and Practice. Alexandria, VA, American Diabetes Association, 2019

75. Klonoff DC, Parkes JL, Kovatchev BP, et al. Investigation of the accuracy of 18 marketed blood glucose monitors. Diabetes Care 2018;41: 1681–1688

76. Beck RW, Riddlesworth T, Ruedy K, et al.; DIAMOND Study Group. Effect of continuous glucose monitoring on glycemic control in adults with type 1 diabetes using insulin injections: the DIAMOND randomized clinical trial. JAMA 2017;317:371–378

77. Visser MM, Charleer S, Fieuws S, et al. Comparing real-time and intermittently scanned continuous glucose monitoring in adults with type 1 diabetes (ALERTT1): a 6-month, prospective, multicentre, randomised controlled trial. Lancet 2021;397:2275–2283

78. Pratley RE, Kanapka LG, Rickels MR, Ahmann A, Aleppo G, Beck R, et al. Effect of continuous glucose monitoring on hypoglycemia in older adults with type 1 diabetes: a randomized clinical Trial. JAMA 2020;323:2397–2406

79. Bergenstal RM, Ahmann AJ, Bailey T, et al. Recommendations for standardizing glucose reporting and analysis to optimize clinical decision making in diabetes: the Ambulatory Glucose Profile (AGP). Diabetes Technol Ther 2013;15:198–211

80. Beck RW, Bergenstal RM. Beyond A1C—standardization of continuous glucose monitoring reporting: why it is needed and how it continues to evolve. Diabetes Spectr 2021;34:102–108

81. Pleus S, Ulbrich S, Zschornack E, Kamann S, Haug C, Freckmann G. Documentation of skin-related issues associated with continuous glucose monitoring use in the scientific literature. Diabetes Technol Ther 2019;21:538–545

82. Herman A, de Montjoye L, Baeck M. Adverse cutaneous reaction to diabetic glucose sensors and insulin pumps: irritant contact dermatitis or allergic contact dermatitis? Contact Dermat 2020;83:25–30

83. Rigo RS, Levin LE, Belsito DV, Garzon MC, Gandica R, Williams KM. Cutaneous reactions to continuous glucose monitoring and continuous subcutaneous insulin infusion devices in type 1 diabetes mellitus. J Diabetes Sci Technol 2021;15:786–791

84. Deiss D, Irace C, Carlson G, Tweden KS, Kaufman FR. Real-world safety of an implantable continuous glucose sensor over multiple cycles of use: a post-market registry study. Diabetes Technol Ther 2020;22:48–52

85. Sanchez P, Ghosh-Dastidar S, Tweden KS, Kaufman FR. Real-world data from the first u.s. commercial users of an implantable continuous glucose sensor. Diabetes Technol Ther 2019;21: 677–681

86. National Institute for Health and Care Excellence. Type 1 diabetes in adults: diagnosis and management. Accessed 10 June 2021. Available from www.nice.org.uk/guidance/ng17

87. Danne T, Matsuhisa M, Sussebach C, et al. Lower risk of severe hypoglycaemia with insulin glargine 300 U/mL versus glargine 100 U/mL in participants with type 1 diabetes: a meta-analysis of 6-month phase 3 clinical trials. Diabetes Obes Metab 2020;22:1880–1885

88. Lane W, Bailey TS, Gerety G, et al.; Group Information; SWITCH 1. Effect of insulin degludec vs insulin glargine u100 on hypoglycemia in patients with type 1 diabetes: the SWITCH 1 randomized clinical trial. JAMA 2017;318:33–44

89. Šoupal J, Petruželková L, Grunberger G, et al. Glycemic outcomes in adults with T1D are impacted more by continuous glucose monitoring than by insulin delivery method: 3 years of follow-up from the COMISAIR study. Diabetes Care 2020;43:37–43

90. Bergenstal RM, Garg S, Weinzimer SA, et al. Safety of a hybrid closed-loop insulin delivery system in patients with type 1 diabetes. JAMA 2016;316:1407–1408

91. Brown SA, Kovatchev BP, Raghinaru D, et al.; iDCL Trial Research Group. Six-month randomized, multicenter trial of closed-loop control in type 1 diabetes. N Engl J Med 2019;381: 1707–1717

92. Gibney MA, Arce CH, Byron KJ, Hirsch LJ. Skin and subcutaneous adipose layer thickness in adults with diabetes at sites used for insulin injections: implications for needle length recommendations. Curr Med Res Opin 2010;26: 1519–1530

93. Kesavadev J, Srinivasan S, Saboo B, Krishna B M, Krishnan G. The do-it-yourself artificial pancreas: a comprehensive review. Diabetes Ther 2020;11:1217–1235

94. Boughton CK, Hovorka R. The artificial pancreas. Curr Opin Organ Transplant 2020;25: 336–342

95. Famulla S, Hövelmann U, Fischer A, et al. Insulin injection into lipohypertrophic tissue: blunted and more variable insulin absorption and action and impaired postprandial glucose control. Diabetes Care 2016;39:1486–1492

96. Blanco M, Hernández MT, Strauss KW, Amaya M. Prevalence and risk factors of lipohypertrophy in insulin-injecting patients with diabetes. Diabetes Metab 2013;39:445–453

97. McGill JB, Peters A, Buse JB, et al. Comprehensive pulmonary safety review of inhaled Technosphere® insulin in patients with diabetes mellitus. Clin Drug Investig 2020; 40:973–983

98. Spaan N, Teplova A, Stam G, Spaan J, Lucas C. Systematic review: continuous intraperitoneal insulin infusion with implantable insulin pumps for diabetes mellitus. Acta Diabetol 2014; 51:339–351

99. Renard E; EVADIAC Group. Implantable insulin pumps. A position statement about their clinical use. Diabetes Metab 2007;33:158–166

100. International Hypoglycaemia Study Group. Glucose concentrations of less than 3.0 mmol/l (54 mg/dl) should be reported in clinical trials: a joint position statement of the American Diabetes Association and the European Association for the Study of Diabetes. Diabetologia 2017; 60:3–6

101. Heinemann L, Freckmann G, Ehrmann D, et al. Real-time continuous glucose monitoring in adults with type 1 diabetes and impaired hypoglycaemia awareness or severe hypoglycaemia treated with multiple daily insulin injections (HypoDE): a multicentre, randomised controlled trial. Lancet 2018;391:1367–1377

102. Renard E, Ikegami H, Daher Vianna AG, et al. The SAGE study: global observational analysis of glycaemic control, hypoglycaemia and diabetes management in T1DM. Diabetes Metab Res Rev. 28 December 2020 [Epub ahead of print]. DOI: 10.1002/dmrr.3430

103. Seaquist ER, Anderson J, Childs B, et al. Hypoglycemia and diabetes: a report of a workgroup of the American Diabetes Association and the Endocrine Society. Diabetes Care 2013;36:1384–1395

104. Cryer PE. Mechanisms of hypoglycemia-associated autonomic failure in diabetes. N Engl J Med 2013;369:362–372

105. Henriksen MM, Andersen HU, Thorsteinsson B, Pedersen-Bjergaard U. Hypoglycemic exposure and risk of asymptomatic hypoglycemia in type 1 diabetes assessed by continuous glucose monitoring. J Clin Endocrinol Metab 2018;103:2329–2335

106. van Beers CAJ, Caris MG, DeVries JH, Serné EH. The relation between HbA1c and hypoglycemia revisited; a secondary analysis from an intervention trial in patients with type 1 diabetes and impaired awareness of hypoglycemia. J Diabetes Complications 2018;32:100–103

107. Gagnum V, Stene LC, Jenssen TG, et al. Causes of death in childhood-onset type 1 diabetes: long-term follow-up. Diabet Med 2017;34:56–63

108. International Hypoglycaemia Study Group. Hypoglycaemia, cardiovascular disease, and mortality in diabetes: epidemiology, pathogenesis, and management. Lancet Diabetes Endocrinol 2019;7:385–396

109. Jacobson AM, Musen G, Ryan CM, et al.; Diabetes Control and Complications Trial/ Epidemiology of Diabetes Interventions and Complications Study Research Group. Long-term effect of diabetes and its treatment on cognitive function. N Engl J Med 2007;356:1842–1852

110. Jacobson AM, Ryan CM, Braffett BH, et al.; DCCT/EDIC Research Group. Cognitive performance declines in older adults with type 1 diabetes: results from 32 years of follow-up in the DCCT and EDIC Study. Lancet Diabetes Endocrinol 2021;9:436–445

111. Chaytor NS, Barbosa-Leiker C, Ryan CM, Germine LT, Hirsch IB, Weinstock RS. Clinically significant cognitive impairment in older adults with type 1 diabetes. J Diabetes Complications 2019;33:91–97

112. Lin YK, Fisher SJ, Pop-Busui R. Hypoglycemia unawareness and autonomic dysfunction in diabetes: Lessons learned and

roles of diabetes technologies. J Diabetes Investig 2020;11:1388–1402

113. Geddes J, Schopman JE, Zammitt NN, Frier BM. Prevalence of impaired awareness of hypoglycaemia in adults with type 1 diabetes. Diabet Med 2008;25:501–504

114. Gold AE, MacLeod KM, Frier BM. Frequency of severe hypoglycemia in patients with type I diabetes with impaired awareness of hypoglycemia. Diabetes Care 1994;17:697–703

115. Mitrakou A, Ryan C, Veneman T, et al. Hierarchy of glycemic thresholds for counterregulatory hormone secretion, symptoms, and cerebral dysfunction. Am J Physiol 1991;260: E67–E74

116. Janssen MM, Snoek FJ, Heine RJ. Assessing impaired hypoglycemia awareness in type 1 diabetes: agreement of self-report but not of field study data with the autonomic symptom threshold during experimental hypoglycemia. Diabetes Care 2000;23:529–532

117. Clarke WL, Cox DJ, Gonder-Frederick LA, Julian D, Schlundt D, Polonsky W. Reduced awareness of hypoglycemia in adults with IDDM. A prospective study of hypoglycemic frequency and associated symptoms. Diabetes Care 1995;18:517–522

118. Pedersen-Bjergaard U, Pramming S, Thorsteinsson B. Recall of severe hypoglycaemia and self-estimated state of awareness in type 1 diabetes. Diabetes Metab Res Rev 2003;19: 232–240

119. Speight J, Barendse SM, Singh H, et al. Characterizing problematic hypoglycaemia: iterative design and preliminary psychometric validation of the Hypoglycaemia Awareness Questionnaire (HypoA-Q). Diabet Med 2016; 33:376–385

120. Hopkins D, Lawrence I, Mansell P, et al. Improved biomedical and psychological outcomes 1 year after structured education in flexible insulin therapy for people with type 1 diabetes: the U.K. DAFNE experience. Diabetes Care 2012;35:1638–1642

121. Little SA, Leelarathna L, Barendse SM, et al. Severe hypoglycaemia in type 1 diabetes mellitus: underlying drivers and potential strategies for successful prevention. Diabetes Metab Res Rev 2014;30:175–190

122. Little SA, Speight J, Leelarathna L, et al. Sustained reduction in severe hypoglycemia in adults with type 1 diabetes complicated by impaired awareness of hypoglycemia: two-year follow-up in the HypoCOMPaSS randomized clinical trial. Diabetes Care 2018;41:1600–1607

123. Iqbal A, Heller SR. The role of structured education in the management of hypoglycaemia. Diabetologia 2018;61:751–760

124. Cranston I, Lomas J, Maran A, Macdonald I, Amiel SA. Restoration of hypoglycaemia awareness in patients with long-duration insulin-dependent diabetes. Lancet 1994;344:283–287

125. Yeoh E, Choudhary P, Nwokolo M, Ayis S, Amiel SA. Interventions that restore awareness of hypoglycemia in adults with type 1 diabetes: a systematic review and meta-analysis. Diabetes Care 2015;38:1592–1609

126. Cox DJ, Gonder-Frederick L, Ritterband L, et al. Blood glucose awareness training: what is it, where is it, and where is it going? Diabetes Spectr 2006;19:43–49

127. Rondags SMPA, de Wit M, Twisk JW, Snoek FJ. Effectiveness of HypoAware, a brief partly web-based psychoeducational intervention for adults with type 1 and insulin-treated type 2 diabetes and problematic hypoglycemia: a cluster randomized controlled trial. Diabetes Care 2016;39:2190–2196

128. Hermanns N, Kulzer B, Krichbaum M, Kubiak T, Haak T. Long-term effect of an education program (HyPOS) on the incidence of severe hypoglycemia in patients with type 1 diabetes. Diabetes Care 2010;33:e36–e36

129. Cryer PE. Hypoglycemia in type 1 diabetes mellitus. Endocrinol Metab Clin North Am 2010;39:641–654

130. Pinsker JE, Bartee A, Katz M, et al. Predictive low-glucose suspend necessitates less carbohydrate supplementation to rescue hypoglycemia: need to revisit current hypo-glycemia treatment guidelines. Diabetes Technol Ther 2021;23:512–516

131. American Diabetes Association. 5. Lifestyle management: *Standards of Medical Care in Diabetes—2019*. Diabetes Care 2019;42(Suppl. 1):S46–S60

132. Bell KJ, Barclay AW, Petocz P, Colagiuri S, Brand-Miller JC. Efficacy of carbohydrate counting in type 1 diabetes: a systematic review and meta-analysis. Lancet Diabetes Endocrinol 2014;2:133–140

133. Schmidt S, Schelde B, Nørgaard K. Effects of advanced carbohydrate counting in patients with type 1 diabetes: a systematic review. Diabet Med 2014;31:886–896

134. Evert AB, Dennison M, Gardner CD, et al. Nutrition therapy for adults with diabetes or prediabetes: a consensus report. Diabetes Care 2019;42:731–754

135. Hermann JM, Meusers M, Bachran R, et al.; DPV initiative. Self-reported regular alcohol consumption in adolescents and emerging adults with type 1 diabetes: a neglected risk factor for diabetic ketoacidosis? Multicenter analysis of 29 630 patients from the DPV registry. Pediatr Diabetes 2017;18:817–823

136. Kerr D, Penfold S, Zouwail S, Thomas P, Begley J. The influence of liberal alcohol consumption on glucose metabolism in patients with type 1 diabetes: a pilot study. QJM 2009; 102:169–174

137. Turner BC, Jenkins E, Kerr D, Sherwin RS, Cavan DA. The effect of evening alcohol consumption on next-morning glucose control in type 1 diabetes. Diabetes Care 2001;24: 1888–1893

138. Pastor A, Conn J, MacIsaac RJ, Bonomo Y. Alcohol and illicit drug use in people with diabetes. Lancet Diabetes Endocrinol 2020;8: 239–248

139. Barnard K, Sinclair JMA, Lawton J, Young AJ, Holt RIG. Alcohol-associated risks for young adults with type 1 diabetes: a narrative review. Diabet Med 2012;29:434–440

140. Barnard KD, Dyson P, Sinclair JMA, et al. Alcohol health literacy in young adults with type 1 diabetes and its impact on diabetes management. Diabet Med 2014;31:1625–1630

141. Engler PA, Ramsey SE, Smith RJ. Alcohol use of diabetes patients: the need for assessment and intervention. Acta Diabetol 2013; 50:93–99

142. Pan A, Wang Y, Talaei M, Hu FB. Relation of smoking with total mortality and cardiovascular events among patients with diabetes mellitus: a meta-analysis and systematic review. Circulation 2015;132:1795–1804

143. Uruska A, Araszkiewicz A, Uruski P, Zozulinska-Ziolkiewicz D. Higher risk of microvascular complications in smokers with type 1 diabetes despite intensive insulin therapy. Microvasc Res 2014;92:79–84

144. Tikkanen-Dolenc H, Wadén J, Forsblom C, et al.; FinnDiane Study Group. Physical activity reduces risk of premature mortality in patients with type 1 diabetes with and without kidney disease. Diabetes Care 2017;40:1727–1732

145. Bohn B, Herbst A, Pfeifer M, et al.; DPV Initiative. Impact of physical activity on glycemic control and prevalence of cardiovascular risk factors in adults with type 1 diabetes: a cross-sectional multicenter study of 18,028 patients. Diabetes Care 2015;38:1536–1543

146. Wu N, Bredin SSD, Guan Y, et al. Cardiovascular health benefits of exercise training in persons living with type 1 diabetes: a systematic review and meta-analysis. J Clin Med 2019;8:253

147. Chimen M, Kennedy A, Nirantharakumar K, Pang TT, Andrews R, Narendran P. What are the health benefits of physical activity in type 1 diabetes mellitus? A literature review. Diabetologia 2012;55:542–551

148. Wadén J, Forsblom C, Thorn LM, et al.; FinnDiane Study Group. Physical activity and diabetes complications in patients with type 1 diabetes: the Finnish Diabetic Nephropathy (FinnDiane) Study. Diabetes Care 2008;31:230–232

149. Moser O, Riddell MC, Eckstein ML, et al. Glucose management for exercise using continuous glucose monitoring (CGM) and intermittently scanned CGM (isCGM) systems in type 1 diabetes: position statement of the European Association for the Study of Diabetes (EASD) and of the International Society for Pediatric and Adolescent Diabetes (ISPAD) endorsed by JDRF and supported by the American Diabetes Association (ADA). Diabetologia 2020;63:2501–2520

150. Lemaster JW, Reiber GE, Smith DG, Heagerty PJ, Wallace C. Daily weight-bearing activity does not increase the risk of diabetic foot ulcers. Med Sci Sports Exerc 2003;35:1093–1099

151. Riddell MC, Gallen IW, Smart CE, et al. Exercise management in type 1 diabetes: a consensus statement. Lancet Diabetes Endocrinol 2017;5:377–390

152. Colberg SR. Older adults. In *Exercise and Diabetes: A Clinician's Guide to Prescribing Physical Activity.* 1st ed. Colberg SR, Ed. Alexandria, VA, American Diabetes Association, 2013, p. 424

153. Reutrakul S, Thakkinstian A, Anothaisintawee T, et al. Sleep characteristics in type 1 diabetes and associations with glycemic control: systematic review and meta-analysis. Sleep Med 2016;23:26–45

154. Denic-Roberts H, Costacou T, Orchard TJ. Subjective sleep disturbances and glycemic control in adults with long-standing type 1 diabetes: the Pittsburgh's Epidemiology of Diabetes Complications study. Diabetes Res Clin Pract 2016;119:1–12

155. van Dijk M, Donga E, van Dijk JG, et al. Disturbed subjective sleep characteristics in adult patients with long-standing type 1 diabetes mellitus. Diabetologia 2011;54:1967–1976

156. American Diabetes Association. 6. Glycemic targets: *Standards of Medical Care in Diabetes—2020.* Diabetes Care 2020;43(Suppl. 1):S66–S76

157. Centers for Disease Control and Prevention. (2020) Managing sick days. Available from www.cdc.gov/diabetes/managing/flu-sick-days.html. Accessed: 16 July 2021

158. Diabetes UK. Diabetes when you're unwell. Accessed 16 July 2021. Available from www.diabetes.org.uk/guide-to-diabetes/life-with-diabetes/illness

159. Graveling AJ, Frier BM. Driving and diabetes: problems, licensing restrictions and recommendations for safe driving. Clin Diabetes Endocrinol 2015;1:8

160. Lorber D, Anderson J, Arent S, et al.; American Diabetes Association. Diabetes and driving. Diabetes Care 2014;37(Suppl. 1):S97–S103

161. Anderson JE, Greene MA, Griffin JW Jr, et al.; American Diabetes Association. Diabetes and employment. Diabetes Care 2014;37(Suppl. 1):S112–S117

162. Sansum Diabetes Research Institute. (2019). Time zones. Accessed 19 February 2021. Available from https://diabetestravel.sansum.org/time-zones/

163. Charlton AR, Charlton JR. World travel with type 1 diabetes using continuous subcutaneous insulin infusion. British Journal of Diabetes 2019; 19:141–146

164. IDF and the Diabetes & Ramadan International Alliance. Diabetes and Ramadan: practical guidelines 2021. Accessed 16 July 2021. Available from https://idf.org/e-library/guidelines/165-idf-dar-practical-guidelines-2021.html

165. de Groot M, Golden SH, Wagner J. Psychological conditions in adults with diabetes. Am Psychol 2016;71:552–562

166. van Duinkerken E, Snoek FJ, de Wit M. The cognitive and psychological effects of living with type 1 diabetes: a narrative review. Diabet Med 2020;37:555–563

167. Speight J, Hendrieckx C, Pouwer F, Skinner TC, Snoek FJ. Back to the future: 25 years of 'Guidelines for encouraging psychological well-being' among people affected by diabetes. Diabet Med 2020;37:1225–1229

168. Fisher L, Polonsky WH, Hessler DM, et al. Understanding the sources of diabetes distress in adults with type 1 diabetes. J Diabetes Complications 2015;29:572–577

169. Hessler DM, Fisher L, Polonsky WH, et al. Diabetes distress is linked with worsening diabetes management over time in adults with type 1 diabetes. Diabet Med 2017;34:1228–1234

170. de Wit M, Trief PM, Huber JW, Willaing I. State of the art: understanding and integration of the social context in diabetes care. Diabet Med 2020;37:473–482

171. Barnard KD, Skinner TC, Peveler R. The prevalence of co-morbid depression in adults with type 1 diabetes: systematic literature review. Diabet Med 2006;23:445–448

172. Hermanns N, Kulzer B, Krichbaum M, Kubiak T, Haak T. Affective and anxiety disorders in a German sample of diabetic patients: prevalence, comorbidity and risk factors. Diabet Med 2005;22:293–300

173. Smith KJ, Béland M, Clyde M, et al. Association of diabetes with anxiety: a systematic review and meta-analysis. J Psychosom Res 2013;74:89–99

174. Snoek FJ, Bremmer MA, Hermanns N. Constructs of depression and distress in diabetes: time for an appraisal. Lancet Diabetes Endocrinol 2015;3:450–460

175. Pouwer F, Schram MT, Iversen MM, Nouwen A, Holt RIG. How 25 years of psychosocial research has contributed to a better understanding of the links between depression and diabetes. Diabet Med 2020;37:383–392

176. Fisher L, Hessler DM, Polonsky WH, et al. Prevalence of depression in type 1 diabetes and the problem of over-diagnosis. Diabet Med 2016;33:1590–1597

177. Sultan S, Epel E, Sachon C, Vaillant G, Hartemann-Heurtier A. A longitudinal study of coping, anxiety and glycemic control in adults with type 1 diabetes. Psychol Health 2008;23:73–89

178. Nefs G, Hendrieckx C, Reddy P, et al. Comorbid elevated symptoms of anxiety and depression in adults with type 1 or type 2 diabetes: results from the international diabetes MILES study. J Diabetes Complications 2019;33:523–529

179. Nano J, Carinci F, Okunade O, et al.; Diabetes Working Group of the International Consortium for Health Outcomes Measurement (ICHOM). A standard set of person-centred outcomes for diabetes mellitus: results of an international and unified approach. Diabet Med 2020;37:2009–2018

180. Krieger T, Zimmermann J, Huffziger S, et al. Measuring depression with a well-being index: further evidence for the validity of the WHO Well-Being Index (WHO-5) as a measure of the severity of depression. J Affect Disord 2014;156:240–244

181. Polonsky WH, Anderson BJ, Lohrer PA, et al. Assessment of diabetes-related distress. Diabetes Care 1995;18:754–760

182. Kroenke K, Spitzer RL, Williams JB. The PHQ-9: validity of a brief depression severity measure. J Gen Intern Med 2001;16:606–613

183. Spitzer RL, Kroenke K, Williams JBW, Löwe B. A brief measure for assessing generalized anxiety disorder: the GAD-7. Arch Intern Med 2006;166:1092–1097

184. Kroenke K, Spitzer RL, Williams JBW. The Patient Health Questionnaire-2: validity of a two-item depression screener. Med Care 2003;41:1284–1292

185. Kroenke K, Spitzer RL, Williams JBW, Löwe B. An ultra-brief screening scale for anxiety and depression: the PHQ-4. Psychosomatics 2009;50: 613–621

186. McGuire BE, Morrison TG, Hermanns N, et al. Short-form measures of diabetes-related emotional distress: the Problem Areas in Diabetes Scale (PAID)-5 and PAID-1. Diabetologia 2010;53: 66–69

187. Fisher L, Glasgow RE, Mullan JT, Skaff MM, Polonsky WH. Development of a brief diabetes distress screening instrument. Ann Fam Med 2008;6:246–252

188. Pouwer F, Snoek FJ, van der Ploeg HM, Adèr HJ, Heine RJ. Monitoring of psychological well-being in outpatients with diabetes: effects on mood, HbA$_{1c}$, and the patient's evaluation of the quality of diabetes care: a randomized controlled trial. Diabetes Care 2001;24:1929–1935

189. Snoek FJ, Kersch NYA, Eldrup E, et al. Monitoring of Individual Needs in Diabetes (MIND)-2: follow-up data from the cross-national

Diabetes Attitudes, Wishes, and Needs (DAWN) MIND study. Diabetes Care 2012;35:2128–2132

190. Wild D, von Maltzahn R, Brohan E, Christensen T, Clauson P, Gonder-Frederick L. A critical review of the literature on fear of hypoglycemia in diabetes: implications for diabetes management and patient education. Patient Educ Couns 2007;68:10–15

191. Snoek FJ, Hajos TRS, Rondags SMPA. Psychological effects of hypoglycaemia. In Hypoglycaemia in Clinical Diabetes. Frier BM, Heller SR, McCrimmon RJ, Eds. Chichester, John Wiley & Sons, 2014, p. 323–333

192. Gonder-Frederick LA, Schmidt KM, Vajda KA, et al. Psychometric properties of the hypoglycemia fear survey-ii for adults with type 1 diabetes. Diabetes Care 2011;34:801–806

193. Jones JM, Lawson ML, Daneman D, Olmsted MP, Rodin G. Eating disorders in adolescent females with and without type 1 diabetes: cross sectional study. BMJ 2000;320:1563–1566

194. Colton PA, Olmsted MP, Daneman D, et al. Eating disorders in girls and women with type 1 diabetes: a longitudinal study of prevalence, onset, remission, and recurrence. Diabetes Care 2015;38:1212–1217

195. Luyckx K, Verschueren M, Palmeroni N, Goethals ER, Weets I, Claes L. Disturbed eating behaviors in adolescents and emerging adults with type 1 diabetes: a one-year prospective study. Diabetes Care 2019;42:1637–1644

196. Wisting L, Reas DL, Bang L, Skrivarhaug T, Dahl-Jørgensen K, Rø Ø. Eating patterns in adolescents with type 1 diabetes: associations with metabolic control, insulin omission, and eating disorder pathology. Appetite 2017;114:226–231

197. d'Emden H, Holden L, McDermott B, et al. Disturbed eating behaviours and thoughts in Australian adolescents with type 1 diabetes. J Paediatr Child Health 2013;49:E317–E323

198. Hill-Briggs F, Adler NE, Berkowitz SA, et al. Social determinants of health and diabetes: a scientific review. Diabetes Care 2021;44:258–279

199. Centers for Disease Control and Prevention. Tools for putting social determinants of health into action. Accessed 18 February 2021. Available from www.cdc.gov/socialdeterminants/tools/index.htm

200. Institute of Medicine. Capturing Social and Behavioral Domains and Measures in Electronic Health Records: Phase 2. Washington, DC, The National Academies Press, 2014

201. American Academy of Family Physicians. Social needs screening tool. Accessed 23 August 2021. Available from www.aafp.org/dam/AAFP/documents/patient_care/everyone_project/hops19-physician-form-sdoh.pdf

202. Giuse NB, Koonce TY, Kusnoor SV, et al. Institute of medicine measures of social and behavioral determinants of health: a feasibility study. Am J Prev Med 2017;52:199–206

203. Walker RJ, Garacci E, Palatnik A, Ozieh MN, Egede LE. The longitudinal influence of social determinants of health on glycemic control in elderly adults with diabetes. Diabetes Care 2020;43:759–766

204. Heller CG, Parsons AS, Chambers EC, Fiori KP, Rehm CD. Social risks among primary care patients in a large urban health system. Am J Prev Med 2020;58:514–525

205. Young-Hyman D, de Groot M, Hill-Briggs F, Gonzalez JS, Hood K, Peyrot M. psychosocial care for people with diabetes: a position statement of the American Diabetes Association. Diabetes Care 2016;39:2126–2140

206. van der Feltz-Cornelis CM, Nuyen J, Stoop C, et al. Effect of interventions for major depressive disorder and significant depressive symptoms in patients with diabetes mellitus: a systematic review and meta-analysis. Gen Hosp Psychiatry 2010;32:380–395

207. De Hert M, Dekker JM, Wood D, Kahl KG, Holt RIG, Möller H-J. Cardiovascular disease and diabetes in people with severe mental illness position statement from the European Psychiatric Association (EPA), supported by the European Association for the Study of Diabetes (EASD) and the European Society of Cardiology (ESC). Eur Psychiatry 2009;24:412–424

208. Stenov V, Joensen LE, Knudsen L, Lindqvist Hansen D, Willaing Tapager I. "Mental health professionals have never mentioned my diabetes, they don't get into that": a qualitative study of support needs in adults with type 1 and type 2 diabetes and severe mental illness. Can J Diabetes 2020;44:494–500

209. Benoit SR, Hora I, Pasquel FJ, Gregg EW, Albright AL, Imperatore G. Trends in emergency department visits and inpatient admissions for hyperglycemic crises in adults with diabetes in the U.S., 2006-2015. Diabetes Care 2020;43:1057–1064

210. Kalscheuer H, Seufert J, Lanzinger S, et al.; DPV Initiative. Event rates and risk factors for the development of diabetic ketoacidosis in adult patients with type 1 diabetes: analysis from the DPV Registry based on 46,966 patients. Diabetes Care 2019;42:e34–e36

211. Ehrmann D, Kulzer B, Roos T, Haak T, Al-Khatib M, Hermanns N. Risk factors and prevention strategies for diabetic ketoacidosis in people with established type 1 diabetes. Lancet Diabetes Endocrinol 2020;8:436–446

212. Kinney GL, Akturk HK, Taylor DD, Foster NC, Shah VN. Cannabis use is associated with increased risk for diabetic ketoacidosis in adults with type 1 diabetes: findings from the T1D Exchange clinic registry. Diabetes Care 2020;43:247–249

213. Hare MJL, Deitch JM, Kang MJY, Bach LA. Clinical, psychological and demographic factors in a contemporary adult cohort with diabetic ketoacidosis and type 1 diabetes. Intern Med J 2021;51:1292–1297

214. Garg SK, Walker AJ, Hoff HK, D'Souza AO, Gottlieb PA, Chase HP. Glycemic parameters with multiple daily injections using insulin glargine versus insulin pump. Diabetes Technol Ther 2004;6:9–15

215. Hoshina S, Andersen GS, Jørgensen ME, Ridderstråle M, Vistisen D, Andersen HU. Treatment modality-dependent risk of diabetic ketoacidosis in patients with type 1 diabetes: Danish adult diabetes database study. Diabetes Technol Ther 2018;20:229–234

216. Danne T, Garg S, Peters AL, et al. International consensus on risk management of diabetic ketoacidosis in patients with type 1 diabetes treated with sodium-glucose cotransporter (SGLT) inhibitors. Diabetes Care 2019;42:1147–1154

217. Goldenberg RM, Gilbert JD, Hramiak IM, Woo VC, Zinman B. Sodium-glucose co-transporter inhibitors, their role in type 1 diabetes treatment and a risk mitigation strategy for preventing diabetic ketoacidosis: The STOP DKA Protocol. Diabetes Obes Metab 2019;21:2192–2202

218. Peters AL, Buschur EO, Buse JB, Cohan P, Diner JC, Hirsch IB. Euglycemic diabetic ketoacidosis: a potential complication of treatment with sodium-glucose cotransporter 2 inhibition. Diabetes Care 2015;38:1687–1693

219. Dhatariya KK, Vellanki P. Treatment of diabetic ketoacidosis (DKA)/hyperglycemic hyperosmolar state (HHS): novel advances in the management of hyperglycemic crises (UK versus USA). Curr Diab Rep 2017;17:33

220. Kitabchi AE, Umpierrez GE, Fisher JN, Murphy MB, Stentz FB. Thirty years of personal experience in hyperglycemic crises: diabetic ketoacidosis and hyperglycemic hyperosmolar state. J Clin Endocrinol Metab 2008;93:1541–1552

221. Savage MW, Dhatariya KK, Kilvert A, et al.; Joint British Diabetes Societies. Joint British Diabetes Societies guideline for the management of diabetic ketoacidosis. Diabet Med 2011;28:508–515

222. Umpierrez G, Korytkowski M. Diabetic emergencies - ketoacidosis, hyperglycaemic hyperosmolar state and hypoglycaemia. Nat Rev Endocrinol 2016;12:222–232

223. Gruessner RWG, Gruessner AC. The current state of pancreas transplantation. Nat Rev Endocrinol 2013;9:555–562

224. Barton FB, Rickels MR, Alejandro R, et al. Improvement in outcomes of clinical islet transplantation: 1999-2010. Diabetes Care 2012;35:1436–1445

225. Niclauss N, Morel P, Berney T. Has the gap between pancreas and islet transplantation closed? Transplantation 2014;98:593–599

226. Bassi R, Fiorina P. Impact of islet transplantation on diabetes complications and quality of life. Curr Diab Rep 2011;11:355–363

227. Thompson DM, Meloche M, Ao Z, et al. Reduced progression of diabetic microvascular complications with islet cell transplantation compared with intensive medical therapy. Transplantation 2011;91:373–378

228. Speight J, Woodcock AJ, Reaney MD, et al. Well, I wouldn't be any worse off, would I, than I am now? A qualitative study of decision-making, hopes, and realities of adults with type 1 diabetes undergoing islet cell transplantation. Transplant Direct 2016;2:e72

229. Gruessner AC, Sutherland DER, Gruessner RWG. Long-term outcome after pancreas transplantation. Curr Opin Organ Transplant 2012;17:100–105

230. Sollinger HW, Odorico JS, Becker YT, D'Alessandro AM, Pirsch JD. One thousand simultaneous pancreas-kidney transplants at a single center with 22-year follow-up. Ann Surg 2009;250:618–630

231. Lehmann R, Graziano J, Brockmann J, et al. Glycemic control in simultaneous islet-kidney versus pancreas-kidney transplantation in type 1 diabetes: a prospective 13-year follow-up. Diabetes Care 2015;38:752–759

232. Kandaswamy R, Sutherland DER. Pancreas versus islet transplantation in diabetes mellitus: How to allocate deceased donor pancreata? Transplant Proc 2006;38:365–367

233. Robertson P, Davis C, Larsen J, Stratta R; American Diabetes Association. Pancreas transplantation in type 1 diabetes. Diabetes Care 2004;27(Suppl. 1):S105

234. Ryan EA, Shandro T, Green K, et al. Assessment of the severity of hypoglycemia and glycemic lability in type 1 diabetic subjects

undergoing islet transplantation. Diabetes 2004; 53:955–962

235. Senior PA, Bellin MD, Alejandro R, et al.; Clinical Islet Transplantation Consortium. Consistency of quantitative scores of hypoglycemia severity and glycemic lability and comparison with continuous glucose monitoring system measures in long-standing type 1 diabetes. Diabetes Technol Ther 2015;17:235–242

236. Bellin MD, Barton FB, Heitman A, et al. Potent induction immunotherapy promotes long-term insulin independence after islet transplantation in type 1 diabetes. Am J Transplant 2012;12:1576–1583

237. Qi M, Kinzer K, Danielson KK, et al. Five-year follow-up of patients with type 1 diabetes transplanted with allogeneic islets: the UIC experience. Acta Diabetol 2014;51:833–843

238. Clinical Islet Transplantation Consortium. Clinical Islet Transplantation Study. Accessed 11 February 2021. Available from www.isletstudy.org/

239. O'Connell PJ, Holmes-Walker DJ, Goodman D, et al.; Australian Islet Transplant Consortium. Multicenter Australian trial of islet transplantation: improving accessibility and outcomes. Am J Transplant 2013;13:1850–1858

240. Brooks AM, Walker N, Aldibbiat A, et al. Attainment of metabolic goals in the integrated UK islet transplant program with locally isolated and transported preparations. Am J Transplant 2013;13:3236–3243

241. Speight J, Reaney MD, Woodcock AJ, Smith RM, Shaw JAM. Patient-reported outcomes following islet cell or pancreas transplantation (alone or after kidney) in type 1 diabetes: a systematic review. Diabet Med 2010;27:812–822

242. Choudhary P, Rickels MR, Senior PA, et al. Evidence-informed clinical practice recommendations for treatment of type 1 diabetes complicated by problematic hypoglycemia. Diabetes Care 2015;38:1016–1029

243. Lablanche S, Vantyghem M-C, Kessler L, et al.; TRIMECO trial investigators. Islet transplantation versus insulin therapy in patients with type 1 diabetes with severe hypoglycaemia or poorly controlled glycaemia after kidney transplantation (TRIMECO): a multicentre, randomised controlled trial. Lancet Diabetes Endocrinol 2018; 6:527–537

244. Snaith JR, Holmes-Walker DJ, Greenfield JR. Reducing type 1 diabetes mortality: role for adjunctive therapies? Trends Endocrinol Metab 2020;31:150–164

245. Liu Y-S, Chen C-N, Chen Z-G, Peng Y, Lin X-P, Xu L-L. Vascular and metabolic effects of metformin added to insulin therapy in patients with type 1 diabetes: a systematic review and meta-analysis. Diabetes Metab Res Rev 2020;36: e3334

246. Petrie JR, Chaturvedi N, Ford I, et al.; REMOVAL Study Group. Cardiovascular and metabolic effects of metformin in patients with type 1 diabetes (REMOVAL): a double-blind, randomised, placebo-controlled trial. Lancet Diabetes Endocrinol 2017;5:597–609

247. Kong MF, King P, Macdonald IA, et al. Infusion of pramlintide, a human amylin analogue, delays gastric emptying in men with IDDM. Diabetologia 1997;40:82–88

248. Kong MF, Stubbs TA, King P, et al. The effect of single doses of pramlintide on gastric emptying

of two meals in men with IDDM. Diabetologia 1998;41:577–583

249. Fineman MS, Koda JE, Shen LZ, et al. The human amylin analog, pramlintide, corrects postprandial hyperglucagonemia in patients with type 1 diabetes. Metabolism 2002;51:636–641

250. Chapman I, Parker B, Doran S, et al. Effect of pramlintide on satiety and food intake in obese subjects and subjects with type 2 diabetes. Diabetologia 2005;48:838–848

251. Whitehouse F, Kruger DF, Fineman M, et al. A randomized study and open-label extension evaluating the long-term efficacy of pramlintide as an adjunct to insulin therapy in type 1 diabetes. Diabetes Care 2002;25:724–730

252. Ratner RE, Want LL, Fineman MS, et al. Adjunctive therapy with the amylin analogue pramlintide leads to a combined improvement in glycemic and weight control in insulin-treated subjects with type 2 diabetes. Diabetes Technol Ther 2002;4:51–61

253. Hollander PA, Levy P, Fineman MS, et al. Pramlintide as an adjunct to insulin therapy improves long-term glycemic and weight control in patients with type 2 diabetes: a 1-year randomized controlled trial. Diabetes Care 2003;26:784–790

254. Ratner RE, Dickey R, Fineman M, et al. Amylin replacement with pramlintide as an adjunct to insulin therapy improves long-term glycaemic and weight control in Type 1 diabetes mellitus: a 1-year, randomized controlled trial. Diabet Med 2004;21:1204–1212

255. von Herrath M, Bain SC, Bode B, et al.; Anti-IL-21–liraglutide Study Group investigators and contributors. Anti-interleukin-21 antibody and liraglutide for the preservation of β-cell function in adults with recent-onset type 1 diabetes: a randomised, double-blind, placebo-controlled, phase 2 trial. Lancet Diabetes Endocrinol 2021;9: 212–224

256. Nauck MA, Meier JJ. GLP-1 receptor agonists in type 1 diabetes: a MAG1C bullet? Lancet Diabetes Endocrinol 2020;8:262–264

257. Mathieu C, Zinman B, Hemmingsson JU, et al.; ADJUNCT ONE Investigators. Efficacy and safety of liraglutide added to insulin treatment in type 1 diabetes: the ADJUNCT ONE treat-to-target randomized trial. Diabetes Care 2016;39:1702–1710

258. Ahrén B, Hirsch IB, Pieber TR, et al.; ADJUNCT TWO Investigators. Efficacy and safety of liraglutide added to capped insulin treatment in subjects with type 1 diabetes: the ADJUNCT TWO randomized trial. Diabetes Care 2016;39: 1693–1701

259. Sheahan KH, Wahlberg EA, Gilbert MP. An overview of GLP-1 agonists and recent cardiovascular outcomes trials. Postgrad Med J 2020;96:156–161

260. Wilding JPH, Batterham RL, Calanna S, et al.; STEP 1 Study Group. Once-weekly semaglutide in adults with overweight or obesity. N Engl J Med 2021;384:989

261. Taylor SI, Blau JE, Rother KI, Beitelshees AL. SGLT2 inhibitors as adjunctive therapy for type 1 diabetes: balancing benefits and risks. Lancet Diabetes Endocrinol 2019;7:949–958

262. Zelniker TA, Wiviott SD, Raz I, et al. SGLT2 inhibitors for primary and secondary prevention of cardiovascular and renal outcomes in type 2 diabetes: a systematic review and meta-analysis of

cardiovascular outcome trials. Lancet 2019;393: 31–39

263. Groop P-H, Dandona P, Phillip M, et al. Effect of dapagliflozin as an adjunct to insulin over 52 weeks in individuals with type 1 diabetes: post-hoc renal analysis of the DEPICT randomised controlled trials. Lancet Diabetes Endocrinol 2020;8:845–854

264. Jensen DM, Korsholm L, Ovesen P, et al. Peri-conceptional A1C and risk of serious adverse pregnancy outcome in 933 women with type 1 diabetes. Diabetes Care 2009;32:1046–1048

265. Abell SK, Boyle JA, de Courten B, et al. Contemporary type 1 diabetes pregnancy outcomes: impact of obesity and glycaemic control. Med J Aust 2016;205:162–167

266. Feig DS, Donovan LE, Corcoy R, et al.; CONCEPTT Collaborative Group. Continuous glucose monitoring in pregnant women with type 1 diabetes (CONCEPTT): a multicentre international randomised controlled trial. Lancet 2017;390:2347–2359

267. Nielsen LR, Pedersen-Bjergaard U, Thorsteinsson B, Johansen M, Damm P, Mathiesen ER. Hypoglycemia in pregnant women with type 1 diabetes: predictors and role of metabolic control. Diabetes Care 2008;31:9–14

268. Sibai BM, Viteri OA. Diabetic ketoacidosis in pregnancy. Obstet Gynecol 2014;123:167–178

269. Roeder HA, Moore TR, Ramos GA. Changes in postpartum insulin requirements for patients with well-controlled type 1 diabetes. Am J Perinatol 2016;33:683–687

270. Davies HA, Clark JD, Dalton KJ, Edwards OM. Insulin requirements of diabetic women who breast feed. BMJ 1989;298:1357–1358

271. WHO. (2015). Medical eligibility criteria wheel for contraceptive use. Accessed 16 July 2021. Available from www.who.int/reproductivehealth/publications/family_planning/mec-wheel-5th/en/

272. American Diabetes Association. 14. Management of Diabetes in Pregnancy: Standards of Medical Care in Diabetes—2021. Diabetes Care 2021;44(Suppl. 1):S200–S210

273. National Institute for Health and Care Excellence. Diabetes in pregnancy: management from preconception to the postnatal period. Published 25 February 2015. Accessed 18 February 2021. Available from www.nice.org.uk/guidance/ng3

274. Leung E, Wongrakpanich S, Munshi MN. Diabetes management in the elderly. Diabetes Spectr 2018;31:245–253

275. Wang PH, Lau J, Chalmers TC. Meta-analysis of effects of intensive blood-glucose control on late complications of type I diabetes. Lancet 1993;341:1306–1309

276. Molitch ME, Adler AI, Flyvbjerg A, et al. Diabetic kidney disease: a clinical update from Kidney Disease: Improving Global Outcomes. Kidney Int 2015;87:20–30

277. Aleppo G, Calhoun P, Foster NC, Maahs DM, Shah VN; T1D Exchange Clinic Network. Reported gastroparesis in adults with type 1 diabetes (T1D) from the T1D Exchange clinic registry. J Diabetes Complications 2017;31:1669–1673

278. The Diabetes Control and Complications Trial Research Group. Early worsening of diabetic retinopathy in the Diabetes Control and Complications Trial. Arch Ophthalmol 1998;116: 874–886

279. Llewelyn JG, Thomas PK, Fonseca V, King RH, Dandona P. Acute painful diabetic neuropathy precipitated by strict glycaemic control. Acta Neuropathol 1986;72:157–163

280. de Ferranti SD, de Boer IH, Fonseca V, et al. Type 1 diabetes mellitus and cardiovascular disease: a scientific statement from the American Heart Association and American Diabetes Association. Diabetes Care 2014;37:2843–2863

281. American Diabetes Association. 15. Diabetes care in the hospital: *Standards of Medical Care in Diabetes—2021*. Diabetes Care 2021;44(Suppl. 1):S211–S220

282. Umpierrez GE, Kitabchi AE. Diabetic ketoacidosis: risk factors and management strategies. Treat Endocrinol 2003;2:95–108

283. Galindo RJ, Umpierrez GE, Rushakoff RJ, et al. Continuous glucose monitors and automated insulin dosing systems in the hospital consensus guideline. J Diabetes Sci Technol 2020;14:1035–1064

284. Mendez CE, Umpierrez GE. Management of type 1 diabetes in the hospital setting. Curr Diab Rep 2017;17:98

285. Bailon RM, Partlow BJ, Miller-Cage V, et al. Continuous subcutaneous insulin infusion (insulin pump) therapy can be safely used in the hospital in select patients. Endocr Pract 2009;15:24–29

286. Cook CB, Boyle ME, Cisar NS, et al. Use of continuous subcutaneous insulin infusion (insulin pump) therapy in the hospital setting: proposed guidelines and outcome measures. Diabetes Educ 2005;31:849–857

287. Nair GG, Tzanakakis ES, Hebrok M. Emerging routes to the generation of functional β-cells for diabetes mellitus cell therapy. Nat Rev Endocrinol 2020;16:506–518

288. Desai T, Shea LD. Advances in islet encapsulation technologies. Nat Rev Drug Discov 2017;16:338–350

289. Hendriks WT, Warren CR, Cowan CA. Genome editing in human pluripotent stem cells: approaches, pitfalls, and solutions. Cell Stem Cell 2016;18:53–65

290. Dayan CM, Korah M, Tatovic D, Bundy BN, Herold KC. Changing the landscape for type 1 diabetes: the first step to prevention. Lancet 2019;394:1286–1296

291. Hughes JW, Bao YK, Salam M, et al. Late-onset T1DM and older age predict risk of additional autoimmune disease. Diabetes Care 2019;42:32–38

292. Milluzzo A, Falorni A, Brozzetti A, et al. Risk for coexistent autoimmune diseases in familial and sporadic type 1 diabetes is related to age at diabetes onset. Endocr Pract 2021;27:110–117

293. Bergenstal RM, Gal RL, Connor CG, et al.; T1D Exchange Racial Differences Study Group. Racial differences in the relationship of glucose concentrations and hemoglobin A1c levels. Ann Intern Med 2017;167:95–102

Consensus Report: Definition and Interpretation of Remission in Type 2 Diabetes

Diabetes Care 2021;44:2438–2444 | https://doi.org/10.2337/dci21-0034

Matthew C. Riddle,[1] William T. Cefalu,[2] Philip H. Evans,[3] Hertzel C. Gerstein,[4] Michael A. Nauck,[5] William K. Oh,[6] Amy E. Rothberg,[7] Carel W. le Roux,[8] Francesco Rubino,[9] Philip Schauer,[10] Roy Taylor,[11] and Douglas Twenefour[12]

[1]Division of Endocrinology, Diabetes, & Clinical Nutrition, Department of Medicine, Oregon Health & Science University, Portland, OR
[2]Division of Diabetes, Endocrinology and Metabolic Diseases, National Institute of Diabetes and Digestive and Kidney Diseases, National Institutes of Health, Bethesda, MD
[3]College of Medicine and Health, University of Exeter, Exeter, U.K.
[4]Population Health Research Institute and Department of Medicine, McMaster University and Hamilton Health Sciences, Hamilton, Ontario, Canada
[5]Diabetes Division, Katholisches Klinikum Bochum gGmbH, St. Josef-Hospital, Ruhr University Bochum, Bochum, Germany
[6]Division of Hematology and Medical Oncology, Tisch Cancer Institute, Icahn School of Medicine at Mount Sinai, New York, NY
[7]Department of Internal Medicine, Michigan Medicine, and Department of Nutritional Sciences, School of Public Health, University of Michigan, Ann Arbor, MI
[8]Diabetes Complications Research Centre, University College Dublin, Dublin, Ireland
[9]Department of Diabetes, School of Life Course Sciences, King's College London, London, U.K.
[10]Pennington Biomedical Research Center, Baton Rouge, LA
[11]Translational and Clinical Research Institute, Newcastle University, Newcastle upon Tyne, U.K.
[12]Diabetes UK, London, U.K.

Corresponding author: Matthew C. Riddle, riddlem@ohsu.edu

Received 17 June 2021 and accepted 17 June 2021

This Consensus Report is jointly published in The Journal of Clinical Endocrinology & Metabolism, published by Oxford University Press on behalf of the Endocrine Society; Diabetologia, published by Springer-Verlag, GmbH, on behalf of the European Association for the Study of Diabetes; Diabetic Medicine, published by Wiley on behalf of Diabetes UK; and Diabetes Care, published by the American Diabetes Association.

A consensus report of a particular topic contains a comprehensive examination and is authored by an expert panel (i.e., consensus panel) and represents the panel's collective analysis, evaluation, and opinion. The need for a consensus report arises when clinicians, scientists, regulators, and/

Improvement of glucose levels into the normal range can occur in some people living with diabetes, either spontaneously or after medical interventions, and in some cases can persist after withdrawal of glucose-lowering pharmacotherapy. Such sustained improvement may now be occurring more often due to newer forms of treatment. However, terminology for describing this process and objective measures for defining it are not well established, and the long-term risks versus benefits of its attainment are not well understood. To update prior discussions of this issue, an international expert group was convened by the American Diabetes Association to propose nomenclature and principles for data collection and analysis, with the goal of establishing a base of information to support future clinical guidance. This group proposed "remission" as the most appropriate descriptive term, and HbA$_{1c}$ <6.5% (48 mmol/mol) measured at least 3 months after cessation of glucose-lowering pharmacotherapy as the usual diagnostic criterion. The group also made suggestions for active observation of individuals experiencing a remission and discussed further questions and unmet needs regarding predictors and outcomes of remission.

The natural history of type 2 diabetes (T2D) is better understood now than previously. It is clearly heterogeneous, with both genetic and environmental factors contributing to its pathogenesis and evolution. Typically, a genetic predisposition is present at birth but the hyperglycemia that defines diabetes appears only gradually and reaches diagnostic levels in adulthood. Environmental factors modulating expression of T2D include availability of various foods; opportunity for and participation in physical activity; stress related to family, work, or other influences; exposure to pollutants and toxins; and access to public health and medical resources. Two common but transitory events can lead to earlier emergence of hyperglycemia in susceptible individuals: pregnancy or short-term therapy with glucocorticoids. Accordingly, people may develop "gestational diabetes" or "steroid diabetes" as conditions that are distinct but nevertheless related to typical T2D (1,2). In these settings, hyperglycemia is provoked by insulin resistance but may not persist, as responses to insulin improve when the baby is delivered or glucocorticoid therapy ceases. Glucose levels can return to normal after the pregnancy, yet an increased risk of later T2D remains (3). Acute illness or other stressful experiences can also provoke temporary hyperglycemia, sometimes called "stress hyperglycemia," in vulnerable individuals. T2D that has developed gradually and independent of these stimuli, but most often accompanying weight gain in midlife, can become easier to control or appear to remit following weight loss in some cases. Moreover, individuals with T2D can unintentionally lose weight due to illness, emotional distress, or unavailability of food related to serious social dislocation. Either voluntary or unexpected decline of weight in T2D may allow or require cessation of glucose-lowering treatment.

These changing patterns of glycemia have important epidemiologic implications. One is that T2D can remit without specific intervention in some cases. Another is that complications specific to diabetes, such as diabetic glomerulopathy, can be found in people without concurrent diabetes who were exposed to chronic hyperglycemia in the past (4). Yet another is a U-shaped relationship between glucose levels and death in T2D, with increased risk at normal or lower levels of hemoglobin A_{1c} (HbA_{1c}). This pattern might be attributed to overtreatment of T2D, leading to an increased risk of hypoglycemia (5), but alternatively could result from weight loss and declining glucose levels due to another serious and potentially fatal illness (6). Thus, both sustained increases and sustained decreases of glucose levels can occur spontaneously or through interventions and can present problems of interpretation.

Therapies targeting metabolic control in T2D have improved greatly in recent years. Short-term pharmacologic therapy at the time of first presentation of T2D in adults can sometimes restore nearly normal glycemic control, allowing therapy to be withdrawn (7–9). Reversal of "glucose toxicity" accompanying restoration of glycemic control is best documented with early intensive insulin therapy but can occur with other interventions. New classes of drugs, the glucagon-like peptide 1 (GLP-1) receptor agonists and sodium–glucose cotransporter inhibitors, can sometimes attain excellent glycemic control with little tendency to cause hypoglycemia. Significant behavioral changes—mainly related to nutrition and weight management—can lead to a return from overt hyperglycemia to nearly normal glucose levels for extended periods of time (10,11). More dramatically, surgical or other enteral interventions can induce both significant

weight loss and further improvement of metabolic control by other mechanisms for prolonged periods (12–14)—5 years or more in some cases. A return to nearly normal glycemic regulation after all these forms of intervention is most likely early in the course of T2D and can involve partial recovery of both insulin secretion and insulin action (15).

Increasingly, experience with sustained improvement of glucose levels into the normal range has prompted a reevaluation of terminology and definitions that may guide current discussions and future research in managing such transitions in glycemia in T2D. In 2009 a consensus statement initiated by the American Diabetes Association (ADA) addressed these issues (16). It suggested that "remission," signifying "abatement or disappearance of the signs and symptoms," be adopted as a descriptive term. Three categories of remission were proposed. "Partial" remission was considered to occur when hyperglycemia below diagnostic thresholds for diabetes was maintained without active pharmacotherapy for at least 1 year. "Complete" remission was described as normal glucose levels without pharmacotherapy for 1 year. "Prolonged" remission could be described when a complete remission persisted for 5 years or more without pharmacotherapy. A level of HbA_{1c} <6.5% (<48 mmol/mol) and/or fasting plasma glucose (FPG) 100–125 mg/dL (5.6 to 6.9 mmol/L) were used to define a partial remission, while "normal" levels of HbA_{1c} and FPG (<100 mg/dL [5.6 mmol/L]) were required for a complete remission.

To build upon this statement and subsequent publications (17) in the context of more recent experience, the ADA convened an international, multidisciplinary expert group. Representatives from the American Diabetes Association, European Association for the Study of Diabetes, Diabetes UK, the Endocrine Society, and the Diabetes Surgery Summit were included. For another perspective, an oncologist

was also part of the expert group. This group met three times in person and conducted additional electronic exchanges between February 2019 and September 2020. The following is a summary of these discussions and conclusions derived from them. This report is not intended to establish treatment guidelines or to favor specific interventions. Instead, based on consensus reached by the authors, it proposes suitable definitions of terms and ways to assess glycemic measurements, to facilitate collection and analysis of data that may lead to future clinical guidance.

OPTIMAL TERMINOLOGY

The choice of terminology has implications for clinical practice and policy decisions. Several terms have been proposed for people who have become free of a previously diagnosed disease state. In T2D, the terms *resolution*, *reversal*, *remission*, and *cure* each have been used to describe a favorable outcome of interventions resulting in a disease-free status. In agreement with the prior consensus group's conclusions (16), this expert panel concluded that diabetes *remission* is the most appropriate term. It strikes an appropriate balance, noting that diabetes may not always be active and progressive yet implying that a notable improvement may not be permanent. It is consistent with the view that a person may require ongoing support to forestall relapse, and regular monitoring to allow intervention should hyperglycemia recur. Remission is a term widely used in the field of oncology (18), defined as a decrease in or disappearance of signs and symptoms of cancer.

A common tendency is to equate remission with "no evidence of disease," allowing a binary choice of diagnosis. However, diabetes is defined by hyperglycemia, which exists on a continuum. The consensus group concluded that "no evidence of diabetes" was not an appropriate term to apply to T2D. One reason for this decision was that the underlying pathophysiology of T2D, including both deficiency of insulin and resistance to insulin's actions, as well as other abnormalities, is rarely completely normalized by interventions (19–21). In addition, any criterion for identifying a remission of diabetes will necessarily be arbitrary, a point on a continuum of glycemic levels. Although the previous consensus statement suggested dividing diabetes remission into partial and complete categories, using different glycemic thresholds (16), this distinction could introduce ambiguity affecting policy decisions related to insurance premiums, reimbursements, and coding of medical encounters. The prior statement's suggestion that a prolonged remission, longer than 5 years, be considered separately did not have an objective basis. The present group doubted that this distinction would assist clinical decisions or processes, at least until more objective information about the frequency of long-term remissions and the medical outcomes associated with them is available. A single definition of remission based on glycemic measurements was thought more likely to be helpful.

The other candidate terms have limitations. Considering a diagnosis of diabetes to be *resolved* suggests either that the original diagnosis was in error or that an entirely normal state has been permanently established. The term *reversal* is used to describe the process of returning to glucose levels below those diagnostic of diabetes, but it should not be equated with the state of remission. The term *cure* seems especially problematic in suggesting that all aspects of the condition are now normalized and that no clinical follow-up or further management will be needed either for a recurrence of hyperglycemia or for additional risks associated with the underlying physiological abnormalities. While cure is a hoped-for outcome, as in cancer patients, the group agreed that the term should be avoided in the context of T2D.

GLYCEMIC CRITERIA FOR DIAGNOSING REMISSION OF T2D

Measures widely used for diagnosis or glycemic management of T2D include HbA_{1c}, FPG, 2-h plasma glucose after an oral glucose challenge, and mean daily

glucose as measured by continuous glucose monitoring (CGM). The group favored HbA_{1c} below the level currently used for initial diagnosis of diabetes, 6.5% (48 mmol/mol), and remaining at that level for at least 3 months without continuation of the usual antihyperglycemic agents as the main defining measurement. Methods used to measure HbA_{1c} must have stringent quality assurance in place and assays must be standardized to criteria aligned to international reference values (22–24).

However, a number of factors can affect HbA_{1c} measurements, including a variant hemoglobin, differing rates of glycation, or alterations of erythrocyte survival that can occur in a variety of disease states. Information on which methods are affected by variant hemoglobins can be found at http://ngsp.org/interf.asp. Thus, in some people a normal HbA_{1c} value may be present when glucose is actually elevated, or HbA_{1c} may be high when mean glucose is normal. In settings where HbA_{1c} may be unreliable, measurement of 24-h mean glucose concentrations by CGM has been proposed as an alternative. A glycated hemoglobin value calculated as equivalent to the observed mean glucose by CGM has been termed the estimated HbA_{1c} (eA1C) (25) or most recently a glucose management indicator (GMI) (26). In cases where the accuracy of HbA_{1c} values is uncertain, CGM can be used to assess the correlation between mean glucose and HbA_{1c} and identify patterns outside the usual range of normal (27,28).

An FPG lower than 126 mg/dL (7.0 mmol/L) can in some settings be used as an alternate criterion for remission, just as a value higher than that level is an alternative for initial diagnosis of T2D. This approach has the disadvantage of requiring sample collection while fasting overnight, together with significant variation between repeated measurements. Testing of 2-h plasma glucose following a 75-g oral glucose challenge seems a less desirable choice, in part because of the added complexity of obtaining it and the high variability between repeated measurements. In addition, metabolic surgical interventions can alter the usual patterns of glycemic response to oral glucose, with early hyperglycemia followed by later hypoglycemia after an oral glucose

challenge, further confounding interpretation of the test.

Considering all alternatives, the group strongly favored use of HbA_{1c} <6.5% (48 mmol/mol) as generally reliable and the simplest and most widely understood defining criterion under usual circumstances. In some circumstances, an eA1C or GMI <6.5% can be considered an equivalent criterion.

CAN REMISSION BE DIAGNOSED WHILE GLUCOSE-LOWERING DRUGS ARE BEING USED?

Diabetes remission may be achieved by a change of lifestyle, other medical or surgical interventions, or—as is often the case—a combination of these approaches. Whether a therapy needs to be discontinued before making a diagnosis of remission depends on the intervention. Alterations of lifestyle involving day-to-day routines related to nutrition and physical activity have health effects that extend well beyond those related to diabetes. Moreover, the possibility of not only achieving diabetes remission but also generally improving health status may have motivated the individual to make these changes in the first place. These considerations also apply to surgical approaches, which, in addition, are not easily reversed. A remission can therefore be diagnosed postoperatively and in the setting of ongoing lifestyle efforts.

Whether a remission can be diagnosed in the setting of ongoing pharmacotherapy is a more complex question. In some cases, excellent glycemic control can be restored by short-term use of one or more glucose-lowering drugs, with persistence of nearly normal levels even after cessation of these agents. If antihyperglycemic drug therapy continues, it is not possible to discern whether a drug-independent remission has occurred. A diagnosis of remission can only be made after all glucose-lowering agents have been withheld for an interval that is sufficient both to allow waning of the drug's effects and to assess the effect of the absence of drugs on HbA_{1c} values.

This criterion would apply to all glucose-lowering drugs including those with other effects. Notably, metformin might be prescribed for weight maintenance, to improve markers of risk for cardiovascular disease or cancer, or for the polycystic ovarian syndrome (29). GLP-1 receptor agonists might be favored to control weight or reduce risk of cardiovascular events, and sodium-glucose cotransporter inhibitors may be prescribed for heart failure or renal protection. If such considerations preclude stopping these drugs, then remission cannot be diagnosed even though nearly normal glycemic levels are maintained. A clinical decision may be made to continue such therapies without testing for remission, and in that case, whether a true remission has been attained remains unknown. The group also recognized that some drugs have a modest glucose-lowering effect but are not indicated for glucose lowering, as in the case of some weight loss drugs. Because these drugs are not used to manage hyperglycemia specifically, they would not need to be stopped before a diagnosis of diabetes remission can be made.

Another concern is the possible role of preventive drug intervention for individuals who have been diagnosed with remission or are otherwise known to be at very high risk of T2D, such as women with prior gestational diabetes. Should such individuals be candidates for treatment with antihyperglycemic therapy, especially with metformin? This is a controversial area, with arguments both for and against. In favor of pharmacotherapy to prevent emergence or re-emergence of overt diabetes is the possibility of safely and inexpensively eliminating a period of undiagnosed yet harmful hyperglycemia (30). On the other side is the argument that protection against β-cell deterioration by pharmacotherapy has yet to be convincingly

proven and preventive intervention has known costs and potential risks (31).

Whether preventive intervention is justified was thought to be beyond the scope of the present statement, except to note that, if it is used, whether a remission is persisting cannot be known. Data systematically collected based on the definitions proposed in this document may help to clarify the roles of the various interventions that might be used in this setting.

TEMPORAL ASPECTS OF DIAGNOSING REMISSION

When intervention in T2D is by pharmacotherapy or surgery, the time of initiation is easily determined and the clinical effects are rapidly apparent (Table 1). When intervention is by alteration of lifestyle, the onset of benefit can be slower, and up to 6 months may be required for stabilization of the effect. A further temporal factor is the approximately 3 months needed for an effective intervention to be entirely reflected by the change of HbA_{1c}, which reflects mean glucose over a period of several months. Considering these factors, an interval of at least 6 months after initiation of a lifestyle intervention is needed before testing of HbA_{1c} can reliably evaluate the response. After a more rapidly effective surgical intervention, an interval of at least 3 months is required while the HbA_{1c} value stabilizes. When the intervention is with temporary pharmacotherapy, or when a lifestyle or metabolic surgery intervention is added to prior pharmacotherapy, an interval of at least 3 months after cessation of any glucose-lowering agent is required. With all interventions leading to remission, subsequent measurements of HbA_{1c} not more often than

every 3 months nor less frequent than yearly are advised to confirm continuation of the remission. In contrast to HbA_{1c}, FPG or eA1C derived from CGM can stabilize at a shorter time after initiation of an intervention, or increase more rapidly if glycemic control worsens later on. When these measurements of glucose are substituted for HbA_{1c}, they can be collected sooner after the intervention and more frequently thereafter, but because they are more variable, a value consistent with onset or loss of a remission should be confirmed by a repeated measurement.

PHYSIOLOGIC CONSIDERATIONS REGARDING REMISSIONS FOLLOWING INTERVENTION WITH PHARMACOTHERAPY, LIFESTYLE, OR METABOLIC SURGERY

When a remission is documented after temporary use of glucose-lowering agents, the direct effects of pharmacotherapy do not persist. Reversal of the adverse effects of poor metabolic control (32) on insulin secretion and action may establish a remission, but other underlying abnormalities persist and the duration of the remission is quite variable. In contrast, when a persistent change of lifestyle leads to remission, the change in food intake, physical activity, and management of stress and environmental factors can favorably alter insulin secretion and action for long periods of time. In this setting, long-term remissions are possible, but not assured. The effects of metabolic surgery are more profound and generally more sustained (33). Structural changes of the gastrointestinal tract lead to a novel hormonal milieu. This includes, among other changes, several-fold greater GLP-1 concentrations in blood after

Table 1—Interventions and temporal factors in determining remission of T2D

Intervention Note: Documentation of remission should include a measurement of HbA_{1c} just prior to intervention	Interval before testing of HbA_{1c} can reliably evaluate the response	Subsequent measurements of HbA_{1c} to document continuation of a remission
Pharmacotherapy	At least 3 months after cessation of this intervention	Not more often than every 3 months nor less frequent than yearly
Surgery	At least 3 months after the procedure *and* 3 months after cessation of any pharmacotherapy	
Lifestyle	At least 6 months after beginning this intervention *and* 3 months after cessation of any pharmacotherapy	

eating, which through interaction with relevant areas of the brain may reduce appetite and food intake and additionally alter peripheral metabolism. Re-establishment of glucose homeostasis by these mechanisms is typically longer lasting. The changes of anatomy and physiology are essentially permanent, but even so the desirable effects on glycemic patterns may not be sustained indefinitely. Partial regain of weight can occur, and continuing decline of β-cell capacity may contribute to rising levels of glucose over time.

ONGOING MONITORING

For the reasons just described, a remission is a state in which diabetes is not present but which nonetheless requires continued observation because hyperglycemia frequently recurs. Weight gain, stress from other forms of illness, and continuing decline of β-cell function can all lead to recurrence of T2D. Testing of HbA_{1c} or another measure of glycemic control should be performed no less often than yearly. Ongoing attention to maintenance of a healthful lifestyle is needed, and pharmacotherapy for other conditions with agents known to promote hyperglycemia, especially glucocorticoids and certain antipsychotic agents, should be avoided.

The metabolic memory, or legacy effect (34), is relevant in this setting. These terms describe the persisting harmful effects of prior hyperglycemia in various tissues. Even after a remission, the classic complications of diabetes—including retinopathy, nephropathy, neuropathy, and enhanced risk of cardiovascular disease—can still occur (35). Hence, people in remission from diabetes should be advised to have regular retinal screening, tests of renal function, foot evaluation, and measurement of blood pressure and weight in addition to ongoing monitoring of HbA_{1c}. At present, there is no long-term evidence indicating that any of the usually recommended assessments for complications can safely be discontinued. Individuals who are in remission should be advised to remain under active medical observation including regular checkups.

In addition to continued gradual progression of established complications of T2D, there is another risk potentially associated with a remission. This is the possibility of an abrupt worsening of microvascular disease following a rapid reduction of glucose levels after a long period of hyperglycemia. In particular, when poor glycemic control is present together with retinopathy beyond the presence of microaneurysms, rapid reduction of glucose levels should be avoided and retinal screening repeated if a rapid decline in blood glucose is observed. This suggestion is based mainly upon experience with worsening of retinopathy after initiation or intensification of insulin therapy, which is seen only if moderate or worse retinopathy is present at baseline (36,37). Worsening of retinopathy can occur with other interventions, although there is some evidence that this risk is less after metabolic surgery (38).

FURTHER QUESTIONS AND UNMET NEEDS

The preceding discussion is based largely on expert opinion. It is not intended to provide guidance regarding how or when glycemic control qualifying as a remission should be sought. It also does not aim to clarify the role of preventive pharmacotherapy after a remission is identified. Rather, it proposes terminology and a structure to facilitate future research and collection of information to support future clinical guidelines. Some of the areas needing further research are listed below.

Validation of Using 6.5% HbA_{1c} as the Defining Measurement
The relative effectiveness of using 6.5% HbA_{1c} (48 mmol/mol) as the cut point for diagnosis of remission, as opposed to 6.0% HbA_{1c} (42 mmol/mol), HbA_{1c} 5.7% (39 mmol/mol), or some other level, in predicting risk of relapse or of microvascular or cardiovascular complications should be evaluated. The use of CGM-derived data to adjust HbA_{1c} target ranges for identifying glycemic remission should be further explored. Use of CGM-derived average glucose judged equivalent to HbA_{1c} <6.5% (<48 mmol/mol) or use of FPG <7.0 mmol/L (<126 mg/dL) instead of HbA_{1c} could be studied.

Validation of the Timing of Glycemic Measurements
Less frequent testing of HbA_{1c} might be possible without altering predictive efficiency. For example, routine measurements at 6 months and 12 months might be sufficient to identify remission and risk of relapse in the short term.

Evaluation of the Effects of Metformin and Other Drugs After Remission Is Established
Metformin's main action affecting glycemic control in diabetes is to improve hepatic responsiveness to portal insulin. Whether it can delay relapse through other mechanisms is unknown. After diagnosis of remission, therapy with metformin or other drugs not used for glycemic indications may delay recurrence of hyperglycemia and/or protect against progression of other metabolic disturbances. Objective information on this point is limited, and more research is clearly required.

Evaluation of Nonglycemic Measures During Remission
Improved glycemic control is not the only aspect of metabolism that may affect long-term outcomes. For example, circulating lipoprotein profiles, peripheral and visceral adiposity, and intracellular fat deposition in the liver and other tissues may all be relevant effects accompanying—or possibly separate from—glycemic remission and could be evaluated. The role of changes in GLP-1 and other peptide mediators after pharmacologic, behavioral, or surgical interventions in altering risks of relapse or medical events remains unknown.

Research on Duration of Remission
The expected duration of a remission induced by various interventions is still not well defined, and factors associated with relapse from remission should be examined more fully.

Documentation of Long-term Outcomes After Remission
Long-term effects of remission on mortality, cardiovascular events, functional capacity, and quality of life are unknown. Metabolic and clinical factors related to these outcomes during remission are poorly understood and could be defined.

Development of Educational Materials for Health Care Professionals and Patients
Development and standardization of educational and screening programs for individuals in remission would facilitate

application of various recommendations to clinical practice.

CONCLUSIONS

A return to normal or nearly normal glucose levels in patients with typical T2D can sometimes be attained by using current and emerging forms of medical or lifestyle interventions or metabolic surgery. The frequency of sustained metabolic improvement in this setting, its likely duration, and its effect on subsequent medical outcomes remain unclear. To facilitate clinical decisions, data collection, and research regarding outcomes, more clear terminology describing such improvement is needed. On the basis of our discussions, we propose the following:

1. The term used to describe a sustained metabolic improvement in T2D to nearly normal levels should be *remission* of diabetes.
2. Remission should be defined as a return of HbA_{1c} to <6.5% (<48 mmol/mol) that occurs spontaneously or following an intervention and that persists for *at least 3 months* in the absence of usual glucose-lowering pharmacotherapy.
3. When HbA_{1c} is determined to be an unreliable marker of chronic glycemic control, *FPG <126 mg/dL (<7.0 mmol/L)* or *eA1C <6.5%* calculated from CGM values can be used as alternate criteria.
4. Testing of HbA_{1c} to document a remission should be performed just prior to an intervention and no sooner than 3 months after initiation of the intervention and withdrawal of any glucose-lowering pharmacotherapy.
5. Subsequent testing to determine long-term maintenance of a remission should be done at least yearly thereafter, together with the testing routinely recommended for potential complications of diabetes.
6. Research based on the terminology and definitions outlined in the present statement is needed to determine the frequency, duration, and effects on short- and long-term medical outcomes of remissions of T2D using available interventions.

Duality of Interest. M.C.R. reports receiving research grant support through Oregon Health & Science University from Eli Lilly & Co., Novo Nordisk, and AstraZeneca and honoraria for consulting from Adocia, Intercept, and Theracos. H.C.G. holds the McMaster-Sanofi Population Health Institute Chair in Diabetes Research and Care and reports research grants from Eli Lilly & Co., AstraZeneca, Merck, Novo Nordisk and Sanofi; honoraria for speaking from AstraZeneca, Boehringer Ingelheim, Eli Lilly & Co., Novo Nordisk, and Sanofi; and consulting fees from Abbott, AstraZeneca, Boehringer Ingelheim, Eli Lilly & Co., Merck, Novo Nordisk, Janssen, Sanofi, and Kowa. M.A.N. has been a member on advisory boards or has consulted for AstraZeneca, Boehringer Ingelheim, Eli Lilly & Co., GlaxoSmithKline, Menarini/Berlin Chemie, Merck, Sharp & Dohme, and Novo Nordisk; has received grant support from AstraZeneca, Eli Lilly & Co., Menarini/Berlin-Chemie, Merck, Sharp & Dohme, and Novo Nordisk; and has served on the speakers' bureau of AstraZeneca, Boehringer Ingelheim, Eli Lilly & Co., Menarini/Berlin Chemie, Merck, Sharp & Dohme, and Novo Nordisk. W.K.O. reports serving as a consultant to Astellas, AstraZeneca, Bayer, Janssen, Sanofi, and Sema4 and has recently taken a role as Chief Medical Science Officer for Sema4. A.E.R. is a member of the advisory board for Rhythm Pharmaceuticals, Inc. and REWIND Co. C.W.I.R. reports serving on advisory boards and receiving honoraria for speaker meetings from Novo Nordisk, GI Dynamics, Johnson & Johnson, Herbalife, Boehringer Ingelheim, Sanofi, Keyron, and AnBio and has received funding from the EU Innovative Medicine Initiative, Science Foundation Ireland, Health Research Board, Irish Research Council, Swedish Research Council, and European Foundation for Study of Diabetes. F.R. reports receiving research grants from Ethicon and Medtronic and consulting fees from Ethicon, Novo Nordisk, and Medtronic and is on the scientific advisory board of GI Dynamics and Keyron. P.S. received grant support from Ethicon, Medtronic, and Pacira and serves as a consultant for Ethicon, Medtronic, GI Dynamics, Persona, Keyron, Mediflix, SE LLC, and Medscape. R.T. reports lecture fees from Lilly and Novartis and consultancy fees from Wilmington Healthcare and is author of the book *Life Without Diabetes*. D.T. declares no personal conflict of interest but has permanent employment with Diabetes UK, who has commercial relationships with various pharmaceutical and food companies. No other potential conflicts of interest relevant to this article were reported.

References

1. Vounzoulaki E, Khunti K, Abner SC, Tan BK, Davies MJ, Gillies CL. Progression to type 2 diabetes in women with a known history of gestational diabetes: systematic review and meta-analysis. BMJ 2020;369:m1361
2. Simmons LR, Molyneaux L, Yue DK, Chua EL. Steroid-induced diabetes: is it just unmasking of type 2 diabetes? ISRN Endocrinol 2012;2012:910905
3. Li Z, Cheng Y, Wang D, et al. Incidence rate of type diabetes mellitus after gestational diabetes mellitus: a systematic review and meta-analysis of 170,139 women. J Diab Res 2020;3076463
4. Selvin E, Ning Y, Steffes MW, et al. Glycated hemoglobin and the risk of kidney disease and retinopathy in adults with and without diabetes. Diabetes 2011;60:298–305
5. Currie CJ, Peters JR, Tynan A, et al. Survival as a function of HbA_{1c} in people with type 2 diabetes: a retrospective cohort study. Lancet 2010;375:481–489
6. Carson AP, Fox CS, McGuire DK, et al. Low hemoglobin A1c and risk of all-cause mortality among US adults without diabetes. Circ Cardiovasc Qual Outcomes 2010;3:661–667
7. Kramer CK, Zinman B, Retnakaran R. Short-term intensive insulin therapy in type 2 diabetes mellitus: a systematic review and meta-analysis. Lancet Diabetes Endocrinol 2013;1:28–34
8. Kramer CK, Zinman B, Choi H, Retnakaran R. Predictors of sustained drug-free diabetes remission over 48 weeks following short-term intensive insulin therapy in early type 2 diabetes. BMJ Open Diabetes Res Care 2016;4:e000270
9. McInnes N, Smith A, Otto R, et al. Piloting a remission strategy in type 2 diabetes: results of a randomized controlled trial. J Clin Endocrinol Metab 2017;102:1596–1605
10. Lean MEJ, Leslie WS, Barnes AC, et al. Durability of a primary care-led weight-management intervention for remission of type 2 diabetes: 2-year results of the DiRECT open-label, cluster-randomised trial. Lancet Diabetes Endocrinol 2019;7:344–355
11. Gregg EW, Chen H, Wagenknecht LE, et al.; Look AHEAD Research Group. Association of an intensive lifestyle intervention with remission of type 2 diabetes. JAMA 2012;308:2489–2496
12. Mingrone G, Panunzi S, De Gaetano A, et al. Metabolic surgery versus conventional medical therapy in patients with type 2 diabetes: 10-year follow-up of an open-label, single-centre, randomised controlled trial. Lancet 2021;397:293–304
13. Rubino F, Nathan DM, Eckel RH, et al.; Delegates of the 2nd Diabetes Surgery Summit. Metabolic surgery in the treatment algorithm for type 2 diabetes: a joint statement by international diabetes organizations. Diabetes Care 2016;39:861–877
14. Schauer PR, Bhatt DL, Kirwan JP, et al.; STAMPEDE Investigators. Bariatric surgery versus intensive medical therapy for diabetes: 5-year outcomes. N Engl J Med 2017;376:641–651
15. White MG, Shaw JAM, Taylor R. Type 2 diabetes: the pathologic basis of reversible β-cell dysfunction. Diabetes Care 2016;39:2080–2088
16. Buse JB, Caprio S, Cefalu WT, et al. How do we define cure of diabetes? Diabetes Care 2009;32:2133–2135
17. Nagi D, Hambling C, Taylor R. Remission of type 2 diabetes: a position statement from the Association of British Clinical Diabetologists (ABCD) and the Primary Care Diabetes Society (PCDS). Br J Diabetes 2019;19:73–76
18. Barnes E. Between remission and cure: patients, practitioners and the transformation of leukaemia in the late twentieth century. Chronic Illn 2007;3:253–264
19. Taylor R, Al-Mrabeh A, Zhyzhneuskaya S, et al. Remission of human type 2 diabetes requires decrease in liver and pancreas fat content but is dependent upon capacity for β cell recovery. Cell Metab 2018;28:547–556.e3

20. Lim EL, Hollingsworth KG, Aribisala BS, Chen MJ, Mathers JC, Taylor R. Reversal of type 2 diabetes: normalisation of beta cell function in association with decreased pancreas and liver triacylglycerol. Diabetologia 2011;54:2506–2514

21. Camastra S, Manco M, Mari A, et al. Beta-cell function in severely obese type 2 diabetic patients: long-term effects of bariatric surgery. Diabetes Care 2007;30:1002–1004

22. Consensus Committee. Consensus statement on the worldwide standardization of the hemoglobin A1C measurement: the American Diabetes Association, European Association for the Study of Diabetes, International Federation of Clinical Chemistry and Laboratory Medicine, and the International Diabetes Federation. Diabetes Care 2007;30:2399–2400

23. Jeppsson J-O, Kobold U, Barr J, et al.; International Federation of Clinical Chemistry and Laboratory Medicine (IFCC). Approved IFCC reference method for the measurement of HbA1c in human blood. Clin Chem Lab Med 2002;40:78–89

24. EurA1c Trial Group. EurA1c: the European HbA1c trial to investigate the performance of HbA1c assays in 2166 laboratories across 17 countries and 24 manufacturers by use of the IFCC model for quality targets. Clin Chem 2018; 64:1183–1192

25. Danne T, Nimri R, Battelino T, et al. International consensus on use of continuous glucose monitoring. Diabetes Care 2017;40:1631–1640

26. Bergenstal RM, Beck RW, Close KL, et al. Glucose management indicator (GMI): a new term for estimating A1C from continuous glucose monitoring. Diabetes Care 2018;41:2275–2280

27. Beck RW, Connor CG, Mullen DM, Wesley DM, Bergenstal RM. The fallacy of average: how using HbA1c alone to assess glycemic control can be misleading. Diabetes Care 2017;40:994–999

28. Shah VN, DuBose SN, Li Z, et al. Continuous glucose monitoring profiles in healthy non-diabetic participants: a multicenter prospective study. J Clin Endocrinol Metab 2019;104: 4356–4364

29. Hundal RS, Inzucchi SE, Metformin: new understandings, new uses. Drugs 2003;63:1879–1894

30. Herman WH, Ratner RE. Metformin should be used to treat prediabetes in selected individuals. Diabetes Care 2020;43:1988–1990

31. Davidson MB. Metformin should not be used to treat prediabetes. Diabetes Care 2020; 43:1983–1987

32. Yki-Järvinen H. Glucose toxicity. Endocr Rev 1992;13:415–431

33. Isaman DJ, Rothberg AE, Herman WH. Reconciliation of type 2 diabetes remission rates in studies of Roux-en-Y gastric bypass. Diabetes Care 2016;39:2247–2253

34. Ceriello A. The emerging challenge in diabetes: the "metabolic memory." Vascul Pharmacol 2012; 57:133–138

35. Murphy R, Jiang Y, Booth M, et al. Progression of diabetic retinopathy after bariatric surgery. Diabet Med 2015;32:1212–1220

36. Arun CS, Pandit R, Taylor R. Long-term pro-gression of retinopathy after initiation of insulin therapy in Type 2 diabetes: an observational study. Diabetologia 2004;47: 1380–1384

37. The Diabetes Control and Complications Trial Research Group. Early worsening of diabetic retinopathy in the Diabetes Control and Complications Trial. Arch Ophthalmol 1998;116:874–886

38. Singh RP, Gans R, Kashyap SR, et al. Effect of bariatric surgery versus intensive medical management on diabetic ophthalmic outcomes. Diabetes Care 2015;38:e32–e33

Multicenter, Head-to-Head, Real-World Validation Study of Seven Automated Artificial Intelligence Diabetic Retinopathy Screening Systems

Diabetes Care 2021;44:1168–1175 | https://doi.org/10.2337/dc20-1877

Aaron Y. Lee,[1,2,3] Ryan T. Yanagihara,[1] Cecilia S. Lee,[1,2] Marian Blazes,[1] Hoon C. Jung,[1,2] Yewlin E. Chee,[1] Michael D. Gencarella,[1] Harry Gee,[4] April Y. Maa,[5,6] Glenn C. Cockerham,[7,8] Mary Lynch,[5,9] and Edward J. Boyko[10,11]

[1]Department of Ophthalmology, University of Washington School of Medicine, Seattle, WA
[2]Department of Ophthalmology, Puget Sound Veteran Affairs, Seattle, WA
[3]eScience Institute, University of Washington, Seattle, WA
[4]Office of Information and Technology, Clinical Imaging, Seattle, WA
[5]Department of Ophthalmology, Emory University School of Medicine, Atlanta, GA
[6]Regional Telehealth Services, Veterans Affairs Southeast Network Veterans Integrated Service Networks (VISN 7), Duluth, GA
[7]Veterans Health Administration, Specialty Care Services, Washington, DC
[8]Ophthalmology Service, Stanford University School of Medicine, Palo Alto, CA
[9]Ophthalmology Section, Atlanta Veterans Affairs Medical Center, Atlanta, GA
[10]Seattle Epidemiologic Research and Information Center, Department of Veterans Affairs Medical Center, Seattle, WA
[11]Department of Medicine, University of Washington, Seattle, WA

Corresponding author: Aaron Y. Lee, leeay@uw.edu

Received 27 July 2020 and accepted 25 October 2020

This article contains supplementary material online at https://doi.org/10.2337/figshare.13148540.

OBJECTIVE

With rising global prevalence of diabetic retinopathy (DR), automated DR screening is needed for primary care settings. Two automated artificial intelligence (AI)–based DR screening algorithms have U.S. Food and Drug Administration (FDA) approval. Several others are under consideration while in clinical use in other countries, but their real-world performance has not been evaluated systematically. We compared the performance of seven automated AI-based DR screening algorithms (including one FDA-approved algorithm) against human graders when analyzing real-world retinal imaging data.

RESEARCH DESIGN AND METHODS

This was a multicenter, noninterventional device validation study evaluating a total of 311,604 retinal images from 23,724 veterans who presented for teleretinal DR screening at the Veterans Affairs (VA) Puget Sound Health Care System (HCS) or Atlanta VA HCS from 2006 to 2018. Five companies provided seven algorithms, including one with FDA approval, that independently analyzed all scans, regardless of image quality. The sensitivity/specificity of each algorithm when classifying images as referable DR or not were compared with original VA teleretinal grades and a regraded arbitrated data set. Value per encounter was estimated.

RESULTS

Although high negative predictive values (82.72–93.69%) were observed, sensitivities varied widely (50.98–85.90%). Most algorithms performed no better than humans against the arbitrated data set, but two achieved higher sensitivities, and one yielded comparable sensitivity (80.47%, $P = 0.441$) and specificity (81.28%, $P = 0.195$). Notably, one had lower sensitivity (74.42%) for proliferative DR ($P = 9.77 \times 10^{-4}$) than the VA teleretinal graders. Value per encounter varied at $15.14–$18.06 for ophthalmologists and $7.74–$9.24 for optometrists.

CONCLUSIONS

The DR screening algorithms showed significant performance differences. These results argue for rigorous testing of all such algorithms on real-world data before clinical implementation.

A major microvascular complication of diabetes mellitus (DM) is diabetic retinopathy (DR), which is the leading cause of preventable blindness in working-age Americans (1,2). If detected and managed at an early stage, irreversible blindness can be avoided (3). Therefore, the American Academy of Ophthalmology Preferred Practice Pattern recommends that patients with DM undergo an annual dilated retinal fundus examination, and the American Diabetes Association recommends dilated examinations every 2 years for patients with type 2 DM without retinopathy (4,5). The global prevalence of DM has tripled over the past 20 years, affecting 151 million in 2000, 463 million in 2019, and a projected 700 million by 2045 (6). At this rate, eye care providers who deliver routine screening will become overwhelmed (7). Despite the effectiveness of teleretinal screening programs, these programs are also costly and labor intensive (2,8,9). Therefore, an inexpensive, accurate, and automated method to triage DR screening fundus photographs in the primary care clinic setting would greatly benefit providers, health care systems, and patients.

Artificial intelligence (AI)–based algorithms may provide promising solutions to alleviate the DR screening burden. Tufail and colleagues (10,11) have shown that when used in DR screening programs, AI algorithms can detect referable DR with high sensitivity and are cost-effective compared with manual grading, the current gold standard. However, these studies predated the era of deep learning, a machine learning technique that has revolutionized retinal image analysis. Currently existing deep learning algorithms have demonstrated performance similar to, or even better than, human experts at various classification tasks in DR (12,13). With significant advances in powerful deep learning algorithms, multiple companies have developed automated DR screening systems that have garnered the attention of the U.S. Food and Drug Administration (FDA), and to date, two AI-based screening algorithms have already been approved for use. As the FDA considers approval of additional automated machine learning algorithms, understanding their performance in real-world, intended-use settings is becoming increasingly important (14). In fact, the Center for Devices and Radiological Health (the FDA division responsible for regulating devices) prioritized the use of big data and real-world evidence for regulatory decision making in its 2019 regulatory science report, citing the need for validated methods of predicting device performance using real-world data (15). In line with this approach, we aimed to compare the performance of existing (either FDA approved or already in clinical use outside the U.S. and/or submitted for FDA approval) fully automated AI-based algorithms when screening for referable DR using real-world clinical data from two U.S. Veterans Affairs (VA) hospitals in geographically and demographically distinct cities. These algorithms were trained on unique, potentially limited data sets, and we hypothesized that their performance might decrease when tested with a large amount of real-world patient data. To our knowledge, this is the largest deep learning validation study to date.

RESEARCH DESIGN AND METHODS

Study Design

This was a multicenter, noninterventional device validation study that used images acquired from the VA Puget Sound Health Care System (HCS) and the Atlanta VA HCS. The institutional review board at the VA Puget Sound HCS approved the trial protocol. A waiver of informed consent was obtained for patient data used in the study. All participants had a diagnosis of DM and were not undergoing active eye care for any eye diseases and so were referred to the VA teleretinal DR screening program from 2006 to 2018. The overall study design is summarized in Supplementary Fig. 1.

Image Acquisition and Grading Process at the VA

At the VA, clinical photographs are stored in the Veterans Health Information System Technology Architecture (VISTA) Imaging system, and corresponding clinical data are deposited in the corporate data warehouse. At each encounter, at least four nonmydriatic or mydriatic color fundus photographs (at least two 45° images, one fovea centered, and at least two peripheral images) as well as an external color photograph for each eye were obtained using a Topcon TRC-NW8 fundus camera (Topcon Medical Systems, Tokyo, Japan). On average, nine photographs were available per encounter, including an average of 3.5 retinal images. All images were stored in JPG format and encapsulated using Digital Imaging and Communications in Medicine per standard VA VISTA processing for routine clinical care, with no perturbations or additional compression. The resolution of the images ranged from 4,000 × 3,000 to 4,288 × 2,848 pixels. The images were manually graded by VA-employed optometrists and ophthalmologists using the International Clinical Diabetic Retinopathy Severity Scale (ICDR) as follows: 0 = no DR, 1 = mild nonproliferative DR (NPDR), 2 = moderate NPDR, 3 = severe NPDR, 4 = proliferative DR (PDR), and 5 = ungradable image quality (16). At the VA, referable DR is defined as the presence of any DR (ICDR 1–4). The only difference in the imaging protocols between the two sites was the regular use of pharmacological pupillary dilation in all patients in Atlanta, which was not routinely performed at the Seattle site.

In this study, all images in the full data set were retrospectively acquired from each VA hospital's respective VISTA Imaging system (with the same image quality and format as available to teleretinal graders) and linked to clinical metadata from national and local VA databases, which include the original VA teleretinal grades for each image (17). None of the images had been used previously to train, validate, or test any automated diagnosis system that participated in this study. Other than removing all patient identifiers, no pre- or postprocessing was applied to any image before analysis by the AI algorithms. There were no changes to the teleretinal DR screening clinical pathway. All images were available to the algorithms regardless of quality, including those that were identified as ungradable by the VA teleretinal graders. The presence of any DR was used as the threshold for referable DR per VA standards (18).

Arbitration Data Set Sampling and Grading

A subset of images was regraded using double-masked arbitration by clinical experts. Two random subsets of the full data set were created for regrading. First, a consecutive sampling of images was used, and second, a balanced set that included 50 images from each retinopathy level and ungradable class by the original VA teleretinal grade (obtained from the Seattle and Atlanta data sets evenly) was sampled. These two data sets were combined (to provide enough data to power the sensitivity analysis for the different disease thresholds described below) and presented to a board-certified comprehensive ophthalmologist and two fellowship-trained retina specialists who were masked to the original grades as well as to one another's classifications and who then graded the encounters independently. Differences in opinion were arbitrated by a retina specialist who had the two differing grades but did not know the identities of the graders to avoid confirmation bias. At no point during the arbitration process did any grader have access to the original VA teleretinal grades. The graders read the images on 22-in. 1080p monitors using the same viewing system as the VA teleretinal graders (certified Picture Archive and Communication System for the storage, viewing, and grading of medical images). The graders were allowed to manipulate the images, including changing the brightness, contrast, and zoom and generating a red-free version. This final arbitrated set of encounters was then used as the reference standard when comparing the performance of the algorithms to the VA teleretinal graders in screening for referable DR.

AI Algorithms
We invited 23 companies with automated AI-based DR screening systems to participate in this study: OphtAI, AEye, AirDoc, Cognizant, D-EYE, Diagnos, DreamUp Vision, Eyenuk, Google, IDX, Intelligent Retinal Imaging Systems, Medios Technologies, Microsoft Corporation, Remidio, Retina-AI Health, RetinAI Medical, RetinaLyze System, Retmarker, Singapore Eye Research Institute, SigTuple Technologies, Spect, VisionQuest Biomedical, and Xtend.AI. The details of the study were provided in a letter sent to each company, including the threshold for referable disease. Of the companies approached, five completed the study: OphtAI, AirDoc, Eyenuk, Retina-AI Health, and Retmarker. A total of seven

algorithms were submitted for evaluation in this study. Each company sent its locked software preloaded on a workstation. Each system was masked to the original VA teleretinal grades and independently screened each image for referable DR defined as any degree of DR (ICDR grades 1–4) or unreadable encounters, without Internet connection. At the end of the study, each workstation was securely erased. As agreed upon before study initiation, the identity of each company was masked along with its submitted algorithms (labeled algorithms A–G). The study methods were provided to the participating companies upon request to give them the opportunity to adjust their software for the VA image acquisition protocol. These details included but were not limited to the camera system, image format, image resolution, aspect ratio, and number of photos per encounter. Each algorithm provided a binary classification output of each encounter as follows: 0 = does not need to be referred or 1 = should be referred for an in-person eye examination because of ungradable image quality or presence of any DR. In addition, all algorithms in the study either already had regulatory approval and/or were in active use in clinical settings around the world.

Statistical Analysis
To evaluate the algorithms, the screening performance of each was calculated using the original VA teleretinal grades from Seattle and Atlanta (combined and independently) as reference values. The screening performance measures included sensitivity, specificity, negative predictive value (NPV), and positive predictive value (PPV). Then, a separate analysis was performed using the arbitrated set of encounters as the reference standard. The sensitivity and specificity of the original VA teleretinal grades and those of each algorithm were compared with the arbitrated data set to evaluate their relative performance using a paired exact binomial test (19). In addition, to measure the sensitivities of the algorithms for different levels of disease severity, their performance was compared with the VA teleretinal graders at different disease thresholds identified in the arbitrated data set, including moderate NPDR or worse, severe NPDR or worse, and PDR.

Since each of the algorithms provided the binary output of no DR versus any DR, we calculated the sensitivity of the image subset for each disease severity without including the ungradable images.

Value-per-Encounter Analysis
Using the arbitrated data set, algorithms that performed no worse than the VA teleretinal graders in detecting referable DR in images marked as moderate NPDR or worse were selected to undergo a value-per-encounter analysis (20). The value per encounter for each individual algorithm was defined as the estimated pricing of each algorithm to make a normal profit (i.e., revenue and costs = 0) if deployed at the VA. This calculation was based on a two-stage scenario in which an AI algorithm would be used initially and then the images that screened negative would not need additional review by an optometrist or ophthalmologist. An average of 10 min per encounter was estimated as the amount of time needed to open, review, and write a report of the findings. The National Plan and Provider Enumeration System National Provider Identifier database and the FedsDataCenter database for fiscal year 2015 were used to determine the mean salary of providers (ophthalmologists or optometrists) per minute. The value per encounter was calculated as follows: value per encounter = [(10 min per encounter) × (mean salary of provider per min) × (encounter not referred)] / (total encounters). The primary outcome of our study was to evaluate the sensitivity and specificity of each algorithm compared with a human grader when determining whether the patient should be referred for an in-person ophthalmic examination on the basis of the DR screening images taken. Secondary end points included measuring the sensitivity of each algorithm against two random subsets of independently regraded images to permit estimation of the value per encounter that was due to lower reliance on expert human graders.

RESULTS
Patient Demographics and Image Characteristics
Patient demographic information and classification grades are summarized

Table 1—Demographic factors and baseline clinical characteristics of the study population

	Seattle	Atlanta	Total
Patients, n	13,439	10,285	23,724
Age (years)			
Mean (SD)	62.20 (10.91)	63.46 (10.14)	62.75 (10.60)
Range	21–97	24–98	21–98
Male sex	12,724 (94.68)	9,795 (95.24)	22,519 (94.92)
Race			
White	9,482 (70.56)	4,678 (45.48)	14,160 (59.69)
African American	1,642 (12.22)	5,085 (49.44)	6,727 (28.35)
Asian	383 (2.85)	34 (0.33)	417 (1.76)
Other	605 (4.50)	90 (0.88)	695 (2.93)
Unknown	1,327 (9.87)	398 (3.87)	1,725 (7.27)
Encounters, n	21,797	13,104	34,901
Retinopathy grade			
No DR	15,270 (70.05)	11,166 (85.21)	26,436 (75.75)
Mild NPDR	2,364 (10.85)	957 (7.31)	3,321 (9.51)
Moderate NPDR	494 (2.27)	311 (2.37)	805 (2.31)
Severe NPDR	110 (0.50)	153 (1.17)	263 (0.75)
PDR	22 (0.10)	193 (1.47)	215 (0.62)
Ungradable	3,537 (16.23)	324 (2.47)	3,861 (11.06)
Images, n	199,142	112,462	311,604

Data are n (%) unless otherwise indicated.

in Table 1. A total of 311,604 retinal images were acquired from 23,724 racially diverse patients. In the Seattle group, there was a higher prevalence of mild NPDR compared with severe NPDR. In contrast, a relatively higher number of patients presented to Atlanta with advanced stages of DR, including severe NPDR (1.17%) and PDR (1.47%), compared with Seattle (0.50% and 0.10%, respectively). More images from Seattle (16.23%) were of ungradable image quality compared with Atlanta (2.47%).

Automated DR Screening Performance
The sensitivity, specificity, NPV, and PPV for each AI screening system were calculated (using the original VA teleretinal grades as the reference standard) and are summarized in Fig. 1. In the full data set (Fig. 1A), sensitivity ranged from 50.98 to 85.90%, specificity from 60.42 to 83.69%, NPV from 82.72 to 93.69%, and PPV from 36.46 to 50.80%. Overall, the algorithms achieved higher NPVs using the Atlanta data set (range 90.71–98.05%) (Fig. 1B) compared with the Seattle data set (77.57–90.66%) (Fig. 1C). In contrast, PPV ranged from 24.80 to 39.07% in the Atlanta data set, which was lower than the Seattle data set (42.04–62.92%).

A subset of 7,379 images from 735 encounters was regraded for the arbitrated data set. Using the arbitrated grades as the new reference standard, the VA teleretinal graders achieved an overall sensitivity and specificity of 82.22% (95% CI 80.80%, 83.63%) and 84.36% (83.02%, 85.70%), respectively (Fig. 2A). When the algorithms were evaluated in this subset, algorithm G was the only one that did not perform significantly worse in terms of both sensitivity (80.47% [79.00%, 81.93%], $P = 0.441$) and specificity (81.28% [79.84%, 82.72%], $P = 0.195$) compared with the VA teleretinal graders. Algorithms E and F achieved higher sensitivities than the VA teleretinal graders (92.71% [91.75%, 93.67%], $P = 1.25 \times 10^{-6}$, and 92.71% [91.75%, 93.67%], $P = 7.29 \times 10^{-7}$, respectively) but were less specific. Algorithm A was the only one that achieved higher specificity (90.00% [88.89%, 91.11%], $P = 2.14 \times 10^{-2}$) than the VA teleretinal graders. In moderate and severe NPDR and PDR, the VA teleretinal graders achieved a sensitivity of 100% in gradable images. In moderate NPDR or worse (Fig. 2B), algorithms E, F, and G performed similarly to the VA teleretinal grader ($P = 0.500, 0.500,$ and 1.000, respectively), whereas algorithms A–C had significantly lower sensitivities ($P < 0.03$). In severe NPDR or worse (Fig. 2C), only algorithms A and B performed worse than the VA teleretinal graders. With PDR, only algorithm A differed significantly from the VA teleretinal grader ($P = 9.77 \times 10^{-4}$) (Fig. 2D).

Value per Encounter
Only algorithms E, F, and G achieved comparable sensitivity to humans in detecting referable disease in encounters with moderate NPDR or worse; we report the value-per-encounter analysis of

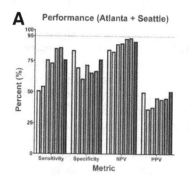
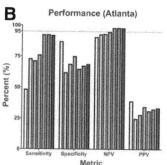
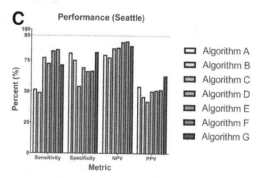

Figure 1—The relative screening performance of AI algorithms. Using the full-image data set (A), the sensitivity, specificity, NPV, and PPV of each algorithm are shown using the original teleretinal grader as the reference standard. These analyses were repeated separately using color fundus photographs obtained from Atlanta (B) and Seattle (C).

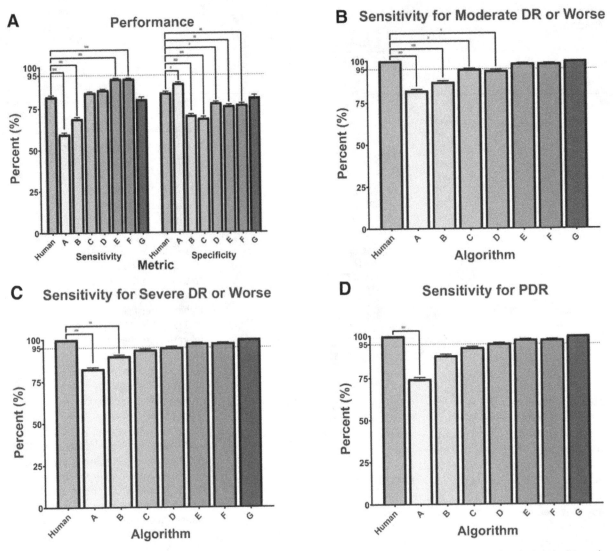

Figure 2—Relative performance of human grader compared with AI algorithms. The relative performance of the VA teleretinal grader (Human) and algorithms A–G in screening for referable DR using the arbitrated data set at different thresholds of DR. *A:* Sensitivity and specificity of each algorithm compared with a human grader with 95% CI bars against a subset of double-masked arbitrated grades in screening for referable DR in images with mild NPDR or worse and ungradable image quality. *B–D:* Only gradable images were used. The VA teleretinal grader is compared with the AI sensitivities, with 95% CIs, at different thresholds of disease, including moderate NPDR or worse (*B*), severe NDPR or worse (*C*), and PDR (*D*). *$P \leq$ 0.05, **$P \leq$ 0.001, ***$P \leq$ 0.0001.

these algorithms only (Fig. 3). The value per encounter of each algorithm was similar regardless of location for both ophthalmologists and optometrists. In the combined Atlanta and Seattle data set, the estimated value per encounter for ophthalmologists was $15.14 (95% CI $12.33, $17.95), $15.35 ($12.50, $18.20), and $18.06 ($14.71, $21.41) for algorithms E, F, and G, respectively. For optometrists, the approximate value of each respective algorithm on the combined data set was $7.74 ($6.43, $9.05), $7.85 ($6.52, $9.18), and $9.24 ($7.67, $10.80).

CONCLUSIONS

In this independent, external, head-to-head automated DR screening algorithm validation study, we found that the screening performance of state-of-the-art algorithms varied considerably, with substantial differences in overall performance, even though all the tested algorithms are currently being used clinically around the world and one has FDA approval. Using the arbitrated data set as the ground truth, the performance of the VA teleretinal graders was excellent, and no case of referable DR in images of moderate NPDR or worse was

missed. In contrast, most of the algorithms performed worse, with only three of seven (42.86%) and one of seven (14.29%) of them having comparable sensitivity and specificity to the VA teleretinal graders, respectively. Only one algorithm (G) had similar performance to that of VA graders.

Overall, the algorithms had low PPVs compared with the human teleretinal grades, especially in the Atlanta data set. Both NPV and PPV should be considered when evaluating the performance of algorithms. For the purpose of screening, high NPV has foremost

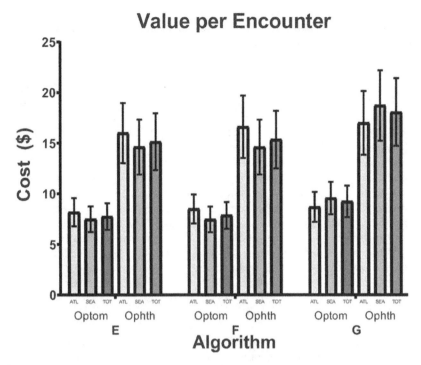

Value per Encounter

Figure 3—Value per encounter of AI algorithms meeting the sensitivity threshold. The value per encounter with 95% CI bars of algorithms E, F, and G. Only algorithms that achieved equivalent sensitivity to the VA teleretinal graders in screening for referable DR in images regraded as moderate NPDR or worse in the arbitrated data set were carried forward. The value per encounter of each algorithm if optometrists (Optom) or ophthalmologists (Ophth) were to implement this system into their clinical practice to make a normal profit on the basis of geographical location or the combined data set is shown. ATL, Atlanta; SEA, Seattle; TOT, total (Atlanta and Seattle).

importance to ensure that negative cases indeed do not have DR, while there should be a low threshold for in-person evaluation for unclear cases, possibly leading to low PPV. The different predictive value results in the two populations may also reflect differences in disease prevalence: 14.79% of the Atlanta population had DR compared with 29.95% of the Seattle population. The lower DR prevalence in Atlanta likely influenced the lower PPV on the basis of Bayes theorem, even though Atlanta had a higher rate of more severe DR.

The algorithms performed better overall on the Atlanta data set compared with Seattle, with fewer ungradable images, which is likely associated with the use of pharmacologic pupillary dilation (21). All patients were routinely dilated before screening in Atlanta (2.47% ungradable) but not in Seattle (16.23% ungradable). The majority of the participating algorithms are designed for nonmydriatic retinal imaging, but dilation requirements may vary between screening centers, and algorithms must be able to generalize.

The difference in the number of ungradable images (fewer in the Atlanta data set) may also be due to the Atlanta VA's imaging protocol, which involves extensive technician training and retaking of poor-quality images. In addition, while the Seattle VA population was predominantly White (70.56%), nearly 50% of the Atlanta patients were African American. Different ethnic backgrounds may have affected the quality of fundus photos because the background retinal and choroidal pigmentation can vary substantially (22). The performance difference between Atlanta and Seattle is significant and highlights the potential lack of generalizability of some algorithms.

Several reasons may explain the discrepancy between our study results and previously reported findings (13,23–28). If studies use training data that are limited to a certain geographic and/or ethnic group, performance can decrease when the algorithm is tested in a different population (26). In addition, many studies process or remove lower-quality images from their analysis

(13,23–25,28). Studies that exclude ungradable images and/or patients with comorbid eye disease (glaucoma, etc.) do not reflect the real-world data set where all images from all patients are analyzed, which can lower the performance of an algorithm (13,27). We made all images available to the algorithms, although some may analyze more images per encounter than others. Details of how most of these algorithms are trained and developed are not publicly available except for the two FDA-approved algorithms, which require two fundus images per eye.

The limited performance of most of the algorithms in our study emphasizes the need for external validation of screening algorithms before their clinical application. One of the seven algorithms in our study has FDA approval, four are in clinical use outside the U.S. and have been submitted to the FDA for approval, and several have a CE marking. Nevertheless, most algorithms performed similarly or even worse than the VA teleretinal graders. The two algorithms (E and F) that achieved superior sensitivities than the VA teleretinal graders had worse specificity for mild DR or worse and ungradable image quality. Additionally, none were better than the human graders in identifying referable disease when analyzed by DR severity. In fact, the performance of algorithm A was significantly worse than that of the VA teleretinal graders at all levels of DR severity. In this group of patients, algorithm A would miss 25.58% of advanced retinopathy cases, an error that can potentially result in severe vision loss. Because most of these algorithms are already in clinical use, these results are concerning. Implementation of such algorithms in a real-world clinical setting would pose a serious patient safety hazard (28).

An important question regarding the clinical implementation of these algorithms is estimating their economic value (29). As an initial screening tool, the appropriately selected algorithm could reduce the burden on human graders by eliminating images without retinopathy; fewer images/encounters requiring evaluation reduces costs. We only performed an economic analysis of the algorithms that did not perform worse than the human VA teleretinal grader (algorithms E, F, and G, which had higher or equivalent sensitivities compared with the teleretinal graders) in screening for referable DR in images regraded as moderate NPDR or worse because the performance of these three algorithms was closest to the current standard of care. In addition, although these models must achieve a level of sensitivity that is safe for clinical use, a model with high specificity translates to additional labor savings that could be interpreted as higher value per encounter. On the basis of the performance of the three best algorithms and the mean salary of eye care providers, we approximated the value of each DR screening encounter to range from $15.14 to $18.06 for a system with ophthalmologists as human graders and from $7.74 to $9.24 when optometrists are the graders. Thus, if there are 100,000 annual cases to be screened for DR, using an acceptable automated algorithm as the first step and relying on ophthalmologists to review only the ungradable and abnormal cases detected by the algorithm, the resulting annual labor savings would be $1,500,000–$1,800,000. Interestingly, we found that the value per encounter did not differ significantly between Seattle and Atlanta, despite the difference in PDR prevalence.

Several limitations exist in our study. First, although the patients were from geographically different sites and had varying ethnic backgrounds, they were predominantly older male (94.68%) veterans, and almost all of them had type 2 DM. These factors may have affected the performance of the algorithms, and additional validation in different populations will be important. Second, it is possible that in clinical practice, images may be graded by both an algorithm and a human grader in a semiautomated fashion. While this setup may improve sensitivity and specificity, the semiautomated system relies on the algorithm to first identify patients who require further screening by the physician; hence, it is important to evaluate its performance independently. Furthermore, each tested algorithm was designed to be fully automated, so we used an all-AI scenario to evaluate the performance and value of each algorithm. Third, the threshold for referable DR in the VA system does not distinguish between mild versus higher levels of DR, while the referral threshold in many health care systems is moderate DR or

worse. The results of the sensitivity analysis for different thresholds of disease, in which several algorithms were equivalent to the human teleretinal graders, indicate that these algorithms would be applicable for health care settings that do not refer for mild DR. In addition, the presence of macular edema is a positive indicator of diabetic disease, but unlike human readers, the tested algorithms do not provide an output for the presence/absence of macular edema. Fourth, the results suggest that the human graders may have had lower sensitivity for mild NPDR compared with the algorithms given that a single microaneurysm or dot-and-blot hemorrhage would cross the threshold into mild NPDR. The use of double-masked, arbitrated expert human grades as the benchmark when comparing the algorithms' performance to the teleretinal graders may be considered as a limitation. However, current accepted reference standards by regulatory bodies, such as the FDA and AI literature, use expert human grading. We used double-masked, arbitrated regrading by experts as our reference standard, and our experts had no access to previous teleretinal grades, the same as with the AI algorithms.

Another limitation of our study was the relatively small number of companies that participated. We agreed to mask the identity of the algorithms to encourage participation, but of the 23 companies we approached, only 5 (21.74%) agreed to participate (providing seven algorithms for evaluation). Studies like ours that validate algorithms using real-world data sets will ultimately accelerate their subsequent performance but will need buy-in from all companies. New reporting guidelines recommend increasing transparency about how AI devices are trained and evaluated, including plans for anticipating and mitigating risks upon implementation (14,30,31). With greater openness and participation, progress in AI efficacy, safety, and science will advance the field, inspire innovation, and benefit the global population.

The value-per-encounter analysis in our study did not factor in fringe benefits and indirect costs for optometrists and ophthalmologists, and costs of graphics processing unit servers were not included. Additionally, the estimated value per encounter is specific to the VA. Although these automated systems are intended for use with the teleretinal screening

system, we did not estimate the cost of adding automated grading to the existing VA teleretinal system, which would include the costs associated with integration and any additional computing hardware needs. Many of the AI companies offer a cloud-based solution so that the latter is less of a concern.

To our knowledge, this is the largest AI-based DR screening algorithm validation study to date, modeling real-world conditions by analyzing 311,604 color fundus photographs from two geographically diverse populations regardless of quality and without any preprocessing or filtering. Our study was powered to evaluate the presence of referable disease in images with undiagnosed PDR. Unlike other studies in which too few severe cases can lead to oversampling of mild disease, our large database did not require balancing since it covers >10 years of clinical data (16). Thus, unlike many studies reported previously (12,13,32), we were able to assess both PPV and NPV and acquire insights into the relative performance of the algorithms in regions with different prevalence rates.

Although some algorithms in our study performed well from a screening perspective, others would pose safety concerns if implemented within the VA. These results demonstrate that automated devices should undergo prospective, interventional trials to evaluate their efficacy as they are integrated into clinical practice, even after FDA approval. Ideally, validation data sets should include real-world data sets representative of where the algorithms will be deployed so that they function well regardless of variables such as race, image quality, dilation practices, and coexisting disease. Automated screening systems are not limited to DR and may be applicable for other conditions, such as age-related macular degeneration and glaucoma, where earlier detection would likely improve clinical outcome. Rigorous pre- and postapproval testing of all such algorithms is needed to sufficiently identify and understand the algorithms' characteristics to determine suitability for clinical implementation.

Funding. A.Y.L. is supported by the FDA. This material is the result of work supported with resources and the use of facilities at VA Puget Sound and the Veterans Health Administration Innovation Ecosystem. This study was supported by National Institutes of Health grants K23-EY-029246 and R01-AG-060942 and an unrestricted grant from Research to Prevent Blindness.

The sponsors/funding organizations had no role in the design or conduct of this research. The contents do not represent the views of the U.S. Department of Veterans Affairs, the FDA, or the United States Government.

Duality of Interest. A.Y.L. reports grants from Santen, Carl Zeiss Meditec, and Novartis and personal fees from Genentech, Topcon, and Verana Health outside the submitted work. A.Y.M. reports consulting fees from Warby Parker and Click Therapeutics outside of the submitted work. E.J.B. reports personal fees from Bayer AG. No other potential conflicts of interest relevant to this article were reported.

Author Contributions. A.Y.L., C.S.L., and E.J.B. conceived and designed the study. A.Y.L. developed and validated the algorithms with C.S.L., Y.E.C., and E.J.B. providing clinical input. A.Y.L., H.C.J., M.D.G., A.Y.M., and M.L. collected and prepared the data. A.Y.L., R.T.Y., C.S.L., and M.B. wrote the initial draft. A.Y.L., R.T.Y., C.S.L., M.B., H.C.J., Y.E.C., M.D.G., H.G., A.Y.M., G.C.C., M.L., and E.J.B. subsequently critically edited the report. All authors read and approved the final report. A.Y.L. is the guarantor of this work and, as such, had full access to all the data in the study and takes responsibility for the integrity of the data and the accuracy of the data analysis.

Prior Presentation. Parts of this study were presented in abstract form at the 38th Annual Scientific Meeting of the American Society of Retina Specialists, Virtual, 24–26 July 2020.

References

1. Lee R, Wong TY, Sabanayagam C. Epidemiology of diabetic retinopathy, diabetic macular edema and related vision loss. Eye Vis (Lond) 2015;2:17

2. Liew G, Michaelides M, Bunce C. A comparison of the causes of blindness certifications in England and Wales in working age adults (16-64 years), 1999-2000 with 2009-2010. BMJ Open 2014;4:e004015

3. Jampol LM, Glassman AR, Sun J. Evaluation and care of patients with diabetic retinopathy. N Engl J Med 2020;382:1629–1637

4. Flaxel CJ, Adelman RA, Bailey ST, et al. Diabetic retinopathy preferred practice pattern®. Ophthalmology 2020;127:66–P145

5. American Diabetes Association. 11. Microvascular complications and foot care: *Standards of Medical Care in Diabetes—2020*. Diabetes Care 2020;43(Suppl. 1):S135–S151

6. International Diabetes Federation. Diabetes Facts & Figures. Accessed 26 April 2020. Available from https://www.idf.org/aboutdiabetes/what-is-diabetes/facts-figures.html

7. Resnikoff S, Felch W, Gauthier T-M, Spivey B. The number of ophthalmologists in practice and training worldwide: a growing gap despite more than 200,000 practitioners. Br J Ophthalmol 2012;96:783–787

8. Kirkizlar E, Serban N, Sisson JA, Swann JL, Barnes CS, Williams MD. Evaluation of telemedicine for screening of diabetic retinopathy in the Veterans Health Administration. Ophthalmology 2013;120:2604–2610

9. Joseph S, Kim R, Ravindran RD, Fletcher AE, Ravilla TD. Effectiveness of teleretinal imaging-based hospital referral compared with universal referral in identifying diabetic retinopathy: a cluster randomized clinical trial. JAMA Ophthalmol 2019;137:786–792

10. Tufail A, Kapetanakis VV, Salas-Vega S, et al. An observational study to assess if automated diabetic retinopathy image assessment software can replace one or more steps of manual imaging grading and to determine their cost-effectiveness. Health Technol Assess 2016;20:1–72

11. Tufail A, Rudisill C, Egan C, et al. Automated diabetic retinopathy image assessment software: diagnostic accuracy and cost-effectiveness compared with human graders. Ophthalmology 2017;124:343–351

12. Ting DSW, Cheung CY-L, Lim G, et al. Development and validation of a deep learning system for diabetic retinopathy and related eye diseases using retinal images from multiethnic populations with diabetes. JAMA 2017;318:2211–2223

13. Abràmoff MD, Lavin PT, Birch M, Shah N, Folk JC. Pivotal trial of an autonomous AI-based diagnostic system for detection of diabetic retinopathy in primary care offices. NPJ Digit Med 2018;1:39

14. Keane PA, Topol EJ. With an eye to AI and autonomous diagnosis. NPJ Digit Med 2018;1:40

15. Center for Devices and Radiological Health. CDRH Regulatory Science Priorities. U.S. Food and Drug Administration, 2019. Accessed 23 July 2020. Available from https://www.fda.gov/medical-devices/science-and-research-medical-devices/cdrh-regulatory-science-priorities

16. Ogunyemi O, Kermah D. Machine learning approaches for detecting diabetic retinopathy from clinical and public health records. AMIA Annu Symp Proc 2015;2015:983–990

17. Kuzmak P, Demosthenes C, Maa A. Exporting diabetic retinopathy images from VA VISTA Imaging for research. J Digit Imaging 2019;32:832–840

18. Conlin PR, Fisch BM, Orcutt JC, Hetrick BJ, Darkins AW. Framework for a national teleretinal imaging program to screen for diabetic retinopathy in Veterans Health Administration patients. J Rehabil Res Dev 2006;43:741–748

19. Stock C, Hielscher T. DTComPair: Comparison of Binary Diagnostic Tests in a Paired Study Design, 2014. Accessed 20 April 2020. Available from https://rdrr.io/cran/DTComPair/man/dtcompair-package.html

20. Xie Y, Nguyen QD, Hamzah H, et al. Artificial intelligence for teleophthalmology-based diabetic retinopathy screening in a national programme: an economic analysis modelling study. Lancet Digit Health 2020;2:e240–e249

21. Wintergerst MWM, Brinkmann CK, Holz FG, Finger RP. Undilated versus dilated monoscopic smartphone-based fundus photography for optic nerve head evaluation. Sci Rep 2018;8:10228

22. Silvar SD, Pollack RH. Racial differences in pigmentation of the fundus oculi. Psychon Sci 1967;7:159–159

23. Abràmoff MD, Lou Y, Erginay A, et al. Improved automated detection of diabetic retinopathy on a publicly available dataset through integration of deep learning. Invest Ophthalmol Vis Sci 2016;57:5200–5206

24. Gulshan V, Peng L, Coram M, et al. Development and validation of a deep learning algorithm for detection of diabetic retinopathy in retinal fundus photographs. JAMA 2016;316:2402–2410

25. Gargeya R, Leng T. Automated identification of diabetic retinopathy using deep learning. Ophthalmology 2017;124:962–969

26. Romero-Aroca P, Verges-Puig R, de la Torre J, et al. Validation of a deep learning algorithm for diabetic retinopathy. Telemed J E Health 2020;26:1001–1009

27. Bhaskaranand M, Ramachandra C, Bhat S, et al. The value of automated diabetic retinopathy screening with the EyeArt system: a study of more than 100,000 consecutive encounters from people with diabetes. Diabetes Technol Ther 2019;21:635–643

28. Natarajan S, Jain A, Krishnan R, Rogye A, Sivaprasad S. Diagnostic accuracy of community-based diabetic retinopathy screening with an offline artificial intelligence system on a smartphone. JAMA Ophthalmol 2019;137:1182–1188

29. Xie Y, Gunasekeran DV, Balaskas K, et al. Health economic and safety considerations for artificial intelligence applications in diabetic retinopathy screening. Transl Vis Sci Technol 2020;9:22

30. Cruz Rivera S, Liu X, Chan A-W, Denniston AK, Calvert MJ; SPIRIT-AI and CONSORT-AI Working Group; SPIRIT-AI and CONSORT-AI Steering Group; SPIRIT-AI and CONSORT-AI Consensus Group. Guidelines for clinical trial protocols for interventions involving artificial intelligence: the SPIRIT-AI extension. Nat Med 2020;26:1351–1363

31. Liu X, Rivera SC, Moher D, Calvert MJ, Denniston AK; SPIRIT-AI and CONSORT-AI Working Group. Reporting guidelines for clinical trial reports for interventions involving artificial intelligence: the CONSORT-AI Extension. BMJ 2020;370:m3164

32. Ranganathan P, Aggarwal R. Common pitfalls in statistical analysis: understanding the properties of diagnostic tests - part 1. Perspect Clin Res 2018;9:40–43

COVID-19 and Type 1 Diabetes: Addressing Concerns and Maintaining Control

Linda A. DiMeglio

Diabetes Care 2021;44:1924–1928 | https://doi.org/10.2337/dci21-0002

The worldwide outbreak of severe acute respiratory syndrome coronavirus 2 (SARS-CoV-2) has been an unprecedented pandemic. Early on, even as the signs and symptoms of coronavirus disease 2019 (COVID-19) were first characterized, significant concerns were articulated regarding its potential impact on people with chronic disease, including type 1 diabetes. Information about the basic and clinical interrelationships between COVID-19 and diabetes has rapidly emerged. Initial rapid reports were useful to provide alerts and guide health care responses and initial policies. Some of these have proven subsequently to have durable findings, whereas others lacked scientific rigor/reproducibility. Many publications that report on COVID-19 and "diabetes" also have not distinguished between type 1 and type 2 [1]. Available evidence now demonstrates that people with type 1 diabetes have been acutely affected by COVID-19 in multiple ways. This includes effects from limited access to health care, particularly during lockdown periods, and increased morbidity/mortality in infected adults with type 1 diabetes compared with peers without diabetes.

MIGHT COVID-19 CAUSE OR ACCELERATE TYPE 1 DIABETES?

At present, there is not convincing evidence that severe acute respiratory syndrome coronavirus 2 (SARS-CoV-2) exacerbates or induces persistent diabetes. A small initial report suggested concerning increases in type 1 diabetes incidence concurrent with the pandemic [2]. Later population-based reporting did not confirm this observation [3]. Rather, data suggest that affected individuals and their caregivers delayed accessing care at the time of diagnosis [4] and that primary care offices were shut down when acute care centers were open, leading to greater numbers of people presenting more acutely to hospital settings. It is possible but not proven that the cytokine storm that is common in coronavirus disease 2019 (COVID-19) may also injure or stun the limited β-cell reserve in individuals nearing stage 3 of type 1 diabetes, accelerating the last weeks of acute disease presentation. Although there were early concerns that the SARS-CoV-2 angiotensin converting enzyme coreceptor (ACE) and the required transmembrane serine protease (TMPRSS) cofactors for cellular entry might be found in insulin-producing β-cells and that these cells might be susceptible to viral infection, later immunohistochemistry pancreatic work did not confirm these findings [5,6]. It is also unlikely that during active infection these receptors are induced in β-cells [7].

Will the pandemic acutely or chronically change epidemiology of type 1 diabetes? This question has been raised since a few viral illnesses have been suspected to induce or accelerate type 1 diabetes. Evidence to date suggests that it is unlikely that the SARS-CoV-2 infection either induces autoimmunity or causes permanent

Division of Pediatric Endocrinology and Diabetology, Department of Pediatrics, Indiana University School of Medicine, Indianapolis, IN

Corresponding author: Linda A. DiMeglio, dimeglio@iu.edu

Received 29 March 2021 and accepted 29 March 2021

This article is part of two special article collections, available at https://care.diabetesjournals.org/collection/diabetes-care-symposium-2021 and https://care.diabetesjournals.org/collection/diabetes-and-COVID19.

See accompanying articles, pp. 1916 and 1929.

β-cell damage (7). However, given that we now recognize many endotypes of type 1 diabetes, further surveillance is needed to determine if a subset of people develops type 1 diabetes after SARS-CoV-2 infection. Decreases in other circulating endemic and seasonal viral infections due to public health guidelines to mask and wash hands might also reduce presentation of autoimmune diseases, although larger future endemic infectious outbreaks are also possible (8).

RISKS FROM COVID-19 FOR PEOPLE WITH TYPE 1 DIABETES

There does not appear to be any increased susceptibility to SARS-CoV-2 infection for individuals with type 1 diabetes (9,10). Generally, people with type 1 diabetes present with similar COVID-19 symptoms as those in the general population: dry cough, nausea, vomiting, fever (11).

Yet, once an adult with type 1 diabetes is infected with SARS-CoV-2, they are at increased disease-related risk. Overall, adults with type 1 diabetes have odds similar to those for people with type 2 diabetes for severity of illness, hospitalization, and in-hospital mortality (12). COVID-19 may initially present with concurrent hyperglycemia and even diabetic ketoacidosis (DKA). Some of the typical COVID-19 symptoms (nausea/vomiting) may also mask the DKA onset, delaying DKA diagnoses and further worsening prognosis (13).

Certain intra-individual factors translate into increased risk for infected individuals with type 1 diabetes. For starters, older age, which also affects the likelihood of long-term complications or death from COVID-19 in the general population, appears to be the greatest risk factor for hospitalization and illness severity for adults with type 1 diabetes. French population-based analyses (the CORONADO study) showed higher mortality in older patients with COVID-19 and type 1 diabetes compared with patients without type 1 diabetes (14). In CORONADO, the risk for younger patients with type 1 diabetes was less; for example, among individuals <55 years of age, 12% of those with type 1 diabetes died or required intubation within the first week of hospitalization compared with 30% of individuals with type 2 diabetes. Another U.S.-based

study (that combined type 1 diabetes and type 2 diabetes) found that illness severity nearly doubled for each 25-year increase in age (12). Additional information about how much of the impact of "older age" is in fact "duration of diabetes" is needed.

No present evidence suggests that youth with type 1 diabetes have higher mortality or morbidity, including risk of hospitalization, than healthy peers (15,16). Reports that suggest otherwise that are based on small sample sizes subject to type I error and publication bias or fail to consider confounders such as acuity of hospitalization (17,18). They should not be used as the basis for public health messaging. Confusion about the difference between "autoimmune" disease and "immune deficiency" has also produced unwarranted concerns.

Glycemic control at the time of infection may also play a role in outcomes. One U.K. study reporting on deaths in 463 individuals (56.6% male) with COVID-19 and type 1 diabetes suggested a higher mortality risk in those with an HbA_{1c} >10% (86 mmol/mol, hazard ratio 2.23 [95% CI 1.5–3.3, $P < 0.0001$] [19]). Poor glycemic control is known to be associated with more serious infection in other settings (20); in individuals with COVID-19, it may amplify the hyperimmune response (21). COVID-19 itself also can impair any remaining endogenous insulin secretion and reduce glucose disposal by inducing inflammation and cytokine production. Additionally, individuals with COVID-19 may be volume depleted, immobilized, treated with steroids, and/or experience acute kidney injury (7)—all of which can also worsen glycemia.

Other factors in adults with type 1 diabetes appear to worsen risks from COVID-19. Those who are non-Hispanic Black, use public insurance, and have hypertension are more likely to be hospitalized for COVID-19 infection (22). Obesity also likely increases the risk (23), whereas insulin pump and continuous glucose monitor use may be mitigating factors (12).

Since HbA_{1c} tends to remain relatively stable in adults over time (24), individuals with higher HbA_{1c} at the time of SARS-CoV-2 infection also have a higher likelihood of longer-term hyperglycemia and concomitant diabetes-related vascular disease. COVID-19

has clear vascular effects. For people with type 1 diabetes and underlying micro- and macrovascular disease, the disease course is likely worsened due to the inflammatory, endothelial dysfunction, and prothrombotic effects of SARS-CoV-2 infection. Indeed, diabetic retinopathy has recently been described to be independently associated with risk of intubation in hospitalized COVD-19 patients (25). The risk of mortality also appears to be increased in individuals with vascular diabetes-associated complications (19,26). This vascular aspect of COVID-19 likely explains why children with type 1 diabetes are relatively protected from severe illness; i.e., children with type 1 diabetes are more like other children from a vascular and risk perspective than they are like adults with long-standing type 1 diabetes.

Increased risk recognition has gradually translated into governmental advice for caution for adults living with type 1 diabetes. The Centers for Disease Control and Prevention has released information on which individuals in the U.S. should take extra precautions related to COVID-19 (27). Initially, that guidance, based on a preponderance of available information from individuals with type 2 diabetes (9) without considering newer information about type 1 diabetes, suggested that people with type 2 diabetes are at increased risk of severe COVID-19 illness, whereas type 1 diabetes "might" increase the risk of severe illness. This policy was revised in late March 2021. In contrast, the U.K. Joint Committee on Vaccination and Immunization SARS-COV-2 vaccine policy more appropriately stated from its start that individuals with both type 1 and type 2 diabetes are considered at clinical risk for more severe disease (28).

CARE CONSIDERATIONS FOR COVID-19 AND TYPE 1 DIABETES

At present, the overall public health advice for people with type 1 diabetes during the pandemic is equivalent to that of the general population: wear masks, follow social distancing guidelines, eschew nonessential travel, and avoid indoor gatherings whenever possible. This is particularly important as more-transmissible and potentially less-vaccine-susceptible SARS-CoV-2 variants are circulating. Additionally, given the association of worse COVID-19 outcomes for people with poorer glycemic control, individuals with type 1 diabetes should do what is possible and necessary to optimize glycemic control, targeting an HbA$_{1c}$ of <7%. Some data suggest worsening of glycemic control in adults with type 1 diabetes during lockdown periods (29), which is potentially associated with greater stress and anxiety, less exercise, and weight gain (30). Additionally, DKA risk during this pandemic time appears to be heightened even for people with type 1 diabetes who are not infected with SARS-CoV-2, most likely due to delays in accessing care (31,32).

The pandemic has also adversely affected research aiming to prevent, cure, and ameliorate type 1 diabetes. The pandemic has put immunotherapy trials seeking to prevent or reverse type 1 diabetes on indefinite hold and reduced participant entry rates into ongoing trials (33) of other agents. As an example, the Type 1 Diabetes Trial-Net network, following advice from its infectious disease committee, has put a prevention study using rituximab (anti-CD20) and abatacept (CTLA-4-Ig) (NCT03929601) on indefinite hold. The funding streams for organizations committed to curing and improving care for people affected by type 1 diabetes have been significantly impacted, with the biggest impact on the not-for-profit organizations American Diabetes Association and JDRF, who have cut funding opportunities and staffing (34,35).

Coronavirus vaccines are being distributed to ever-widening groups of individuals around the nation and the world. People with diabetes (not distinguishing between type 1 and type 2) were included in all the major trials without suggestions of decreased vaccine effectiveness for individuals with diabetes (36,37). With the advent of this public health advance comes a series of decisions and concerns given the limited rate of vaccine distributions, and many efforts to prioritize the highest-risk groups. The Centers for Disease Control and Prevention initial guidance indicating differences in risk of COVID-19 by type of diabetes led to some states inappropriately excluding people with type 1 diabetes from the high-risk categories of individuals getting access to vaccine. Advocacy around improving access to the vaccine for

people with type 1 diabetes is critical and actively underway (38). In general, people with type 1 diabetes should seek out and receive effective vaccines as soon as possible and permitted based on local guidelines.

LOOKING TO THE FUTURE

There have been some bright spots in this pandemic for the care of people with type 1 diabetes. The pandemic provided an incentive for considerable expansion of telemedicine (39). Data suggest that telemedicine can be beneficial for management of children and adults with type 1 diabetes (40). Although at first virtual visits were performed out of urgent necessity to provide care, over time they have become part of the fabric of diabetes centers. Even after this pandemic, telemedicine offers an opportunity to provide additional touchpoints for the highest-risk people with diabetes and provide more clinical care without taxing further limited physical clinical space. Telemedicine may also ultimately increase the efficiency and cost-effectiveness of the care. Full incorporation of telemedicine will require advocacy for maintained payor coverage of virtual care, deliberate planning to permit interstate care delivery, intentional work to offer this to people with type 1 diabetes with limited technology access, and general acceptance of glycemic metrics that can be obtained by remote downloads (e.g., time in range, glucose management indicators) as an alternative quality measure to laboratory measures of HbA$_{1c}$.

The pandemic also accelerated the use of continuous glucose monitor based remote monitoring of glycemia. In the hospital, it began to be used more routinely for people with diabetes who were being cared for to reduce care provider exposure to virus (41). In the ambulatory care setting, it permitted remote monitoring of care when patients were unable to attend in-person clinical visits. Concomitant with this is an apparent rise in the "literacy" of both patients and caregivers to download devices and upload reports from home. Ongoing technical support will be needed for patients and providers lest this ability for remote monitoring widens the observed racial and

socioeconomic disparities in care for persons with type 1 diabetes (42).

An additional pivot that has happened amid this pandemic is the change to virtual scientific meetings. This includes the change of several large diabetes meetings where scientists and others who care for people with type 1 diabetes gather to exchange data and ideas. Although this pivot has certainly had its downsides, particularly for junior faculty who are not able to network as readily with senior scientists in their fields, it has also permitted wider audiences for some meetings and has enabled people with other obligations (e.g., child care) that might have prevented them from being able to attend remote meetings in person to be engaged. Early data suggest that a move to virtual meetings may have improved representation of women as session chairs and invited speakers (43).

Although there were initial concerns about access to needed supplies and insulin, overall, children and adults with type 1 diabetes without COVID-19 who were in "lockdown" at home did not experience acute deterioration in their glycemic control or overall care, and some even saw improvements. Some of this was likely due to increased time for attention to diabetes (44), some due to more consistent food and sleep intake, and some due to lower physical activity (45); some may have been due to fewer circulating viruses and less intercurrent illness. Other data, particularly for children, suggest improvements in glycemic control in some groups, potentially due to greater parental/caregiver supervision of care (46).

CONCLUSIONS

It is essential that we continue to both evaluate and report on outcomes of people with type 1 diabetes during this unprecedented pandemic period and that we base public health recommendations on the best available quality data. This is especially critical for advocating clearly about the need for all with type 1 diabetes to be vaccinated while still deliberately and clearly messaging to parents and caregivers about the more limited risks to our youngest patients as we work to optimize their glycemic control. We need to continue to work to ensure everyone worldwide with type 1 diabetes has access to insulin and other needed diabetes supplies, even when health care systems are stressed by waves of affected individuals and supply-chain disruptions. We should also continue to monitor for the possibility of particular "long COVID" effects for people who also live with type 1 diabetes (47). Efforts such as the CoviDiab Registry (CoviDiab.e-dendrite.com) are critical. As always, we should work with patients and their families to nurture their resilience and coping skills, even in the face of significant challenges.

As of this writing, hope is on the horizon. Mass vaccination efforts for adults are ramping up worldwide. Trials to evaluate safety and efficacy for vaccines in younger children are ongoing. Ultimately, more research is needed on the acute and long-term effects of COVID-19 on people with type 1 diabetes, as well as how the pandemic and the accompanying changes in environmental and infectious disease exposures impact future rates of presentation of autoimmune conditions such as diabetes.

Acknowledgments. The author thanks Heather Conner of the Indiana University School of Medicine for administrative support.
Duality of Interest. No potential conflicts of interest relevant to this article were reported.

References

1. Tenforde MW, Billig Rose E, Lindsell CJ, et al.; CDC COVID-19 Response Team. Characteristics of adult outpatients and inpatients with COVID-19—11 academic medical centers, United States, March–May 2020. MMWR Morb Mortal Wkly Rep 2020;69:841–846
2. Unsworth R, Wallace S, Oliver NS, et al. New-onset type 1 diabetes in children during COVID-19: multicenter regional findings in the UK. Diabetes Care 2020;43:e170–e171
3. Tittel SR, Rosenbauer J, Kamrath C, et al.; DPV Initiative. Did the COVID-19 lockdown affect the incidence of pediatric type 1 diabetes in Germany? Diabetes Care 2020;43:e172–e173
4. Dayal D, Gupta S, Raithatha D, Jayashree M. Missing during COVID-19 lockdown: children with onset of type 1 diabetes. Acta Paediatr 2020;109:2144–2146
5. Coate KC, Cha J, Shrestha S, et al. SARS-CoV-2 cell entry factors ACE2 and TMPRSS2 are expressed in the microvasculature and ducts of human pancreas but are not enriched in β cells. Cell Metab 2020;32:1028–1040.e4
6. Kusmartseva I, Wu W, Syed F, et al. Expression of SARS-CoV-2 entry factors in the pancreas of normal organ donors and individuals with COVID-19. Cell Metab 2020;32:1041–1051.e6
7. Accili D. Can COVID-19 cause diabetes? Nat Metab 2021;3:123–125

8. Baker RE, Park SW, Yang W, Vecchi GA, Metcalf CJE, Grenfell BT. The impact of COVID-19 nonpharmaceutical interventions on the future dynamics of endemic infections. Proc Natl Acad Sci U S A 2020;117:30547–30553
9. Apicella M, Campopiano MC, Mantuano M, Mazoni L, Coppelli A, Del Prato S. COVID-19 in people with diabetes: understanding the reasons for worse outcomes. Lancet Diabetes Endocrinol 2020;8:782–792
10. d'Annunzio G, Maffeis C, Cherubini V, et al. Caring for children and adolescents with type 1 diabetes mellitus: Italian Society for Pediatric Endocrinology and Diabetology (ISPED) statements during COVID-19 pandemia. Diabetes Res Clin Pract 2020;168:108372
11. Nassar M, Nso N, Baraka B, et al. The association between COVID-19 and type 1 diabetes mellitus: a systematic review. Diabetes Metab Syndr 2021;15:447–454
12. Gregory JM, Slaughter JC, Duffus SH, et al. COVID-19 severity is tripled in the diabetes community: a prospective analysis of the pandemic's impact in type 1 and type 2 diabetes. Diabetes Care 2021;44:526–532
13. Buonsenso D, Onesimo R, Valentini P, et al.; pedCOVID-team. Children's healthcare during corona virus disease 19 pandemic: the Italian experience. Pediatr Infect Dis J 2020;39:e137–e140
14. Wargny M, Gourdy P, Ludwig L, et al.; CORONADO investigators. Type 1 diabetes in people hospitalized for COVID-19: new insights from the CORONADO study. Diabetes Care 2020;43:e174–e177
15. DiMeglio LA, Albanese-O'Neill A, Muñoz CE, Maahs DM. COVID-19 and children with diabetes—updates, unknowns, and next steps: first, do no extrapolation. Diabetes Care 2020;43:2631–2634
16. Cardona-Hernandez R, Cherubini V, Iafusco D, Schiaffini R, Luo X, Maahs DM. Children and youth with diabetes are not at increased risk for hospitalization due to COVID-19. Pediatr Diabetes 2021;22:202–206
17. Gregory J. T1D and T2D dramatically increase COVID-19 risks. Discover (Vanderbilt University Medical Center). Accessed 11 April 2021. Available from https://discover.vumc.org/mms/mar-2021-peds-diabetes/
18. The Endocrine Society. Poor diabetes control in children tied to high risk for COVID-19 complications, death. Published 20 March 2021. Accessed 11 April 2021. Available from https://www.endocrine.org/news-and-advocacy/news-room/featured-science-from-endo-2021/poor-diabetes-control-in-children-tied-to-high-risk-for-covid19-complications-death#:~:text=Children%20with%20poorly%20controlled%20type,the%20Endocrine%20Society's%20annual%20meeting
19. Holman N, Knighton P, Kar P, et al. Risk factors for COVID-19-related mortality in people with type 1 and type 2 diabetes in England: a population-based cohort study. Lancet Diabetes Endocrinol 2020;8:823–833
20. Critchley JA, Carey IM, Harris T, DeWilde S, Hosking FJ, Cook DG. Glycemic control and risk of infections among people with type 1 or type 2 diabetes in a large primary care cohort study. Diabetes Care 2018;41:2127–2135
21. Sattar N, McInnes IB, McMurray JJV. Obesity is a risk factor for severe COVID-19 infection: multiple potential mechanisms. Circulation 2020;142:4–6

22. O'Malley G, Ebekozien O, Desimone M, et al. COVID-19 hospitalization in adults with type 1 diabetes: results from the T1D Exchange multicenter surveillance study. J Clin Endocrinol Metab 2021;106:e936–e942
23. Stefan N, Birkenfeld AL, Schulze MB. Global pandemics interconnected - obesity, impaired metabolic health and COVID-19. Nat Rev Endocrinol 2021;17:135–149
24. Alderisio A, Bozzetto L, Franco L, Riccardi G, Rivellese AA, Annuzzi G. Long-term body weight trajectories and metabolic control in type 1 diabetes patients on insulin pump or multiple daily injections: a 10-year retrospective controlled study. Nutr Metab Cardiovasc Dis 2019;29:1110–1117
25. Corcillo A, Cohen S, Li A, Crane J, Kariyawasam D, Karalliedde J. Diabetic retinopathy is independently associated with increased risk of intubation: a single centre cohort study of patients with diabetes hospitalised with COVID-19. Diabetes Res Clin Pract 2021;171:108529
26. Barron E, Bakhai C, Kar P, et al. Associations of type 1 and type 2 diabetes with COVID-19-related mortality in England: a whole-population study. Lancet Diabetes Endocrinol 2020;8:813–822
27. Centers for Disease Control and Prevention. Certain medical conditions and risk for severe COVID-19 illness. Accessed 14 April 2021. Available from https://www.cdc.gov/coronavirus/2019-ncov/need-extra-precautions/people-with-medical-conditions.html
28. Department of Health and Social Care. Priority groups for coronavirus (COVID-19) vaccination: advice from the JCVI, 30 December 2020. Accessed 29 March 2021. Available from https://www.gov.uk/government/publications/priority-groups-for-coronavirus-covid-19-vaccination-advice-from-the-jcvi-30-december-2020
29. Barchetta I, Cimini FA, Bertoccini L, et al. Effects of work status changes and perceived stress onglycaemiccontrol in individuals with type 1 diabetes during COVID-19 lockdown in Italy. Diabetes Res Clin Pract 2020;170:108513
30. Ruissen MM, Regeer H, Landstra CP, et al. Increased stress, weight gain and less exercise in relation to glycemic control in people with type 1 and type 2 diabetes during the COVID-19 pandemic. BMJ Open Diabetes Res Care 2021;9:e002035
31. Beliard K, Ebekozien O, Demeterco-Berggren C, et al. Increased DKA at presentation among newly diagnosed type 1 diabetes patients with or without COVID-19: data from a multi-site surveillance registry. J Diabetes 2021;13:270–272
32. Rabbone I, Schiaffini R, Cherubini V, Maffeis C; Diabetes Study Group of the Italian Society for Pediatric Endocrinology and Diabetes. Has COVID-19 delayed the diagnosis and worsened the presentation of type 1 diabetes in children? Diabetes Care 2020;43:2870–2872
33. Haller MJ, Jacobsen LM, Posgai AL, Schatz DA. How do we move type 1 diabetes immunotherapies forward during the current COVID-19 pandemic? Diabetes 2021;70:1021–1028
34. American Diabetes Association. Pathway to Stop Diabetes. Accessed 11 April 2021. Available from https://professional.diabetes.org/meetings/pathway-stop-diabetes%C2%AE
35. JDRF Grant Center. Project concepts (strategic research agreement). Accessed 11 April 2021. Available from https://grantcenter.jdrf.org/rfa/project-concepts-strategic-research-agreement/

36. Polack FP, Thomas SJ, Kitchin N, et al.; C4591001 Clinical Trial Group. Safety and efficacy of the BNT162b2 mRNA Covid-19 vaccine. N Engl J Med 2020;383:2603–2615

37. Baden LR, El Sahly HM, Essink B, et al.; COVE Study Group. Efficacy and safety of the mRNA-1273 SARS-CoV-2 vaccine. N Engl J Med 2021;384:403–416

38. JDRF. COVID-19 vaccine access guide. Accessed 29 March 2021. Available from https://www.jdrf.org/blog/2021/01/22/answering-your-questions-about-the-covid-19-vaccines/

39. Garg SK, Rodbard D, Hirsch IB, Forlenza GP. Managing new-onset type 1 diabetes during the COVID-19 pandemic: challenges and opportunities. Diabetes Technol Ther 2020;22:431–439

40. Predieri B, Leo F, Candia F, et al. Glycemic control improvement in Italian children and adolescents with type 1 diabetes followed through telemedicine during lockdown due to the COVID-19 pandemic. Front Endocrinol (Lausanne) 2020;11:595735

41. Shehav-Zaltzman G, Segal G, Konvalina N, Tirosh A. Remote glucose monitoring of hospitalized, quarantined patients with diabetes and COVID-19. Diabetes Care 2020;43:e75–e76

42. Addala A, Auzanneau M, Miller K, et al. A decade of disparities in diabetes technology use and HbA$_{1c}$ in pediatric type 1 diabetes: a transatlantic comparison. Diabetes Care 2021;44:133–140

43. Dunne J, Maizel JL, Posgai AL, Atkinson MA, DiMeglio LA. The women's leadership gap in diabetes: a call for equity and excellence. Diabetes Care 2021;44:1734–1743

44. Prabhu Navis J, Leelarathna L, Mubita W, et al. Impact of COVID-19 lockdown on flash and real-time glucose sensor users with type 1 diabetes in England. Acta Diabetol 2021;58:231–237

45. Assaloni R, Pellino VC, Puci MV, et al. Coronavirus disease (Covid-19): how does the exercise practice in active people with type 1 diabetes change? A preliminary survey. Diabetes Res Clin Pract 2020;166:108297

46. Di Dalmazi G, Maltoni G, Bongiorno C, et al. Comparison of the effects of lockdown due to COVID-19 on glucose patterns among children, adolescents, and adults with type 1 diabetes: CGM study. BMJ Open Diabetes Res Care 2020;8:8

47. Hoskins M. 'Long haul' Covid-19 and type 1 diabetes. Published 11 March 2021. Accessed 27 March 2021. Available from https://www.healthline.com/diabetesmine/ long-haul-covid-type1-diabetes

Adult-Onset Type 1 Diabetes: Current Understanding and Challenges

Diabetes Care 2021;44:2449–2456 | https://doi.org/10.2337/dc21-0770

R. David Leslie,[1]
Carmella Evans-Molina,[2,3]
Jacquelyn Freund-Brown,[4]
Raffaella Buzzetti,[5] Dana Dabelea,[6]
Kathleen M. Gillespie,[7] Robin Goland,[8]
Angus G. Jones,[9] Mark Kacher,[4]
Lawrence S. Phillips,[10] Olov Rolandsson,[11]
Jana L. Wardian,[12] and Jessica L. Dunne[4]

Recent epidemiological data have shown that more than half of all new cases of type 1 diabetes occur in adults. Key genetic, immune, and metabolic differences exist between adult- and childhood-onset type 1 diabetes, many of which are not well understood. A substantial risk of misclassification of diabetes type can result. Notably, some adults with type 1 diabetes may not require insulin at diagnosis, their clinical disease can masquerade as type 2 diabetes, and the consequent misclassification may result in inappropriate treatment. In response to this important issue, JDRF convened a workshop of international experts in November 2019. Here, we summarize the current understanding and unanswered questions in the field based on those discussions, highlighting epidemiology and immunogenetic and metabolic characteristics of adult-onset type 1 diabetes as well as disease-associated comorbidities and psychosocial challenges. In adult-onset, as compared with childhood-onset, type 1 diabetes, HLA-associated risk is lower, with more protective genotypes and lower genetic risk scores; multiple diabetes-associated autoantibodies are decreased, though GADA remains dominant. Before diagnosis, those with autoantibodies progress more slowly, and at diagnosis, serum C-peptide is higher in adults than children, with ketoacidosis being less frequent. Tools to distinguish types of diabetes are discussed, including body phenotype, clinical course, family history, autoantibodies, comorbidities, and C-peptide. By providing this perspective, we aim to improve the management of adults presenting with type 1 diabetes.

[1]Centre for Immunobiology, Blizard Institute, Queen Mary University of London, London, U.K.
[2]Departments of Pediatrics and Medicine and Center for Diabetes and Metabolic Diseases, Indiana University School of Medicine, Indianapolis, IN
[3]Richard L. Roudebush VA Medical Center, Indianapolis, IN
[4]JDRF, New York, NY
[5]Department of Experimental Medicine, Sapienza University of Rome, Rome, Italy
[6]Lifecourse Epidemiology of Adiposity & Diabetes Center, Colorado School of Public Health, and Departments of Epidemiology and Pediatrics, University of Colorado Anschutz Medical Campus, Aurora, CO
[7]Translational Health Sciences, Bristol Medical School, University of Bristol, Bristol, U.K.
[8]Naomi Berrie Diabetes Center, Columbia University, New York, NY
[9]Institute of Biomedical and Clinical Science, University of Exeter, Exeter, U.K.
[10]Atlanta VA Medical Center and Division of Endocrinology, Metabolism, and Lipids, Department of Medicine, Emory University School of Medicine, Atlanta, GA
[11]Department of Public Health and Clinical Medicine, Umeå University, Umeå, Sweden
[12]College of Medicine, University of Nebraska Medical Center, Omaha, NE

Corresponding author: Carmella Evans-Molina, cevansmo@iu.edu, or R. David Leslie, r.d.g. leslie@qmul.ac.uk

Received 7 April 2021 and accepted 12 August 2021

Clinically, it has been relatively easy to distinguish the acute, potentially lethal, childhood-onset diabetes from the less aggressive condition that affects adults. However, experience has taught us that not all children with diabetes are insulin dependent and not all adults are non–insulin dependent. Immune, genetic, and metabolic analysis of these two, apparently distinct, forms of diabetes revealed inconsistencies, such that insulin-dependent and immune-mediated diabetes was redefined as type 1 diabetes, while most other forms were relabeled as type 2 diabetes. Recent data suggest a further shift in our thinking, with the recognition that more than half of all new cases of type 1 diabetes occur in adults. However, many adults may not require insulin at diagnosis of type 1 diabetes and have a more gradual onset of hyperglycemia, often leading to misclassification and inappropriate care. Indeed, misdiagnosis occurs in nearly 40% of adults with new type 1 diabetes, with the risk of error increasing with age (1,2). To consider this important issue, JDRF convened a workshop of international experts in November 2019 in New York, NY. In this Perspective, based on that workshop, we outline the evidence for a new viewpoint, suggesting future directions of research and ways to alter disease management to help adults living with type 1 diabetes.

UNDERSTANDING ADULT-ONSET TYPE 1 DIABETES

Incidence of Type 1 Diabetes Among Adults Worldwide

Adult-onset type 1 diabetes is more common than childhood-onset type 1 diabetes, as shown from epidemiological data from both high-risk areas such as Northern Europe and low-risk areas such as China (3–8). In southeastern Sweden, the disease incidence among individuals aged 0–19 years is similar to that among individuals 40–100 years of age (37.8 per 100,000 persons per year and 34.0/100,000/year, respectively) (3). Given that the comparable incidence spans only two decades in children, it follows that adult-onset type 1 diabetes is more prevalent. Similarly, analysis of U.S. data from commercially insured individuals demonstrated an overall lower incidence in individuals 20–64 years of age (18.6/100,000/year) than in youth aged 0–19 years (34.3/100,000/year), but the total number of new cases in adults over a 14-year period was 19,174 compared with 13,302 in youth (4). Despite the incidence of childhood-onset type 1 diabetes in China being among the lowest in the world, prevalence data show similar trends across the life span. From 2010–2013, the incidence was 1.93/100,000 among individuals aged 0–14 years and 1.28/100,000 among those 15–29 years of age versus 0.69/100,000 among older adults (5). In aggregate, adults comprised 65.3% of all clinically defined newly diagnosed type 1 diabetes cases in China, which is similar to estimates using genetically stratified data from the population-based UK Biobank using a childhood-onset polygenic genetic risk score (GRS) (6). It is important to note that the proportion would likely be higher if autoimmune cases not requiring insulin initially were classified as type 1 diabetes. For example, in a clinic-based European study, the proportion of adults with diabetes not initially requiring insulin yet with type 1 diabetes–associated autoantibodies was even higher than those started on insulin at diagnosis with a defined type 1 diabetes diagnosis (9). Moreover, in an adult population-based

study in China, the fraction (8.6%) with diabetes not requiring insulin yet with type 1 diabetes–associated autoantibodies was similar to that in Europe, implying that there could be over 6 million Chinese with adult-onset type 1 diabetes (10). While there is a wide range in the incidence of type 1 diabetes across different ethnic groups, even using differing methods of case identification (7), these data support the notion that, worldwide, over half of all new-onset type 1 diabetes cases occur in adults.

Natural History Studies of Type 1 Diabetes

Our understanding of the natural history of type 1 diabetes has been informed by a number of longitudinal and cross-sectional studies. At one end of the spectrum are prospective birth cohort studies, such as the BABYDIAB study in Germany and The Environmental Determinants of Diabetes in the Young (TEDDY) study, which includes sites in Germany, Finland, Sweden, and the U.S. While these studies now have the potential to explore the pathogenesis of islet autoimmunity by being extended into adulthood, they have primarily focused on events occurring in childhood (11). Clinical centers in North America, Europe, and Australia collaborate within Type 1 Diabetes TrialNet, a study that identifies autoantibody-positive adults and children in a cross-sectional manner to examine the pathogenesis of type 1 diabetes and to perform clinical trials on those at high risk in order to preserve β-cell function (12). At the other end of the spectrum, the European Prospective Investigation into Cancer and Nutrition (EPIC)-InterAct study is a case-cohort study nested in the U.K. prospective adult population-based EPIC study (13), while the clinical, immunogenetic, and metabolic characteristics of autoimmune adult-onset type 1 diabetes have been extensively studied in large American, European, and Chinese studies, including UK Prospective Diabetes Study (UKPDS), Action LADA, Scandia, Non Insulin Requiring Autoimmune Diabetes (NIRAD), and LADA China (9,14–19). Based on these cross-sectional and prospective studies, considerable data have been generated to define differences within type 1 diabetes according to the age at onset. Here, we highlight key aspects of age-related genetic, immune, and metabolic heter-ogeneity in type 1 diabetes. Of note,

the term latent autoimmune diabetes in adults (LADA) has been used to describe adults with slowly progressive autoimmunity, sometimes exhibiting features overlapping with those of type 2 diabetes (9,14,18). At the outset of the workshop and for the purposes of this Perspective, LADA was not considered a unique entity; rather, we considered the classification of type 1 diabetes to include all individuals with evidence of autoimmunity, regardless of the trajectory of disease development (i.e., rapid or slowly progressive) or other associated demographic and/or clinical features (e.g., obesity).

Age-Related Genetic Heterogeneity

Type 1 diabetes shows heterogeneity across a broad range of clinical, genetic, immune, histological, and metabolic features (20). Childhood-onset type 1 diabetes is most often attributed to susceptibility alleles in human leukocyte antigen (HLA), which contribute ~50% of the disease heritability. Whereas ethnic differences exist, notably for specific HLA genotypes, several broad principles apply. Compared with childhood-onset disease, adult-onset type 1 diabetes cases show lower type 1 diabetes concordance rates in twins (21), less high-risk HLA heterozygosity (19), lower HLA class I (14), more protective genotypes (14,15), and lower GRS (6,22), which are calculated by summing the odds ratios (OR) for disease-risk alleles.

Diabetes-Associated Immune Changes

Adult-onset type 1 diabetes, like childhood-onset type 1 diabetes, is associated with the presence of serum autoantibodies against β-cell antigens. Serum glutamic acid decarboxylase (GADA) autoantibodies may be useful as a predictor of type 1 diabetes in adults, as adult-onset cases most often present with GADA positivity (9,10,15,17,18,20,22) and possess an HLA-DR3 genotype (9,14,15, 20,21,23). In one prospective study of a general population, the hazard risk of incident diabetes in those with a high type 1 diabetes GRS and GADA positivity was 3.23 compared with all other individuals, suggesting that 1.8% of incident diabetes in adults was attributable to that combination of risk factors (13). In adult-onset type 1 diabetes, multiple diabetes-associated autoantibodies tend to be less prevalent with increasing age at diagnosis (1,8), yet GADA remains the dominant autoantibody irrespective of the need for insulin treatment at diagnosis and irrespective of ethnicity (9,17,18,24, 25), even despite a paucity of HLA DR3, as in Japan and China (17,18). In contrast, childhood-onset type 1 diabetes cases often have insulin autoantibodies and an HLA-DR4 genotype, higher identical twin disease concordance, more HLA heterozygosity, and higher GRS (20). Taken together, these data indicate that type 1 diabetes is heterogeneous across the spectrum of diagnoses, suggesting that pathogenesis and optimal therapy are also diverse.

Data from the TrialNet Pathway to Prevention cohort demonstrated lower risk of progression to type 1 diabetes in adults than children, even when both show multiple autoantibodies on a single occasion and are monitored over 10 years (12). One recent analysis found that the 5-year rate of progression to diabetes in multiple autoantibody–positive adults was only ~15%, with a number of them remaining diabetes-free for decades (26). A combined cohort study, known as the Slow or Nonprogressive Autoimmunity to the Islets of Langerhans (SNAIL) study, is following such "slow progressors" with multiple autoantibodies who have yet to progress to stage 3 type 1 diabetes (i.e., clinical diagnosis) over at least a 10-year period (27). Many of these slow progressors lose disease-associated autoantibodies over time, adding complexity to cross-sectional classification (28). Based on estimates from natural history studies, slow progressors, even if identified when young, cannot account for all autoimmune adult-onset diabetes, indicating that autoantibodies must develop at all ages (11). However, little is known about those who initially develop autoimmunity as adults, mostly due to the lack of longitudinal studies focusing on this population.

People with type 1 diabetes, in contrast to the majority of those with type 2 diabetes, have altered adaptive immunity (i.e., islet autoantibodies and T-cell activation), while innate immune changes, including cytokine changes, are common to both (29). Increased T-cell activation by islet proteins has also been found in a proportion of adults with initially non-insulin-requiring diabetes, even when they lack diabetes autoantibodies (30).

However, there is a paucity of immune studies on adult-onset type 1 diabetes and few histologic studies. An analysis of tissues from the Network for Pancreatic Organ Donors with Diabetes (nPOD) showed no relationship between age at diabetes onset and the frequency of islet insulitis (31). The composition of islet insulitis differs in very young children compared with older individuals, with the former having an increased frequency of B cells in islet infiltrates (32). However, relating pancreatic histological changes to changes in peripheral blood remains a challenge.

Adults with new-onset type 1 diabetes are at increased risk of other autoimmune conditions. About 30% of individuals with adult-onset type 1 diabetes have thyroid autoimmunity (27,29). In addition, adults with type 1 diabetes who possess high-titer GADA and/or multiple islet autoantibodies are at increased risk of progression to hypothyroidism (24,33). In a large population-based Chinese study, the prevalence of adult-onset type 1 diabetes was 6% among initially non-insulin-requiring diabetes cases, and 16.3% of them had thyroid autoimmunity (OR 2.4) (10). Of note, those with islet antigen 2 autoantibodies had a high risk of tissue transglutaminase autoantibodies, a marker for celiac disease (OR 19.1) (10). Thus, in the clinical setting, there should be a high index of suspicion for other autoimmune conditions in individuals with adult-onset type diabetes, and associated autoimmunity should be screened where clinically indicated.

Metabolic Characteristics of Adult-Onset Type 1 Diabetes

Age-related differences in type 1 diabetes extend to metabolic parameters. C-peptide at diagnosis is higher in adults than children, driven in part by higher BMI (34). Analysis of U.K., TrialNet, and Chinese cohorts has identified two distinct phases of C-peptide decline in stage 3 disease: an initial exponential fall followed by a period of relative stability. Along with initial differences at the time of clinical diagnosis, the rate of decline over 2–4 years was inversely related to age at onset (10,34–36). Furthermore, the U.S. T1D Exchange Study found that glycemic control was better in adults with type 1 diabetes than in children and adolescents with type 1 diabetes (37). The American Diabetes

Association (ADA) targets for glycemia are higher in children, so that in this same cohort, 17% of children, compared with 21% of adults, achieved the ADA hemoglobin A_{1c} (HbA_{1c}) goal of <7.5% and <7.0%, respectively (37). Other factors confound this relationship between age at diagnosis and metabolic control. First, individuals with adult-onset type 1 diabetes are more likely to have residual insulin-producing β-cells and persistent measurable C-peptide in disease of long duration, the latter of which has been linked to improved glycemic control (38,39). Second, individuals with adult-onset type 1 diabetes, initially not on insulin therapy, tend to have worse metabolic control than people with type 2 diabetes, even when receiving insulin treatment (9,40). The sole exception is the LADA China study, where worse control was noted only among those with a high GAD titer (18). Metabolic differences between adults and children extend beyond C-peptide. Adults with autoantibody positivity who progressed to type 1 diabetes were less likely than very young children to exhibit elevated proinsulin/C-peptide ratios prior to stage 3 disease onset (41). In addition, in individuals with disease of long duration, those diagnosed at an older age had evidence of improved proinsulin processing and nutrient-induced proinsulin secretory capacity (42).

Diagnosis and Management of Adult-Onset Type 1 Diabetes

Correctly identifying diabetes etiology and type is difficult, and misclassification may occur in up to 40% of adults presenting with type 1 diabetes (1,2). Reasons underlying misclassification are multiple and include *1*) lack of awareness that the onset of type 1 diabetes is not limited to children; *2*) the overwhelming majority of people developing diabetes as older adults have type 2 diabetes, contributing to a confirmation bias (2); *3*) typical clinical criteria, such as BMI and metabolic syndrome, can be poor discriminators, especially as rates of obesity in the overall population increase (9,43); *4*) clinical characteristics of adult-onset type 1 diabetes can masquerade as type 2 diabetes, given their slow metabolic progression and risk of metabolic syndrome (which occurs in about 40%), so that the distinction between types of diabetes may be blurred (43–45); and 5) lack of awareness of and accessibility to biomarkers that may serve as tools to distinguish type 1 diabetes and type 2 diabetes.

Tools to distinguish type 1 and type 2 diabetes are under active development. For example, classification models integrating up to five prespecified predictor variables, including clinical features (age of diagnosis and BMI) and clinical biomarkers (autoantibodies and GRS) in a White European population, had high accuracy to identify adults with recently diagnosed diabetes with rapid insulin requirement despite using GRS derived from childhood-onset type 1 diabetes. While GRS have the potential to assist diagnosis of type 1 diabetes in uncertain cases, they are not yet widely available in clinical practice. Moreover, it is important to note that while the model was optimized with the inclusion of all five variables, the addition of GRS had only a modest effect on overall model performance (22).

Classification can be aided by the measurement of autoantibodies and C-peptide. Recommended autoantibodies to assay at the time of diagnosis include those to insulin (insulin autoantibody), glutamate decarboxylase isoform 65 (GAD65A), insulinoma antigen 2, and zinc transporter isoform 8 (Znt8A), with GAD65A being the most prevalent autoantibody among adults. High levels or the presence of more than one antibody increases the likelihood of type 1 diabetes. However, it is important to realize that islet autoantibodies are a continuous marker that can also occur in the population without diabetes. As with many other tests, an abnormal test is usually based on a threshold signal from control populations without diabetes, usually the 97.5th or the 99th centile. Therefore, false-positive results with these assays can occur and can be reduced by using higher-specificity assays or thresholds and targeting testing toward those with clinical features suggestive of type 1 diabetes (46). Finally, since antibody levels can wane over time in established type 1 diabetes, the absence of autoantibodies does not rule out the possibility of a diagnosis of type 1 diabetes.

Measurement of C-peptide, paired with a blood glucose in the same sample, provides an estimate of endo-genous insulin production and has the most

utility in disease of long duration when levels fall below 300 pmol/L (39,47). However, C-peptide levels are typically higher at presentation and may be difficult to distinguish from levels in type 2 diabetes, which are usually >600 pmol/L. Thus, thresholds of C-peptide that clearly delineate type 1 diabetes from type 2 diabetes at diagnosis cannot be categorically defined, and C-peptide must be interpreted within the context of other clinical and laboratory features. Measurement of a random nonfasting C-peptide is superior to fasting C-peptide in identifying type 1 diabetes (48) and is well correlated with stimulated C-peptide levels measured during a mixed-meal tolerance test, which is considered the gold standard assessment of insulin secretory function in established type 1 diabetes (49). A recent analysis found that concomitant blood glucose $\geq$144 mg/dL (8 mmol/L) increased the specificity of random C-peptide in predicting a stimulated C-peptide level <600pmol/L, suggesting this is a reasonable threshold of blood glucose to employ for C-peptide interpretation (49).

C-peptide also can be used to guide therapy (50). Individuals with a random C-peptide level $\leq$300 pmol/L should be managed mainly with insulin. For those with random C-peptide levels >300 pmol/L, insulin could be combined with other diabetes therapies, although evidence about safety and efficacy is limited. It is generally agreed that sulfonylureas should be avoided because of the potential to hasten β-cell failure (50). There is concern for increased risk of diabetic ketoacidosis (DKA) with sodium–glucose cotransporter 1 (SGLT1) and SGLT2 inhibitors when these agents are used in type 1 diabetes, especially in nonobese individuals who may need only low dosages of insulin (51). All other agents could be considered for therapy in those not requiring insulin initially. In individuals with random C-peptide levels exceeding 600 pmol/L, management can be much as recommended for type 2 diabetes, with the caveats outlined above (50). An important consideration is that loss of β-cell function may be rapid in autoimmune diabetes. As such, individuals treated without insulin should be closely monitored.

In the absence of prospectively validated decision support tools that have

been tested in multiethnic populations, we suggest, as an approach to aid the practicing physician, assessment of age, autoimmunity, body habitus/BMI, background, control, and comorbidities, using the acronym AABBCC (Table 2). This approach includes the clinical consideration of autoimmunity and other clinical features suggestive of type 1 diabetes, including age at diagnosis, low BMI, an unexplained or rapid worsening of clinical course manifesting as a lack of response or rising HbA$_{1c}$ with type 2 diabetes medications, and a rapid requirement for insulin therapy, especially within 3 years of diagnosis. It should be emphasized that among these features, age at diagnosis (<40 years), low BMI (<25 kg/m^2), and rapid need for insulin therapy are the most discriminatory (43). We recommend measurement of islet antibodies and C-peptide be considered in all older people with clinical features that suggest type 1 diabetes, with islet autoantibodies being the initial test of choice in short-duration disease (<3 years) and C-peptide the test of choice at longer durations.

Diabetes-Associated Comorbidities and Complications

DKA

The U.S. SEARCH for Diabetes in Youth study reported that nearly 30% of youth with newly diagnosed type 1 diabetes age <20 years presented with DKA (52). The frequency of DKA among adults at diagnosis with type 1 diabetes is unknown but is believed to be lower given that they often have higher C-peptide levels at diagnosis and a slower decline in β-cell function over time, even in those requiring insulin initially (34). Among childhood-onset type 1 diabetes, most episodes of DKA beyond diagnosis are associated with insulin omission, pump failure, or treatment error (53). However, for adults with type 1 diabetes, the primary risk factors are noncompliance and infections (54), the former sometimes due to the cost of insulin (55). Thus, there is a need to further understand DKA in adults, not least because it is associated with long-term worsening glycemic control (56).

Hypoglycemia

Fear of hypoglycemia remains a major problem in the clinical management of adults with type 1 diabetes (57), influencing quality of life and glycemic control. The effect of diabetes duration or age at diagnosis on hypoglycemia risk is not consistent among different studies. However, α-cell responses to hypoglycemia and hypoglycemia risk are both lower in individuals with higher C-peptide levels (38). Because residual C-peptide is more likely to be observed in those with a later age of onset, hypoglycemia risk may be different between those with childhood- and adult-onset diabetes. While insulin pumps and continuous glucose monitors are associated with improved glycemic control and reduced hypoglycemia (37), adults may show reluctance or inertia in adopting newer technologies. In the T1D Exchange study population, 63% of adults used an insulin pump while only 30% used a continuous glucose monitor, and use of these technologies tended to be lower in adults than in children (37).

Factors that dictate use of these technologies are multiple and may include reduced access to or acceptance of wearable technology, challenges with insurance coverage, especially in the context of past misclassification, and/or inadequate education about hypoglycemia risk (58). A better understanding of potential barriers to technology use in adult-onset type 1 diabetes is needed. Furthermore, little is known about changes in hypoglycemia risk across the life span of individuals with adult-onset disease, representing an important gap in knowledge.

Microvascular and Macrovascular Disease Complications
Despite the prevalence of adult-onset type 1 diabetes, there is a paucity of data on the burden of microvascular complications in this population. Current knowledge is largely based on small, cross-sectional studies. In aggregate, these studies suggest that the prevalence of nephropathy and retinopathy are lower in adult-onset type 1 than in type 2 diabetes, but this conclusion is potentially confounded by diabetes duration. For example, the prevalence of nephropathy and retinopathy was lower in Chinese individuals with adult-onset type 1 diabetes than in those with type 2, but only in those with a disease duration <5 years, while in the Botnia Study, retinopathy risk in adult-onset type 1 diabetes increased, as expected, with disease duration (59). Two substantial prospective studies recently reported that those adults with diabetes enrolled in the UKPDS who were also GADA positive (i.e., presumably with type 1 diabetes) compared with those who were GADA negative (with type 2 diabetes) showed a higher prevalence of retinopathy and lower prevalence of cardiovascular

Table 1—Knowledge gaps

Area of focus	Description
Eliminating cultural bias in order to understand what impacts disease development	Most large-scale studies of adult type 1 diabetes have been done in Europe, North America, and China. There is a pressing need to extend these studies to other continents and to diverse racial and ethnic groups. Such studies could help us identify and understand the nature and implications of diversity, whether in terms of pathogenesis, cultural differences, or health care disparity. In addition, prospective childhood studies of high-risk birth cohorts could be extended into adulthood and new studies initiated to better understand mechanisms behind disease development and whether there is a differentiation in the disease process between young and adult type 1 diabetes.
Population screening	At present, universal childhood screening programs are being developed in many countries. Research will be needed to develop strategies for the follow-up of autoantibody-positive populations throughout adulthood.
Disease-modifying therapies in early-stage disease	Trials of disease-modifying therapies have generally shown better efficacy in children (12). There are likely to be important differences in agent selection between adult and pediatric populations, and these differences require study.
Diagnosis and misclassification	There is a need to build a diagnostic decision tree to aid in diabetes classification. Tools are needed to estimate individual-level risk.
Adjunctive therapies	There is a need to better understand the benefits and risks of using therapies that are adjunctive to insulin in adult-onset type 1 diabetes. To this end, large-scale drug trials need to be performed, and therapeutic decision trees are required to help health care professionals and endocrinologists select such therapies.
Post-diagnosis education and support	Improving education and support post-diagnosis is vital and should include psychosocial support, health care provision, and analysis of long-term outcomes (including complications) in adult-onset type 1 diabetes. Current knowledge is limited with respect to complications, especially related to the complex mechanisms contributing to macrovascular disease in adult-onset type 1 diabetes. Surveillance efforts based on larger and representative cohorts of patients with clear and consistent case definitions are needed to better understand the burden and risk of diabetes-related chronic complications in this large population.

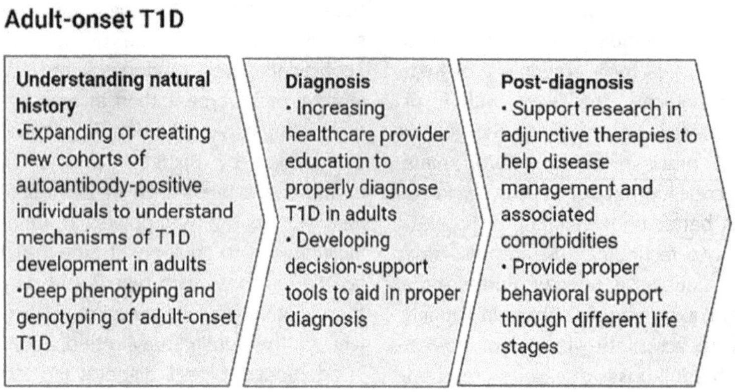

Adult-onset T1D

Figure 1—Proposed roadmap to better understand, diagnose, and care for adults with type 1 diabetes (T1D). Created in BioRender (BioRender.com).

events (60,61). These results are consistent with people with adult-onset type 1 diabetes compared with those with type 2 diabetes, showing a general tendency to higher HbA_{1c} levels (40,44,60,61) as well as reduced traditional cardiovascular risk factors, including reduced adiposity (BMI and waist circumference), metabolic (lipid levels), and vascular (blood pressure) profiles (9,24,62). Nevertheless, all-cause mortality and cardiovascular mortality rates in such individuals with adult-onset type 1 diabetes (59) are still higher than those among individuals without diabetes. In addition, there are discrepancies across studies, likely related to differences in populations under study (i.e., age, race/ethnicity, and diabetes duration), lack of consistent case definitions (i.e., adult-onset type 1 diabetes or LADA cases), and different outcomes, as well as small sample sizes with insufficient events on which to base strong recommendations.

Psychosocial Challenges

Negative stressors, including pressure to achieve target HbA_{1c} levels, lifestyle considerations, and fear of complications, are factors leading to the increased frequency of mood disorders, attempted suicide, and psychiatric care in adults with diabetes (63). In individuals who have experienced misclassification, additional stress derives from conflicting messages about the nature of their diabetes. Among adults with type 1 diabetes, those with high psychological coping skills (e.g., self-efficacy, self-esteem, and optimism) and adaptive skills may buffer the negative effect of stress and should be cultivated (64). Relationship challenges, including sexual intimacy, starting a family, caring for children, and relational stress, are major stressors for adults with

type 1 diabetes (65). In addition, there is the looming threat of complications, including blindness and amputations (65). Adults with type 1 diabetes describe a sense of powerlessness, fear of hypoglycemia, and the challenges of both self-management and appropriate food management (66). A common misunderstanding is that while they face the same life choices associated with type 2 diabetes (e.g., weight loss, exercise, and limiting intake of simple sugars), adults with type 1 diabetes may require different management skills (67). Moreover, there is a strong association in adults with type 1 diabetes between chronic, stressful life events and fluctuating HbA_{1c}, possibly due to indirect mechanisms, including adherence to diabetes management (68).

Whether these risks differ between those diagnosed as children or as adults is unclear and requires additional study.

CLOSING

In this Perspective, we have summarized the current understanding of adult-onset type 1 diabetes while identifying many knowledge gaps (Table 1). Epidemiological data from diverse ethnic groups show that adult-onset type 1 diabetes is often more prevalent than childhood-onset type 1 diabetes. However, our understanding of type 1 diabetes presenting in adults is limited. This striking shortfall in knowledge (Table 1) results in frequent misclassification, which may negatively impact disease management. Here, we outline a roadmap for addressing these deficiencies (Fig. 1). A cornerstone of this roadmap is a renewed emphasis on the careful consideration of the underlying etiology of diabetes in every adult presenting with diabetes.

In the absence of data-driven classification tools capable of estimating individual-level risk, we offer a simple set of questions, incorporating what we have termed the AABBCCs of diabetes classification and management (Table 2). In parallel, we invite the research community to join together in addressing key gaps in knowledge through studies aimed at defining the genetic, immunologic, and metabolic phenotype of adult-onset type 1 diabetes with the goal of using this

Table 2—AABBCC approach to diabetes classification

Parameter	Description
Age	Autoimmune diabetes is most prevalent in patients aged <50 years at diagnosis. Those aged <35 years at diagnosis should be considered for maturity-onset diabetes of the young as well as type 1 diabetes
Autoimmunity	Does this individual have islet autoantibodies or a history of autoimmunity (i.e., thyroid disease, celiac disease)? Is there a goiter or vitiligo on exam?
Body habitus/BMI	Is the body habitus or BMI inconsistent with a diagnosis of type 2 diabetes, especially if BMI <25 kg/m²?
Background	What is the patient's background? Is there a family history of autoimmunity and/or type 1 diabetes? Are they from a high-risk ethnic group?
Control	Are diabetes control and HbA_{1c} worsening on noninsulin therapies? Has there been an accelerated change in HbA_{1c}? Is the C-peptide low, that is, ≤300 pmol/L (especially <200 pmol/L), or is there clinical evidence that β-cell function is declining? Was there a need for insulin therapy within 3 years of diabetes diagnosis?
Comorbidities	Irrespective of immunogenetic background, coexistent cardiac or renal disease and their risk factors impact the approach to therapy and HbA_{1c} targets.

knowledge to develop improved approaches for disease management and prevention (Fig. 1).

Acknowledgments. Sharon Saydah, Division of Diabetes Translation, National Center for Chronic Disease Prevention and Health Promotion, Centers for Disease Control and Prevention, attended the workshop and participated in subsequent discussions of the manuscript. Elizabeth Seaquist, Division of Diabetes, Endocrinology, and Metabolism at the University of Minnesota, participated in the workshop. The authors acknowledge Marilyn L. Wales for her assistance with formatting the manuscript.

Funding and Duality of Interest. This manuscript is the result of a one-day meeting held at JDRF headquarters in New York, NY. Financial support for the workshop was provided by JDRF and Janssen Research and Development, LLC. Financial support from Janssen Research and Development, LLC, for the workshop was in an unrestricted grant to JDRF. JDRF provided participants with transportation, lodging, and meals to attend the workshop. No additional support was provided for the writing of the manuscript. R.D.L. is supported by a grant from the European Union (contract no. QLGi-CT-2002-01886). C.E.-M. is supported by National Institute for Health Research grants R01 DK093954, R21DK119800, U01DK127786, R01DK127308, and P30DK097512; VA Merit Award I01BX001733; JDRF grant 2-SRA-2019-834-S-B; and gifts from the Sigma Beta Sorority, the Ball Brothers Foundation, and the George and Frances Ball Foundation. R.B. is supported in part by the Italian Ministry of University and Research (project code 20175L9H7H). A.G.J. is funded by a National Institute for Health Research (NIHR) Clinician Scientist fellowship (CS-2015-15-018). L.S.P. is supported in part by U.S. Department of Veterans Affairs (VA) awards CSP #2008, I01 CX001899, I01 CX001737, and Health Services Research & Development IIR 07-138; National Institute for Health Research awards R21 DK099716, R18 DK066204, R03 AI133172, R21 AI156161, U01 DK091958, U01 DK098246, and UL1 TR002378; and Cystic Fibrosis Foundation award PHILLI12A0.

R.D.L. received unrestricted educational grants from Novo Nordisk, Sanofi, MSD, and AstraZeneca. C.E.-M. has participated in advisory boards for Dompé Pharmaceuticals, Provention Bio, MaiCell Technologies, and ISLA Technologies. C.E.M. is the recipient of in-kind research support from Nimbus Pharmaceuticals and Bristol Myers Squibb and an investigator-initiated research grant from Eli Lilly and Company. J.F.-B. and J.L.D. were employed by JDRF during the workshop and early stages of writing. J.F.-B. is currently an employee of Provention Bio, and J.L.D. is currently an employee of Janssen Research and Development, LLC. R.B. participated in advisory boards for Sanofi and Eli Lilly and received honoraria for speaker bureaus from Sanofi, Eli Lilly, AstraZeneca, Novo Nordisk, and Abbott. L.S.P. has served on scientific advisory boards for Janssen and has or had research support from Merck, Pfizer, Eli Lilly, Novo Nordisk, Sanofi, PhaseBio, Roche, AbbVie, Vascular Pharmaceuticals, Janssen, GlaxoSmithKline, and the Cystic Fibrosis Foundation. L.S.P. is also a cofounder and officer and board member and stockholder for a company, Diasyst, Inc., that markets software aimed to help improve diabetes management. No other potential conflicts of interest relevant to this article were reported.

The sponsors had no role in the design and conduct of the study, collection, management, analysis, and interpretation of the data, and preparation, review, or approval of the manuscript. This work is not intended to reflect the official opinion of the VA or the U.S. Government.

Author Contributions. R.D.L., C.E.M., J.F.-B., and J.L.D. conceived of the article and wrote and edited the manuscript. All other authors were involved in the writing and editing of the manuscript. R.D.L. and C.E.-M. are guarantors of this work and, as such, had full access to all the data in the study and take responsibility for the integrity of the data and the accuracy of the data analysis.

References

1. Muñoz C, Floreen A, Garey C, et al. Misdiagnosis and diabetic ketoacidosis at diagnosis of type 1 diabetes: patient and caregiver perspectives. Clin Diabetes 2019;37:276–281

2. Thomas NJ, Lynam AL, Hill AV, et al. Type 1 diabetes defined by severe insulin deficiency occurs after 30 years of age and is commonly treated as type 2 diabetes. Diabetologia 2019;62:1167–1172

3. Thunander M, Petersson C, Jonzon K, et al. Incidence of type 1 and type 2 diabetes in adults and children in Kronoberg, Sweden. Diabetes Res Clin Pract 2008;82:247–255

4. Rogers MAM, Kim C, Banerjee T, Lee JM. Fluctuations in the incidence of type 1 diabetes in the United States from 2001 to 2015: a longitudinal study. BMC Med 2017;15:199

5. Weng J, Zhou Z, Guo L, et al.; T1D China Study Group. Incidence of type 1 diabetes in China, 2010-13: population based study. BMJ 2018;360:j5295

6. Thomas NJ, Jones SE, Weedon MN, Shields BM, Oram RA, Hattersley AT. Frequency and phenotype of type 1 diabetes in the first six decades of life: a cross-sectional, genetically stratified survival analysis from UK Biobank. Lancet Diabetes Endocrinol 2018;6:122–129

7. Diaz-Valencia PA, Bougnères P, Valleron AJ. Global epidemiology of type 1 diabetes in young adults and adults: a systematic review. BMC Public Health 2015;15:255

8. Gorham ED, Barrett-Connor E, Highfill-McRoy RM, et al. Incidence of insulin-requiring diabetes in the US military. Diabetologia 2009;52:2087–2091

9. Hawa MI, Kolb H, Schloot N, et al.; Action LADA Consortium. Adult-onset autoimmune diabetes in Europe is prevalent with a broad clinical phenotype: Action LADA 7. Diabetes Care 2013;36:908–913

10. Xiang Y, Huang G, Zhu Y, et al.; China National Diabetes and Metabolic Disorders Study Group. Identification of autoimmune type 1 diabetes and multiple organ-specific autoantibodies in adult-onset non-insulin-requiring diabetes in China: a population-based multicentre nationwide survey. Diabetes Obes Metab 2019;21:893–902

11. Ziegler AG, Rewers M, Simell O, et al. Seroconversion to multiple islet autoantibodies and risk of progression to diabetes in children. JAMA 2013;309:2473–2479

12. Wherrett DK, Chiang JL, Delamater AM, et al.; Type 1 Diabetes TrialNet Study Group. Defining pathways for development of disease-modifying therapies in children with type 1 diabetes: a consensus report. Diabetes Care 2015;38:1975–1985

13. Rolandsson O, Hampe CS, Sharp SJ, et al. Autoimmunity plays a role in the onset of diabetes after 40 years of age. Diabetologia 2020;63:266–277

14. Mishra R, Åkerlund M, Cousminer DL, et al. Genetic discrimination between LADA and childhood-onset type 1 diabetes within the MHC. Diabetes Care 2020;43:418–425

15. Zhu M, Xu K, Chen Y, et al. Identification of novel T1D risk loci and their association with age and islet function at diagnosis in autoantibody-positive T1D individuals: based on a two-stage genome-wide association study. Diabetes Care 2019;42:1414–1421

16. Buzzetti R, Di Pietro S, Giaccari A, et al.; Non Insulin Requiring Autoimmune Diabetes Study Group. High titer of autoantibodies to GAD identifies a specific phenotype of adult-onset autoimmune diabetes. Diabetes Care 2007;30:932–938

17. Yasui J, Kawasaki E, Tanaka S, et al.; Japan Diabetes Society Committee on Type 1 Diabetes Mellitus Research. Clinical and genetic characteristics of non-insulin-requiring glutamic acid decarboxylase (GAD) autoantibody-positive diabetes: a nationwide survey in Japan. PLoS One 2016;11:e0155643

18. Zhou Z, Xiang Y, Ji L, et al.; LADA China Study Group. Frequency, immunogenetics, and clinical characteristics of latent autoimmune diabetes in China (LADA China study): a nationwide, multicenter, clinic-based cross-sectional study. Diabetes 2013;62:543–550

19. Howson JM, Rosinger S, Smyth DJ, Boehm BO; ADBW-END Study Group. Genetic analysis of adult-onset autoimmune diabetes. Diabetes 2011;60:2645–2653

20. Battaglia M, Ahmed S, Anderson MS, et al. Introducing the endotype concept to address the challenge of disease heterogeneity in type 1 diabetes. Diabetes Care 2020;43:5–12

21. Redondo MJ, Yu L, Hawa M, et al. Heterogeneity of type I diabetes: analysis of monozygotic twins in Great Britain and the United States. Diabetologia 2001;44:354–362

22. Lynam A, McDonald T, Hill A, et al. Development and validation of multivariable clinical diagnostic models to identify type 1 diabetes requiring rapid insulin therapy in adults aged 18-50 years. BMJ Open 2019;9:e031586

23. Cousminer DL, Ahlqvist E, Mishra R, et al.; Bone Mineral Density in Childhood Study. First genome-wide association study of latent autoimmune diabetes in adults reveals novel insights linking immune and metabolic diabetes. Diabetes Care 2018;41:2396–2403

24. Zampetti S, Capizzi M, Spoletini M, et al.; NIRAD Study Group. GADA titer-related risk for organ-specific autoimmunity in LADA subjects subdivided according to gender (NIRAD study 6). J Clin Endocrinol Metab 2012;97:3759–3765

25. Balcha SA, Demisse AG, Mishra R, et al. Type 1 diabetes in Africa: an immunogenetic study in the Amhara of North-West Ethiopia. Diabetologia 2020;63:2158–2168

26. Jacobsen LM, Bocchino L, Evans-Molina C, et al. The risk of progression to type 1 diabetes is highly variable in individuals with multiple autoantibodies following screening. Diabetologia 2020;63:588–596

27. Long AE, Wilson IV, Becker DJ, et al. Characteristics of slow progression to diabetes in multiple islet autoantibody-positive individuals from five longitudinal cohorts: the SNAIL study. Diabetologia 2018;61:1484–1490

28. Hanna SJ, Powell WE, Long AE, et al. Slow progressors to type 1 diabetes lose islet autoantibodies over time, have few islet antigen-specific CD8+ T cells and exhibit a distinct CD95hi B cell phenotype. Diabetologia 2020;63:1174–1185

29. Schloot NC, Pham MN, Hawa MI, et al.; Action LADA Group. Inverse relationship between organ-specific autoantibodies and systemic immune mediators in type 1 diabetes and type 2 diabetes: Action LADA 11. Diabetes Care 2016;39:1932–1939

30. Brooks-Worrell BM, Palmer JP. Setting the stage for islet autoimmunity in type 2 diabetes: obesity-associated chronic systemic inflammation and endoplasmic reticulum (ER) stress. Diabetes Care 2019;42:2338–2346

31. Campbell-Thompson M, Fu A, Kaddis JS, et al. Insulitis and β-cell mass in the natural history of type 1 diabetes. Diabetes 2016;65:719–731

32. Leete P, Willcox A, Krogvold L, et al. Differential insulitic profiles determine the extent of β-cell destruction and the age at onset of type 1 diabetes. Diabetes 2016;65:1362–1369

33. Fleiner HF, Bjøro T, Midthjell K, Grill V, Åsvold BO. Prevalence of thyroid dysfunction in autoimmune and type 2 diabetes: the population-based HUNT study in Norway. J Clin Endocrinol Metab 2016;101:669–677

34. Greenbaum CJ, Beam CA, Boulware D, et al.; Type 1 Diabetes TrialNet Study Group. Fall in C-peptide during first 2 years from diagnosis: evidence of at least two distinct phases from composite Type 1 Diabetes TrialNet data. Diabetes 2012;61:2066–2073

35. Gong S, Wu C, Zhong T, et al. Complicated curve association of body weight at diagnosis with C-peptide in children and adults with new-onset type 1 diabetes. Diabetes Metab Res Rev 2020;36:e3285

36. Hao W, Gitelman S, DiMeglio LA, Boulware D; Type 1 Diabetes TrialNet Study Group. Fall in c-peptide during first 4 years from diagnosis of type 1 diabetes: variable relation to age, HbA1c, and insulin dose. Diabetes Care 2016;39:1664–1670

37. Foster NC, Beck RW, Miller KM, et al. State of type 1 diabetes management and outcomes from the T1D exchange in 2016-2018. Diabetes Technol Ther 2019;21:66–72

38. Rickels MR, Evans-Molina C, Bahnson HT, et al.; T1D Exchange β-Cell Function Study Group. High residual C-peptide likely contributes to glycemic control in type 1 diabetes. J Clin Invest 2020;130:1850–1862

39. Davis AK, DuBose SN, Haller MJ, et al.; T1D Exchange Clinic Network. Prevalence of detectable C-peptide according to age at diagnosis and duration of type 1 diabetes. Diabetes Care 2015;38:476–481

40. Andersen CD, Bennet L, Nyström L, et al. Worse glycaemic control in LADA patients than in those with type 2 diabetes, despite a longer time on insulin therapy. Diabetologia 2013;56:252–258

41. Sims EK, Chaudhry Z, Watkins R, et al. Elevations in the fasting serum proinsulin-to-C-peptide ratio precede the onset of type 1 diabetes. Diabetes Care 2016;39:1519–1526

42. Sims EK, Bahnson HT, Nyalwidhe J, et al.; T1D Exchange Residual C-Peptide Study Group. Proinsulin secretion is a persistent feature of type 1 diabetes. Diabetes Care 2019;42:258–264

43. Shields BM, Peters JL, Cooper C, et al. Can clinical features be used to differentiate type 1 from type 2 diabetes? A systematic review of the literature. BMJ Open 2015;5:e009088

44. Ahlqvist E, Storm P, Käräjämäki A, et al. Novel subgroups of adult-onset diabetes and their association with outcomes: a data-driven cluster analysis of six variables. Lancet Diabetes Endocrinol 2018;6:361–369

45. Hawa MI, Thivolet C, Mauricio D, et al.; Action LADA Group. Metabolic syndrome and autoimmune diabetes: action LADA 3. Diabetes Care 2009;32:160–164

46. Jones AG, McDonald TJ, Shields BM, Hagopian W, Hattersley AT. Latent autoimmune diabetes of adults (LADA) is likely to represent a mixed population of autoimmune (type 1) and nonautoimmune (type 2) diabetes. Diabetes Care 2021dc202834

47. Jones AG, Hattersley AT. The clinical utility of C-peptide measurement in the care of patients with diabetes. Diabet Med 2013;30:803–817

48. Berger B, Stenström G, Sundkvist G. Random C-peptide in the classification of diabetes. Scand J Clin Lab Invest 2000;60:687–693

49. Hope SV, Knight BA, Shields BM, Hattersley AT, McDonald TJ, Jones AG. Random non-fasting C-peptide: bringing robust assessment of endogenous insulin secretion to the clinic. Diabet Med 2016;33:1554–1558

50. Buzzetti R, Tuomi T, Mauricio D, et al. Management of latent autoimmune diabetes in adults: a consensus statement from an international expert panel. Diabetes 2020;69:2037–2047

51. Danne T, Garg S, Peters AL, et al. International consensus on risk management of diabetic keto-acidosis in patients with type 1 diabetes treated with sodium-glucose cotransporter (SGLT) inhibitors. Diabetes Care 2019;42:1147–1154

52. Dabelea D, Rewers A, Stafford JM, et al.; SEARCH for Diabetes in Youth Study Group. Trends in the prevalence of ketoacidosis at diabetes diagnosis: the SEARCH for diabetes in youth study. Pediatrics 2014;133:e938–e945

53. Rewers A. Acute metabolic complications in diabetes. In *Diabetes in America*. 3rd ed. Bethesda, MD, National Institute of Diabetes and Digestive and Kidney Diseases, 2018; pp. 1–19

54. Umpierrez GE, Kitabchi AE. Diabetic ketoac-idosis: risk factors and management strategies. Treat Endocrinol 2003;2:95–108

55. Randall L, Begovic J, Hudson M, et al. Recurrent diabetic ketoacidosis in inner-city minority patients: behavioral, socioeconomic, and psychosocial factors. Diabetes Care 2011;34:1891–1896

56. Duca LM, Reboussin BA, Pihoker C, et al. Diabetic ketoacidosis at diagnosis of type 1 diabetes and glycemic control over time: the SEARCH for diabetes in youth study. Pediatr Diabetes 2019;20:172–179

57. Martyn-Nemeth P, Schwarz Farabi S, Mihailescu D, Nemeth J, Quinn L. Fear of hypoglycemia in adults with type 1 diabetes: impact of therapeutic advances and strategies for prevention – a review. J Diabetes Complications 2016;30:167–177

58. Engler R, Routh TL, Lucisano JY. Adoption barriers for continuous glucose monitoring and their potential reduction with a fully implanted system: results from patient preference surveys. Clin Diabetes 2018;36:50–58

59. Isomaa B, Almgren P, Henricsson M, et al. Chronic complications in patients with slowly progressing autoimmune type 1 diabetes (LADA). Diabetes Care 1999;22:1347–1353

60. Maddaloni E, Coleman RL, Agbaje O, Buzzetti R, Holman RR. Time-varying risk of microvascular complications in latent autoimmune diabetes of adulthood compared with type 2 diabetes in adults: a post-hoc analysis of the UK Prospective Diabetes Study 30-year follow-up data (UKPDS 86). Lancet Diabetes Endocrinol 2020;8:206–215

61. Maddaloni E, Coleman RL, Pozzilli P, Holman RR. Long-term risk of cardiovascular disease in individuals with latent autoimmune diabetes in adults (UKPDS 85). Diabetes Obes Metab 2019;21:2115–2122

62. Tuomi T, Carlsson A, Li H, et al. Clinical and genetic characteristics of type 2 diabetes with and without GAD antibodies. Diabetes 1999;48:150–157

63. Robinson ME, Simard M, Larocque I, Shah J, Nakhla M, Rahme E. Risk of psychiatric disorders and suicide attempts in emerging adults with diabetes. Diabetes Care 2020;43:484–486

64. Yi JP, Vitaliano PP, Smith RE, Yi JC, Weinger K. The role of resilience on psychological adjustment and physical health in patients with diabetes. Br J Health Psychol 2008;13:311–325

65. Trief PM, Sandberg JG, Dimmock JA, Forken PJ, Weinstock RS. Personal and relationship challenges of adults with type 1 diabetes: a qualitative focus group study. Diabetes Care 2013;36:2483–2488

66. Fisher L, Polonsky WH, Hessler DM, et al. Understanding the sources of diabetes distress in adults with type 1 diabetes. J Diabetes Complications 2015;29:572–577

67. Hilliard ME, Yi-Frazier JP, Hessler D, Butler AM, Anderson BJ, Jaser S. Stress and A1c among people with diabetes across the lifespan. Curr Diab Rep 2016;16:67

68. Lloyd CE, Dyer PH, Lancashire RJ, Harris T, Daniels JE, Barnett AH. Association between stress and glycemic control in adults with type 1 (insulin-dependent) diabetes. Diabetes Care 1999;22:1278–1283

The Evolution of Hemoglobin A$_{1c}$ Targets for Youth With Type 1 Diabetes: Rationale and Supporting Evidence

Maria J. Redondo,[1] Ingrid Libman,[2] David M. Maahs,[3,4,5] Sarah K. Lyons,[1] Mindy Saraco,[6] Jane Reusch,[7] Henry Rodriguez,[8] and Linda A. DiMeglio[9]

Diabetes Care 2021;44:301–312 | https://doi.org/10.2337/dc20-1978

The American Diabetes Association 2020 *Standards of Medical Care in Diabetes* (Standards of Care) recommends a hemoglobin A$_{1c}$ (A1C) of <7% (53 mmol/mol) for many children with type 1 diabetes (T1D), with an emphasis on target personalization. A higher A1C target of <7.5% may be more suitable for youth who cannot articulate symptoms of hypoglycemia or have hypoglycemia unawareness and for those who do not have access to analog insulins or advanced diabetes technologies or who cannot monitor blood glucose regularly. Even less stringent A1C targets (e.g., <8%) may be warranted for children with a history of severe hypoglycemia, severe morbidities, or short life expectancy. During the "honeymoon" period and in situations where lower mean glycemia is achievable without excessive hypoglycemia or reduced quality of life, an A1C <6.5% may be safe and effective. Here, we provide a historical perspective of A1C targets in pediatrics and highlight evidence demonstrating detrimental effects of hyperglycemia in children and adolescents, including increased likelihood of brain structure and neurocognitive abnormalities, microvascular and macrovascular complications, long-term effects, and increased mortality. We also review data supporting a decrease over time in overall severe hypoglycemia risk for youth with T1D, partly associated with the use of newer insulins and devices, and weakened association between lower A1C and severe hypoglycemia risk. We present common barriers to achieving glycemic targets in pediatric diabetes and discuss some strategies to address them. We aim to raise awareness within the community on Standards of Care updates that impact this crucial goal in pediatric diabetes management.

Twenty-seven years ago, the Diabetes Control and Complications Trial (DCCT) first demonstrated in a randomized clinical trial that intensive insulin treatment aiming to lower glucose levels closer to the normal range, beyond that necessary to control symptoms of hyperglycemia, reduced the risk of microvascular (1) and long-term (2) diabetes complications. Increased severe hypoglycemia risk was an adverse effect of intensive therapy. In addition, there was fear that intensive treatment could increase the risk of macrovascular complications due to hyperinsulinemia, and significant real-world impediments to feasibility of and accessibility to the diabetes care required to achieve the study results were noted in the initial report almost three decades ago (3).

Since its 1993 landmark publication, the DCCT and many other studies have progressively provided overwhelming evidence that near-normal glucose control diminishes the risks of retinopathy, nephropathy, neuropathy, and macrovascular complications (4). The development of insulin analogs, more sophisticated insulin delivery systems (e.g., insulin pumps), continuous glucose monitoring (CGM), and,

[1]Texas Children's Hospital, Baylor College of Medicine, Houston, TX
[2]Division of Pediatric Endocrinology, Diabetes and Metabolism, UPMC Children's Hospital of Pittsburgh, Pittsburgh, PA
[3]Division of Pediatric Endocrinology and Diabetes, Stanford University, Stanford, CA
[4]Stanford Diabetes Research Center, Stanford University, Stanford, CA
[5]Health Research and Policy (Epidemiology), Stanford University, Stanford, CA
[6]American Diabetes Association, Arlington, VA
[7]University of Colorado and Rocky Mountain Regional VA Medical Center, Aurora, CO
[8]USF Diabetes and Endocrinology Section, University of South Florida, Tampa, FL
[9]Division of Pediatric Endocrinology and Diabetology and Wells Center for Pediatric Research, Indiana University School of Medicine, Indianapolis, IN

Corresponding author: Maria J. Redondo, redondo@bcm.edu

Received 7 August 2020 and accepted 8 November 2020

This article contains supplementary material online at https://doi.org/10.2337/figshare.13235495.

more recently, integrated systems (e.g., sensor-augmented insulin pumps, predictive low-glucose suspend systems, and closed-loop control systems) greatly enhanced the feasibility of maintaining glucose levels within a prespecified target range. These advances have also contributed to lessening hypoglycemia risk and have diminished the relationship of significant or severe hypoglycemia with lower glycemic targets in people with T1D. Consideration of emerging evidence relevant to pediatrics has prompted the American Diabetes Association (ADA) to revise its hemoglobin A_{1c} (A1C) targets in pediatric T1D several times through the years.

The ADA's Professional Practice Committee updates the *Standards of Medical Care in Diabetes* (Standards of Care) (5) annually "to ensure that clinicians, health plans, and policy makers can continue to rely on it as the most authoritative source for current guidelines for diabetes care" (6). With the 2020 Standards of Care (5), the ADA issued a new recommendation for children with T1D: "A1C goals must be individualized and reassessed over time. An A1C of <7% (53 mmol/mol) is appropriate for many children" (recommendation 13.21, evidence grade B) (7). The previous version, published in January 2019, had recommended a goal of 7.5% for most children (8).

In this Perspective, we review the history of pediatric A1C targets and the evidence supporting the 2020 revision. Barriers to achieving pediatric A1C targets are discussed, as are proposed strategies to address them. With this article, we aim to raise awareness within the diabetes community of the updated 2020 A1C recommendations to the Standards of Care.

HISTORICAL PERSPECTIVE OF A1C GOALS IN PEDIATRIC T1D

The 2003 Standards of Care established that, while the general A1C goal for individuals with diabetes was <7%, a "less stringent treatment goal may be appropriate for . . . very young children." In 2005, the ADA issued a statement with age-specific A1C goals for pediatric T1D. A range of 7.5% to 8.5% was recommended for children <6 years of age, <8% for children 6–12 years old (≤8 stated in the narrative), and <7.5% for adolescents 13–19 years old. The 2011 Standards of Care introduced the concept that lower A1C targets for children with T1D were

reasonable if achievable without significant hypoglycemia (see Table 1 for goals). In 2015, the Standards of Care recommended a goal of <7.5% across all pediatric age-groups, <7% if achievable without excessive hypoglycemia, with premeal and bedtime/overnight plasma blood glucose ranges also recommended. The 2020 Standards of Care recommends an A1C goal of <7% for many children with T1D (recommendation 13.21, evidence grade B). A higher target of <7.5% may be more appropriate for youth who cannot articulate symptoms of hypoglycemia or have hypoglycemia unawareness, as well as those who do not have access to analog insulins, cannot monitor their blood glucose regularly, or do not have access to advanced diabetes technologies, including insulin pumps and CGM (recommendation 13.22, evidence grade B). Individuals who have nonglycemic factors that increase A1C, such as higher erythrocyte life span, or are high glycators (i.e., those who, for the same level of glucose, have consistently higher A1C) may also need a higher target such as <7.5% (recommendation 13.22, evidence grade B). Similar to that for adults with diabetes, a target of <8% is recommended for youth with a history of severe hypoglycemia, severe morbidities, or short life expectancy (recommendation 13.23, evidence grade B). A lower A1C target, such as <6.5%, may be appropriate during the partial remission period (or "honeymoon") or in persons with longer-standing T1D if achievable without excessive hypoglycemia, poor quality of life, or undue burden of care (recommendation 13.24, evidence grade B).

The 2020 revision aligns the A1C goals in pediatric T1D and type 2 diabetes (T2D). Table 1 illustrates a summary of the history of ADA's guidelines for A1C targets in youth with T1D or T2D since 2000. Supplementary Table 1 provides significant narrative information on goals and additional details such as specific changes from year to year, whether guidance was labeled as a recommendation, and level of evidence as graded by the ADA.

The emphasis on glycemic target individualization has been a constant through the years in the ADA clinical guidelines. Age-specific goals were recommended between 2005 and 2015. The 2020 Standards of Care recommends considering a less stringent A1C goal if, based on the individual's circumstances, the risks (such as increased risk of hypoglycemia, increased burden of care,

or decreased feasibility) exceed potential benefits or when A1C is not a reliable indicator of mean glucose concentrations (recommendation 13.22, evidence grade B, and recommendation 13.23, evidence grade B). On the other hand, in selected children, a lower target (e.g., <6.5%) is reasonable (recommendation 13.24, evidence grade B).

Besides A1C goals, the premeal/bedtime/overnight glucose targets have also been adjusted empirically through the years to reflect A1C goal changes. Yet specific evidence on ways to achieve A1C goals is currently sparse, reflecting a need for more data.

EVIDENCE SUGGESTING DETRIMENTAL EFFECTS OF HYPERGLYCEMIA IN CHILDREN AND ADOLESCENTS

Structural and Neurocognitive Effects on the Central Nervous System

The negative effects of hypoglycemia on the brain have long been established, with those of chronic hyperglycemia appreciated more recently. Reported relationships between dysglycemia-associated neurocognitive and brain structure changes have varied by study design and differing clinical populations. Barnea-Goraly et al. (9) studied 127 children aged 4 to <10 years with T1D and 67 age-matched control subjects and found abnormalities in axial diffusivity (a measure that reflects fiber coherence), reduced radial diffusivity (a measure of fiber integrity and myelination), and fractional anisotropy (reflecting the degree of diffusion anisotropy, which is determined by fiber diameter and density, myelination, extracellular diffusion, interaxonal spacing, and fiber tract coherence). These changes correlated with earlier onset of diabetes, longer diabetes duration, and higher A1C. A Diabetes Research in Children Network (DirecNet) longitudinal study (10) in 142 children with T1D and 65 age-matched control subjects (4–10 years of age at study entry) observed slower hippocampal growth in the span of 18 months associated with higher A1C and greater glycemic variability, as assessed by CGM. A separate analysis from this DirecNet study pediatric population (11) incorporated high-resolution structural MRI combined with neurocognitive testing, finding that both hyperglycemia and glucose variability (but not hypoglycemia), were associated with slower growth in specific

Table 1—History of ADA guidance for A1C targets for youth with diabetes since 2000. Years when glycemic target changed are illustrated. Specific changes from the previous goal are indicated in boldface type. A more detailed version of this table is provided as Supplementary Table 1.

Date and publication	Type 1 diabetes	Type 2 diabetes
2000: Type 2 Diabetes in Children and Adolescents (Consensus Statement)(70)		**All children: <7%**
2003: Standards of Medical Care for Patients With Diabetes Mellitus (71)	**Very young children: less stringent treatment goals than the <7% recommended for other individuals**	
2005: Care of Children and Adolescents With Type 1 Diabetes: A Statement of the American Diabetes Association (72)	**Children <6 years: between 7.5% and 8.5%** **Children 6–12 years: <8% (≤8 in the narrative)** **Adolescents (13–19 years): <7.5%**	

2005: Standards of Medical Care in Diabetes (73)	**Plasma blood glucose and A1C goals:**
	Toddlers and preschoolers (<6 years)
	    Before meals: 100–180 mg/dL
	    Bedtime/overnight: 110–200 mg/dL
	    A1C: ≤8.5 (but ≥7.5%)
	School age (6–12 years)
	    Before meals: 90–180 mg/dL
	    Bedtime/overnight: 100–180 mg/dL
	    A1C: <8%
	Adolescents and young adults (13–19 years)
	    Before meals: 90–130 mg/dL
	    Bedtime/overnight: 90–150 mg/dL
	    A1C: <7.5% (a lower goal [<7%] is reasonable if it can be achieved without excessive hypoglycemia)	

2006: Standards of Medical Care in Diabetes (74)	Plasma blood glucose and A1C goals:
	Toddlers and preschoolers (0–6 years)
	    Before meals: 100–180 mg/dL
	    Bedtime/overnight: 110–200 mg/dL
	    A1C: **<8.5% (but >7.5%)**
	School age (6–12 years)
	    Before meals: 90–180 mg/dL
	    Bedtime/overnight: 100–180 mg/dL
	    A1C: <8%
	Adolescents & young adults (13–19 years)
	    Before meals: 90–130 mg/dL
	    Bedtime/overnight: 90–150 mg/dL
	    A1C: <8% (a lower goal [<7.0%] is reasonable if it can be achieved without excessive hypoglycemia)	

2007: Standards of Medical Care in Diabetes (75)	Plasma blood glucose and A1C goals:
	Toddlers and preschoolers (0–6 years)
	    Before meals: 100–180 mg/dL
	    Bedtime/overnight: 110–200 mg/dL
	    A1C: <8.5% (but >7.5%)
	School age (6–12 years)
	    Before meals: 90–180 mg/dL
	    Bedtime/overnight: 100–180 mg/dL
	    A1C: <8%
	Adolescents & young adults (13–19 years)
	    Before meals: 90–130 mg/dL
	    Bedtime/overnight: 90–150 mg/dL
	    A1C: **<7.5%** (a lower goal [<7.0%] is reasonable if it can be achieved without excessive hypoglycemia)	

Continued on p. 304

Table 1—Continued

Date and publication	Type 1 diabetes	Type 2 diabetes

2011: Standards of Medical Care in Diabetes (76)	Plasma blood glucose and A1C goals:
	 Toddlers and preschoolers (0–6 years)
	   Before meals: 100–180 mg/dL
	   Bedtime/overnight: 110–200 mg/dL
	   A1C: <8.5% **(a lower goal [<8.0%] is reasonable if it can be achieved without excessive hypoglycemia)**
	 School age (6–12 years)
	   Before meals: 90–180 mg/dL
	   Bedtime/overnight: 100–180 mg/dL
	   A1C: <8% **(a lower goal [<7.5%] is reasonable if it can be achieved without excessive hypoglycemia)**
	 Adolescents and young adults (13–19 years)
	   Before meals: 90–130 mg/dL
	   Bedtime/overnight: 90–150 mg/dL
	   A1C: <7.5% (a lower goal [<7.0%] is reasonable if it can be achieved without excessive hypoglycemia)	

2015: Standards of Medical Care in Diabetes (77)	**An A1C goal of <7.5% is recommended across all pediatric age-groups.** Plasma blood glucose and A1C goals **across all pediatric** age-groups: **Before meals: 90–130 mg/dL (5.0–7.2 mmol/L** **Bedtime/overnight: 90–150 mg/dL (5.0–8.3 mmol/L)** **A1C: <7.5% (a lower goal [<7.0%] is reasonable if it can be achieved without excessive hypoglycemia)**	
2016: Standards of Medical Care in Diabetes (78)	An A1C goal of <7.5% (58 mmol/mol) is recommended across all pediatric age-groups. **Blood** glucose across all pediatric age-groups: Before meals: 90–130 mg/dL (5.0–7.2 mmol/L) Bedtime/overnight: 90–150 mg/dL (5.0–8.3 mmol/L) A1C: <7.5% (58 mmol/mol) (a lower goal [<7.0%] is reasonable if it can be achieved without excessive hypoglycemia)	
2018: Evaluation and Management of Youth-Onset Type 2 Diabetes: A Position Statement by the American Diabetes Association (79)		<7% (most youth). **More stringent A1C goals (such as <6.5%) may be appropriate for selected individual patients if they can be achieved without significant hypoglycemia or other adverse effects of treatment. Appropriate patients might include those with short duration of diabetes and lesser degrees of β-cell dysfunction and patients treated with lifestyle or metformin only who achieve significant weight improvement. E**
2019: Standards of Medical Care in Diabetes (8)		Incorporated the recommendations in the 2018 Position Statement

Continued on p. 305

Table 1—Continued

Date and publication	Type 1 diabetes	Type 2 diabetes
2020: Standards of Medical Care in Diabetes (7)	**Recommendation 13.21: A1C goals must be individualized and reassessed over time. An A1C of <7% (53 mmol/mol) is appropriate for many children. B** **Recommendation 13.22: Less stringent A1C goals (such as <7.5% [58 mmol/mol]) may be appropriate for patients who cannot articulate symptoms of hypoglycemia; have hypoglycemia unawareness; lack access to analog insulins, advanced insulin delivery technology, and/or continuous glucose monitors; cannot check blood glucose regularly; or have nonglycemic factors that increase A1C (e.g., high glycators). B** **Recommendation 13.23: Even less stringent A1C goals (such as <8% [64 mmol/mol]) may be appropriate for patients with a history of severe hypoglycemia, limited life expectancy, or extensive comorbid conditions. B** **Recommendation 13.24: Providers may reasonably suggest more stringent A1C goals (such as <6.5% [48 mmol/mol]) for selected individual patients if they can be achieved without significant hypoglycemia, negative impacts on well-being, or undue burden of care, or in those who have nonglycemic factors that decrease A1C (e.g., lower erythrocyte life span). Lower targets may also be appropriate during the honeymoon phase. B**	<7% (53 mmol/mol) (most youth); <6.5% (48 mmol/mol) (selected youth as specified in 2019 Standards of Care). **Less stringent A1C goals (such as 7.5% [58 mmol/mol]) may be appropriate if there is increased risk of hypoglycemia.**

regions of gray (left precuneus, right temporal, frontal, and parietal lobes and right medial-frontal cortex) and white (splenium of the corpus callosum, bilateral superior-parietal lobe, bilateral anterior forceps, and inferior-frontal fasciculus) matter areas over the 18 months of the study. However, no differences in cognitive and executive function scores between groups were observed. Perantie et al. (12) analyzed a cohort of 108 children 7–17 years old with T1D and 51 healthy sibling control subjects; hyperglycemia was associated with smaller gray matter volume in the right cuneus and precuneus, smaller white matter volume in a right posterior parietal region, and larger gray matter volume in a right prefrontal region, while a history of severe hypoglycemia was associated with smaller gray matter volume in the left superior temporal region. A further study (13) in a subset of the DirecNet cohort of children aged 3 to <10 years with T1D ($n = 22$) and age- and sex-matched healthy control subjects ($n = 14$) demonstrated that

higher time-weighted A1C values were significantly correlated with lower overall intellectual functioning measured by the full-scale intelligence quotient and, within the diabetes group, there was a significant, positive correlation between time-weighted A1C and radial diffusivity. In a recent study, children with T1D performed worse on visuospatial working memory tasks and showed greater increase in activation with higher working memory load (i.e., compensatory modulation of activation) as measured by functional MRI (14).

A meta-analysis on executive function in T1D, including 17 studies and 1,619 pooled participants, determined that inhibition, working memory, set shifting, and overall executive function were lower in adolescents and young adults with T1D than in control subjects (15). A systematic review of 500 youth concluded that repeated episodes of acute hyperglycemia, e.g., diabetic ketoacidosis (DKA), is detrimental to the brain in children and adolescents (16).

Overall, evidence indicates that both hyperglycemia (chronic and acute) and hypoglycemia are associated with structural brain changes, brain function adaptation, and neurocognitive dysfunction in children. More studies are needed on the underlying pathophysiology that can be leveraged for preventive and treatment purposes as well as on optimal glycemic range/glucose variability targets for brain development and growth.

Microvascular and Macrovascular Complications

The DCCT demonstrated that intensive diabetes treatment diminished the risk and rate of development of diabetic complications in individuals with T1D aged 13 to 39 years (1,2). In a subanalysis of the adolescents between the ages of 13 and 17 years at DCCT study entry ($n = 125$), who were followed for a mean of 7.4 years (range 4–9 years), those in the intensive treatment group attained a mean A1C of 8.06% (SE 0.13) and had significantly lower risk of microalbuminuria as well as retinopathy appearance or progression compared with participants in the conventional treatment group with a mean A1C of 9.76% (SE 0.12). These results were consistent with the risk reduction observed in adults.

In a longitudinal Australian cohort of adolescents with T1D, a mean decrease in A1C from 9.1% to 8.5% was associated with lower rate of retinopathy (17). The Vascular Diabetic Complications in Southeast Sweden (VISS) study observed 451 individuals diagnosed with T1D before age 35 years and found that no one with long-term weighted mean A1C <7.6% (60 mmol/mol) developed proliferative retinopathy or persistent macroalbuminuria, compared with 51% of individuals with long-term weighted mean A1C >9.5% (60 mmol/mol) (18). A population-based Swedish National Diabetes Registry cohort study of 10,398 children and adults with T1D between 1998 and 2017 observed that, while A1C under 6.5% increased the risk of hypoglycemia, the risk of any retinopathy and nephropathy progressively increased with A1C above 6.5% (19) (Fig. 1).

Data from the Pittsburgh Epidemiology of Diabetes Complications (EDC) study, including 658 subjects with childhood-onset (<17 years old) T1D diagnosed between 1950 and 1980, evaluated at baseline between 1986 and 1988 and then followed biennially, showed that A1C was an independent risk factor for fatal coronary artery disease (20). Moreover, the longitudinal A1C trajectory was associated with 25-year cardiovascular disease incidence in this cohort; associations were similar across the specific manifestations of cardiovascular disease (21).

Long-term Effects on the Risk of Complications ("Metabolic Memory")

The Epidemiology of Diabetes Interventions and Complications (EDIC) study was launched to follow adult and pediatric participants after conclusion of the DCCT and evaluate the long-term effects of the DCCT interventions. Over 90% of DCCT participants participated in the EDIC study. After 30 years of diabetes, the cumulative incidences of proliferative retinopathy, nephropathy, and cardiovascular disease were much lower (21%, 9%, and 9%) in the DCCT intensive therapy group compared with 50%, 25%, and 14% in the DCCT in the conventional

group (22) despite similar A1C after the DCCT concluded. An analysis restricted to pediatric participants ($n = 175$) observed that, although the mean A1C trajectories of the intensive and conventional groups converged, the risk of retinopathy progression decreased by 74–78% over the next 4 years in the intensive treatment group compared with the conventional group (23). Longitudinal observation of this cohort of adolescents aged 13–18 years at randomization demonstrated that, although none developed diabetic retinopathy requiring treatment while <18 years of age, there were three cases of proliferative diabetic retinopathy in participants <21 years of age, all females in the conventional therapy arm (24). More long-term DCCT/EDIC outcome studies are needed, especially for the pediatric cohort.

Early good glycemic control may also beget long-term improved control. Glucose control tracking has been demonstrated in a longitudinal study (25) of 1,146 children and adolescents in Austria and Germany where prepubertal A1C predicted metabolic control in young adulthood after adjustment for confounders. Similarly, the Swedish pediatric diabetes quality registry and the Swedish National Diabetes Register analyzed data from 1,543 youth and found that higher A1C close to diagnosis was associated with higher A1C in adult life as well as risk of microalbuminuria and retinopathy (26). Although more research is needed in this area, it is clear that achieving the best glucose control possible as early as feasible after diagnosis is an important pediatric goal.

Mortality

Mortality is increased for persons diagnosed with T1D during childhood and is associated with glycemic control. The Swedish National Diabetes Register studied 27,195 individuals with T1D registered between 1998 and 2012 and 135,178 matched general population control subjects. This study found the highest excess risks compared with the control subjects of both all-cause mortality and cardiovascular disease in individuals who were diagnosed with T1D at <10 years of age, adjusting for diabetes duration, with risk over fourfold for all-cause mortality, over sevenfold for cardiovascular mortality, and over elevenfold for cardiovascular disease. In comparison, the corresponding hazard ratios in individuals diagnosed

with T1D between 26 and 30 years of age were 2.83, 3.64, and 3.85 (27). Therefore, earlier age at T1D diagnosis is associated with higher risk of mortality and cardiovascular disease, suggesting the importance of early risk factor control. These findings are in direct contradiction to the historical wisdom that the clock determining risk of complications does not start until puberty. An analysis of 12,652 individuals in the Swedish pediatric diabetes quality registry from 2006 to 2014 showed that higher mortality in young people (<30 years of age) was associated with higher A1C during childhood (28).

EVIDENCE OF DECREASE IN HYPOGLYCEMIA RISK—AN EVOLUTION SINCE DCCT

Historically, the increased risk of hypoglycemia associated with lower A1C led to establishing guidelines with higher glycemic targets for youth. At the individual level, fear of hypoglycemia leads persons with T1D, caregivers of children with T1D, and diabetes care providers to adopt strategies to maintain hyperglycemia to mitigate this risk (29). While increased risk of hypoglycemia was a major adverse effect in the intensive treatment group in the DCCT study, this study started recruitment in 1983 and concluded follow-up of participants in 1993. The incidence of hypoglycemia has been declining over the almost three decades since then.

The Danish Adult Diabetes Database (DADD) documented an annual decrease of 8.4% in the incidence rate of severe hypoglycemia (30). An analysis of temporal trends in children diagnosed with T1D <15 years of age from 1995 to 2016 from the longitudinal, prospective, population-based German/Austrian Diabetes Patient History Documentation (Diabetes Patienten Verlaufsdokumenation, DPV) ($N = 59,883$) and Western Australian Children's Diabetes Database (WACDD) ($N = 2,595$) diabetes registries demonstrated concurrent improvements in A1C and decreasing severe hypoglycemia rates (31) between 1995 and 2016. The relationship of A1C and severe hypoglycemia has also changed in the 27 years that have elapsed since the DCCT report. In children and adolescent participants in the U.S. T1D Exchange ($N = 7,102$), German/Austrian DPV ($N = 18,887$), or WACDD ($N = 865$) diabetes registries between 2011 and 2012, rates

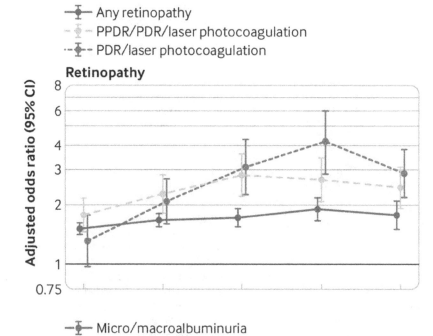

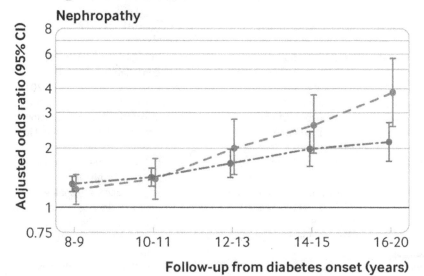

Figure 1—Adjusted odds ratios (95% CI) for retinopathy and nephropathy for 10 mmol/mol increase in A1C area under the curve in the Swedish National Diabetes Registry (19), which collected data between 1 January 1998 and 31 December 2017. Whiskers represent 95% CI. PDR, proliferative diabetic retinopathy; PPDR, preproliferative diabetic retinopathy.

the risk of severe hypoglycemia was not different between the children with A1C ≤6.7% and those with higher A1C after adjusting for confounders (35). In the DADD cohort, the risk of severe hypoglycemia associated with a lower A1C decreased between the time periods of 1995–2003 and 2004–2012 (36). A further analysis of data from 17,230 older teenagers (>16 years old) and adults with T1D in the DADD between 2006 and 2012 found that the association between hypoglycemia and A1C was nonlinear, with a much more marked *increase* for hypoglycemia risk with A1C above 7.6% (60 mmol/mol) than below that level (30).

Newer Treatment Modalities and Hypoglycemic Risk

A plausible explanation for the observed decline in hypoglycemia rates is the increased use of insulin analogs and diabetes technology. The rapid succession of newer and better insulins that started with the approval of the first rapid-acting insulin analog, lispro, in 1996 has been followed by dramatic falls in the rates of hypoglycemia at night and after meals (37).

Advances in technology to administer insulin and monitor glucose have been shown to improve glucose control in T1D. In the study by Cooper et al. (34) with 1,770 children (<16 years of age) followed between 2000 and 2011, children utilizing insulin pumps had lower risk of severe hypoglycemia than children using insulin injections. The study of 8,806 children <15 years of age in the four Nordic countries between 2008 and 2012 showed that pump use was associated with lower risk of severe hypoglycemia (35). In a case-controlled, nonrandomized study, Johnson et al. (38) observed that use of insulin pumps reduced A1C by 0.6% and lowered the risk of severe hypoglycemia by 50%. In the DPV population-based cohort study with over 30,000 pediatric participants with T1D between 2011 and 2015 in Germany, Austria, and Luxembourg, pump therapy was associated with lower A1C and lower rates of severe hypoglycemia and DKA (39).

The recent CGM Intervention in Teens and Young Adults with T1D (CITY) study randomized 153 adolescents and young adults (ages 14–24 years old) with T1D to CGM or blood glucose monitoring (usual care) and demonstrated a significant

of severe hypoglycemia per 100 patient-years were not associated with lower A1C overall or with source registry, treatment regimen, or age-group (32). These results are consistent with a previous analysis of 37,539 participants aged 1 to 20 years old with T1D in the DPV study in Germany and Austria that observed a weakening of the association between lower A1C and severe hypoglycemia (33). A more recently analysis of the DPV and WACDD cohorts confirmed the decreases in A1C

and severe hypoglycemia rate and found similarly low severe hypoglycemia rates in all A1C categories (Fig. 2) (31). Similarly, in a study (34) of 1,770 children (<16 years of age) followed between 2000 and 2011, those with A1C <7% did not have higher rates of hypoglycemia compared with children with A1C 8–9%. A study of 8,806 children <15 years of age (n = 8,806) in Nordic countries Denmark, Iceland, Norway, and Sweden between 2008 and 2012 showed that

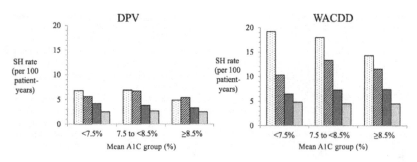

Figure 2—A1C and rates of severe hypoglycemia, adjusted for sex, age at diagnosis, and diabetes duration, observed in the longitudinal, prospective DPV (German-Austrian) and WACDD (Austrialian) cohorts since 1991 (31). The rates of severe hypoglycemia (SH) decreased since 1991 and were similar across A1C groups (i.e., <7.5%, 7.5 to <8.5%, and ≥8.5%), particularly in the last time period (2012–2016). Severe hypoglycemia was defined as a hypoglycemic episode resulting in loss of consciousness and/or seizure. White bar with dots represent 1991–2001; striped bar, 2002–2006; dark gray bar, 2007–2011; and light gray bar, 2012–2016.

improvement in glucose control (A1C, time in range) and mean time in hypoglycemia and higher glucose monitoring satisfaction over the 26 weeks of the study (40). This is in contrast with a 2008 study where an early-generation CGM system improved A1C in adult patients (>25 years of age) but not in younger participants, who also had lower device wear times (41). This difference reflects that later-generation devices are better tolerated and have improved in ease of placement and accuracy, leading to greater wear time.

Sensor-augmented insulin pump therapy with the threshold-suspend feature (i.e., predictive low-glucose suspend system) reduced nocturnal hypoglycemia in a randomized trial with 247 participants (42). In a pediatric randomized clinical trial, Ly et al. (43) demonstrated that the predictive low-glucose suspend system significantly reduced time in hypoglycemia although, as expected since the system does not address hyperglycemia, A1C did not decrease.

Closed-loop control systems have been developed to address both hypo- and hyperglycemia. A randomized clinical trial with a total of 168 participants between 14 and 71 years old found 11% significantly higher mean adjusted time in range in participants on the closed-loop system than in those on sensor-augmented pump therapy (control group) (44). A recent study demonstrated that switching to a predictive low-glucose suspend system reduced time in range and increased A1C compared with participants who stayed on a closed-loop system, while time in hypoglycemia did not change (45).

A systematic review and meta-analysis conducted with data up to January 2017

that included 27 comparisons from 24 studies and a total of 585 participants (219 in adult studies, 265 in pediatric studies, and 101 in combined studies) concluded that time in target was 12.59% higher with artificial pancreas systems (95% CI 9.02–16.16; $P < 0.0001$) (46). Similar conclusions were reached by others (47).

Overall, these results support the concept that in the future hypoglycemia rates will continue to decline and time in range will continue to increase. Diabetes technology has consistently demonstrated that it has the potential to improve glucose control in pediatric and adult individuals with T1D. This evidence supports the ADA Standards of Care statement that CGM should be considered for all children and adolescents with T1D (recommendation 7.12, evidence grade B) (5). Studies are needed to translate the interventions proven efficacious in research trials into real-world settings.

A1C and Continuous Glucose Monitoring as Measures of Glycemic Control

Utilization of A1C as an indicator of glycemic control must acknowledge potential nonglycemic confounders. These include factors that lower the measured A1C, e.g., lower erythrocyte life span, and those that increase it, e.g., untreated iron deficiency anemia (48). High or low "glycator" individuals will have, respectively, higher or lower A1C levels than expected based on their glucose levels. In addition, there are significant racial differences in the relationship between glucose levels and A1C, with Black individuals having A1C that is on average 0.4

percentage points (95% CI 0.2–0.6) higher than that in White individuals for a given mean glucose concentration. Of note, this phenomenon was not observed with glycated albumin or fructosamine (49). To overcome the potential risk of error when estimating average glucose from measured A1C, when feasible clinicians can use recent CGM data to document time above and below target range prior to lowering an individual's A1C target. In addition, CGM allows estimation of time in range and, in particular within close-loop systems, minimization of hypoglycemia and hyperglycemic excursions (50). A1C and CGM-derived measures provide complementary assessments of glucose control. Besides widespread accessibility and acceptability of CGM across all population subsets, studies are needed comparing the ability of A1C and CGM-derived measures of glucose control to predict long-term outcomes in individuals with diabetes.

INTERNATIONAL A1C TARGET RECOMMENDATIONS

The International Society for Pediatric and Adolescent Diabetes (ISPAD) Clinical Practice Consensus Guidelines in 2018 (51) recommended a target of <7% for children and youth >5 years old. However, aiming for <7.5% was endorsed for those who cannot articulate symptoms of hypoglycemia or have hypoglycemia unawareness, have a history of severe hypoglycemia, lack access to analogs, are unable to monitor blood glucose regularly, or lack access to advanced insulin delivery technology or CGMs and in high glycators. A target of <6.5% was deemed optimal in situations where this target is attainable without excessive hypoglycemia, poor quality of life, or undue burden of care, and lower targets may be appropriate during the honeymoon period.

The National Institute for Health Care and Excellence (NICE) in the U.K. recommended in 2015 that providers explain to children and young people with T1D and their family members or caregivers (as appropriate) that an A1C target level of 48 mmol/mol (6.5%) or lower is ideal to minimize the risk of long-term complications (52).

The Swedish National Diabetes Register 2018 report revised A1C targets from <57 mmol/mol (<7.4%) to <48 mmol/mol (<6.5%) in May 2017, based on the results from the population-based cohort

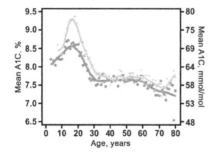

Figure 3—Higher A1C in the 2016–2018 period compared with 2010–2012 across all ages, with particular elevation in adolescents and young adults (56) in the T1D Exchange Clinical Registry, which collected data from multiple clinical centers across the U.S.

analysis between 1998 and 2017 (19). Of note, this decrease in A1C target was followed by a sharp decline in average A1C in children to 54.7 mmol/mol (7.2%).

COMMON BARRIERS TO ACHIEVING A1C TARGETS IN T1D IN YOUTH AND STRATEGIES TO ADDRESS THEM

Although near-normalization of A1C in children is associated with better diabetes outcomes during childhood and beyond, there are numerous barriers to achieving this goal. A major one is the fear of hypoglycemia on the part of persons with diabetes, their caregivers, and their clinical care providers (53). However, as detailed in the previous sections, the previously reported correlation between hypoglycemia and A1C is not observed with contemporary therapies and technology. The use of insulin analogs and diabetes technologies has increased the feasibility of achieving near-normal glycemia and demonstrably lowered the risk of severe hypoglycemia for children with T1D. It is expected that ongoing studies on the impact of the newest devices and systems on hypoglycemia and other diabetes-relevant outcomes including or focusing on pediatric participants (e.g., NCT04084171 in preschoolers, NCT02129868 in children and adolescents, NCT02302963, NCT02844517, and others; ClinicalTrials.gov) will demonstrate further risk reductions. Weight gain is another potential concern with intensive control, as the DCCT reports showed greater weight gain in persons in the intensive group (54). However, a subsequent pediatric study of children in four cohorts (1999, 2002, 2006, and 2009) found that, although use of intensive therapy increased, prevalence of overweight or obesity remained stable

over time (55). In addition, in this study there was no relationship between A1C and BMI z-score after adjusting for potential confounders. Working with children and their parents to prevent weight gain is crucial in this population.

There are multiple levels where barriers to optimal glucose control may exist: biological (e.g., lack of residual β-cell function), behavioral (e.g., burnout), familial (e.g., burden of care), societal (e.g., lack of health insurance), as well as at the health care provider level (e.g., therapeutic inertia). An interplay of influences may result in marked worsening in glucose control, such as during adolescence, when puberty and growth hormones that promote gluconeogenesis and insulin resistance compound with the normal psychological process of striving for independence. Therefore, overcoming hurdles to optimal glucose control will require combinations of strategies. While diabetes technology has been demonstrated to lower A1C, the recent rise in A1C in the pediatric cohort of the T1D Exchange (56) (Fig. 3), despite increased technology adoption, emphasizes the need for multilayer approaches, including strategies that preserve β-cell function after T1D onset (57), improve quality of life, promote adherence to evidence-based recommendations and ongoing treatment plans, provide education to caregivers, advocate for policy changes, and combat therapeutic inertia, among others. The long-term tracking of glucose control from the time of onset (25,26) supports efforts to optimize modifiable factors as close to diagnosis as possible.

Wide disparities exist in A1C and other health outcomes among youth with T1D. Socioeconomically disadvantaged children and those from racial/ethnic minority backgrounds have worse glycemic control, more frequent comorbidities (58–60), more frequent diabetes complications (61), and higher diabetes-associated costs (62). Strategies are needed that address the potentially modifiable factors that underlie disparities at multiple levels, including less access to care and technology, lower health education, and higher frequency of comorbidities (e.g., obesity, hypertension, dyslipidemia) (63). Racial and ethnic disparities in health outcomes are apparent from stage 3 diabetes onset, when African Americans are more likely to present in DKA and less likely to experience a partial remission period, and continue during the first years after diagnosis, with higher A1Cs and

more frequent severe hypoglycemia and cardiovascular risk factors (64). Therefore, intervention approaches that are delivered early in the disease course among socioeconomically disadvantaged youth are needed to promote optimal T1D management and prevent costly complications.

Unfortunately, not every child worldwide has access to modern insulins, diabetes supplies, and even food. Similarly, diabetes technologies are not equally accessible to everyone. Studies demonstrate disparities in their use based on factors related to socioeconomics, health insurance type, age, access to care, race/ethnicity, education, and geography, among others (59). Trials to translate efficacious interventions into real-world settings, cost analyses, and advocacy are needed to help close the gaps in access to diabetes technology.

Mean A1C is higher in the U.S. than in some European countries. A comparison of eight high-income countries for glucose control in youth with T1D, with adjustment for sex, age, diabetes duration, and racial/ethnic minority status, found the lowest A1C in Sweden, where variation within centers was also lowest (65) (Fig. 4). Although all registries in this study reported International Federation of Clinical Chemistry and Laboratory Medicine (IFCC)-aligned values, differences in methodology across the different laboratories could have contributed to the variation observed. However, supporting international differences in A1C, a decline in A1C levels was observed in Sweden after lowering the target, unlike in the U.S., where a 2014 decrease in A1C target did not modify the upward temporal trend of A1C in youth with T1D. Participation in a quality improvement collaborative was a significantly differential factor between centers that experienced a decrease in A1C and others that did not between 2010 and 2014 in Sweden (66). In the U.S., the T1D Exchange Quality Improvement Collaborative (T1DX-QI) was established in 2016, initially with 10 U.S. participating diabetes clinics, and has since expanded with the goal to share data and best practices to improve care delivery in T1D (67).

CONCLUSIONS AND FUTURE DIRECTIONS

The 2020 Standards of Care recommends adopting an A1C goal of <7% (53 mmol/

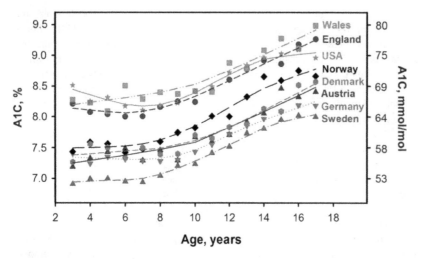

Figure 4—Comparison of mean A1C by age across eight high-income countries (69) in the Pediatric Diabetes Quality Registry, which collected data from Austria, Denmark, England, Germany, Norway, Sweden, the U.S., and Wales between 2013 and 2014.

mol) for many children with T1D, with an emphasis on individualized targets based on the individual risk-benefit ratio (recommendation 13.21, evidence grade B). This recommendation is driven by the overwhelming evidence of the deleterious influences of both chronic and acute hypoglycemia and hyperglycemia (e.g., brain structure changes, neurocognitive defects, long-lasting effects on the risk of microvascular and macrovascular complications), the decrease in overall incidence of severe hypoglycemia, the waning association between lower A1C target and hypoglycemia, and newer insulins and technological advances that have increased the feasibility of minimizing out-of-range glucose levels. The recent adaptation of a lower target for children by the ADA reflects similar guidance from other societies worldwide. Specifically, ISPAD proposed <7% in 2018 (51), NICE in the U.K. <6.5% in 2015 (52), and the Swedish National Diabetes Register 6.5% in 2018 (68).

Current gaps in knowledge include the risk factors for poor diabetes outcomes and hypoglycemia that allow identification of high-risk individuals for targeted interventions. Additionally, it will be important to understand the pathophysiology of the deleterious consequences of hypo- and hyperglycemia (e.g., effects on the brain, relative contribution of the degree and duration of hyperglycemia) that can be leveraged for prevention and treatment. A key gap area is socioeconomic and racial/ethnic disparities in diabetes outcomes and inequality in access to diabetes care and technology; this recognized need is fueling multiple initiatives at the research level, including trials to translate efficacious interventions to real-world settings, advocacy, and public policy. Furthermore, the implementation of strategies proven effective to optimize diabetes outcomes will be facilitated by ongoing behavioral research to address lack of adherence to treatment plans, concerns about quality of life, undue burden of care, and therapeutic inertia. International data indicate that lower A1C can be achieved safely in pediatrics, and there are ongoing efforts to utilize quality improvement methodology to implement proven efficacious strategies to optimize A1C in the U.S.

Funding. D.M.M. was supported by National Institute of Diabetes and Digestive and Kidney Diseases grant P30DK116074.
Duality of Interest. No potential conflicts of interest relevant to this article were reported.
Author Contributions. M.J.R. wrote the first draft of the manuscript. I.L., D.M.M., S.K.L., M.S., J.R., H.R., and L.A.D. contributed to the discussion and manuscript review and edits.

References

1. Reichard P, Nilsson BY, Rosenqvist U. The effect of long-term intensified insulin treatment on the development of microvascular complications of diabetes mellitus. N Engl J Med 1993;329: 304–309
2. Diabetes Control and Complications Trial Research Group; Nathan DM, Genuth S, Lachin J, et al. The effect of intensive treatment of diabetes on the development and progression of long-term complications in insulin-dependent diabetes mellitus. N Engl J Med 1993;329: 977–986
3. Lasker RD. The Diabetes Control and Complications Trial. Implications for policy and practice. N Engl J Med 1993;329:1035–1036
4. Nathan DM, Cleary PA, Backlund J-YC, et al.; Diabetes Control and Complications Trial/Epidemiology of Diabetes Interventions and Complications (DCCT/EDIC) Study Research Group. Intensive diabetes treatment and cardiovascular disease in patients with type 1 diabetes. N Engl J Med 2005; 353:2643–2653
5. American Diabetes Association. *Standards of Medical Care in Diabetes—2020.* Diabetes Care 2020;43(Suppl. 1):S1–S212
6. American Diabetes Association. Introduction: *Standards of Medical Care in Diabetes—2020.* Diabetes Care 2020;43(Suppl. 1):S1–S2
7. American Diabetes Association. 13. Children and adolescents: *Standards of Medical Care in Diabetes—2020.* Diabetes Care 2020;43(Suppl. 1):S163–S182
8. American Diabetes Association. 13. Children and adolescents: *Standards of Medical Care in Diabetes—2019.* Diabetes Care 2019;42(Suppl. 1):S148–S164
9. Barnea-Goraly N, Raman M, Mazaika P, et al.; Diabetes Research in Children Network (DirecNet). Alterations in white matter structure in young children with type 1 diabetes. Diabetes Care 2014;37:332–340
10. Foland-Ross LC, Buckingam B, Mauras N, et al.; Diabetes Research in Children Network (DirecNet). Executive task-based brain function in children with type 1 diabetes: An observational study. PLoS Med 2019;16:e1002979
11. Mauras N, Mazaika P, Buckingham B, et al.; Diabetes Research in Children Network (DirecNet). Longitudinal assessment of neuroanatomical and cognitive differences in young children with type 1 diabetes: association with hyperglycemia. Diabetes 2015;64:1770–1779
12. Perantie DC, Wu J, Koller JM, et al. Regional brain volume differences associated with hyperglycemia and severe hypoglycemia in youth with type 1 diabetes. Diabetes Care 2007;30:2331–2337
13. Aye T, Barnea-Goraly N, Ambler C, et al. White matter structural differences in young children with type 1 diabetes: a diffusion tensor imaging study. Diabetes Care 2012;35:2167–2173
14. Foland-Ross LC, Tong G, Mauras N, et al.; Diabetes Research in Children Network (DirecNet). Brain function differences in children with type 1 diabetes: a functional MRI study of working memory. Diabetes 2020;69:1770–1778
15. Broadley MM, White MJ, Andrew B. A systematic review and meta-analysis of executive function performance in type 1 diabetes mellitus. Psychosom Med 2017;79:684–696
16. Pourabbasi A, Tehrani-Doost M, Qavam SE, Arzaghi SM, Larijani B. Association of diabetes mellitus and structural changes in the central nervous system in children and adolescents: a systematic review. J Diabetes Metab Disord 2017;16:10
17. Downie E, Craig ME, Hing S, Cusumano J, Chan AKF, Donaghue KC. Continued reduction in the prevalence of retinopathy in adolescents with type 1 diabetes: role of insulin therapy and glycemic control. Diabetes Care 2011;34: 2368–2373

18. Nordwall M, Abrahamsson M, Dhir M, Fredrikson M, Ludvigsson J, Arnqvist HJ. Impact of HbA$_{1c}$, followed from onset of type 1 diabetes, on the development of severe retinopathy and nephropathy: the VISS Study (Vascular Diabetic Complications in Southeast Sweden). Diabetes Care 2015;38:308–315

19. Lind M, Pivodic A, Svensson A-M, Ólafsdóttir AF, Wedel H, Ludvigsson J. HbA$_{1c}$ level as a risk factor for retinopathy and nephropathy in children and adults with type 1 diabetes: Swedish population based cohort study. BMJ 2019;366:l4894

20. Conway B, Costacou T, Orchard T. Is glycaemia or insulin dose the stronger risk factor for coronary artery disease in type 1 diabetes? Diab Vasc Dis Res 2009;6:223–230

21. Miller RG, Anderson SJ, Costacou T, Sekikawa A, Orchard TJ. Hemoglobin A$_{1c}$ level and cardiovascular disease incidence in persons with type 1 diabetes: an application of joint modeling of longitudinal and time-to-event data in the Pittsburgh Epidemiology of Diabetes Complications Study. Am J Epidemiol 2018;187:1520–1529

22. Diabetes Control and Complications Trial/Epidemiology of Diabetes Interventions and Complications (DCCT/EDIC) Research Group; Nathan DM, Zinman B, Cleary PA, et al. Modern-day clinical course of type 1 diabetes mellitus after 30 years' duration: the diabetes control and complications trial/epidemiology of diabetes interventions and complications and Pittsburgh epidemiology of diabetes complications experience (1983-2005). Arch Intern Med 2009;169:1307–1316

23. White NH, Cleary PA, Dahms W, Goldstein D, Malone J, Tamborlane WV; Diabetes Control and Complications Trial (DCCT)/Epidemiology of Diabetes Interventions and Complications (EDIC) Research Group. Beneficial effects of intensive therapy of diabetes during adolescence: outcomes after the conclusion of the Diabetes Control and Complications Trial (DCCT). J Pediatr 2001;139:804–812

24. Gubitosi-Klug RA, Bebu I, White NH, et al.; Diabetes Control and Complications Trial (DCCT)/Epidemiology of Diabetes Interventions and Complications (EDIC) Research Group. Screening eye exams in youth with type 1 diabetes under 18 years of age: Once may be enough? Pediatr Diabetes 2019;20:743–749

25. Hofer SE, Raile K, Fröhlich-Reiterer E, et al.; Austrian/German Diabetes Patienten Verlaufsdokumentation DPV Initiative; German Competence Network for Diabetes Mellitus. Tracking of metabolic control from childhood to young adulthood in type 1 diabetes. J Pediatr 2014;165:956–961.e1–2

26. Samuelsson U, Steineck I, Gubbjornsdottir S. A high mean-HbA1c value 3-15 months after diagnosis of type 1 diabetes in childhood is related to metabolic control, macroalbuminuria, and retinopathy in early adulthood—a pilot study using two nation-wide population based quality registries. Pediatr Diabetes 2014;15:229–235

27. Rawshani A, Sattar N, Franzén S,, et al. Excess mortality and cardiovascular disease in young adults with type 1 diabetes in relation to age at onset: a nationwide, register-based cohort study. Lancet 2018;392:477–486

28. Samuelsson J, Samuelsson U, Hanberger L, Bladh M, Åkesson K. Poor metabolic control in childhood strongly correlates to diabetes-related premature death in persons <30 years of age—a population-based cohort study. Pediatr Diabetes 2020;21:479–485

29. Van Name MA, Hilliard ME, Boyle CT, et al. Nighttime is the worst time: parental fear of hypoglycemia in young children with type 1 diabetes. Pediatr Diabetes 2018;19:114–120

30. Ishtiak-Ahmed K, Carstensen B, Pedersen-Bjergaard U, Jørgensen ME. Incidence trends and predictors of hospitalization for hypoglycemia in 17,230 adult patients with type 1 diabetes: a Danish register linkage cohort study. Diabetes Care 2017;40:226–232

31. Haynes A, Hermann JM, Clapin H, et al.; WACDD and DPV registries. Decreasing trends in mean HbA$_{1c}$ are not associated with increasing rates of severe hypoglycemia in children: a longitudinal analysis of two contemporary population-based pediatric type 1 diabetes registries from Australia and Germany/Austria between 1995 and 2016. Diabetes Care 2019;42:1630–1636

32. Haynes A, Hermann JM, Miller KM, et al.; T1D Exchange; WACDD and DPV registries. Severe hypoglycemia rates are not associated with HbA1c: a cross-sectional analysis of 3 contemporary pediatric diabetes registry databases. Pediatr Diabetes 2017;18:643–650

33. Karges B, Rosenbauer J, Kapellen T, et al. Hemoglobin A1c Levels and risk of severe hypoglycemia in children and young adults with type 1 diabetes from Germany and Austria: a trend analysis in a cohort of 37,539 patients between 1995 and 2012. PLoS Med 2014;11:e1001742

34. Cooper MN, O'Connell SM, Davis EA, Jones TW. A population-based study of risk factors for severe hypoglycaemia in a contemporary cohort of childhood-onset type 1 diabetes. Diabetologia 2013;56:2164–2170

35. Birkebaek NH, Drivvoll AK, Aakeson K, et al. Incidence of severe hypoglycemia in children with type 1 diabetes in the Nordic countries in the period 2008-2012: association with hemoglobin A$_{1c}$ and treatment modality. BMJ Open Diabetes Res Care 2017;5:e000377

36. Karges B, Kapellen T, Wagner VM, et al.; DPV Initiative. Glycated hemoglobin A1c as a risk factor for severe hypoglycemia in pediatric type 1 diabetes. Pediatr Diabetes 2017;18:51–58

37. Bulsara MK, Holman CDJ, Davis EA, Jones TW. The impact of a decade of changing treatment on rates of severe hypoglycemia in a population-based cohort of children with type 1 diabetes. Diabetes Care 2004;27:2293–2298

38. Johnson SR, Cooper MN, Jones TW, Davis EA. Long-term outcome of insulin pump therapy in children with type 1 diabetes assessed in a large population-based case-control study. Diabetologia 2013;56:2392–2400

39. Karges B, Schwandt A, Heidtmann B, et al. Association of insulin pump therapy vs insulin injection therapy with severe hypoglycemia, ketoacidosis, and glycemic control among children, adolescents, and young adults with type 1 diabetes. JAMA 2017;318:1358–1366

40. Laffel LM, Kanapka LG, Beck RW, et al.; CGM Intervention in Teens and Young Adults with T1D (CITY) Study Group. Effect of continuous glucose monitoring on glycemic control in adolescents and young adults with type 1 diabetes: a randomized clinical trial. JAMA 2020;323:2388–2396

41. Juvenile Diabetes Research Foundation Continuous Glucose Monitoring Study Group; Tamborlane WV, Beck RW, Bode BW, et al. Continuous glucose monitoring and intensive treatment of type 1 diabetes. N Engl J Med 2008;359:1464–1476

42. Bergenstal RM, Klonoff DC, Garg SK, et al.; ASPIRE In-Home Study Group. Threshold-based insulin-pump interruption for reduction of hypoglycemia. N Engl J Med 2013;369:224–232

43. Ly TT, Nicholas JA, Retterath A, Lim EM, Davis EA, Jones TW. Effect of sensor-augmented insulin pump therapy and automated insulin suspension vs standard insulin pump therapy on hypoglycemia in patients with type 1 diabetes: a randomized clinical trial. JAMA 2013;310:1240–1247

44. Brown SA, Kovatchev BP, Raghinaru D, et al.; iDCL Trial Research Group. Six-month randomized, multicenter trial of closed-loop control in type 1 diabetes. N Engl J Med 2019;381:1707–1717

45. Brown SA, Beck RW, Raghinaru D, et al.; iDCL Trial Research Group. Glycemic outcomes of use of CLC versus PLGS in type 1 diabetes: a randomized controlled trial. Diabetes Care 2020;43:1822–1828

46. Weisman A, Bai J-W, Cardinez M, Kramer CK, Perkins BA. Effect of artificial pancreas systems on glycaemic control in patients with type 1 diabetes: a systematic review and meta-analysis of outpatient randomised controlled trials. Lancet Diabetes Endocrinol 2017;5:501–512

47. Steineck I, Ranjan A, Nørgaard K, Schmidt S. Sensor-augmented insulin pumps and hypoglycemia prevention in type 1 diabetes. J Diabetes Sci Technol 2017;11:50–58

48. Wright LA-C, Hirsch IB. Metrics beyond hemoglobin A1C in diabetes management: time in range, hypoglycemia, and other parameters. Diabetes Technol Ther 2017;19(S2):S16–S26

49. Bergenstal RM, Gal RL, Connor CG, et al.; T1D Exchange Racial Differences Study Group. Racial differences in the relationship of glucose concentrations and hemoglobin A1c levels. Ann Intern Med 2017;167:95–102

50. Pease A, Lo C, Earnest A, Kiriakova V, Liew D, Zoungas S. Time in range for multiple technologies in type 1 diabetes: a systematic review and network meta-analysis. Diabetes Care 2020;43:1967–1975

51. DiMeglio LA, Acerini CL, Codner E, et al. ISPAD Clinical Practice Consensus Guidelines 2018: Glycemic control targets and glucose monitoring for children, adolescents, and young adults with diabetes. Pediatr Diabetes 2018;19(Suppl. 27):105–114

52. National Institute for Health and Care Excellence (NICE). Diabetes (type 1 and type 2) in children and young people: diagnosis and management. NICE guideline [NG18], 2015. Accessed 30 October 2020. Available from https://www.nice.org.uk/guidance/ng18

53. Haugstvedt A, Wentzel-Larsen T, Graue M, Søvik O, Rokne B. Fear of hypoglycaemia in mothers and fathers of children with Type 1 diabetes is associated with poor glycaemic control and parental emotional distress: a population-based study. Diabet Med 2010;27:72–78

54. Fullerton B, Jeitler K, Seitz M, Horvath K, Berghold A, Siebenhofer A. Intensive glucose control versus conventional glucose control

for type 1 diabetes mellitus. Cochrane Database Syst Rev 2014;2:CD009122

55. Baskaran C, Volkening LK, Diaz M, Laffel LM. A decade of temporal trends in overweight/obesity in youth with type 1 diabetes after the Diabetes Control and Complications Trial. Pediatr Diabetes 2015;16:263–270

56. Foster NC, Beck RW, Miller KM, et al. State of type 1 diabetes management and outcomes from the T1D Exchange in 2016-2018. Diabetes Technol Ther 2019;21:66–72

57. Haller MJ, Long SA, Blanchfield JL, et al.; Type 1 Diabetes TrialNet ATG-GCSF Study Group. Low-dose anti-thymocyte globulin preserves C-Peptide, reduces HbA$_{1c}$, and increases regulatory to conventional T-cell ratios in new-onset type 1 diabetes: two-year clinical trial data. Diabetes 2019;68:1267–1276

58. Hamman RF, Bell RA, Dabelea D, et al.; SEARCH for Diabetes in Youth Study Group. The SEARCH for Diabetes in Youth study: rationale, findings, and future directions. Diabetes Care 2014;37:3336–3344

59. Willi SM, Miller KM, DiMeglio LA, et al.; T1D Exchange Clinic Network. Racial-ethnic disparities in management and outcomes among children with type 1 diabetes. Pediatrics 2015;135:424–434

60. Mayer-Davis EJ, Beyer J, Bell RA, et al.; SEARCH for Diabetes in Youth Study Group. Diabetes in African American youth: prevalence, incidence, and clinical characteristics: the SEARCH for Diabetes in Youth Study. Diabetes Care 2009;32(Suppl. 2):S112–S122

61. Lado JJ, Lipman TH. Racial and ethnic disparities in the incidence, treatment, and outcomes of youth with type 1 diabetes. Endocrinol Metab Clin North Am 2016;45:453–461

62. Glantz NM, Duncan I, Ahmed T, et al. Racial and ethnic disparities in the burden and cost of diabetes for US Medicare beneficiaries. Health Equity 2019;3:211–218

63. Agarwal S, Kanapka LG, Raymond JK, et al. Racial-ethnic inequity in young adults with type 1 diabetes. J Clin Endocrinol Metab 2020;105:dgaa236

64. Redondo MJ, Libman I, Cheng P, et al.; Pediatric Diabetes Consortium. Racial/ethnic minority youth with recent-onset type 1 diabetes have poor prognostic factors. Diabetes Care 2018;41:1017–1024

65. Charalampopoulos D, Hermann JM, Svensson J, et al. Exploring variation in glycemic control across and within eight high-income countries: a cross-sectional analysis of 64,666 children and adolescents with type 1 diabetes. Diabetes Care 2018;41:1180–1187

66. Samuelsson U, Åkesson K, Peterson A, Hanas R, Hanberger L. Continued improvement of metabolic control in Swedish pediatric diabetes care. Pediatr Diabetes 2018;19:150–157

67. Alonso GT, Corathers S, Shah A, et al. Establishment of the T1D Exchange Quality Improvement Collaborative (T1DX-QI). Clin Diabetes 2020;38:141–151

68. Åkesson K, Eriksson E, Samuelsson U, et al. Swediabkids - Swedish national quality registry for diabetes in children and adolescents, annual report 2018. Accessed 30 October 2020. Available from https://www.ndr.nu/pdfs/Yearreport_Swediabkids_2018_Eng.pdf

69. Anderzén J, Hermann JM, Samuelsson U, et al. International benchmarking in type 1 diabetes: large difference in childhood HbA1c between eight high-income countries but similar rise during adolescence-A quality registry study. Pediatr Diabetes 2020;21:621–627

70. American Diabetes Association. Type 2 diabetes in children and adolescents. Diabetes Care 2000;23:381–389

71. American Diabetes Association. Standards of medical care for patients with diabetes mellitus. Diabetes Care 2003;26(Suppl. 1):S33–S50

72. Silverstein J, Klingensmith G, Copeland K, et al.; American Diabetes Association. Care of children and adolescents with type 1 diabetes: a statement of the American Diabetes Association. Diabetes Care 2005;28:186–212

73. American Diabetes Association. Standards of medical care in diabetes. Diabetes Care 2005;28(Suppl. 1):S4–S36

74. American Diabetes Association. Standards of medical care in diabetes—2006. Diabetes Care 2006;29(Suppl. 1):S4–S42

75. American Diabetes Association. Standards of medical care in diabetes—2007. Diabetes Care 2007;30(Suppl. 1):S4–S41

76. American Diabetes Association. Standards of medical care in diabetes—2011. Diabetes Care 2011;34(Suppl. 1):S11–S61

77. American Diabetes Association. *Standards of Medical Care in Diabetes—2015*. Diabetes Care 2015;38(Suppl. 1):S1–S93

78. American Diabetes Association. 11. Children and adolescents. Diabetes Care 2016;39(Suppl. 1):S86–S93

79. Arslanian S, Bacha F, Grey M, Marcus MD, White NH, Zeitler P. Evaluation and management of youth-onset type 2 diabetes: a position statement by the American Diabetes Association. Diabetes Care 2018;41:2648–2668

Diabetes and Overweight/Obesity Are Independent, Nonadditive Risk Factors for In-Hospital Severity of COVID-19: An International, Multicenter Retrospective Meta-analysis

Diabetes Care 2021;44:1281–1290 | https://doi.org/10.2337/dc20-2676

Danielle K. Longmore,[1,2,3]
Jessica E. Miller,[1,4] Siroon Bekkering,[1,5]
Christoph Saner,[1,6] Edin Mifsud,[1,7]
Yanshan Zhu,[8] Richard Saffery,[1,4]
Alistair Nichol,[9,10,11] Graham Colditz,[12]
Kirsty R. Short,[8] and David P. Burgner,[1,3,4,13]
on behalf of the International BMI-COVID
consortium*

[1]Murdoch Children's Research Institute, The Royal
Children's Hospital, Parkville, Victoria, Australia
[2]Menzies School of Health Research, Charles
Darwin University, Darwin, Australia
[3]Infectious Diseases Unit, Department of General
Medicine, The Royal Children's Hospital, Parkville, Victoria, Australia
[4]Department of Paediatrics, Melbourne University, Parkville, Victoria, Australia
[5]Department of Internal Medicine and Radboud
Institute for Molecular Life Sciences, Radboud University Medical Center, Nijmegen, the Netherlands
[6]Pediatric Endocrinology, Diabetology and Metabolism, Department of Pediatrics, University
Hospital Inselspital, University of Bern, Bern,
Switzerland
[7]World Health Organization Collaborating Centre for Reference and Research on Influenza,
Doherty Institute, Melbourne, Australia
[8]School of Chemistry and Molecular Biosciences,
The University of Queensland, Brisbane, Australia
[9]Department of Intensive Care, Alfred Health,
Melbourne, Australia
[10]Australian and New Zealand Intensive Care
Research Centre, Monash University, Melbourne,
Australia
[11]University College Dublin Clinical Research Centre, St Vincent's Hospital, Dublin, Ireland
[12]Washington University, St. Louis, MO
[13]Department of Paediatrics, Monash University,
Clayton, Victoria, Australia

Corresponding authors: David P. Burgner, david.
burgner@mcri.edu.au, and Danielle K. Longmore,
danielle.longmore@mcri.edu.au

Received 29 October 2020 and accepted 14
January 2021

This article contains supplementary material online
at https://doi.org/10.2337/figshare.13616024.

D.K.L. and J.E.M. contributed equally as first
authors, and K.R.S. and D.P.B. contributed
equally as senior authors.

*A complete list of International BMI-COVID con-
sortium members is included in the supplementary material online.

This article is part of a special article collection
available at https://care.diabetesjournals.org/
collection/diabetes-and-COVID19.

OBJECTIVE

Obesity is an established risk factor for severe coronavirus disease 2019 (COVID-19), but the contribution of overweight and/or diabetes remains unclear. In a multicenter, international study, we investigated if overweight, obesity, and diabetes were independently associated with COVID-19 severity and whether the BMI-associated risk was increased among those with diabetes.

RESEARCH DESIGN AND METHODS

We retrospectively extracted data from health care records and regional databases of hospitalized adult patients with COVID-19 from 18 sites in 11 countries. We used standardized definitions and analyses to generate site-specific estimates, modeling the odds of each outcome (supplemental oxygen/noninvasive ventilatory support, invasive mechanical ventilatory support, and in-hospital mortality) by BMI category (reference, overweight, obese), adjusting for age, sex, and prespecified comorbidities. Subgroup analysis was performed on patients with preexisting diabetes. Site-specific estimates were combined in a meta-analysis.

RESULTS

Among 7,244 patients (65.6% overweight/obese), those with overweight were more likely to require oxygen/noninvasive ventilatory support (random effects adjusted odds ratio [aOR] 1.44; 95% CI 1.15–1.80) and invasive mechanical ventilatory support (aOR 1.22; 95% CI 1.03–1.46). There was no association between overweight and in-hospital mortality (aOR 0.88; 95% CI 0.74–1.04). Similar effects were observed in patients with obesity or diabetes. In the subgroup analysis, the aOR for any outcome was not additionally increased in those with diabetes and overweight or obesity.

CONCLUSIONS

In adults hospitalized with COVID-19, overweight, obesity, and diabetes were associated with increased odds of requiring respiratory support but were not associated with death. In patients with diabetes, the odds of severe COVID-19 were not increased above the BMI-associated risk.

In the first 6 months of the coronavirus disease 2019 (COVID-19) pandemic (until 30 June 2020), >10 million people had been infected with severe acute respiratory syndrome coronavirus 2 (SARS-CoV-2) and >500,000 COVID-19–related deaths had been recorded (1), but striking variation in clinical severity and outcomes remains. Identifying risk factors associated with more severe COVID-19 is essential for optimizing individual treatment and resource allocation and prioritizing immunization distribution. Obesity has emerged as an important risk factor for severe COVID-19 (2), but several key questions remain unanswered (3).

First, most studies to date have focused on individuals with obesity (BMI ≥30 kg/m^2) (4), but the specific contribution of overweight (BMI between ≥25 and <30) to severe COVID-19 has only been investigated in a few studies, which have reported inconsistent results (5–10). This is a significant knowledge gap, because 40% of the global population is overweight, in addition to the 13% living with obesity (11). Second, most studies are single-center analyses and are unlikely to be globally representative, given the marked intercountry variation in overweight and obesity (12). This shortcoming has partially been addressed by meta-analyses, but these rarely include individuals who are overweight (2). Finally, both overweight and obesity frequently occur with other comorbidities, particularly type 2 diabetes (13). However, many studies have either not adjusted for these covariables or the regression models used did not allow clinical translation of findings (3). Specifically, a key clinical question is whether patients with both diabetes and higher BMI have a higher risk of severe COVID-19 compared with those with diabetes and BMI in the normal range.

In the present study, we aimed to address these unresolved questions by performing an international, retrospective, multisite analysis of 7,244 hospitalized patients with COVID-19 from 18 sites in 11 countries. We used common definitions and analyses to delineate whether overweight, obesity, and diabetes are independent risk factors for respiratory support and in-hospital mortality. In patients with diabetes, we also investigated the association between BMI category and COVID-19 severity.

RESEARCH DESIGN AND METHODS
Study Design
We conducted an international, multicenter, retrospective analysis of hospitalized patients with COVID-19 from a total of 69 hospitals in 11 countries (Supplementary Table 1) from 17 January 2020 to 2 June 2020. Data from 69 hospitals were collated to form 18 sites that each provided site-specific outcomes and estimates. We modeled the odds of in-hospital respiratory support (supplemental oxygen/noninvasive ventilatory support, invasive mechanical ventilatory support) and in-hospital mortality by BMI category, adjusting for age, sex, and prespecified comorbidities, as described later in this section. A protocol was finalized on 20 April 2020 (see Statistical Analysis Plan [SAP] in Supplementary Material) prior to commencement of the study. The study was conducted in accordance with Good Clinical Practice guidelines, local regulations, and the ethical principles described in the Declaration of Helsinki. Ethical approval was obtained at the coordinating center (Murdoch Children's Research Institute [MCRI], Royal Children's Hospital, Melbourne, Australia; approval no. HREC 63887), and local approvals were obtained at participating sites, depending on local regulations. Informed consent was not required.

Data Source
We analyzed deidentified data from existing collections of hospital data and regional databases, including the Norwegian Intensive Care and Pandemic Registry, Norway, and Washington University, St. Louis, Missouri (see Supplementary Material for participating sites and investigators). Data from smaller contributing hospitals were collected for clinical auditing processes approved by local hospitals and in accordance with local regulations. Each site followed a standardized protocol for data coding and analysis to generate site-specific estimates for each study population (see SAP in Supplementary Material). Deidentified data from hospitals in Austria, Singapore, the Netherlands, Switzerland, and Indonesia were exported to the coordinating center (MCRI) for generation of site-specific estimates. All transfer of data and site-specific estimates to the MCRI was subject to a data transfer agreement. Statisticians at the MCRI completed the meta-analyses.

Data Collection
Study participants were aged ≥18 years, admitted to hospital with COVID-19 (confirmed by PCR for SARS-CoV-2), and had height and weight recorded on admission to participating sites with local approval to participate. The period for data collection from individual sites varied (Supplementary Table 1).

Information regarding participant demographic variables (age, sex), BMI, preexisting medical conditions, clinical variables including intensive care unit admission, and treatment including oxygen and noninvasive ventilatory support and mechanical ventilatory support were identified. Supplemental oxygen was defined as the provision of oxygen via nasal canulae or face mask. Noninvasive ventilatory support was defined as the use of a device providing continuous positive airway pressure or bilevel positive airway pressure. Cardiovascular disease was defined as preexisting, physician-diagnosed coronary heart disease, ischemic stroke, heart failure, and/or peripheral vascular disease. Diabetes was defined as preexisting diabetes (including type 1 or 2). In all countries, type 2 diabetes was diagnosed according to the American Diabetes Association guidelines or local guidelines with the same diagnostic criteria as the American Diabetes Association guidelines. For three sites only (Cape Town, South Africa; Lausanne, Switzerland; and Ticino, Switzerland), a small number of patients were included who were first diagnosed with diabetes during their admission with COVID-19. Preexisting respiratory conditions and hypertension were defined as physician-diagnosed and currently on treatment. Data cleaning was performed for out-of-range values, inconsistent data, and repeated participant entries. Central source data verification was not feasible for this study, because coding was performed by the individual participating centers.

Statistical Analysis
All analyses were conducted as outlined in our protocol (see SAP in Supplementary Material). Participant data are presented as frequency (percent). Each site (or the MCRI) followed a standardized protocol for data coding and analysis to generate site-specific estimates from each study population, modeling the odds of each outcome by BMI (calculated

as weight [kg] divided by height squared [m^2]) category (see SAP in Supplementary Material). BMI was categorized as underweight ($\geq$12 to <18), normal ($\geq$18 to <25 [reference]), overweight ($\geq$25 to <30), and obese ($\geq$30). In sensitivity analyses for Asian populations, respective BMI categories were based on the following ranges: $\geq$12 to <18.5, $\geq$18.5 to <24 (reference), $\geq$24 to <28, and $\geq$28 (14). Logistic regression was used to model the association between BMI category and the use of in-hospital respiratory therapies (supplemental oxygen/noninvasive ventilation, mechanical ventilation) and in-hospital mortality.

All models estimated crude (unadjusted) and adjusted odds ratios. Two levels of adjustments were made. The first level, available for all sites, included age, sex, preexisting cardiovascular disease, diabetes, preexisting respiratory conditions, and hypertension. The second level of adjustments included the first level of adjustments plus current smoking status and/or race/ethnicity, depending on data availability. The second level was available for only five sites. The crude and adjusted (first-level) models were run on data from a subgroup of patients with preexisting diabetes. No adjustment was made for multiple comparisons. Covariables had few missing data and no imputations were warranted. Site-specific adjusted estimates for BMI category, each independent covariable included in the adjusted models, and the diabetes subgroup estimates were combined in meta-analyses.

Summarized estimates included fixed and random effects models (15). Random effects estimates are presented in the text. Of note, the Los Angeles, New York, and Cape Town sites were not included in analysis of supplemental oxygen/noninvasive ventilatory support, because nearly all hospitalized patients received supplemental oxygen per local policies. Data on supplemental oxygen were not available for Austria, Norway, or Amphia (the Netherlands). Variations to the preplanned analysis were made because there were insufficient data available from the majority of sites. The outcomes not analyzed included intensive care unit length of stay, hospital length of stay, and extracorporeal membrane oxygenation use (see SAP in Supplementary Material). Site-specific analyses were performed

in SAS (SAS Institute, Cary, NC), Stata (StataCorp College Station, TX), or R studio (PBC, Boston, MA) (16). Meta-analyses were performed in Stata SE, version 16.0 (17).

RESULTS

Characteristics of Patients Included in the Study

A total of 7,244 patients from 18 sites (n = 69 hospitals) in 11 countries were included in this study of hospitalized patients with COVID-19 (Supplementary Tables 1 and 3). Among these, 60.1% were male and 51.7% were older than 65 years. Overall, 34.8% were overweight and 30.8% obese; however, there was considerable variability across different individual countries and sites. Prevalence of obesity for each site country is provided in Supplementary Table 2. The rates of comorbidities and the frequency of outcomes varied across sites (Supplementary Tables 3 and 4). Prevalence of diabetes varied from 7% in Guangdong Province, China, to 46% in St. Louis, Missouri. Prevalence of diabetes among those of normal weight ranged from 6% in Milan Sacco, Italy, to 39% in Cape Town, South Africa. Prevalence of diabetes among those who were overweight or obese ranged from 7% and 5%, respectively, in Guangdong Province, China, to 47% and 53%, respectively, in St. Louis, Missouri.

Association of Overweight, Obesity With Supplemental Oxygen/Noninvasive Ventilatory Support, Mechanical Ventilatory Support, and In-Hospital Death

Compared with normal weight, overweight and obesity were associated with increased odds of supplemental oxygen/noninvasive ventilatory support (random effects adjusted odds ratio (aOR) 1.44 [95% CI 1.15–1.80], P = 0.02; and aOR 1.75 [95% CI 1.33–2.30], P < 0.01), respectively (Fig. 1). Obesity was associated with a 73% increase in odds for invasive mechanical ventilatory support (aOR 1.73; 95% CI 1.29–2.32; P < 0.01) (Fig. 2), and a more modest association was observed for overweight (aOR 1.22; 95% CI 1.03–1.46; P = 0.02). Data on this outcome were not available from Amphia (the Netherlands).

Overweight was not associated with an increase in odds for in-hospital mortality (aOR 0.88; 95% CI 0.74–1.04; P = 0.13) (Fig. 3). Obesity was also not associated with an increase in odds of in-hospital mortality, with confidence

limits including the null (aOR 1.23; 95% CI 0.92–1.64; P = 0.17). The low number of participants in the underweight group (n = 162) precluded calculation of robust odds ratios. The I^2 statistic, which describes the percentage of variation across studies that is due to heterogeneity rather than chance, was 43.6% and 53.7% among the obese groups for invasive mechanical ventilatory support and in-hospital mortality, respectively, suggesting modest heterogeneity across studies. Unadjusted site-specific odds ratios are presented in Figs. 1–3.

For the Chinese, Indonesian, and Singaporean sites, odds ratios varied slightly depending on whether the standard or Asian country–specific BMI categories were used. The variation did not meaningfully affect the summarized meta-analysis estimates (Supplementary Table 4). Additional adjustments for current smoking and race/ethnicity, where data were available, had little impact on the odds ratios (Supplementary Table 5).

Association of Diabetes With Supplemental Oxygen/Noninvasive Ventilatory Support, Mechanical Ventilatory Support, and In-Hospital Death

Compared with patients without diabetes, those with diabetes had an increased odds of needing mechanical ventilatory support in random effects models adjusted for all covariables, including BMI category and comorbidities (aOR 1.21; 95% CI 1.03–1.41; P = 0.02) (Supplementary Fig. 1). There was no increase in odds of noninvasive respiratory support or in-hospital mortality in those with diabetes (Supplementary Fig. 1). In addition to diabetes, other host factors previously associated with severe COVID-19 (i.e., increased age, male sex, preexisting cardiovascular disease, and chronic respiratory disease) (18) were each independently associated with an increased risk of one or more of the selected study outcomes (Supplementary Figs. 2–4).

Among Patients With Diabetes, Increased BMI Did Not Increase the Risk of Severe COVID-19 Outcomes

To further inform patient care, we next performed a subgroup analysis of individuals with diabetes. Specifically, we investigated if BMI category among those with diabetes was associated with the selected COVID-19 outcomes. Strikingly, there was no association between

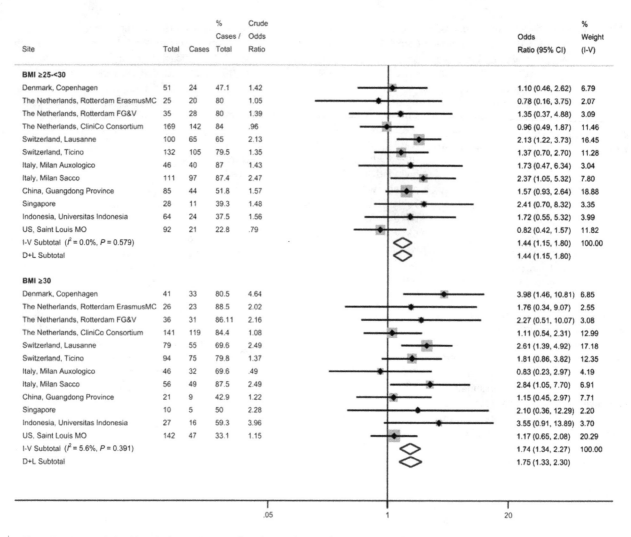

Figure 1—Meta-analysis odds ratios for requirement of supplemental oxygen/noninvasive ventilatory support by BMI category. Models were adjusted for age (<65, ≥65 years), sex (male/female), preexisting cardiovascular disease (yes/no), diabetes (yes/no), preexisting respiratory conditions (yes/no), and hypertension (yes/no). The reference BMI is ≥18 to <25. The 95% CIs of the odds ratios were not adjusted for multiple testing and should not be used to infer definitive effects. Data from Norway; Amphia (in the Netherlands); Austria; South Africa; University of California, Los Angeles, California; and Cornell University, Ithaca, New York, were not included in this model because data were either not available for this outcome or all patients received the therapy. D+L, DerSimonian and Laird random effects model; FG&V, Franciscus Gasthuis & Vlietland; I-V, inverse-variance weighted fixed effects model; MC, medical center.

overweight or obesity and supplemental oxygen use/noninvasive ventilatory support (aOR 1.04 [95% CI 0.54–2.00], P = 0.91; and 1.29 [95% CI 0.68–2.46], P = 0.44, respectively), invasive mechanical ventilatory support (aOR 0.67 [95% CI 0.40–1.12], P = 0.10; and 1.25 [95% CI 0.62–2.53], P = 0.73, respectively), or in-hospital mortality (aOR 0.79 [95% CI 0.52–1.20], P = 0.28; and 1.14 [95% CI 0.61–2.13], P = 0.52, respectively) in those with preexisting diabetes (Fig. 4). In this subgroup analysis, the sample size was reduced and resulted in wide CIs.

CONCLUSIONS

In this large, international, multicenter study of patients hospitalized with

COVID-19, overweight was associated overall with an increased requirement of respiratory support. The association between overweight and in-hospital mortality was not statistically significant. Similar trends were observed in patients with obesity. In addition to the associations with BMI, diabetes was independently associated with increased COVID-19 severity but not death. Importantly, among patients with diabetes, overweight/obesity were not associated with an increased risk of severe COVID-19.

The data presented here are consistent with those of previous studies that reported not only obesity but also advanced age, male sex, and preexisting cardiovascular, metabolic, and respiratory

disease were associated with worse outcomes with COVID-19 (19). In the present study, neither overweight/obesity nor diabetes was associated with in-hospital mortality. Although previous analyses have suggested that obesity increases the mortality risk associated with COVID-19 (4,8,20), these studies did not necessarily make adjustments for age, sex, and other comorbidities as we did in the present study, or only found an effect on death for those with more severe obesity (BMI >35) (21). The data presented here are consistent with previous findings that an elevated BMI is associated with an increased requirement for respiratory support (5,22–24) and that diabetes in patients with COVID-19 is not

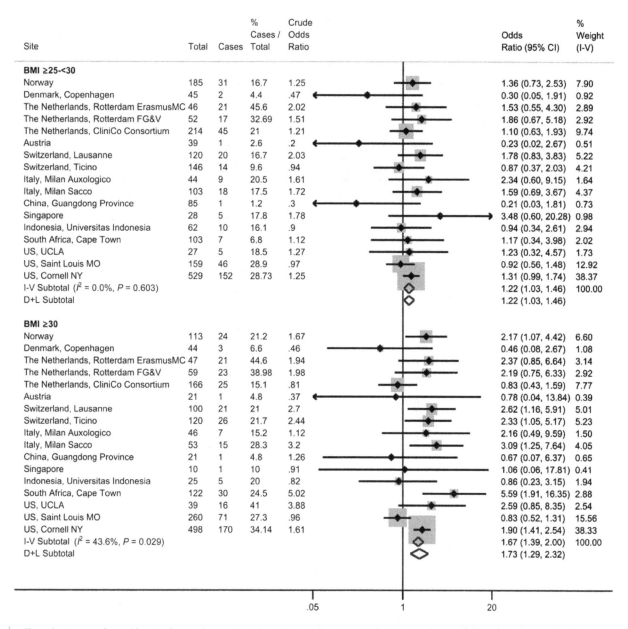

Figure 2—Meta-analysis odds ratios for invasive mechanical ventilatory support by BMI category. Models were adjusted for age (<65, ≥65 years), sex (male/female), preexisting cardiovascular disease (yes/no), diabetes (yes/no), preexisting respiratory conditions (yes/no), and hypertension (yes/no). The reference BMI is ≥18 to <25. The 95% CIs of the odds ratios have not been adjusted for multiple testing and should not be used to infer definitive effects. Data from Amphia (in the Netherlands) were not available for invasive mechanical ventilatory support. D+L, DerSimonian and Laird random effects model; FG&V, Franciscus Gasthuis & Vlietland; I-V, inverse-variance weighted fixed effects model; UCLA, University of California, Los Angeles, California.

significantly associated with in-hospital mortality after appropriate adjustment (25).

The mechanisms underlying the association between BMI and COVID-19 severity likely reflect a dysregulated host response, resulting in heightened inflammation and/or a suboptimal antiviral response. There are a number of relevant immunomodulatory effects of overweight/obesity, including chronic systemic inflammation (26), reduced production of type I interferons (27), reduced antigen

presentation (28), complement activation (29), and/or suboptimal T-cell responses (30). Moreover, these immunomodulatory effects may be compounded by the reduced functional respiratory capacity in individuals with overweight/obesity, which may lead to a lower threshold for noninvasive or invasive respiratory support (31).

It is likely that the independent role identified for diabetes in COVID-19 severity reflects the role of hyperglycemia in severe respiratory disease. Indeed,

data from Denmark suggest that each 1 mmol/L increase in plasma glucose level is associated with a 6% increased risk of hospitalization for pneumonia (32). Elevated blood glucose levels are also associated with altered activity of transporters responsible for clearing the lung of interstitial edema and for maintaining the integrity of the pulmonary epithelial–endothelial barrier (33–35), both of which are likely to be important in determining the clinical outcome of SARS-CoV-2 infection. This hypothesis is

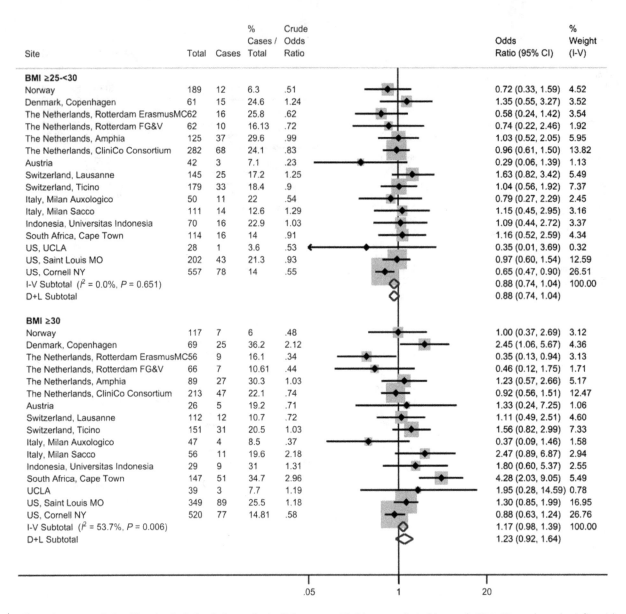

Figure 3—Meta-analysis odds ratios for in-hospital mortality by BMI category. Models were adjusted for age (<65, ≥65 years), sex (male/female), preexisting cardiovascular disease (yes/no), diabetes (yes/no), preexisting respiratory conditions (yes/no), and hypertension (yes/no). The reference BMI is ≥18 to <25. The 95% CIs of the odds ratios were not adjusted for multiple testing and should not be used to infer definitive effects. Data from Guandong Province, China, and Singapore were not available for in-hospital mortality. D+L, DerSimonian and Laird random effects model; FG&V, Franciscus Gasthuis & Vlietland; I-V, inverse-variance weighted fixed effects model; UCLA, University of California, Los Angeles, California.

consistent with observations that well-controlled blood glucose levels correlated with improved clinical outcomes in patients with COVID-19 who also had diabetes (36). More severe COVID-19, however, may also be associated with elevated glucose levels (37). With respect to the relationship between longer-term glucose control and COVID-19 severity, an elevated hemoglobin A_{1c} is associated with increased risk of hospital admission due to COVID-19 in those with diabetes (38). Additional studies investigating the mechanistic roles of both BMI and diabetes in COVID-19 severity are warranted.

Currently, it is estimated that ~90% of patients with type 2 diabetes are overweight or obese (39). Previous studies have suggested that among patients with COVID-19 who have diabetes, nonsurvivors had a greater prevalence of comorbidities compared with survivors (25). Given the clear independent role of BMI in COVID-19 severity, we reasoned that patients with both diabetes and an elevated BMI may be at increased risk of severe disease outcomes compared with patients with diabetes and a BMI in the normal range. Surprisingly, BMI was not associated with the risk of in-hospital

respiratory support or death among patients with both COVID-19 and diabetes. Larger studies will be needed to confirm these findings; however, this finding may reflect a "threshold effect" of susceptibility to severe COVID-19 in these conditions. This hypothesis will require clinical and experimental evaluation.

Our data will inform public policy, particularly for risk-stratification of severe COVID-19 disease. The U.S. Centers for Disease Control and Prevention identifies individuals with obesity (BMI ≥30) as being at increased risk for severe disease, as well as those with cardiovascular

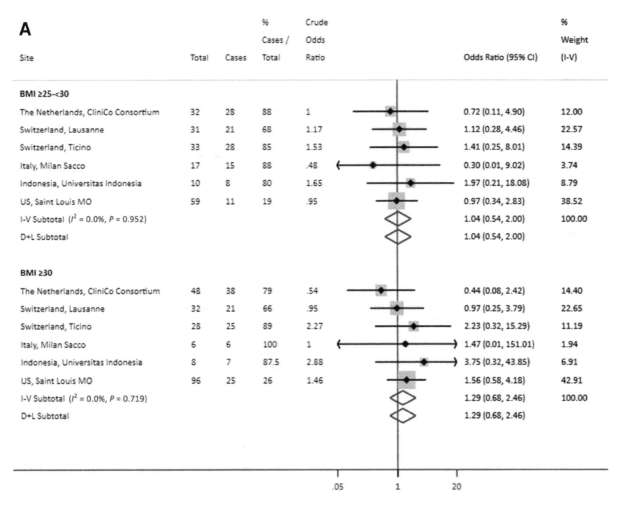

Figure 4—Meta-analysis odds ratios for supplemental oxygen/noninvasive ventilatory support (*A*), invasive mechanical ventilatory support (*B*), and in-hospital mortality by BMI category in patients with preexisting diabetes (*C*). Models were adjusted for age (<65, ≥65 years), sex (male/female), preexisting cardiovascular disease (yes/no), preexisting respiratory conditions (yes/no), and hypertension (yes/no). The reference BMI is ≥18 to <25. The 95% CI of the odds ratios have not been adjusted for multiple testing and should not be used to infer definitive effects. Data from New York were not available for this subgroup analysis. D+L, DerSimonian and Laird random effects model; FG&V, Franciscus Gasthuis & Vlietland; I-V, inverse-variance weighted fixed effects model.

disease, and has recently outlined that individuals who are overweight may be at increased risk (40). Similarly, the most recent guidelines from Public Health England consider overweight and obesity as risk factors for severe COVID-19 (41), in contrast to more conservative guidelines from the U.K. National Health Service that suggested an increased risk only for a BMI ≥40 (42). The World Health Organization now considers obesity a risk factor for severe COVID-19 disease (43). Inconsistent recommendations may impede optimal patient care and compromise clear public health messaging. To our knowledge, there is currently no clinical guidance on the role of BMI in COVID-19 risk stratification of patients with diabetes.

We acknowledge limitations of our study. Data on socioeconomic status were not available, limiting the interpretation of these findings, particularly because there may be important relationships among BMI, race/ethnicity, and socioeconomic status (44). Adjustment for confounders including smoking and race/ethnicity was only possible for five sites, with no difference in odds ratio observed. Supplemental oxygen use varied; oxygen was administered to all hospitalized patients at a limited number of sites, affecting our ability to determine the influence of host comorbidities on this outcome. There may also be varying and unmeasurable differences in thresholds for escalating care in those with overweight and obesity.

Given that this analysis involves patients admitted to hospital with COVID-19 only, we also were unable to assess whether patients with diabetes and obesity were more likely to experience out-of-hospital death due to COVID-19 infection. These patients were not captured in the data, and this may have resulted in an underestimation of overall mortality. At some sites, BMI was not consistently recorded during the study period, which may have introduced site-specific bias. Because of the relatively small numbers of patients at some sites, we were unable to stratify BMI categories to include underweight (BMI <18.5) or BMI >40, so we were unable to report specific odds ratios for these groups. We were unable to

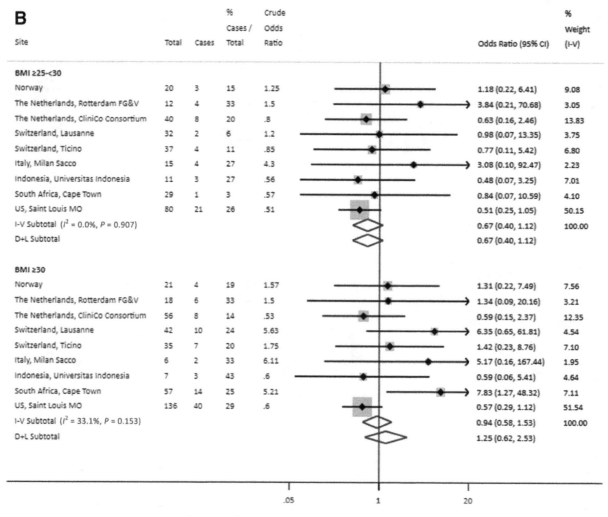

			% Cases /	Crude Odds			% Weight
Site	Total	Cases	Total	Ratio		Odds Ratio (95% CI)	(I-V)
BMI ≥25–<30							
Norway	20	3	15	1.25		1.18 (0.22, 6.41)	9.08
The Netherlands, Rotterdam FG&V	12	4	33	1.5		3.84 (0.21, 70.68)	3.05
The Netherlands, CliniCo Consortium	40	8	20	.8		0.63 (0.16, 2.46)	13.83
Switzerland, Lausanne	32	2	6	1.2		0.98 (0.07, 13.35)	3.75
Switzerland, Ticino	37	4	11	.85		0.77 (0.11, 5.42)	6.80
Italy, Milan Sacco	15	4	27	4.3		3.08 (0.10, 92.47)	2.23
Indonesia, Universitas Indonesia	11	3	27	.56		0.48 (0.07, 3.25)	7.01
South Africa, Cape Town	29	1	3	.57		0.84 (0.07, 10.59)	4.10
US, Saint Louis MO	80	21	26	.51		0.51 (0.25, 1.05)	50.15
I-V Subtotal (I^2 = 0.0%, P = 0.907)						0.67 (0.40, 1.12)	100.00
D+L Subtotal						0.67 (0.40, 1.12)	
BMI ≥30							
Norway	21	4	19	1.57		1.31 (0.22, 7.49)	7.56
The Netherlands, Rotterdam FG&V	18	6	33	1.5		1.34 (0.09, 20.16)	3.21
The Netherlands, CliniCo Consortium	56	8	14	.53		0.59 (0.15, 2.37)	12.35
Switzerland, Lausanne	42	10	24	5.63		6.35 (0.65, 61.81)	4.54
Switzerland, Ticino	35	7	20	1.75		1.42 (0.23, 8.76)	7.10
Italy, Milan Sacco	6	2	33	6.11		5.17 (0.16, 167.44)	1.95
Indonesia, Universitas Indonesia	7	3	43	.6		0.59 (0.06, 5.41)	4.64
South Africa, Cape Town	57	14	25	5.21		7.83 (1.27, 48.32)	7.11
US, Saint Louis MO	136	40	29	.6		0.57 (0.29, 1.12)	51.54
I-V Subtotal (I^2 = 33.1%, P = 0.153)						0.94 (0.58, 1.53)	100.00
D+L Subtotal						1.25 (0.62, 2.53)	

.05   1   20

Figure 4—*Continued*.

differentiate between type 1 and type 2 diabetes from the data available. Notwithstanding, the majority of patients with diabetes included would be expected to have type 2 diabetes, given the expected prepandemic relative prevalence (25). Moreover, type 1 diabetes has not been associated with increased severity of COVID-19 (45); therefore, we believe the findings for patients with diabetes predominantly represent those with type 2 diabetes. It is important to note that the modest sample size of this study precludes precise estimates of risk, particularly with respect to the associations among the subgroup of patients with diabetes. We acknowledge that the number of deaths likely decreased over the period of the study, which may have altered results dependent on dates of data collection and the timing of COVID-

19 surges in different countries. Given that improvements in clinical care did not occur uniformly in all countries, however, we were unable to adjust for this in our analysis. Finally, although we enrolled multiple sites, our findings should not be considered regionally or globally representative and the study population was underrepresented for low- and middle-income countries, which may limit generalizability.

Notwithstanding, to our knowledge, this study remains one of the largest multinational studies to date on the risk factors associated with severe COVID-19. Inclusion of individuals from low- and middle-income countries and disadvantaged or higher-risk populations in such analyses is essential, and it is hoped that as the pandemic progresses and more data become available, data

from these populations can be added to our ongoing analysis; potential collaborators are encouraged to contact the corresponding authors.

In conclusion, our findings highlight the importance of maintaining a healthy BMI, because patients with either overweight or obesity are at risk for severe COVID-19. Although reducing the current levels of overweight and obesity is unlikely in the short term to have an impact on the COVID-19 pandemic, doing so may contribute to reducing disease burden in future viral pandemics (41,46). Furthermore, the absence of an association between overweight/obesity and COVID-19 severity among those with diabetes should guide additional exploration of mechanistic pathways and may inform risk stratification and appropriate patient treatment. Finally, our findings

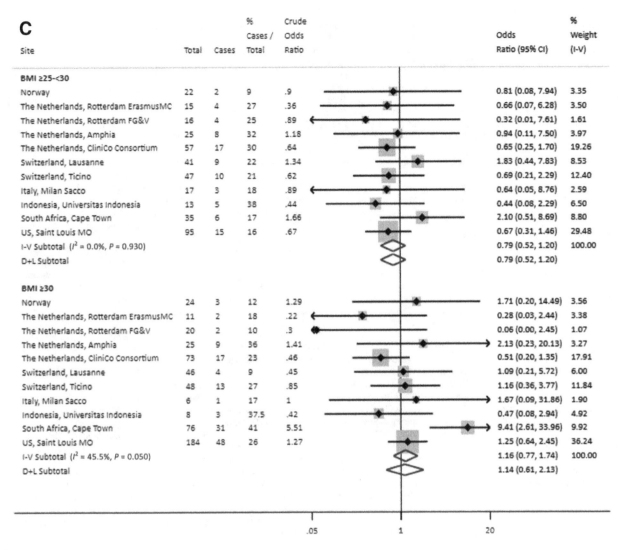

Figure 4—*Continued.*

may inform immunization prioritization for higher-risk groups.

Acknowledgments. Authors from several sites wish to extend acknowledgments: Those at Aux-ilogico, Milan, Italy, acknowledge Drs. Irene Campi, Iacopo Chiodini, Luca Giovanelli, Giovanni Perego, Francesca Heilbron, Roberto Menè, Andrea Cas-cella, Stefano Vicini, and all nurses; those at the University of California, Los Angeles, acknowledge Dr. Paul C. Adamson; those in Cape Town, South Africa, acknowledge doctors and nurses working in COVID-19 inpatient service; those in Indonesia thank the patients, doctors, nurses, pharmacists, other health care workers, and research admin-istrators at all the participating sites. Authors in Ticino, Switzerland, acknowledge Lorenzo Ruinelli; those in Lausanne, Switzerland, acknowledge Oriol Manuel, Desgranges Florian, Filippidis Paraskevas, Kampouri Eleftheria-Evdokia, Tschopp Jonathan, and Viala Benjamin; those at Amphia, the Nether-lands, acknowledge A.G. Loman and B.W. Driessen; those at Franciscus Gasthuis & Vlietland, Rotter-dam, the Netherlands, acknowledge Dr. Bianca M. Boxma-de Klerk; those at Washington University,

St. Louis, Missouri, acknowledge Drs. Albert Lai and Randi Foraker of the Institute for Informatics at Washington University School of Medicine. The main writing group acknowledges patients and their families and health care providers worldwide.

Funding. There was no specific project funding for the study. Individual investigators were funded as follows: J.E.M. was supported by a fellowship from the DHB Foundation, Australia; S.B. is supported by the Dutch Heart Foundation (Dekker grant 2018-T028); E.M. is supported by the World Health Organization Collaborating Centre for Reference and Research on Influ-enza, funded by the Australian Commonwealth Government, Department of Health. K.R.S. was supported by the Australian Research Council (grant DE180100512); A.N. is supported by a Health Research Board of Ireland Clinical Trail Network award (grant CTN-2014-012); and D.P.B. was supported by a National Health and Medical Research Council Australian Investigator grant (GTN1175744). Research at the Murdoch Children's Research Institute is supported by the Victorian Government's Operational Infrastructure Support Program.

The funders had no role in study design, data collection, data analysis, data interpretation, or writing of the report.

Duality of Interest. No potential conflicts of interest relevant to this article were reported.

Author Contributions. Authors had full access to their corresponding site's data in the study and had final responsibility for the decision to submit for publication. D.K.L., E.M., Y.Z., K.R.S., and D.P.B. contributed to data interpretation and wrote the first draft of the manuscript. J.E.M., S.B., and C.S. performed the data analysis, contributed to data interpretation, and reviewed the manu-script. R.S., A.N., and G.C. contributed to the data interpretation and reviewed the manuscript. J.E.M. and D.P.B. are the guarantors of this work and, as such, had full access to all the data in the study and take responsibility for the integrity of the data and the accuracy of the data analysis.

References

1. World Health Organization. *Coronovirus Dis-ease (COVID-19) Situation Report -162.* Geneva, World Health Organization, 2020, p. 17
2. Popkin BM, Du S, Green WD, et al. Individuals with obesity and COVID-19: a global perspective

on the epidemiology and biological relationships. Obes Rev 2020;21:e13128

3. Selvin E, Juraschek SP. Diabetes epidemiology in the COVID-19 pandemic. Diabetes Care 2020; 43:1690–1694

4. Rottoli M, Bernante P, Belvedere A, et al. How important is obesity as a risk factor for respiratory failure, intensive care unit admission and death in hospitalised COVID-19 patients? Results from a single Italian centre. Eur J Endocrinol 2020;183: 389–397

5. Simonnet A, Chetboun M, Poissy J, et al.; LICORN and the Lille COVID-19 and Obesity study group. High prevalence of obesity in severe acute respiratory syndrome coronavirus-2 (SARS-CoV-2) requiring invasive mechanical ventilation. Obesity (Silver Spring) 2020;28:1195–1199

6. Halasz G, Leoni ML, Villani GQ, Nolli M, Villani M. Obesity, overweight and survival in critically ill patients with SARS-CoV-2 pneumonia: is there an obesity paradox? Preliminary results from Italy. Eur J Prev Cardiol. 7 July 2020 [Epub ahead of print]. DOI: 10.1177/2047487320939675

7. Hamer M, Gale CR, Kivimäki M, Batty GD. Overweight, obesity, and risk of hospitalization for COVID-19: a community-based cohort study of adults in the United Kingdom. Proc Natl Acad Sci U S A 2020;117:21011–21013

8. Tartof SY, Qian L, Hong V, et al. Obesity and mortality among patients diagnosed with COVID-19: results from an integrated health care organization. Ann Intern Med 2020;173:773–781

9. Nakeshbandi M, Maini R, Daniel P, et al. The impact of obesity on COVID-19 complications: a retrospective cohort study. Int J Obes 2020;44: 1832–1837

10. Petrilli CM, Jones SA, Yang J, et al. Factors associated with hospital admission and critical illness among 5279 people with coronavirus disease 2019 in New York City: prospective cohort study. BMJ 2020;369:m1966

11. World Health Organization. Obesity and overweight, 2020. Accessed 17 October 2020. Available from https://www.who.int/news-room/fact-sheets/detail/obesity-and-overweight

12. World Health Organization. Prevalence of obesity among adults, BMI >= 30 (crude estimate) (%). 2017. Accessed 19 October 2020. Available from https://www.who.int/data/gho/data/indicators/indicator-details/GHO/prevalence-of-obesity-among-adults-bmi-=-30-(crude-estimate)-(-)

13. Smith KB, Smith MS. Obesity statistics. Prim Care 2016;43:121–135, ix

14. World Health Organization Expert Consultation. Appropriate body-mass index for Asian populations and its implications for policy and intervention strategies. Lancet 2004;363:157–163

15. Harris R, Bradburn M, Deeks J, Harbord R, Altman D, Sterne J. metan: Fixed- and random-effects meta-analysis. Stata J 2008;8:3–28

16. RStudio. Integrated Development for R. RStudio, 2020. Accessed 3 September 2020. Available from https://www.rstudio.com/

17. Statacorp. Stata Statistical Software: release 16. College Station, TX, StataCorp LLC, 2019

18. Zaki N, Alashwal H, Ibrahim S. Association of hypertension, diabetes, stroke, cancer, kidney disease, and high-cholesterol with COVID-19 disease severity and fatality: a systematic review. Diabetes Metab Syndr 2020;14:1133–1142

19. Williamson EJ, Walker AJ, Bhaskaran K, et al. Factors associated with COVID-19-related death using OpenSAFELY. Nature 2020;584:430–436

20. Anderson MR, Geleris J, Anderson DR, et al. Body mass index and risk for intubation or death in SARS-CoV-2 infection: a retrospective cohort study. Ann Intern Med 2020;173:782–790

21. Klang E, Kassim G, Soffer S, Freeman R, Levin MA, Reich DL. Severe obesity as an independent risk factor for COVID-19 mortality in hospitalized patients younger than 50. Obesity (Silver Spring) 2020;28:1595–1599

22. Watanabe M, Caruso D, Tuccinardi D, et al. Visceral fat shows the strongest association with the need of intensive care in patients with COVID-19. Metabolism 2020;111:154319

23. Monteiro AC, Suri R, Emeruwa IO, et al. Obesity and smoking as risk factors for invasive mechanical ventilation in COVID-19: a retrospective, observational cohort study. PLoS One 2020; 15:e0238552

24. Cariou B, Hadjadj S, Wargny M, et al.; CORONADO Investigators. Phenotypic characteristics and prognosis of inpatients with COVID-19 and diabetes: the CORONADO study. Diabetologia 2020;63:1500–1515

25. Shi Q, Zhang X, Jiang F, et al. Clinical characteristics and risk factors for mortality of COVID-19 patients with diabetes in Wuhan, China: a two-center, retrospective study. Diabetes Care 2020;43:1382–1391

26. Suganami T, Tanaka M, Ogawa Y. Molecular mechanisms underlying obesity-induced chronic inflammation. In *Chronic Inflammation: Mechanisms and Regulation*. Miyasaka M, Takatsu K, Eds. Tokyo, Springer Japan, 2016, pp. 291–298

27. Siegers JY, Novakovic B, Hulme KD, et al. A high-fat diet increases influenza A virus-associated cardiovascular damage. J Infect Dis 2020; 222:820–831

28. Smith AG, Sheridan PA, Tseng RJ, Sheridan JF, Beck MA. Selective impairment in dendritic cell function and altered antigen-specific CD8+ T-cell responses in diet-induced obese mice infected with influenza virus. Immunology 2009;126:268–279

29. Lockhart SM, O'Rahilly S. When two pandemics meet: why is obesity associated with increased COVID-19 mortality? Med (N Y) 2020;1: 33–42

30. Paich HA, Sheridan PA, Handy J, et al. Overweight and obese adult humans have a defective cellular immune response to pandemic H1N1 influenza A virus. Obesity (Silver Spring) 2013;21: 2377–2386

31. Kassir R. Risk of COVID-19 for patients with obesity. Obes Rev 2020;21:e13034

32. Benfield T, Jensen JS, Nordestgaard BG. Influence of diabetes and hyperglycaemia on infectious disease hospitalisation and outcome. Diabetologia 2007;50:549–554

33. Yamashita T, Umeda F, Hashimoto T, et al. Effect of glucose on Na, K-ATPase activity in cultured bovine aortic endothelial cells. Endocrinol Jpn 1992;39:1–7

34. Rivelli JF, Amaiden MR, Monesterolo NE, et al. High glucose levels induce inhibition of Na,K-ATPase via stimulation of aldose reductase, formation of microtubules and formation of an acetylated tubulin/Na,K-ATPase complex. Int J Biochem Cell Biol 2012;44:1203–1213

35. Hulme KD, Yan L, Marshall RJ, et al. High glucose levels increase influenza-associated damage to the pulmonary epithelial-endothelial barrier. eLife 2020;9:e56907

36. Zhu L, She Z-G, Cheng X, et al. Association of blood glucose control and outcomes in patients with COVID-19 and pre-existing type 2 diabetes. Cell Metab 2020;31:1068–1077.e3

37. Coppelli A, Giannarelli R, Aragona M, et al.; Pisa COVID-19 Study Group. Hyperglycemia at hospital admission is associated with severity of the prognosis in patients hospitalized for COVID-19: the Pisa COVID-19 Study. Diabetes Care 2020; 43:2345–2348

38. Merzon E, Green I, Shpigelman M, et al. Haemoglobin A1c is a predictor of COVID-19 severity in patients with diabetes. Diabetes Metab Res Rev. 27 August 2020 [Epub ahead of print]. DOI: 10.1002/dmrr.3398

39. Public Health England. *Adult Obesity and Type 2 Diabetes*. London, Public Health England, 2014, pp. 39

40. Centers for Disease Control and Prevention. People with certain medical conditions, 2020. Accessed 26 October 2020. Available from https://www.cdc.gov/coronavirus/2019-ncov/need-extra-precautions/people-with-medical-conditions.html

41. Blackshaw J, Feeley A, Mabbs L, et al. *Excess Weight and COVID-19: Insights from New Evidence*. London, Public Health England, 2020

42. National Health Service. Coronavirus (COVID-19): Shielded patients list, 2020. Accessed 13 July 2020. Available from https://digital.nhs.uk/coronavirus/shielded-patient-list#risk-criteria

43. World Health Organization. COVID-19: vulnerable and high risk groups, 2020. Accessed 12 July 2020. Available from https://www.who.int/westernpacific/emergencies/covid-19/information/high-risk-groups

44. McLaren L. Socioeconomic status and obesity. Epidemiol Rev 2007;29:29–48

45. Vangoitsenhoven R, Martens PJ, van Nes F, et al. No evidence of increased hospitalization rate for COVID-19 in community-dwelling patients with type 1 diabetes. Diabetes Care 2020; 43:e118–e119

46. Short KR, Kedzierska K, van de Sandt CE. Back to the future: lessons learned from the 1918 influenza pandemic. Front Cell Infect Microbiol 2018;8:343

COVID-19, Hyperglycemia, and New-Onset Diabetes

Kamlesh Khunti,[1] Stefano Del Prato,[2] Chantal Mathieu,[3] Steven E. Kahn,[4] Robert A. Gabbay,[5,6] and John B. Buse[7]

Diabetes Care 2021;44:2645–2655 | https://doi.org/10.2337/dc21-1318

Certain chronic comorbidities, including diabetes, are highly prevalent in people with coronavirus disease 2019 (COVID-19) and are associated with an increased risk of severe COVID-19 and mortality. Mild glucose elevations are also common in COVID-19 patients and associated with worse outcomes even in people without diabetes. Several studies have recently reported new-onset diabetes associated with COVID-19. The phenomenon of new-onset diabetes following admission to the hospital has been observed previously with other viral infections and acute illnesses. The precise mechanisms for new-onset diabetes in people with COVID-19 are not known, but it is likely that a number of complex interrelated processes are involved, including previously undiagnosed diabetes, stress hyperglycemia, steroid-induced hyperglycemia, and direct or indirect effects of severe acute respiratory syndrome coronavirus 2 (SARS-CoV-2) on the β-cell. There is an urgent need for research to help guide management pathways for these patients. In view of increased mortality in people with new-onset diabetes, hospital protocols should include efforts to recognize and manage acute hyperglycemia, including diabetic ketoacidosis, in people admitted to the hospital. Whether new-onset diabetes is likely to remain permanent is not known, as the long-term follow-up of these patients is limited. Prospective studies of metabolism in the setting of postacute COVID-19 will be required to understand the etiology, prognosis, and treatment opportunities.

The severe acute respiratory syndrome coronavirus 2 (SARS-CoV-2) that results in the clinical disease coronavirus disease 2019 (COVID-19) was first reported in December 2019 in Wuhan, China, and has claimed over 2 million lives globally (1). Certain chronic comorbidities, such as hypertension, cardiovascular disease, obesity, diabetes, and kidney disease, are highly prevalent in people with COVID-19. While these comorbidities do not appear to increase the risk of developing COVID-19, they are associated with an increased risk of a more severe case of the condition as well as mortality (2).

HYPERGLYCEMIA AND NEW-ONSET DIABETES ASSOCIATED WITH COVID-19

Severe hyperglycemia is common in critically ill patients and is often seen as a marker of disease severity (3). Several studies over the course of the pandemic have reported that COVID-19 is associated with hyperglycemia in people with and without known diabetes (4,5). One study from Wuhan of hospitalized, mainly elderly COVID-19 patients reported that 21.6% had a history of diabetes, and, based on the first glucose measurement upon admission, 20.8% were newly diagnosed with diabetes (fasting admission glucose ≥7.0 mmol/L and/or

[1]Diabetes Research Centre, University Hospitals of Leicester NHS Trust, Leicester General Hospital, Leicester, U.K.
[2]Section of Diabetes, Department of Clinical and Experimental Medicine, University of Pisa, Pisa, Italy
[3]Laboratory for Clinical and Experimental Endocrinology, Department of Chronic Diseases and Metabolism, KU Leuven, Leuven, Belgium
[4]VA Puget Sound Health Care System and University of Washington, Seattle, WA
[5]Harvard Medical School, Boston, MA
[6]American Diabetes Association, Arlington, VA
[7]Division of Endocrinology and Metabolism, University of North Carolina School of Medicine, Chapel Hill, NC

Corresponding author: Kamlesh Khunti, kk22@leicester.ac.uk

Received 24 June 2021 and accepted 3 September 2021

This article is part of a special article collection available at https://care.diabetesjournals.org/collection/diabetes-and-COVID19.

HbA$_{1c}$ $\geq$6.5%), and 28.4% were diagnosed with dysglycemia (fasting glucose 5.6–6.9 mmol/L and/or HbA$_{1c}$ 5.7–6.4%) (5).

A number of studies have reported new-onset diabetes (that phenotypically could be classified as either type 1 diabetes [T1D] or type 2 diabetes [T2D]) as being associated with the presence of COVID-19 (Table 1). A study from London, U.K., reported 30 children aged 23 months to 16.8 years with new-onset T1D (6). Of these, 70% presented with diabetic ketoacidosis (DKA), 52% with severe DKA, and 15% with a positive COVID-19 test (6). The authors concluded that this represented an 80% increase in new-onset T1D during the pandemic compared with previous years (6). Further, it would also appear that the severity of presentation of youth with T1D is increased (7). Conflicting results have also been reported, however, with data from 216 pediatric diabetes centers in Germany showing no increase in the number of children diagnosed with T1D during the early months of the pandemic (8). However, the same centers reported data on 532 children and adolescents with newly diagnosed T1D and found significant increases in DKA and severe ketoacidosis at diagnosis during the same time period (9).

A few studies have also observed that DKA and hyperosmolar hyperglycemic state are unusually common in COVID-19 patients with known diabetes (10–13). In a Chinese study, 42 patients had COVID-19 and ketoacidosis, and 27 had no prior diagnosis of diabetes (12). A study from London, U.K., included 35 patients with COVID-19 who presented with DKA (31.4%), mixed DKA and hyperosmolar hyperglycemic state (HSS; 31.7%), HSS (5.7%), or hyperglycemic ketoacidosis (25.7%) (14). Overall, 80% had T2D. Of those with T2D, the prevalence of DKA was high, indicating insulinopenia in people with COVID-19. In addition, 5.7% of the 35 patients with COVID-19 had newly diagnosed diabetes. DKA was protracted in people with COVID-19 compared with previous reports of those with non–COVID-19 DKA (35 h vs. 12 h), and they had a higher insulin requirement (14). Another recent U.S. study of 5,029 patients (mean age 47 years) from 175 hospitals found that patients with COVID-19 had higher BMI, higher insulin requirement,

prolonged time to resolution of DKA, and higher mortality than those without COVID-19 (15). A U.K. study reported that children presented more frequently with DKA than during the prepandemic period (10% severe prepandemic vs. 47% during the first wave of the pandemic) and had higher HbA$_{1c}$ (13% vs. 10.4%) (7).

A number of studies have also reported that preexisting diabetes as well as newly diagnosed diabetes with a first glucose measurement on hospital admission are both associated with an increased risk of all-cause mortality in hospitalized patients with COVID-19. In a systematic review of 3,711 COVID-19 patients from 8 studies (492 patients with new-onset diabetes), the pooled prevalence of new-onset diabetes was 14.4% (95% CI 5.9–25.8%) from a random-effect meta-analysis (16). Worryingly, the risk of mortality appears to be higher in people with new-onset diabetes than with COVID-19 patients with known diabetes (5,17). An Italian study of 271 people admitted with COVID-19, 20.7% of whom had preexisting diabetes, found that hyperglycemia was independently associated with mortality (hazards ratio [HR] 1.80, 95% CI 1.03–3.15). The study also showed that people with diabetes and hyperglycemia had worse inflammatory profiles (18). In a study from Wuhan, China, patients with newly diagnosed diabetes were more likely to be admitted to the intensive care unit, require invasive mechanical ventilation, have a high prevalence of acute respiratory distress syndrome, acute kidney injury, or shock, and have the longest hospital stays (5). The study also reported data showing that glucose levels at hospital admission in people with newly diagnosed diabetes and in those with a history of diabetes were both associated with the increased risk of all-cause mortality (5). Patients with newly diagnosed diabetes had a higher mortality than COVID-19 patients with known diabetes, hyperglycemia (fasting glucose 5.6–6.9 mmol/L and/or HbA$_{1c}$ 5.7–6.4%) or normal glucose (HR 9.42, 95% CI 2.18–40.7). This is one of a few studies where HbA$_{1c}$ was measured on admission to determine whether newly diagnosed diabetes was present in asymptomatic patients prior to admission or whether those who developed it did so following admission (5).

TYPE OF DIABETES

It is currently unclear whether the new-onset diabetes associated with COVID-19 is type 1, type 2, or a complex subtype of diabetes. Although in T1D insulin deficiency is usually the result of an autoimmune process, in SARS-CoV-2 infection it could be due to destruction of the β-cells. Unfortunately, studies of islet cell antibodies in people with new-onset diabetes have been limited to a few case reports (19,20). Multiple studies have reported a high number of incidents of DKA in people with and without COVID-19, suggesting a direct effect of SARS-CoV-2 on pancreatic β-cells. One study of hospitalized patients with SARS-CoV-1 infection showed that immunostaining for angiotensin-converting enzyme 2 (ACE2) protein was strong in pancreatic islets but weak in exocrine tissues (21). However, a recent study from India compared new-onset diabetes in hospitalized patients prior to COVID-19 with new-onset diabetes during COVID-19 and found worse glycemic parameters in new-onset diabetes during COVID-19 and diabetes but no difference in symptoms, phenotype, or C-peptide levels (22).

POTENTIAL MECHANISMS FOR NEW-ONSET DIABETES

The precise mechanisms behind the development of new-onset diagnosis in people with COVID-19 are not known, but it is likely that a number of complex, interrelated etiologies are responsible, including impairments in both glucose disposal and insulin secretion, stress hyperglycemia, preadmission diabetes, and steroid-induced diabetes (Fig. 1). One recent article reported an increase in the number of children admitted to pediatric intensive care unit with new-onset T1D with severe DKA and a smaller increase in incidence of new-onset T1D (23). Overall, 7/20 (35%) of the children diagnosed in 2020 were tested for SAR-CoV-2, with all being negative. The authors suggested that the increase in incidence and severity were due to altered presentation during the pandemic rather than direct effects of COVID-19. Current data also suggest a bidirectional relationship between T2D and COVID-19 (24), but whether there is a bidirectional relationship between hyperglycemia and COVID-19

Table 1—Studies reporting new-onset diabetes

Reference	Country	Design	Population	Results
Li et al. (5)	China	Retrospective observational	453 patients with laboratory-confirmed SARS-CoV-2 infection aged 61 (IQR 49, 68) years	94 patients (21%) were newly diagnosed with diabetes (fasting admission glucose ≥7.0 mmol/L and/or HbA_{1c} ≥6.5%)
Unsworth et al. (6)	U.K.	Cross-sectional	33 children aged 10.9 (IQR 6.8) years, 68% male, 36% White European	30 children (91%) presented with new-onset T1D; 5 children tested positive for SARS-CoV-2; 70% presented with DKA and 52% with severe DKA
Ebekozien et al. (17)	U.S.	Cross-sectional	64 children and adults aged 20.9 (SD 14.84) years, 61% female, 48.4% non-Hispanic White	6 patients (9.8%) had new-onset T1D, with 5 (15.6%) in the COVID-19–positive group
Tittel et al. (8)	Germany	Prospective study	Pediatric T1D patients with onset age between 6 months and <18 years diagnosed between 13 March and 13 May in each year between 2011 and 2020 (from German Diabetes Registry data)	T1D incidence (per 100,000 patient-years) increased from 16.4 in 2011 to 22.2 in 2019; the incidence in 2020 (23.4) did not significantly differ from the predicted value
Armeni et al. (14)	U.K.	Retrospective case series	35 patients with SARS-CoV-2 infection aged 60 (IQR 45, 70) years, 22.9% female, 20% Caucasian; inclusion criteria were 1) hospitalization with confirmed COVID-19 diagnosis, 2) DKA and/or hyperosmolar hyperglycemic state at presentation, 3) known or new diagnosis of diabetes and presence of ketonemia, and 4) Glasgow coma scale of at least 12 on admission	28 (80%) patients had T2D, and 2 (5.7%) were new presentations of diabetes
Sathish et al. (16)	China, Italy, U.S.	Systematic review and meta-analysis	From 8 studies, 3,711 COVID-19 patients, aged between 47 and 64.9 years, 53.3–80.0% male	492 patients had newly diagnosed diabetes, and random-effect meta-analysis estimated a pooled prevalence of new-onset diabetes of 14.4% (95% CI 5.9–25.8%)
Wang et al. (64)	China	Retrospective study	605 patients with SARS-CoV-2 infection, aged 59.0 (IQR 47.0, 68.0) years, 46.8% female; exclusion criteria were 1) no definitive 28-day outcome since transfer to another hospital, 2) missing key clinical information, 3) no FBG data available at admission, and 4) having previously diagnosed diabetes	176 patients (29.1%) with new-onset/newly detected diabetes

Continued on p. 2648

Table 1—Continued

Reference	Country	Design	Population	Results
Yang et al. (65)	China	Retrospective cohort study	69 patients with laboratory-confirmed SARS-CoV-2 infection aged 61 (IQR 52, 57) years, 49.3% male; exclusion criteria were patients receiving glucocorticoid treatment or with a history of diabetes, myocardial infarction, heart failure, dialysis, renal transplant, or cirrhosis and patients missing basic medical information	In critical and moderate + severe patients the prevalence of new-onset diabetes was 53.85% and 13.95%, respectively
Fadini et al. (66)	Italy	Retrospective study	413 patients with SARS-CoV-2 infection aged 64.9 (SD 15.4) years, 59.3% male	21 patients (5%) with new-onset/newly detected diabetes
Wu et al. (46)	Australia	Retrospectively analyzed	8 patients with T2D were admitted to the intensive care unit with COVID-19; 5 had preexisting diabetes	Within patients with newly diagnosed diabetes, C-peptide levels and negative anti-GAD antibodies were found, consistent with T2D, and HbA_{1c} ranged from 11.1% to 12.4% (98 to 112 mmol/mol)
Ghosh et al. (22)	India	Retrospective cohort	555 patients with new-onset diabetes were included, with 282 with new-onset diabetes prior to the COVID-19 pandemic (19 September to 20 February) and 273 with new-onset diabetes during COVID-19 (April–October 20)	Patients with new-onset diabetes during the COVID-19 pandemic had higher fasting and postprandial blood glucose, glycated hemoglobin levels, and C-peptide vs. patients with new-onset diabetes prior to pandemic; no differences were seen in C-peptide or glycemic outcomes in the patients with new-onset diabetes between those who tested positive or negative for COVID-19 (antibody test)
Zhang et al. (67)	China	Retrospective study	312 patients with COVID-19 with a mean age of 57 (IQR 38, 66) years; 55% were female, 84 had diabetes, and 36 were new diagnoses (57 had fasting glucose levels ≥7.0 mmol/L, including 30 without and 27 with a known history of diabetes); exclusion criteria included no positive COVID-19 test, patients remaining in hospital, and missing information on clinical outcomes because of transfer to other hospitals	Diabetes at admission was associated with higher risks of adverse outcomes among patients with COVID-19 (irrespective of whether or not the diagnosis was new)

Continued on p. 2649

Table 1—Continued

Reference	Country	Design	Population	Results
Smith et al. (68)	U.S.	Retrospective study	184 patients hospitalized for COVID-19, aged 64.4 years (range 21–100), 67.7% female	6 patients without diabetes and with normal HbA$_{1c}$ levels also had repeatedly elevated fasting blood glucose; these 29 patients had fasting blood glucose levels consistent with new-onset diabetes and temporally associated with recent acquisition of SARS-CoV-2 infection
Liu et al. (69)	China	Retrospective study	In total, 233 patients were included in the final analysis; 80 (34.3%) patients had diabetes, among whom 44 (55.0%) were previously diagnosed and 36 (45.0%) were newly defined as having undiagnosed diabetes with an HbA$_{1c}$ level ≥6.5% (48 mmol/mol) at admission	Risk of in-hospital death was significantly increased in all patients with diabetes (HR 3.80, 95% CI 1.71–8.47), those with diagnosed diabetes (HR 4.03, 95% CI 1.64–9.91), and those with undiagnosed diabetes who were newly defined by HbA$_{1c}$ testing at admission (HR 1.89, 95% CI 1.18–3.05) compared with those without diabetes

IQR, interquartile range.

is not known (Fig. 2). The following sections give more detailed discussions of some of the proposed mechanisms for new-onset diabetes associated with COVID-19.

Preexisting Undiagnosed Diabetes
One reason for new-onset diabetes is that these patients may have had undetected diabetes prior to admission, potentially as a consequence of recent weight gain due to changes in lifestyle and worsening of hyperglycemia mainly due to self-isolation, social distancing, reduced physical activity, and poor diets as a result of mental health issues. For example, a recent survey of 155 countries showed that 53% of individuals had reduced their preventative- and service-level access for noncommunicable diseases either partly or completely (25). These lifestyle changes could lead to insulin resistance, which would further trigger inflammatory pathways, leading to new-onset diabetes.

Stress Hyperglycemia and New-Onset Diabetes Following Acute Illness
The phenomenon of hyperglycemia and new-onset diabetes following admission

to the hospital with acute illness is not new and was previously observed during the SARS-CoV-1 outbreak, where new-onset diabetes without glucocorticoid use on admission was also associated with increased mortality (26). Stress hyperglycemia is a sign of relative insulin deficiency, which is associated with increased lipolysis and increased circulating free fatty acids seen in acute illness such as myocardial infarction or severe infections (27). In COVID-19, stress hyperglycemia may be even more severe due to the cytokine storm.

Studies have shown that patients with newly diagnosed diabetes have higher levels of inflammatory markers such as C-reactive protein, erythrocyte sedimentation rate, and white blood cells (5). Acute inflammation seen in cytokine storm may worsen insulin resistance (10), with one study showing neutrophils, D-dimers, and inflammatory markers being significantly higher in those with hyperglycemia than in those with normal glucose (18). People with obesity are also at risk for diabetes and severe outcomes related to COVID-19 (28), with adiposity being a driver for impaired glucose metabolism, immune responses, and inflammation (10).

Previous studies have reported stress hyperglycemia after several acute conditions, including myocardial infarction. However, there have been difficulties in interpretation of these studies due to the variable definitions used to define new-onset diabetes and stress hyperglycemia. One systematic review of 15 studies of patients admitted with myocardial infarction without diabetes with a glucose level in the range 6.1–8.2 mmol/L was associated with a 3.5-fold (95% CI 2.9–5.4) higher risk of death than that for patients without diabetes with lower glucose concentrations (27). This meta-analysis also reported that glucose values in the range of 8.0–10.0 mmol/L on admission were associated with an increased risk of congestive heart failure or cardiogenic shock in people without diabetes (27), and the risk of death was increased by 70% (relative risk 1.7, 95% CI 1.2–2.4) (27). Stress hyperglycemia following myocardial infarction has also been shown to be associated with an increased risk of in-hospital mortality in patients with and without diabetes (27). Another systematic review of 43 studies totaling 536,476 patients showed that stress

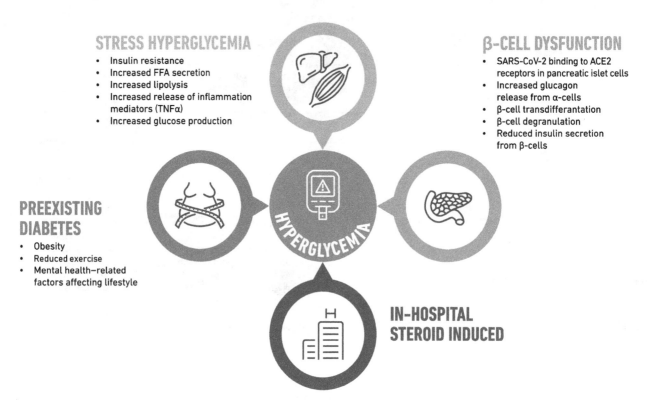

Figure 1—Potential mechanisms for development of new-onset diabetes in people with COVID-19.

hyperglycemia was associated with increased mortality, intensive care unit admission, hospital length of stay, and mechanical ventilation (29).

Although stress-related hyperglycemia in acutely ill hospitalized patients occurs in many settings, the data related to new-onset diabetes due to SARS-CoV-2 seem to suggest that the prevalence is disproportionate compared with data from populations admitted with other acute illnesses (16). A number of studies have reported stress hyperglycemia following critical acute illness; however, only a few studies have followed these patients beyond hospitalization to determine if the stress hyperglycemia is transient or indicative of new-onset diabetes. One meta-analysis of four cohort studies with 2,923 participants included 698 (23.9%) people with stress hyperglycemia. On follow-up more than 3 months after hospital discharge, 131 cases or 18.8% of people with stress hyperglycemia were identified with

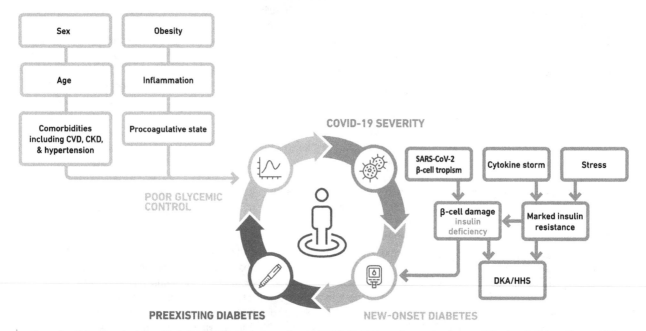

Figure 2—Bidirectional relationship between T2D, hyperglycemia, and COVID-19. CVD, cardiovascular disease; CKD, chronic kidney disease; HHS, hyperosmolar hyperglycemic syndrome.

newly diagnosed diabetes, and stress hyperglycemia was associated with an increased incidence of diabetes (odds ratio [OR] 3.48, 95% CI 2.02–5.98) (30). However, three studies defined stress hyperglycemia as blood glucose of ≥7.8 mmol/L, and one database study defined it as a glucose of >11.1 mmol/L. Furthermore, the timing of glucose measurement was not reported in any of these studies.

Viral Infections and New-Onset Diabetes

Viral infections may have a direct or indirect effect on the pancreas. Previous studies have reported acute inflammation in the pancreas due to other viruses, such as human immunodeficiency virus, mumps, measles, cytomegalovirus virus, herpes simplex virus, and hepatitis virus (13). A meta-analysis of 24 case-control studies showed that enterovirus infection was significantly associated with T1D-related autoimmunity (OR 3.7, 95% CI 2.1–6.8) and clinical T1D (OR 9.8, 95% CI 5.5–17.4) (31). Another meta-analysis of 34 studies showed that there was a significantly increased risk of T2D with hepatitis C viral infection compared with noninfected control subjects in both retrospective (OR 1.68, 95% CI 1.15–2.20) and prospective (OR 1.67, 95% CI 1.28–2.06) studies. The excess risk was also observed compared with hepatitis B virus–infected control subjects (OR 1.80, 95% CI 1.20–1.40) (32). Studies of human islet cells have shown that coxsackie B viruses cause functional impairment or β-cell death (33).

Acute hyperglycemia with coronavirus infection has been linked to the binding of the coronavirus to the ACE2 receptor in the pancreatic islet cells (30). ACE2 expression has been shown to be higher in the pancreas than the lungs and expressed in both exocrine glands and the islets of the pancreas, including β-cells (34,35). However, the evidence for ACE2 expression in pancreatic cells is conflicting, with studies suggesting ACE2 expression in a limited subset of β-cells (36). Data from human pancreatic tissues identified ACE2 expression in pancreatic ductal epithelium and microvasculature and concluded that SARS-CoV-2 infection of pancreatic endocrine cells (including β-cells) is unlikely to be a central mechanism related to diabetes (37). Alternatively, the proinflammatory cytokines and acute-phase reactants due to COVID-19 could directly cause inflammation and damage to pancreatic β-cells (38).

A cytokine storm in people infected with SARS-CoV-2 is a prothrombotic, highly inflammatory pathological state that can have direct and indirect effects on pancreatic β-cells. An autopsy study of three patients who died of COVID-19 in China reported they had degeneration of islets (39). A study from Wuhan of 121 COVID-19 patients showed that even patients with mild COVID-19 had increased levels of amylase and lipase (1.85%), although people with severe COVID-19 had much higher levels (17%) (34). Some patients also had symptoms of acute pancreatitis. In this study, computed tomography scans of people with severe COVID-19 showed changes in the pancreas that comprised mainly enlargement of the pancreas or dilation of the pancreatic duct without acute necrosis (34). A recent study of gene and protein expression in live human pancreatic cultures and postmortem pancreatic tissue from COVID-19 patients observed that SARS-CoV-2 can infect pancreatic cells and indicated that endocrine islets and exocrine acinar and ductal cells within the pancreas allow SARS-CoV-2 entry (40). Another study reported that the SARS-CoV-2 receptor and ACE2 and related entry factors are expressed in the pancreatic β-cells, and in COVID-19 patients they infect β-cells, attenuate pancreatic insulin levels and secretion, and induce β-cell apoptosis (41).

In-Hospital Steroid-Induced Hyperglycemia

Steroid-induced hyperglycemia is common in hospitalized patients. Previous studies show that 53–70% of individuals without diabetes develop steroid-induced hyperglycemia (42). An Australian study of 80 hospitalized people without diabetes reported that 70% of subjects had at least one blood glucose measurement of ≥10 mmol/L (43). A meta-analysis of 13 studies showed that overall, 32.3% of people developed glucocorticoid-induced hyperglycemia and 18.6% developed diabetes (44). Use of steroids, particularly following the publication of the RECOVERY trial with the use of dexamethasone in people admitted to the hospital with COVID-19, may therefore also be associated with an increased risk of developing diabetes, which again could be directly related to steroid-induced abnormalities with delayed or blunted recovery of βcell damage (10).

MANAGEMENT OF PEOPLE WITH NEW-ONSET DIABETES FOLLOWING COVID-19

As the precise mechanisms and epidemiology of new-onset diabetes related to COVID-19 are not known, it is difficult to guide management pathways for these patients. However, in view of increased mortality in people with new-onset diabetes and in those with elevated glucose at admission, hospital protocols should include management of acute hyperglycemia. It is also imperative to recognize new-onset diabetes and manage DKA in people admitted to the hospital to improve outcomes. These patients frequently also require higher doses of insulin than those with acute illness caused by other conditions or non–COVID-19 DKA (18,45,46).

Whether hospital admission of new-onset diabetes is likely to remain permanent is not known, as long-term follow-up of these patients is limited. People with stress hyperglycemia may revert to normoglycemia following the recovery from acute illness and, therefore, may not be classed as having diabetes or requiring any glucose-lowering medication; they will require follow-up to determine if the new-onset diabetes is indeed permanent.

Although there are no data on follow-up of newly diagnosed people with diabetes related to COVID-19, one systematic review of four cohort studies with a 3-month follow-up reported 18.8% with newly diagnosed diabetes in those who were diagnosed with in-hospital hyperglycemia. However, studies differed in their definitions of stress hyperglycemia, participants included, and follow-up (30). In another prospective study, 181 consecutive patients admitted with myocardial infarction in Sweden with an admission glucose of ≥11.1 mmol/L had a 75-g oral glucose tolerance test at 3 months postdischarge (47). Overall, 35% and 40% of patients, respectively, had impaired glucose tolerance at discharge and at 3 months postdischarge, and 31% and 25%, respectively, had new-onset diabetes (47).

A recent case series from India reported that three individuals who had

COVID-19 and developed acute-onset diabetes and DKA initially responded to treatment with intravenous fluid and insulin. They were then transitioned to multiple doses of subcutaneous insulin, and, at follow-up of 4–6 weeks, all had their insulin stopped and were initiated on oral glucose-lowering agents (20). Two patients had GAD antibody measured and were both negative. Although new-acute-onset diabetes with DKA in adults would normally indicate T1D, these case data suggest that these patients have had a transient insulinopenia.

Persistent diabetes in COVID-19 patients may also be related to "long COVID," also known as post–COVID-19 syndrome or post-acute sequelae of COVID-19 (PASC), defined as persistence of symptoms beyond 3 months postinfection. It frequently affects multiple organ systems and is estimated to affect 10% of COVID-19 patients (48,49). Long COVID is complex due to varying symptoms and pathophysiology (48,49) but may be due to immune and inflammatory responses seen in many severe acute viral infections (49). The risks of cardiorenal complications are high in people admitted with COVID-19, and a meta-analysis of 44 studies showed that the prevalence of cardiorenal complications is high in people with long COVID, with acute cardiac injury occurring in 15%, venous thromboembolism in 15%, and acute kidney injury in 6% (50).

As risk factors for poor outcomes in people with COVID-19 include obesity, hyperglycemia, and cardiovascular and renal disease, glucose-lowering agents that improve metabolic function without weight gain would be preferable for long-term management of people following acute COVID-19 infection and sustained symptoms (i.e., long COVID). Novel therapeutic options include sodium–glucose cotransporter 2 inhibitors (SGLT2i) and glucagon-like peptide 1 receptor agonists (GLP-1RAs), particularly as cardiovascular outcome trials in people with T2D have confirmed benefits on weight, glycemic control, and cardiovascular events, including cardiovascular death and renal outcomes (51). SGLT2i have also been shown to reduce hospitalization for heart failure and may reduce the risk of death from noncardiovascular causes (51). However, data for these therapies in management of patients with long COVID are lacking.

The DARE-19 study investigating the safety of dapagliflozin in people admitted to the hospital with COVID-19 have recently been reported (52). The study showed that the primary end points were not achieved; namely, dapagliflozin did not prevent organ dysfunction (pulmonary, cardiac, or renal) or death and did not improve clinical recovery within 30 days following commencing the medication. However, DKA was reported in two patients with T2D of the 625 patients in the dapagliflozin arm, with the events being nonsevere and resolving after study medication discontinuation. Other therapeutic trials are ongoing with dipeptidyl peptidase 4 inhibitors, pioglitazone, and the GLP-1RA semaglutide (53–58).

Long-term follow-up of patients with COVID-19 and hyperglycemia will therefore be required to determine whether they would still need glucose-lowering agents. A recent study from China reported new-onset diabetes in 3.3% of 1,733 people at 6 months following discharge from hospital with COVID-19 (59). Another study from England of 47,780 people discharged from hospital following admission for COVID-19 showed 4.9% developed diabetes at a mean follow-up of 140 days (60). Another study using a national health care database of the U.S. Department of Veterans Affairs reported a higher burden of new-onset diabetes 6 months following COVID-19 (61). However, none of these studies reported any further details regarding new-onset diabetes, including type of diabetes. COVID-19–related hyperglycemia and new-onset diabetes are new findings and of great interest globally. However, it remains to be seen if hyperglycemia associated with COVID-19 is indeed associated with a higher prevalence of new-onset diabetes after acute and chronic illness. The diagnosis of diabetes will need to be based on fasting glucose, 2-h post–oral glucose tolerance test, or HbA$_{1c}$ as recommended by international guidelines (62). Previous studies have demonstrated that new-onset diabetes is associated with the level of in-hospital hyperglycemia. One systematic review of 18 studies (111,078 patients) admitted with acute or chronic illness reported new-onset diabetes in 4% (95% CI 2–7%), 12% (95% CI 9–15%), and 28% (95% CI 18–39%) of patients with in-hospital normoglycemia, mild hyperglycemia, and severe hyperglycemia,

respectively (3). Studies in the meta-analysis had a mean follow-up of 3–60 months without significant effect on diabetes incidence.

It will also be important to continue long-term surveillance of people with new-onset diabetes to ensure their risk factors are managed and that they achieve good glycemic control, as many may also have other symptoms of long COVID. Stress hyperglycemia due to acute critical illness may also identify patients who are already at high risk of diabetes, and therefore early diagnosis, interventions, and long-term follow-up of complications are essential for these patients. Whether screening everyone following a diagnosis of COVID-19 for diabetes and prediabetes would identify a significant number of people or is cost-effective remains to be seen. However, there may be a case for this, as many international guidelines recommend screening high-risk populations for diabetes and prediabetes and, if identified, to then manage people with diabetes according to international guidelines or lifestyle intervention of people with prediabetes. In view of the associated cardiovascular and renal damage following COVID-19, these patients should have regular monitoring of cardiovascular and kidney risk factors with a view to tight risk factor control. These patients may also benefit from regular screening for microvascular and macrovascular complications.

FUTURE RESEARCH RECOMMENDATIONS

New-onset diabetes in relation to COVID-19 is a new phenomenon and provides an opportunity to observe these patients longer term and conduct research studies that include epidemiological and interventional approaches. An international group of researchers have already established a global registry of patients with new-onset COVID-19–related diabetes, called the CoviDIAB Project, and will report on findings in future (63). However, further international collaborative research programs are urgently needed to understand the natural disease epidemiology of COVID-19.

Recommendations for future studies should include the following:
• Multicenter prospective cohort studies following these patients for several

years to assess the trajectory of new-onset diabetes with COVID-19 and quantify whether the risks of admission-related hyperglycemia and new-onset diabetes with COVID-19 are different from usual-onset diabetes.

- Investigation of pathophysiology by cross-sectional and prospective studies to assess β-cell function and insulin resistance in people with COVID-19 related to new-onset diabetes.
- Experimental studies of direct effects of SARS-CoV-2 on pancreatic β-cells and other islet cell types.
- Assessment of inflammatory markers to get full understanding of new-onset COVID-19–related diabetes.
- Development and validation of methods of screening for diabetes in people who have developed COVID-19–related hyperglycemia.
- Modeling of cost-effectiveness of targeted screening of people following COVID-19.
- Evaluation of management plans and models of care that may be appropriate to this phenomenon.
- Determination of prevalence and impact of long COVID in people with new-onset diabetes.
- Comparisons of longer-term outcomes of people with COVID-19–related new-onset diabetes with new-onset diabetes due to other acute illnesses (such as other infections and myocardial infarction).
- Understanding of the benefits and cost-effectiveness of use of different therapeutic options, including novel therapies such as SGLT2i and GLP-1RAs.

CONCLUSIONS

Recently published studies suggest that COVID-19 is associated with new-onset diabetes; therefore, there is potential to identify and manage these people early, with the aim of improving long-term outcomes. Whether elevated glucose concentrations (in a non-diabetes range) or new-onset diabetes is due to immune-mediated and inflammatory responses, the direct effect of SARS-CoV-2 on β-cells, or a complex combination of mechanisms, is not known. The majority of studies have mainly assessed patients who have been hospitalized with COVID-19, and there are no or limited data on patients with milder illness managed in

the community. There are also no data on long-term outcomes of people with diabetes and COVID-19 and their risk of long COVID. New-onset diabetes with SARS-CoV-2 infection also appears to be a complex syndrome associated with a number of pathophysiological mechanisms and, given we are still in the midst of a global COVID-19 pandemic, are likely to see even larger numbers of people globally with new-onset diabetes. International efforts need to be established to study COVID-19–associated new-onset diabetes with follow-up of large numbers of patients.

Funding. K.K. is supported by the National Institute for Health Research (NIHR) Applied Research Collaboration East Midlands and the NIHR Leicester Biomedical Research Centre. J.B.B. is supported by grants from the National Institutes of Health (UL1TR002489 and P30DK124723). S.E.K. is supported by the United States Department of Veterans Affairs.

The views expressed are those of the authors and not necessarily those of the NIHR, National Health Service, or the Department of Health and Social Care.

Duality of Interest. K.K. has acted as a consultant or speaker or received grants for investigator-initiated studies for AstraZeneca, Novartis, Novo Nordisk, Sanofi, Lilly and Merck Sharp & Dohme, Boehringer Ingelheim, Bayer, Berlin-Chemie AG/Menarini Group, Janssen, and Napp. S.D.P. has served on the advisory panel for AstraZeneca, Boehringer Ingelheim, Eli Lilly and Co., GlaxoSmithKline, Merck & Co., Novartis Pharmaceuticals, Novo Nordisk, Sanofi, and Takeda Pharmaceuticals. He received research support from AstraZeneca and Boehringer Ingelheim. C.M. serves or has served on the advisory panel for Novo Nordisk, Sanofi, Merck Sharp & Dohme, Eli Lilly and Co., Novartis, AstraZeneca, Boehringer Ingelheim, Roche, Medtronic, ActoBio Therapeutics, Pfizer, Insulet, and Zealand Pharma. Financial compensation for these activities has been received by KU Leuven. KU Leuven has received research support for C.M. from Medtronic, Novo Nordisk, Sanofi, and ActoBio Therapeutics. C.M. serves or has served on the speakers bureau for Novo Nordisk, Sanofi, Eli Lilly and Co., Boehringer Ingelheim, Astra Zeneca, and Novartis. Financial compensation for these activities has been received by KU Leuven. S.E.K. has served as a consultant and on advisory boards for Bayer, Boehringer Ingelheim, Casma Therapeutics, Eli Lilly and Co., Intarcia, Merck, Novo Nordisk, Pfizer, and Third Rock Ventures and as a speaker for Boehringer Ingelheim and Merck. R.A.G. is an advisor to Onduo, Vida Health, Lark, and HealthReveal. J.B.B.'s contracted consulting fees and travel support for contracted activities are paid to the University of North Carolina by Adocia, Novo Nordisk, Senseonics, and vTv Therapeutics, as well as grant support from Dexcom, NovaTarg, Novo Nordisk, Sanofi,

Tolerion, and vTv Therapeutics. He is also a consultant to Anji, AstraZeneca, Boehringer Ingelheim, Cirius Therapeutics Inc., Eli Lilly and Co., Fortress Biotech, Glycadia, Glyscend, Janssen, Mellitus Health, Moderna, Pendulum Therapeutics, Praetego, Stability Health, and Zealand Pharma. He holds stock/options in Glyscend, Mellitus Health, Pendulum Therapeutics, Phase-Bio, Praetego, and Stability Health.

Author Contributions. K.K. researched the data for this review. K.K. wrote the first draft of this manuscript, and all other authors contributed to and provided critical feedback and edits on the manuscript. K.K. is the guarantor of this work and, as such, had full access to all the data in the study and takes responsibility for the integrity of the review and its conclusions.

References

1. Worldometer. Worldometer COVID-19 data. Accessed 27 July 2020. Available from https://www.worldometers.info/coronavirus/about
2. Singh AK, Gillies CL, Singh R, et al. Prevalence of co-morbidities and their association with mortality in patients with COVID-19: a systematic review and meta-analysis. Diabetes Obes Metab 2020;22:1915–1924
3. Jivanji CJ, Asrani VM, Windsor JA, Petrov MS. New-onset diabetes after acute and critical illness: a systematic review. Mayo Clin Proc 2017;92:762–773
4. Bode B, Garrett V, Messler J, et al. Glycemic characteristics and clinical outcomes of COVID-19 patients hospitalized in the United States. J Diabetes Sci Technol 2020;14:813–821
5. Li H, Tian S, Chen T, et al. Newly diagnosed diabetes is associated with a higher risk of mortality than known diabetes in hospitalized patients with COVID-19. Diabetes Obes Metab 2020;22:1897–1906
6. Unsworth R, Wallace S, Oliver NS, et al. New-onset type 1 diabetes in children during COVID-19: multicenter regional findings in the U.K. Diabetes Care 2020;43:e170–e171
7. McGlacken-Byrne SM, Drew SEV, Turner K, Peters C, Amin R. The SARS-CoV-2 pandemic is associated with increased severity of presentation of childhood onset type 1 diabetes mellitus: a multi-centre study of the first COVID-19 wave. Diabet Med 2021;38:e14640
8. Tittel SR, Rosenbauer J, Kamrath C, et al.; DPV Initiative. Did the COVID-19 lockdown affect the incidence of pediatric type 1 diabetes in Germany? Diabetes Care 2020;43:e172–e173
9. Kamrath C, Mönkemöller K, Biester T, et al. Ketoacidosis in children and adolescents with newly diagnosed type 1 diabetes during the COVID-19 pandemic in Germany. JAMA 2020; 324:801–804
10. Accili D. Can COVID-19 cause diabetes? Nat Metab 2021;3:123–125
11. Alraddadi BM, Watson JT, Almarashi A, et al. Risk factors for primary Middle East respiratory syndrome coronavirus illness in humans, Saudi Arabia, 2014. Emerg Infect Dis 2016;22:49–55
12. Li J, Wang X, Chen J, Zuo X, Zhang H, Deng A. COVID-19 infection may cause ketosis and ketoacidosis. Diabetes Obes Metab 2020;22: 1935–1941

13. Rawla P, Bandaru SS, Vellipuram AR. Review of infectious etiology of acute pancreatitis. Gastroenterol Res 2017;10:153–158

14. Armeni E, Aziz U, Qamar S, et al. Protracted ketonaemia in hyperglycaemic emergencies in COVID-19: a retrospective case series. Lancet Diabetes Endocrinol 2020;8:660–663

15. Pasquel FJ, Messler J, Booth R, et al. Characteristics of and mortality associated with diabetic ketoacidosis among US patients hospitalized with or without COVID-19. JAMA Netw Open 2021;4:e211091

16. Sathish T, Kapoor N, Cao Y, Tapp RJ, Zimmet P. Proportion of newly diagnosed diabetes in COVID-19 patients: a systematic review and meta-analysis. Diabetes Obes Metab 2021;23:870–874

17. Ebekozien OA, Noor N, Gallagher MP, Alonso GT. Type 1 diabetes and COVID-19: preliminary findings from a multicenter surveillance study in the U.S. Diabetes Care 2020;43:e83–e85

18. Coppelli A, Giannarelli R, Aragona M, et al.; Pisa COVID-19 Study Group. Hyperglycemia at hospital admission is associated with severity of the prognosis in patients hospitalized for COVID-19: the Pisa COVID-19 study. Diabetes Care 2020;43:2345–2348

19. Hollstein T, Schulte DM, Schulz J, et al. Autoantibody-negative insulin-dependent diabetes mellitus after SARS-CoV-2 infection: a case report. Nat Metab 2020;2:1021–1024

20. Kuchay MS, Reddy PK, Gagneja S, Mathew A, Mishra SK. Short term follow-up of patients presenting with acute onset diabetes and diabetic ketoacidosis during an episode of COVID-19. Diabetes Metab Syndr 2020;14:2039–2041

21. Yang JK, Lin SS, Ji XJ, Guo LM. Binding of SARS coronavirus to its receptor damages islets and causes acute diabetes. Acta Diabetol 2010;47:193–199

22. Ghosh A, Anjana RM, Shanthi Rani CS, et al. Glycemic parameters in patients with new-onset diabetes during COVID-19 pandemic are more severe than in patients with new-onset diabetes before the pandemic: NOD COVID India study. Diabetes Metab Syndr 2021;15:215–220

23. Salmi H, Heinonen S, Hästbacka J, et al. New-onset type 1 diabetes in Finnish children during the COVID-19 pandemic. Arch Dis Child 27 May 2021 [Epub ahead of print]. DOI: https://doi.org/10.1136/archdischild-2020-321220

24. Muniangi-Muhitu H, Akalestou E, Salem V, Misra S, Oliver NS, Rutter GA. Covid-19 and diabetes: a complex bidirectional relationship. Front Endocrinol (Lausanne) 2020;11:582936

25. World Health Organization. COVID-19 significantly impacts health services for noncommunicable diseases. Published 1 June 2020. Accessed 12 March 2021. Available from https://www.who.int/news/item/01-06-2020-covid-19-significantly-impacts-health-services-for-noncommunicable-diseases

26. Yang JK, Feng Y, Yuan MY, et al. Plasma glucose levels and diabetes are independent predictors for mortality and morbidity in patients with SARS. Diabet Med 2006;23:623–628

27. Capes SE, Hunt D, Malmberg K, Gerstein HC. Stress hyperglycaemia and increased risk of death after myocardial infarction in patients with and without diabetes: a systematic overview. Lancet 2000;355:773–778

28. Seidu S, Gillies C, Zaccardi F, et al. The impact of obesity on severe disease and mortality in people with SARS-CoV-2: a systematic review and meta-analysis. Endocrinol Diabetes Metab 2020;e00176:e00176

29. Olariu E, Pooley N, Danel A, Miret M, Preiser JC. A systematic scoping review on the consequences of stress-related hyperglycaemia. PLoS One 2018;13:e0194952

30. Ali Abdelhamid Y, Kar P, Finnis ME, et al. Stress hyperglycaemia in critically ill patients and the subsequent risk of diabetes: a systematic review and meta-analysis. Crit Care 2016;20:301

31. Yeung WC, Rawlinson WD, Craig ME. Enterovirus infection and type 1 diabetes mellitus: systematic review and meta-analysis of observational molecular studies. BMJ 2011;342:d35

32. White DL, Ratziu V, El-Serag HB. Hepatitis C infection and risk of diabetes: a systematic review and meta-analysis. J Hepatol 2008;49:831–844

33. Roivainen M, Rasilainen S, Ylipaasto P, et al. Mechanisms of coxsackievirus-induced damage to human pancreatic beta-cells. J Clin Endocrinol Metab 2000;85:432–440

34. Liu F, Long X, Zhang B, Zhang W, Chen X, Zhang Z. ACE2 expression in pancreas may cause pancreatic damage after SARS-CoV-2 infection. Clin Gastroenterol Hepatol 2020;18:2128–2130.e2

35. Fignani D, Licata G, Brusco N, et al. SARS-CoV-2 receptor angiotensin I-converting enzyme type 2 (ACE2) is expressed in human pancreatic β-cells and in the human pancreas microvasculature. Front Endocrinol (Lausanne) 2020;11:596898

36. Atkinson MA, Powers AC. Distinguishing the real from the hyperglycaemia: does COVID-19 induce diabetes? Lancet Diabetes Endocrinol 2021;9:328–329

37. Kusmartseva I, Wu W, Syed F, et al. Expression of SARS-CoV-2 entry factors in the pancreas of normal organ donors and individuals with COVID-19. Cell Metab 2020;32:1041–1051.e6

38. Ahlqvist E, Storm P, Käräjämäki A, et al. Novel subgroups of adult-onset diabetes and their association with outcomes: a data-driven cluster analysis of six variables. Lancet Diabetes Endocrinol 2018;6:361–369

39. Yao XH, Li TY, He ZC, et al. [A pathological report of three COVID-19 cases by minimal invasive autopsies]. Zhonghua Bing Li Xue Za Zhi 2020;49:411–417

40. Shaharuddin SH, Wang V, Santos RS, et al. Deleterious effects of SARS-CoV-2 infection on human pancreatic cells. Front Cell Infect Microbiol 2021;11:678482

41. Wu CT, Lidsky PV, Xiao Y, et al. SARS-CoV-2 infects human pancreatic β cells and elicits β cell impairment. Cell Metab 2021;33:1565–1576.e5

42. Cheung NW. Steroid-induced hyperglycaemia in hospitalised patients: does it matter? Diabetologia 2016;59:2507–2509

43. Fong AC, Cheung NW. The high incidence of steroid-induced hyperglycaemia in hospital. Diabetes Res Clin Pract 2013;99:277–280

44. Liu XX, Zhu XM, Miao Q, Ye HY, Zhang ZY, Li YM. Hyperglycemia induced by glucocorticoids in nondiabetic patients: a meta-analysis. Ann Nutr Metab 2014;65:324–332

45. Bornstein SR, Rubino F, Khunti K, et al. Practical recommendations for the management of diabetes in patients with COVID-19. Lancet Diabetes Endocrinol 2020;8:546–550

46. Wu L, Girgis CM, Cheung NW. COVID-19 and diabetes: insulin requirements parallel illness severity in critically unwell patients. Clin Endocrinol (Oxf) 2020;93:390–393

47. Norhammar A, Tenerz A, Nilsson G, et al. Glucose metabolism in patients with acute myocardial infarction and no previous diagnosis of diabetes mellitus: a prospective study. Lancet 2002;359:2140–2144

48. Dennis A, Wamil M, Kapur S, et al. Multi-organ impairment in low-risk individuals with long COVID. medRxiv. 16 October 2020 [preprint]. DOI: https://doi.org/10.1101/2020.10.14.20212555

49. Altmann DM, Boyton RJ. Decoding the unknowns in long COVID. BMJ 2021;372:n132

50. Potere N, Valeriani E, Candeloro M, et al. Acute complications and mortality in hospitalized patients with coronavirus disease 2019: a systematic review and meta-analysis. Crit Care 2020;24:389

51. Zelniker TA, Wiviott SD, Raz I, et al. Comparison of the effects of glucagon-like peptide receptor agonists and sodium-glucose cotransporter 2 inhibitors for prevention of major adverse cardiovascular and renal outcomes in type 2 diabetes mellitus. Circulation 2019;139:2022–2031

52. Kosiborod MN, Esterline R, Furtado RHM, et al. Dapagliflozin in patients with cardiometabolic risk factors hospitalised with COVID-19 (DARE-19): a randomised, double-blind, placebo-controlled, phase 3 trial. Lancet Diabetes Endocrinol 2021;9:586–594

53. U.S. National Library of Medicine. Effects of DPP4 inhibition on COVID-19. ClinicalTrials.gov identifier NCT04341935. Published 10 April 2020. Accessed 9 April 2021. Available from https://clinicaltrials.gov/ct2/show/NCT04341935

54. U.S. National Library of Medicine. Efficacy and safety of dipeptidyl peptidase-4 inhibitors in diabetic patients with established COVID-19. ClinicalTrials.gov identifier NCT04371978. Published 1 May 2020. Accessed 9 April 2021. Available from https://clinicaltrials.gov/ct2/show/NCT04371978

55. U.S. National Library of Medicine. The effect of sitagliptin treatment in COVID-19 positive diabetic patients (SIDIACO). ClinicalTrials.gov identifier NCT04365517. Published 28 April 2020. Accessed 9 April 2021. Available from https://clinicaltrials.gov/ct2/show/NCT04365517

56. U.S. National Library of Medicine. Metformin glycinate in patients with MS or DM2, hospitalized with COVID-19 and SARS secondary to SARS-CoV-2 (DMMETCOV19). ClinicalTrials.gov identifier NCT04626089. Published 12 November 2020. Accessed 9 April 2021. Available from https://clinicaltrials.gov/ct2/show/NCT04626089

57. U.S. National Library of Medicine. Effect of pioglitazone on T2DM patients with COVID-19 (PIOQ8). ClinicalTrials.gov identifier NCT04604223. Published 27 October 2020. Accessed 9 April 2021. Available from https://clinicaltrials.gov/ct2/show/NCT04604223

58. U.S. National Library of Medicine. Semaglutide to reduce myocardial injury in patients with COVID-19 (SEMPATICO). ClinicalTrials.gov identifier NCT04615871. Published 4 November 2020. Accessed 9 April 2021. Available from https://clinicaltrials.gov/ct2/show/NCT04615871

59. Huang C, Huang L, Wang Y, et al. 6-Month consequences of COVID-19 in patients discharged from hospital: a cohort study. Lancet 2021;397:220–232

60. Ayoubkhani D, Khunti K, Nafilyan V, et al. Post-covid syndrome in individuals admitted to hospital with COVID-19: retrospective cohort study. BMJ 2021;372:n693

61. Al-Aly Z, Xie Y, Bowe B. High-dimensional characterization of post-acute sequelae of COVID-19. Nature 2021;594:259–264

62. American Diabetes Association. 2. Classification and diagnosis of diabetes: *Standards of Medical Care in Diabetes—2020*. Diabetes Care 2020;43(Suppl. 1):S14–S31

63. Rubino F, Amiel SA, Zimmet P, et al. New-onset diabetes in Covid-19. N Engl J Med 2020;383:789–790

64. Wang S, Ma P, Zhang S, et al. Fasting blood glucose at admission is an independent predictor for 28-day mortality in patients with COVID-19 without previous diagnosis of diabetes: a multi-centre retrospective study. Diabetologia 2020;63:2102–2111

65. Yang J-K, Jin J-M, Liu S, et al. New onset COVID-19–related diabetes: an indicator of mortality. medRxiv. 26 June 2020 [preprint]. DOI: 10.1101/2020.04.08.20058040.

66. Fadini GP, Morieri ML, Boscari F, et al. Newly-diagnosed diabetes and admission hyperglycemia predict COVID-19 severity by aggravating respiratory deterioration. Diabetes Res Clin Pract 2020;168:108374

67. Zhang J, Kong W, Xia P, et al. Impaired fasting glucose and diabetes are related to higher risks of complications and mortality among patients with coronavirus disease 2019. Front Endocrinol (Lausanne) 2020;11:525

68. Smith SM, Boppana A, Traupman JA, et al. Impaired glucose metabolism in patients with diabetes, prediabetes, and obesity is associated with severe COVID-19. J Med Virol 2021;93: 409–415

69. Liu Y, Lu R, Wang J, et al. Diabetes, even newly defined by HbA1c testing, is associated with an increased risk of in-hospital death in adults with COVID-19. BMC Endocr Disord 2021;21:56

Historical HbA$_{1c}$ Values May Explain the Type 2 Diabetes Legacy Effect: UKPDS 88

Marcus Lind,[1,2] Henrik Imberg,[3] Ruth L. Coleman,[4] Olle Nerman,[3] and Rury R. Holman[4]

Diabetes Care 2021;44:2231–2237 | https://doi.org/10.2337/dc20-2439

OBJECTIVE

Type 2 diabetes all-cause mortality (ACM) and myocardial infarction (MI) glycemic legacy effects have not been explained. We examined their relationships with prior individual HbA$_{1c}$ values and explored the potential impact of instituting earlier, compared with delayed, glucose-lowering therapy.

RESEARCH DESIGN AND METHODS

Twenty-year ACM and MI hazard functions were estimated from diagnosis of type 2 diabetes in 3,802 UK Prospective Diabetes Study participants. Impact of HbA$_{1c}$ values over time was analyzed by weighting them according to their influence on downstream ACM and MI risks.

RESULTS

Hazard ratios for a one percentage unit higher HbA$_{1c}$ for ACM were 1.08 (95% CI 1.07–1.09), 1.18 (1.15–1.21), and 1.36 (1.30–1.42) at 5, 10, and 20 years, respectively, and for MI was 1.13 (1.11–1.15) at 5 years, increasing to 1.31 (1.25–1.36) at 20 years. Imposing a one percentage unit lower HbA$_{1c}$ from diagnosis generated an 18.8% (95% CI 21.1–16.0) ACM risk reduction 10–15 years later, whereas delaying this reduction until 10 years after diagnosis showed a sevenfold lower 2.7% (3.1–2.3) risk reduction. Corresponding MI risk reductions were 19.7% (22.4–16.5) when lowering HbA$_{1c}$ at diagnosis, and threefold lower 6.5% (7.4–5.3%) when imposed 10 years later.

CONCLUSIONS

The glycemic legacy effects seen in type 2 diabetes are explained largely by historical HbA$_{1c}$ values having a greater impact than recent values on clinical outcomes. Early detection of diabetes and intensive glucose control from the time of diagnosis is essential to maximize reduction of the long-term risk of glycemic complications.

[1]Institute of Medicine, Sahlgrenska Academy, University of Gothenburg, Gothenburg, Sweden
[2]Department of Medicine, NU-Hospital Group, Uddevalla, Sweden
[3]Department of Mathematical Sciences, Chalmers University of Technology and University of Gothenburg, Gothenburg, Sweden
[4]Diabetes Trials Unit, Radcliffe Department of Medicine, University of Oxford, Oxford, U.K.

Corresponding author: Marcus Lind, marcus.lind@gu.se

Received 2 October 2020 and accepted 3 May 2021

This article contains supplementary material online at https://doi.org/10.2337/figshare.14575173.

This article is featured in a podcast available at https://www.diabetesjournals.org/content/diabetes-core-update-podcasts.

This article is part of a special article collection available at https://care.diabetesjournals.org/collection/long-term-effects-of-earlier-glycemic-control.

See accompanying articles, pp. 2212, 2216, and 2225.

The UK Prospective Diabetes Study (UKPDS) demonstrated that intensive glycemic control, which achieved 0.9% lower HbA$_{1c}$ levels on average compared with conventional glycemic control, lowered the risk of microvascular complications in patients with type 2 diabetes (T2D) (1). The risks for all-cause mortality (ACM) and myocardial infarction (MI) were not reduced, although the 16% numerical MI risk reduction was borderline statistically significant ($P = 0.052$). A subsequent patient-level meta-analysis of Action to Control Cardiovascular Risk in Diabetes (ACCORD), Action in Diabetes and Vascular Disease: Preterax and Diamicron MR Controlled

Evaluation (ADVANCE), UKPDS, and Veterans Affairs Diabetes Trial (VADT), however, confirmed a 15% MI risk reduction for a 0.88% lower HbA_{1c} (2).

Ten-year posttrial monitoring of surviving UKPDS participants, with virtually no glycemic differences between those randomized previously to intensive or conventional glycemic strategies, revealed relative risk reductions of 16% for ACM ($P = 0.007$) and 15% for MI ($P = 0.01$) (3). These findings, suggesting there is a "legacy" effect conferred by earlier improved glycemic control with increasingly beneficial effects on ACM and MI risks over time (3), have helped influence guidelines to advocate early more intensive postdiagnosis glucose-lowering therapy. Many patients, however, still do not reach their glycemic targets (4–6). Because significant resources are required to promote early diabetes detection (e.g., screening large populations) and to optimize glycemic control after diagnosis, it is essential for care givers, patients, and decision makers to know to what extent early intensive glycemic control can reduce the risk of long-term complications.

In this UKPDS analysis, we examine the degree to which relationships between individual historical HbA_{1c} values over time and downstream risks of ACM and MI may explain the T2D glycemic legacy effect.

RESEARCH DESIGN AND METHODS

Population
The UKPDS design and results have been described previously (1,3,7,8). Briefly, participants were stratified by ideal body weight (<120% vs. ≥120%) (8), with nonoverweight participants assigned randomly to an intensive (insulin or sulfonylurea) or conventional (diet) glycemic management strategy. Overweight participants assigned to the intensive glycemic strategy could also be allocated to metformin (8). The aim for all participants was a fasting plasma glucose <6.0 mmol/L, with second-line glucose-lowering therapy permitted only if fasting plasma glucose values became >15 mmol/L or unacceptable signs of hyperglycemia developed.

After UKPDS closeout, all surviving participants entered a 10-year posttrial monitoring period and were returned to routine care, with no attempt made to

maintain trial-allocated treatment regimens (3). They were seen annually at UKPDS centers for the first 5 years with collection of standardized data, including HbA_{1c}. Thereafter, participants were monitored remotely by means of annual participant- and general practitioner-completed questionnaires.

In this analysis, only those assigned originally to an intensive glycemic strategy with a sulfonylurea or insulin, or to a conventional glycemic strategy with diet, were evaluated. HbA_{1c} values were measured annually in the UKPDS. Participants were excluded if they had a missing baseline HbA_{1c} value or did not have at least one follow-up HbA_{1c} value recorded during the 2 years preceding ACM or MI. HbA_{1c} values, measured as % (7), have been converted to mmol/mol according to guidelines (9).

Relationship of Historical HbA_{1c} Values to Downstream ACM and MI Risks
Time-to-event analysis of diabetes complications and HbA_{1c} is commonly performed using baseline or updated mean HbA_{1c} values (10–13). However, none of these HbA_{1c} metrics consider how HbA_{1c} values, measured at different historical time points, may vary in their individual contribution to the downstream risk of diabetes-related complications. Accordingly, we used a model in which historical HbA_{1c} values were weighted unequally to allow for different risk contributions at each time point. This was done using a multivariable regression model where optimal weights for historical HbA_{1c} values were estimated simultaneously with the effect of the influence weighted HbA_{1c} variable and coefficients for other covariates (14,15). The overall temporal relationship of HbA_{1c} with ACM and MI was investigated by estimating the degree to which the instantaneous risk (hazard) of ACM and MI at 15 and 20 years after diagnosis could be ascribed to HbA_{1c} values measured at previous time points.

ACM and MI Hazard Ratios in Relation to HbA_{1c}
The impact of HbA_{1c} values on diabetes-related complications has commonly been estimated by calculating hazard ratios (HRs) in relation to a one percentage unit (11 mmol/mol) difference in

HbA_{1c} (10,13–15). We estimated ACM and MI HRs at 5, 10, 15, and 20 years after diagnosis of diabetes, assuming a one percentage unit (11 mmol/mol) higher HbA_{1c} from diagnosis onward. To further understand the impact of historical HbA_{1c} levels on downstream ACM and MI risks (legacy effects), we also estimated ACM and MI HRs at 10–20 years after diagnosis in relation to a one percentage unit (11 mmol/mol) lower HbA_{1c}, imposed at diagnosis of diabetes or delayed until 5 or 10 years later. These estimations were repeated for HbA_{1c} decrements of 0.5% (5.5 mmol/mol) and 2.0% (22 mmol/mol).

ACM and MI Relative Risks Relating to Historical HbA_{1c} Values
To study how prior HbA_{1c} values might influence the incidence of downstream ACM and MI over a longer time period, we estimated ACM and MI relative risks at 0–10, 10–15, and 10–20 years after diagnosis when a lower HbA_{1c} was imposed immediately compared with delaying this until 5 or 10 years later.

Impact of UKPDS Randomized Glycemic Strategies
To evaluate whether factors other than glycemic control might explain differences in outcomes, we investigated the extent to which assignment to an intensive or conventional glycemic control strategy, irrespective of achieved HbA_{1c} values, affected the incidence of ACM and MI.

Statistical Analyses
We used a multivariable Poisson regression model that included HbA_{1c}, age, sex, and diabetes duration with the total follow-up period for each patient subdivided into small intervals of 0.2 years, for each of which a constant hazard was assumed. HbA_{1c} was included in the model as a time-dependent weighted integral of all prior HbA_{1c} values, with values weighted unequally to allow for a potential different risk contribution at each time point. The influence-weighted HbA_{1c} variable was computed by first creating a continuous HbA_{1c} curve using linear interpolation between observed HbA_{1c} values, which was then weighted by a piecewise exponential weight function with one knot. The optimal HbA_{1c} weight function parameters were estimated simultaneously with the coefficients of the

covariates in the model using maximum likelihood estimation.

Likelihood ratio tests were used to assess the significance of individual model parameters, with corresponding CIs computed by test inversion (16). Estimates and CIs for influence-weighted HbA_{1c} HRs at various follow-up times and for relative risks associated with imposed immediate or delayed HbA_{1c} reductions were computed from the corresponding regression coefficient, fixing the HbA_{1c} weight function parameters at their estimated values. Model fit was assessed by comparing observed and expected event numbers for various age categories and follow-up times. Additional model and statistical methodology details can be found here (14,15) and in the Supplementary Material (additional statistical analysis details).

Data and Resource Availability
Data may be accessed after a written research proposal and support from investigators and upon request and an appropriate data transfer agreement is in place.

RESULTS

Patient Characteristics
Requisite UKPDS data were available for 3,802 participants with 775 ACM events and for 3,219 participants with 662 MI events. Their mean age at diagnosis of diabetes was 53.3 (SD 8.6) years, and 38.8% were women. For ACM and MI analyses, there were 3,321 (87%) and 3,219 (85%) participants, respectively, monitored for >5 years. The number of participants included in the analyses

with follow-up of >10 and 15 years for ACM were 2,742 (72%) and 1,299 (34%), respectively, and for MI were 2,544 (67%) and 1,156 (30%), respectively.

ACM and MI HRs in Relation to HbA_{1c}
Higher HbA_{1c} values were associated significantly with both higher ACM and MI risks (both $P < 0.0001$). HRs for ACM and MI in relation to imposed 0.5% (5 mmol/mol), 1% (11 mmol/mol), and 2% (22 mmol/mol) higher HbA_{1c} values during the first 5, 10, 15, or 20 years after the diagnosis of diabetes are presented in Table 1. Each 1% (11 mmol/mol) higher HbA_{1c} was related to steadily higher HRs over time for ACM and MI, suggesting increasingly harmful effects of earlier hyperglycemia. HRs for ACM per 1% (11 mmol/mol) higher HbA_{1c} value were 1.08 (95% CI 1.07–1.09), 1.18 (1.15–1.21), and 1.36 (1.30–1.42) at 5, 10, and 20 years of follow-up, respectively, while MI HRs increased from 1.13 (1.11–1.15) at 5 years to 1.31 (1.25–1.36) at 20 years.

Imposing a one percentage unit (11 mmol/mol) lower HbA_{1c} from the diagnosis of diabetes significantly lowered the instantaneous risk (hazard) of ACM or MI events 15 and 20 years later, compared with reducing HbA_{1c} by the same amount from 10 years after diagnosis (Fig. 1). ACM HRs (95% CI) at 15 and 20 years after diagnosis when reducing HbA_{1c} from diagnosis, compared with from 10 years after diagnosis, were, respectively, 0.78 (0.76–0.81) vs. 0.93 (0.92–0.94) and 0.73 (0.70–0.77) vs. 0.84 (0.82–0.87). Corresponding MI HRs were, respectively, 0.79 (0.76–0.82) vs. 0.88

(0.87–0.90) and 0.76 (0.73–0.80) vs. 0.82 (0.80–0.85). HRs calculated when HbA_{1c} lowering was delayed approached those of immediate HbA_{1c} lowering somewhat more rapidly for MI than for ACM (Fig. 1). Similar relationships over time were found for ACM and MI when HbA_{1c} was lowered by one-half or two percentage units (Supplementary Figs. 2 and 3).

Relative Risks of ACM and MI 10–20 Years After Diagnosis in Relation to Early or Delayed Imposed Lowering of HbA_{1c}
To study glucose-lowering legacy effects over longer time periods, we estimated the effect of imposing immediate or delayed HbA_{1c} reductions on ACM and MI risks between 0–10, 10–15, and 10–20 years after diagnosis. The estimated ACM relative risk reduction was 18.8% (95% CI 21.1–16.0) at 10–15 years per one percentage unit lower HbA_{1c} when imposed from diagnosis, but sevenfold smaller at 2.7% (3.1–2.3) when imposed 10 years after diagnosis. The corresponding MI estimates showed a threefold smaller relative risk reduction comparing delayed with immediate imposition of a lower HbA_{1c} (Table 2). For the period 10–20 years after diagnosis, delayed compared with immediate imposition HbA_{1c} lowering by one percentage unit (11 mmol/mol) resulted in an approximately threefold smaller ACM relative risk reduction and a two-fold smaller MI relative risk reduction (Table 2). Similar legacy effects for ACM and MI risks were seen with imposed

Table 1—HRs for ACM and MI per one-half, one, and two percentage unit (5.5, 11, and 22 mmol/mol) higher HbA_{1c} (%) values over the first 5, 10, 15, and 20 years after the diagnosis of T2D

Years after diagnosis	HR (95% CI) per 0.5 percentage units higher	HR (95% CI) per 1 percentage units higher	HR (95% CI) per 2 percentage units higher
ACM			
5	1.04 (1.03–1.04)	1.08 (1.07–1.09)	1.16 (1.14–1.19)
10	1.09 (1.07–1.10)	1.18 (1.15–1.21)	1.40 (1.33–1.47)
15	1.13 (1.11–1.15)	1.28 (1.23–1.32)	1.64 (1.51–1.75)
20	1.17 (1.14–1.19)	1.36 (1.30–1.42)	1.86 (1.68–2.03)
MI			
5	1.06 (1.05–1.07)	1.13 (1.11–1.15)	1.28 (1.22–1.33)
10	1.10 (1.08–1.12)	1.22 (1.17–1.25)	1.48 (1.38–1.57)
15	1.13 (1.10–1.15)	1.27 (1.22–1.32)	1.62 (1.49–1.75)
20	1.14 (1.12–1.17)	1.31 (1.25–1.36)	1.71 (1.55–1.86)

All HRs are statistically significant with $P < 0.0001$. The hazard ratio per z-units increase in HbA_{1c} during t years after diagnosis is given by Eq. 5 in the Supplementary Material. The model coefficients of the HbA_{1c} weight function and covariates included in the model are presented in Supplementary Table 1.

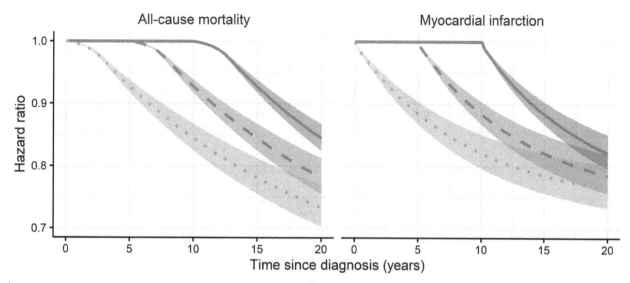

Figure 1—Time-dependent HRs for all cause-mortality (left) and myocardial infarction (right) from 0 to 20 years after diagnosis of type 2 diabetes, assuming a one percentage unit lower HbA$_{1c}$ from diagnosis (green dotted lines), and when the same degree of HbA$_{1c}$ lowering was imposed from 5 years (blue dashed lines), and from 10 years (red solid lines) after diagnosis. The shaded regions represent 95% confidence limits. HRs were calculated according to Eq. 6 in the Supplementary Material.

0.5% and 2.0% lower HbA$_{1c}$ values (Supplementary Table 2).

Relationship of Historical HbA$_{1c}$ Values to Downstream ACM and MI Risks

The overall temporal relationships of HbA$_{1c}$ with ACM and MI are shown in Fig. 2. HbA$_{1c}$ values measured during the first 10 years after diagnosis contributed to 69% (95% CI 60–75) of the HbA$_{1c}$ total effect on ACM risk 15 years after diagnosis and to 45% (33–54) at 20 years (Fig. 2). The corresponding MI estimates were 49% (95% CI 37–56) and 27% (16–35).

Impact of Age, Sex, and Assigned Glycemic Control Strategy

Older age and male sex were associated significantly (both $P < 0.0001$) with increased ACM and MI risks (Supplementary Table 1). When HbA$_{1c}$ was included in the model, the glycemic control strategy assignment (intensive versus conventional) effect was attenuated and not associated with ACM ($P = 0.15$) or MI ($P = 0.07$).

Model Checks

Details of the final model estimated parameters, including coefficients of the HbA$_{1c}$ weight function, are provided in Supplementary Table 1. Several model checks were performed, with no lack-of-fit detected. The model-predicted cumulative number of UKPDS participants

experiencing an ACM or MI event was similar to that observed (Supplementary Fig. 4). A sensitivity analysis to assess the impact of baseline HbA$_{1c}$, which excluded HbA$_{1c}$ values and deaths during the first 4 years after diagnosis, showed similar time associations between HbA$_{1c}$ and ACM. Similar patterns were also seen when an interaction term for time and HbA$_{1c}$ was included in the model.

CONCLUSIONS

Principal Findings

In this analysis of the UKPDS and its posttrial monitoring period, we found that historical HbA$_{1c}$ values were associated with strong legacy effects for the downstream incidence of ACM and MI. Analyses exploring the impact of delaying the imposition of a 1% lower HbA$_{1c}$ until 10 years after diagnosis of diabetes, compared with doing this immediately, showed a sevenfold lower risk reduction for ACM at 10–15 years. At 10–20 years after diagnosis, the risk of death was reduced by threefold when HbA$_{1c}$ was lowered from diagnosis. Similar time-dependent effects were observed for MI, but HbA$_{1c}$ legacy effects were numerically greater for ACM than MI. The impact on ACM and MI risks of delaying imposition of improved glycemic control after the diagnosis of diabetes increased steadily with time. Thus, a one percentage unit (11 mmol/mol) higher HbA$_{1c}$ level was associated with an 8% greater ACM

risk at 5 years, increasing to 36% at 20 years. The risks for ACM and MI were captured by HbA$_{1c}$, whereas the assigned glycemic strategy group was not significant when HbA$_{1c}$ was included in the model. This finding strongly supports the fact that the long-term ACM and MI risk reductions seen in the UKPDS intensive glycemic strategy group are driven by the early introduction of improved glycemic control (1,3). The somewhat stronger legacy effect we see for ACM, compared with MI, reflects the increased ACM risk reduction from 6% to 13% during UKPDS posttrial monitoring, while the degree of MI risk reduction was essentially unchanged (16% vs. 15%) (3).

Other Studies

The existence of a strong legacy effect of earlier glycemic control on cardiovascular disease is supported by findings from studies of patients with type 1 diabetes. In the Epidemiology of Diabetes Interventions and Complications (EDIC) follow-up of the Diabetes Control and Complications Trial (DCCT) study, participants previously assigned to intensive glycemic therapy had fewer cardiovascular disease events, even though the glycemic difference between the intensive and conventional groups was not maintained (17,18). ACM and MI reductions were not seen with intensive glycemic therapy in any of the three large-scale glucose-lowering

Table 2—Estimated relative risks of ACM and MI between 0–10, 10–15, and 10–20 years after diagnosis assuming a one percentage unit (11 mmol/mol) lower HbA$_{1c}$ from diagnosis, and when the same HbA$_{1c}$ lowering was imposed from 5 and from 10 years after diagnosis

Years after diagnosis	HbA$_{1c}$ lowered at diagnosis	HbA$_{1c}$ lowered 5 years after diagnosis	HbA$_{1c}$ lowered 10 years after diagnosis
ACM			
0–10	0.928 (0.919–0.939)	0.987 (0.985–0.989)	1.00
10–15	0.812 (0.789–0.840)	0.885 (0.870–0.902)	0.973 (0.969–0.977)
10–20	0.785 (0.758–0.815)	0.848 (0.829–0.871)	0.928 (0.919–0.939)
MI			
0–10	0.893 (0.877–0.911)	0.968 (0.963–0.973)	1.00
10–15	0.803 (0.776–0.835)	0.851 (0.830–0.876)	0.935 (0.926–0.947)
10–20	0.788 (0.760–0.823)	0.826 (0.803–0.855)	0.893 (0.877–0.911)

Data are presented as relative risk (95% CI) per one percentage unit lower HbA$_{1c}$. The relative risk of an event in a time interval 0–10, 10–15, or 10–20 years after diagnosis was calculated according to Eq. 11 in the Supplementary Material.

studies performed over 3–5 years in patients with generally long-standing T2D (19–21). This may reflect the initially smaller risk reductions with improved HbA$_{1c}$ or the late introduction of improved glycemic control in patients with diabetes of long duration. Minimizing hyperglycemia plays a major role in reducing the risk of diabetic complications, particularly microvascular complications (1,3,8), while other glucose-lowering drugs, such as metformin, glucagon-like peptide 1 (GLP-1) receptor analogs, and sodium–glucose cotransporter 2 inhibitors, likely also act via additional nonglucose-lowering mechanisms to reduce ACM and MI risks (8,22,23). Nonetheless, while the risks of MI and death have reduced over time,

these remain substantially higher for people with T2D (24,25).

Explanations and Interpretations
The legacy effect of earlier hyperglycemia on diabetic complications appears to explain the increasing impact of historical HbA$_{1c}$ values on ACM and MI risks over time. Legacy effects in T2D and "metabolic memory" in type 1 diabetes have been the subject of much debate (3,17,26–29). Certain pathways associated with diabetes complications may be active later but initiated from earlier increases in glucose, where reactive oxygen species have been proposed to play an essential role (26,30). The reason legacy effects are somewhat greater for ACM than MI is speculative.

It is possible that to some extent, death may occur in a time-delayed fashion from several diabetes-related complications (including MI), a fact that may explain how HbA$_{1c}$ affects death and MI with time. Early hyperglycemia leading to nephropathy, initiating processes increasing future risks of ACM and MI, including hypertension, altered lipid metabolism, and inflammatory processes, may also be a major contributor (31,32). In multiple studies, renal complications have been major risk factors for future cardiovascular disease and mortality (13,31–33).

Implications
Although early more intensive glycemic control in UKPDS participants with newly diagnosed T2D has shown ACM

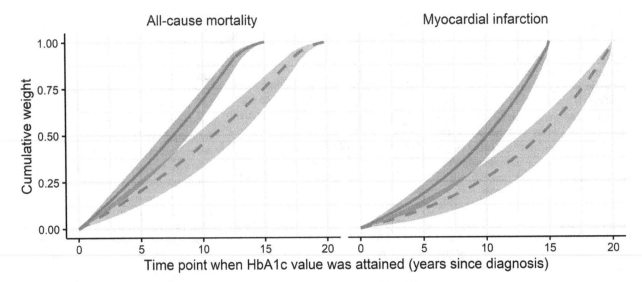

Figure 2—Contribution of historical HbA$_{1c}$ values to their impact on the instantaneous risk (hazard) of all-cause mortality (left) and myocardial infarction (right) at 15 years (red solid lines) and 20 years (blue dashed lines) after diagnosis. The legacy effect of historical HbA$_{1c}$ values on diabetes complications was more pronounced for ACM than for MI. The shaded regions represent 95% confidence limits. Details on the calculations may be found in Eq. 7 in the Supplementary Material.

and MI risk reductions in the longer-term, associations with individual historical HbA_{1c} values and their long-term effects have not been studied. Here we show that imposing a lower HbA_{1c} immediately after the diagnosis of T2D is associated with severalfold greater risk reductions in ACM and MI 10–20 years later compared with delayed HbA_{1c} lowering. T2D is a worldwide epidemic affecting >463 million individuals and causing a large proportion of severe renal, visual, and cardiovascular disease events as well as amputations and shorter life expectancy (34). In addition, many people have undetected diabetes (34). Our results imply that societies should focus even more on early T2D detection and glucose optimization. Moreover, programs in both children and adults without diabetes could prevent or delay diabetes onset and thereby minimize glycemic exposure at an even earlier time period.

Guidelines today recommend screening high risk groups (e.g., obese individuals and first-degree relatives of individuals with T2D) (4,5), but few structural programs exist in many countries. If T2D remains undetected, glucose levels can increase over many years without symptoms but with elevated HbA_{1c} values that are associated with greatly increased risk, as we have shown here; for example, a 2% (22 mmol/mol) higher HbA_{1c} increases ACM risk by 40% after 10 years and by 86% after 20 years.

Another implication is that glycemic control contributes more to risk of ACM and MI than previously thought. Our study found an ACM risk increase of >30% at 20 years per unit HbA_{1c} increase compared with 10–20% in previous studies (10–13). The difference is due to the increasing effects over time, which likely will increase even more for many patients over a lifetime horizon. Besides the need for early detection of diabetes and glycemic optimization, our findings support the need for strict glycemic control when treating people with T2D in clinical practice. Effects of glucose-lowering treatments in cardiovascular outcome trials have likely underestimated the effects of glycemic control because the beneficial effects, according to the current results, increase over at least 15–20 years and thus far beyond the duration of most

studies, which have generally been 3–5 years (19–23,28,29). The increasing and larger risk reductions seen here over time need to be considered when making treatment decisions in clinical practice, writing guidelines, and performing health care economic analyses.

These results are also of interest in light of the current coronavirus disease 2019 pandemic. Individuals with T2D with a high mortality risk after coronavirus disease 2019 infection are generally those with advanced diabetes complications (35,36). To help minimize such risks in future viral epidemics, our findings highlight the crucial need for early implementation of intensive glycemic control in people with newly diagnosed T2D to reduce end-organ damage.

Strengths and Limitations

Strengths of our study include the UKPDS long-term follow-up with detailed HbA_{1c} and adjudicated complication data. Also, participants were monitored from the diagnosis of T2D, which is essential to capture as much information as possible on early hyperglycemic effects. The model we used has previously shown a better fit than traditional models and variables used for describing HbA_{1c} in relation to diabetic complications (10,14,15). Although it shows a good fit here, we cannot exclude residual confounding due to the study's observational nature. In particular, partial confounding may exist between the studied HbA_{1c} variable, which varies nonlinearly with time since diagnosis, and nonlinear effects of diabetes duration. None of the conducted sensitivity analyses, however, revealed any such patterns. Because the current analyses focused on the relative impact of historical HbA_{1c} values, we did not evaluate risk factors other than age, sex, and treatment group. Moreover, it should be noted that healthy living habits, which may be associated with improved glycemic control and were not controlled for in the current analysis, can also influence the risk of MI and mortality. For future estimations of the probability of ACM or MI for individuals, it will be essential to include other risk factors and covariates. However, HbA_{1c} is already known to be an independent risk factor for MI and ACM, as shown in multiple studies, including the UKPDS (11–13). In the

current study, intraindividual HbA_{1c} values (i.e., for each participant) were evaluated to determine their relative contributions over time to MI and ACM. While it would be of interest to determine and also adjust for time-dependent effects of other risk factors (smoking, weight, blood pressure, and lipid profiles), they did not vary greatly over time in UKPDS, and such analyses would be complex to perform.

The use of statins and renin-angiotensin-aldosterone system inhibitors in UKPDS were confined primarily to the posttrial monitoring period. It is possible that by reducing overall cardiovascular risk, they might to some extent influence the effect ascribed to historical HbA_{1c} values but not fundamentally change the relationship between HbA_{1c} and complications.

In conclusion, the adverse effects of HbA_{1c} on ACM and MI increase over time. Strong HbA_{1c} legacy effects exist for both of these outcomes but appear greater for ACM. Given these large legacy effects, early detection of T2D (screening) and glycemic optimization needs greater emphasis in guidelines, by health care providers, and in clinical practice to more effectively prevent long-term complications and achieve a more normal life-expectancy for people with T2D.

Acknowledgments. The authors want to thank all participating sites and participants for making the UKPDS trial possible. The authors thank Anders Odén (Chalmers University of Technology) for important contributions to the current work.
Funding. This study was supported by the Swedish State (ALF grant). R.R.H. is an Emeritus National Institute for Health Research Senior Investigator.
Duality of Interest. M.L. has received research grants from DexCom and Novo Nordisk and been a consultant for AstraZeneca, Boehringer Ingelheim, DexCom, Eli Lilly, MSD, and Novo Nordisk. R.R.H. reports research support from AstraZeneca, Bayer, and Merck Sharp & Dohme, and personal fees from Anji Pharmacueticals, Bayer, Intarcia, Merck Sharp & Dohme, Novartis, and Novo Nordisk. No other potential conflicts of interest relevant to this article were reported.
Author Contributions. M.L. wrote a first draft of the manuscript. M.L., H.I., R.L.C., O.N., and R.R.H. were involved in analyses and interpretations of data and revising the manuscript. M.L. and R.R.H. are the guarantors of this work and, as such, had full access to all the data in the study and take responsibility for the integrity of the data and the accuracy of the data analysis.

References

1. UK Prospective Diabetes Study (UKPDS) Group. Intensive blood-glucose control with sulphonylureas or insulin compared with conventional treatment and risk of complications in patients with type 2 diabetes (UKPDS 33). Lancet 1998;352:837–853

2. Turnbull FM, Abraira C, Anderson RJ, et al.; Control Group. Intensive glucose control and macrovascular outcomes in type 2 diabetes [published correction appears in Diabetologia 2009;52:2470]. Diabetologia 2009;52:2288–2298

3. Holman RR, Paul SK, Bethel MA, Matthews DR, Neil HA. 10-year follow-up of intensive glucose control in type 2 diabetes. N Engl J Med 2008;359:1577–1589

4. American Diabetes Association. Introduction: *Standards of Medical Care in Diabetes—2020.* Diabetes Care 2020;43(Suppl. 1):S1–S2

5. National Institute for Health and Care Excellence. Type 2 diabetes in adults: management. NICE guideline [NG28]. Published 2 December 2015. Accessed 2 October 2020. Available from https://www.nice.org.uk/guidance/ng28

6. Swedish National Diabetes Register. Region Västra Götaland: Centre of Registers. Accessed 2 October 2020. Available from www.ndr.nu

7. UK Prospective Diabetes Study Group. UK Prospective Diabetes Study (UKPDS). VIII. Study design, progress and performance. Diabetologia 1991;34:877–890

8. UK Prospective Diabetes Study (UKPDS) Group. Effect of intensive blood-glucose control with metformin on complications in overweight patients with type 2 diabetes (UKPDS 34). Lancet 1998;352:854–865

9. Hanås R, John G; International HBA1c Consensus Committee. 2010 consensus statement on the worldwide standardization of the hemoglobin A1C measurement. Diabetes Care 2010;33:1903–1904

10. Lind M, Odén A, Fahlén M, Eliasson B. A systematic review of HbA1c variables used in the study of diabetic complications. Diabetes Metab Syndr 2008;2:282–293

11. Selvin E, Marinopoulos S, Berkenblit G, et al. Meta-analysis: glycosylated hemoglobin and cardiovascular disease in diabetes mellitus. Ann Intern Med 2004;141:421–431

12. Stratton IM, Adler AI, Neil HA, et al. Association of glycaemia with macrovascular and microvascular complications of type 2 diabetes (UKPDS 35): prospective observational study. BMJ 2000;321:405–412

13. Tancredi M, Rosengren A, Svensson AM, et al. Excess mortality among persons with type 2 diabetes. N Engl J Med 2015;373:1720–1732

14. Lind M, Odén A, Fahlén M, Eliasson B. The true value of HbA1c as a predictor of diabetic complications: simulations of HbA1c variables. PLoS One 2009;4:e4412

15. Lind M, Odén A, Fahlén M, Eliasson B. The shape of the metabolic memory of HbA1c: re-analysing the DCCT with respect to time-dependent effects. Diabetologia 2010;53:1093–1098

16. Casella G, Berger RL. Statistical Inference. 2nd ed. Pacific Grove, Duxbury, 2002

17. Nathan DM, Cleary PA, Backlund JY, et al.; Diabetes Control and Complications Trial/Epidemiology of Diabetes Interventions and Complications (DCCT/EDIC) Study Research Group. Intensive diabetes treatment and cardiovascular disease in patients with type 1 diabetes. N Engl J Med 2005;353:2643–2653

18. Nathan DM, Genuth S, Lachin J, et al.; Diabetes Control and Complications Trial Research Group. The effect of intensive treatment of diabetes on the development and progression of long-term complications in insulin-dependent diabetes mellitus. N Engl J Med 1993;329:977–986

19. Gerstein HC, Miller ME, Byington RP, et al.; Action to Control Cardiovascular Risk in Diabetes Study Group. Effects of intensive glucose lowering in type 2 diabetes. N Engl J Med 2008;358:2545–2559

20. Patel A, MacMahon S, Chalmers J, et al.; ADVANCE Collaborative Group. Intensive blood glucose control and vascular outcomes in patients with type 2 diabetes. N Engl J Med 2008;358:2560–2572

21. Duckworth W, Abraira C, Moritz T, et al.; VADT Investigators. Glucose control and vascular complications in veterans with type 2 diabetes. N Engl J Med 2009;360:129–139

22. Zinman B, Wanner C, Lachin JM, et al.; EMPA-REG OUTCOME Investigators. Empagliflozin, cardiovascular outcomes, and mortality in type 2 diabetes. N Engl J Med 2015;373:2117–2128

23. Marso SP, Daniels GH, Brown-Frandsen K, et al.; LEADER Steering Committee; LEADER Trial Investigators. Liraglutide and cardiovascular outcomes in type 2 diabetes. N Engl J Med 2016;375:311–322

24. Lind M, Garcia-Rodriguez LA, Booth GL, et al. Mortality trends in patients with and without diabetes in Ontario, Canada and the UK from 1996 to 2009: a population-based study. Diabetologia 2013;56:2601–2608

25. Tancredi M, Rosengren A, Svensson A-M, et al. Glycaemic control and excess risk of major coronary events in patients with type 2 diabetes: a population-based study. Open Heart 2019;6: e000967

26. Ceriello A, Ihnat MA, Thorpe JE. Clinical review 2: The "metabolic memory": is more than just tight glucose control necessary to prevent diabetic complications? J Clin Endocrinol Metab 2009;94:410–415

27. Intine RV, Sarras MP Jr. Metabolic memory and chronic diabetes complications: potential role for epigenetic mechanisms. Curr Diab Rep 2012;12:551–559

28. Reaven PD, Emanuele NV, Wiitala WL, et al.; VADT Investigators. Intensive glucose control in patients with type 2 diabetes—15-year follow-up. N Engl J Med 2019;380:2215–2224

29. Laiteerapong N, Ham SA, Gao Y, et al. The legacy effect in type 2 diabetes: impact of early glycemic control on future complications (The Diabetes & Aging Study). Diabetes Care 2019;42:416–426

30. Shah MS, Brownlee M. Molecular and cellular mechanisms of cardiovascular disorders in diabetes. Circ Res 2016;118:1808–1829

31. Gansevoort RT, Correa-Rotter R, Hemmelgarn BR, et al. Chronic kidney disease and cardiovascular risk: epidemiology, mechanisms, and prevention. Lancet 2013;382:339–352

32. Go AS, Chertow GM, Fan D, McCulloch CE, Hsu CY. Chronic kidney disease and the risks of death, cardiovascular events, and hospitalization. N Engl J Med 2004;351:1296–1305

33. Tancredi M, Rosengren A, Olsson M, et al. The relationship between three eGFR formulas and hospitalization for heart failure in 54 486 individuals with type 2 diabetes. Diabetes Metab Res Rev 2016;32:730–735

34. International Diabetes Federation. IDF Diabetes Atlas. 9th ed. Brussels, Belgium, International Diabetes Federation, 2019

35. Holman N, Knighton P, Kar P, et al. Risk factors for COVID-19-related mortality in people with type 1 and type 2 diabetes in England: a population-based cohort study. Lancet Diabetes Endocrinol 2020;8:823–833

36. Apicella M, Campopiano MC, Mantuano M, et al. COVID-19 in people with diabetes: understanding the reasons for worse outcomes. Lancet Diabetes Endocrinol 2020;8:782–792

Paradigm Shifts in the Management of Diabetes in Pregnancy: The Importance of Type 2 Diabetes and Early Hyperglycemia in Pregnancy

The 2020 Norbert Freinkel Award Lecture

David Simmons

Diabetes Care 2021;44:1075–1081 | https://doi.org/10.2337/dci20-0055

For over 50 years, the diagnosis of gestational diabetes mellitus (GDM) has been based upon an oral glucose tolerance test at 24–28 weeks' gestation. This is the time during pregnancy when insulin resistance is increasing and hyperglycemia develops among those with insufficient insulin secretory capacity to maintain euglycemia. The Hyperglycemia and Adverse Pregnancy Outcomes (HAPO) study and the two major randomized controlled trials of treating GDM are based upon recruitment of women at this time during pregnancy. Meanwhile, the increasing prevalence of type 2 diabetes in pregnancy, with its significant risk of adverse pregnancy outcomes, has led to a need to identify undiagnosed diabetes as near to conception as possible. Screening for undiagnosed diabetes early in pregnancy also identifies women with hyperglycemia less than overt diabetes, yet at increased risk of adverse pregnancy outcomes. Such women are more insulin resistant—with higher blood pressure, triglycerides, perinatal mortality, and neonatal hypoglycemia with a greater need for insulin treatment—than those with GDM diagnosed at 24–28 weeks' gestation. Currently, there is uncertainty over how to diagnose GDM early in pregnancy and the benefits and harms from using the current management regimen. Randomized controlled trials testing the criteria for, and treatment of, GDM early in pregnancy are urgently needed to address this existing equipoise. In the meantime, the importance of early or "prevalent GDM" (i.e., mild hyperglycemia present from early [before] pregnancy) warrants interim criteria and thresholds for medication, which may differ from those in use for GDM diagnosed at 24–28 weeks' gestation.

For over 50 years, the diagnosis of gestational diabetes mellitus (GDM) has been based upon an oral glucose tolerance test (OGTT) at 24–28 weeks' gestation (1). This time in gestation is when insulin resistance is increasing with the development of hyperglycemia among those with insufficient insulin secretory capacity to maintain euglycemia (2). In Freinkel's iconic Banting Lecture in 1980, building upon the Pederson hypothesis (3, 4), hyperglycemia was described as causing short- and long-term harm to the growing fetus through "fuel-mediated teratogenesis" (5). Different time-dependent impacts of hyperglycemia on the fetus, shown in Fig. 1,

Macarthur Clinical School, Western Sydney University, Campbelltown, New South Wales, Australia

Corresponding author: David Simmons, da.simmons@westernsydney.edu.au

The 2020 Norbert Freinkel Award Lecture was presented at the American Diabetes Association's 80th Scientific Sessions (Virtual Meeting), 13 June 2020.

include first trimester effects on organs (leading to congenital malformations), effects on brain development (with behavioral ramifications) across the trimesters, and anthropometric and metabolic effects from the late second trimester onward. At that time, GDM was considered usually to commence at 24–28 weeks, type 2 diabetes in pregnancy was uncommon, and the importance of obesity during pregnancy was largely undescribed. In 1979, 1984, and 1990, three International Workshop Conferences on GDM occurred, "cementing in" approaches to screening (risk factors, then 50-g glucose challenge test [GCT]), diagnosing (100-g, 3-h oral glucose tolerance test [OGTT]), and managing GDM (nutritional counseling; glucose monitoring with targets of <105 mg/dL [5.8 mmol/L] and <120 mg/dL [6.7 mmol/L] pre-/postmeals; insulin therapy if diet "fails"; fetal surveillance and postpartum testing for dysglycemia using a 75-g OGTT) (6).

It is now 40 years since Freinkel's lecture. This 2020 lecture reflects on the changes and paradigm shifts that have occurred since that time and proposes, in particular, the recognition that hyperglycemia is often present early in pregnancy and that the effects of maternal hyperglycemia at conception, versus those at 24–28 weeks in pregnancy, on fetal development need to be assessed separately. GDM may be divided into mild hyperglycemia already present at the beginning of pregnancy ("prevalent GDM") and that arising de novo during pregnancy ("incident GDM"). Such recognition should lead to further major changes in our approaches to treating and managing GDM.

A Paradigm Shift Toward the Importance of Type 2 Diabetes in Pregnancy

In the 1980s, most women with pregestational diabetes had type 1 diabetes. Evidence for a high prevalence of type 2 diabetes among women of reproductive age of non-European descent emerged from studies among indigenous and Pacific populations from the 1960s (7) to other non-European populations, including South Asians (8). Inevitably, growing reports emerged of significant numbers of women with type 2 diabetes in pregnancy (9). For example, between 1994 and 2004 across the U.S.,

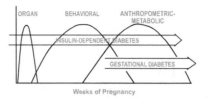

Figure 1—Freinkel's iconic schematic from the Banting Lecture in 1980 (5) of how hyperglycemia affects fetal development and the stage during pregnancy when the hyperglycemia commenced.

the nationwide prevalence of type 1 diabetes in pregnancy increased from 0.24% to 0.33%, an increase of ~33% (10). At the same time, the prevalence of type 2 diabetes in pregnancy increased from 0.09% to 0.42%, an increase of ~367% (10). This led to a shift in pregestational diabetes from a preponderance (73%) of women with type 1 diabetes to a majority (56%) with type 2 diabetes. The growing presence of type 2 diabetes in pregnancy is not simply a case of "mild diabetes." Pregnancies complicated by type 2 diabetes often have comparable rates of congenital malformations, stillbirths, and other adverse pregnancy outcomes (9), requiring the same degree of obstetric monitoring (and intervention) as pregnancies complicated by type 1 diabetes. There are also additional risks from fetal exposure to potentially harmful antihyperglycemic agents, along with a greater prevalence of actually or potentially teratogenic pharmacological agents to manage components of the metabolic syndrome (e.g., antihypertensives and antilipid agents) (11). There are maternal threats from the progression of retinopathy, nephropathy, and cardiovascular disease.

The management of women with type 2 diabetes in pregnancy is often complicated by severe insulin resistance. While this can reflect coexisting obesity, there is often a need for substantial quantities of insulin. Metformin can help reduce insulin requirements in type 2 diabetes (12) (e.g., from 155.29 ± 134.01 units/day to 109.76 ± 105.1 units/day), but the insulin dose remains sizeable and the broad variance reflects some women needing a substantially higher dose. A small 1:2 case-control study (13) in South Auckland, New Zealand (n = 90, 93% Polynesian) was the first to use continuous subcutaneous insulin infusion (CSII) to overcome the

insulin resistance–associated hyperglycemia for women with either preexisting type 2 diabetes (33%) or GDM requiring >100 units/day of insulin (69% >200 units/day). The women on CSII required a median (range) of 246 (116–501) units/day or 2.68 units/kg booking (first antenatal) weight. Glycemia had improved among 79% of the women within 1–2 weeks. Outcomes were similar in terms of birth weight (3,790 vs. 3,720 g), proportion of babies <3,000 g (10.2% vs. 11.8%), and babies ≥4,000 g (34.4% vs. 40.0%). While other obstetric outcomes were comparable, the proportion admitted to the special care baby unit (56.3% vs. 25.0%) was higher in those treated with CSII. No reason is given for these excess admissions, and this finding may be a flag that we need to be "balanced" in our efforts to reduce fetal exposure to hyperglycemia.

In the Metformin in Women With Type 2 Diabetes in Pregnancy Trial (MiTy) (12), metformin therapy was associated with a much lower insulin requirement, alongside a 0.18% lower "last HbA$_{1c}$ in pregnancy," 0.1 kg lower weekly weight gain, and 1.77 kg less overall weight gain. This mix of metformin therapy, less weight gain, and less hyperglycemia (the mean last HbA$_{1c}$ [5.9%] was still higher than the pregnancy HbA$_{1c}$ target of 5.6% [14]) was associated with 0.59-fold (95% CI 0.36–0.98) less extreme large-for-gestational-age (LGA) babies born but a 2.07-fold (95% CI 1.16–3.71) greater proportion of small-for-gestational-age (SGA) babies. While the need for high-level neonatal care >24 h was comparable, the need to "balance" diabetes management with avoiding fetal undernutrition (and the potential for long-term metabolic risks [15]) clearly requires further research. The mechanism behind the SGA remains unclear, with potential contributions from metformin exposure, less gestational weight gain, more mild hypoglycemia episodes/week, and current early pregnancy glycemic targets.

The Emerging Importance of Undiagnosed Type 2 Diabetes in Pregnancy—Enter "Overt Diabetes in Pregnancy" and How To Detect It!

Of course, type 2 diabetes often remains undiagnosed. This growing problem was fully acknowledged by the International Association of the Diabetes and

Pregnancy Study Groups (IADPSG) in their recommendations for the new diagnostic classification for hyperglycemia in pregnancy (16). The IADPSG divided GDM into two on clinical grounds, with likely undiagnosed type 2 diabetes as "overt diabetes in pregnancy" (ODIP) and GDM as "hyperglycemia first detected in pregnancy less than overt diabetes." This classification was subsequently adopted by the World Health Organization, changing its name to "diabetes in pregnancy" (17). This clinical classification thereby allows triaging into those who require, e.g., retinal and renal screening and more intensive management (women with ODIP) and those requiring more limited management (GDM). Although unrelated to the process to define criteria for GDM from the Hyperglycemia and Adverse Pregnancy Outcomes (HAPO) OGTT results at 24–28 weeks (18), this new clinical classification addressed the important paradigm shift in clinical care that had occurred with the growing numbers of women of reproductive age with diagnosed and undiagnosed type 2 diabetes at conception.

The IADPSG recommended that ODIP be diagnosed using the criteria for diabetes in nonpregnant adults, with either a fasting glucose (FBG) ≥ 7.0 mmol/L (126 mg/dL), HbA$_{1c}$ $\geq 6.5\%$ (48 mmol/mol), and/or a random glucose (RBG) (with confirmation) ≥ 11.1 mmol/L (200 mg/dL) (16). Pregnancy complications of ODIP are indeed increased (19). One key finding is that not all women with ODIP are found to have type 2 diabetes postpartum (20). Whether this is due to their antenatal lifestyle changes and other aspects of diabetes in pregnancy management or simply an issue with glycemic variance is unclear.

Screening for ODIP can have its own challenges, and this was exposed by the social distancing required during the coronavirus disease 2019 (COVID-19) pandemic (21, 22). Attending for an FBG can require many women to visit a pathology collection center concurrently. To space out attendance through the day, HbA$_{1c}$ and/or RBG have been recommended, but their test characteristics demonstrate their limitations. In a retrospective analysis of 17,852 pregnancies (19), with a universal RBG around the initial antenatal visit, the area under the receiver operator curve for RBG to detect ODIP was 0.86 (95% CI 0.80–0.92), validating its use as a screening test in that population. Testing for ODIP using HbA$_{1c}$ in early pregnancy has good reproducibility, but its utility is influenced by the variability in half-life between individuals and other nonglycemic factors (23). Even the 6.5% (48 mmol/mol) threshold is only 50% sensitive for ODIP by OGTT (24). For screening for ODIP, a threshold of 5.9% (41 mmol/mol) (24) is associated with two- to fourfold increased risk of adverse pregnancy outcomes, but test characteristics have not been shown. A slightly lower threshold of 5.7% (39 mmol/mol), as used by the American Diabetes Association for prediabetes, is a poor predictor of adverse pregnancy outcomes among obese European women when there is little ODIP (25) (e.g., adjusted odds ratios for birth weight >4 kg, preeclampsia, and cesarean section were 0.94, 0.77, and 0.55, respectively). The OGTT therefore remains the best test for hyperglycemia in pregnancy as it detects both fasting and postprandial hyperglycemia, although reproducibility, convenience, and potentially social distancing issues remain. Further studies are needed to identify the best screening regimen early in pregnancy if the OGTT is not to be used.

A Problem With Screening for ODIP in the First and Early Second Trimesters: Should We Manage Hyperglycemia Less Than ODIP?

Besides the question of how best to test for ODIP, the shift to screening for undiagnosed diabetes has revealed another issue that has been simmering away since Norbert Freinkel's time. In 1988, Maureen Harris asked whether GDM was simply preexisting impaired glucose tolerance rather than newly developed hyperglycemia (26). The potential for GDM (that is not ODIP) to be prevalent in the first half of pregnancy, and to be of importance, was not reflected in Freinkel's iconic 1980 figure.

The existence of hyperglycemia less than ODIP (GDM) early in pregnancy raises a multitude of questions:

- Is the etiological mechanism for GDM from early pregnancy the same as GDM developing later on?

- Is there a difference in the impact of GDM developing earlier and later on pregnancy outcomes and fetal programming?

- What tests and diagnostic thresholds should be used to "diagnose" GDM in early pregnancy? Should different criteria be used early and later in pregnancy?

- Is the treatment of GDM detected in early pregnancy of benefit? Could associated early medication, lower glucose levels including hypoglycemia, and/or insufficient weight gain cause harm?

Is the Etiological Mechanism for This GDM From Early Pregnancy the Same as for GDM Developing Later?

Depending on the setting, screening approach, and diagnostic criteria used, a high proportion (15–70%) of women with GDM have hyperglycemia detectable in early pregnancy (27). Women who develop GDM in early pregnancy appear to be more insulin resistant, with greater waist circumference, higher blood pressure, and higher triglycerides (28), than women who develop GDM later in pregnancy (29). Most importantly, a meta-analysis of 13 cohort studies showed that perinatal mortality (relative risk [RR] 3.58 [95% CI 1.91–6.71]), neonatal hypoglycemia (RR 1.61 [1.02–2.55]), and insulin use (RR 1.71 [1.45–2.03]) were greater among women with early GDM compared with those with GDM diagnosed later in the pregnancy (27). This was despite their GDM receiving standard treatment. The question arises why outcomes were worse in spite of treatment: longer/greater exposure to hyperglycemia and/or similar pathophysiology but with greater severity, and/or a different etiological mechanism?

The proposition that GDM is heterogenous (including early vs. late) is important, as it may suggest different GDM preventive and treatment strategies for different types of GDM. Besides the small numbers of those progressing to type 1 diabetes, monogenic "diabetes" (including maturity-onset diabetes of the young [MODY] 2), and forms associated with other genetic conditions, GDM is proposed to be associated with three different phenotypes (by definition, all have insufficient insulin secretion for their needs) (30). These include reduced insulin sensitivity with normal insulin secretion, normal insulin sensitivity with reduced insulin secretion alone, and reduced insulin sensitivity with reduced insulin secretion (30). The initial studies were in late pregnancy, but the same heterogeneity is shown in early pregnancy, with the reduced insulin sensitivity forms predominant (31). There may be differences in pregnancy outcomes with the less-insulin-sensitive being at greater risk of LGA and cesarean section (30, 31). Perhaps management should differ between these phenotypes as well as between GDM diagnosed earlier and later in pregnancy.

How Should We Diagnose and Manage GDM From Early Pregnancy?

Prior to HAPO and the development of the IADPSG GDM diagnostic criteria, criteria were based upon prediction of future maternal type 2 diabetes (1), complications among nonpregnant adults (World Health Organization), or "glycemic distribution" (32). The IADPSG process took the three-point, 2-h, 75-g OGTT data from the HAPO study and gained broad (but, alas, incomplete) agreement over GDM diagnostic thresholds based upon the linear relationship between glucose and adverse pregnancy outcomes (16). An odds ratio of 1.75-fold risk of adverse outcomes at each of the three time points using the HAPO data was chosen. This approach to equilibrate adverse pregnancy outcome risk at different OGTT time points revealed discordance between existing and proposed fasting (needed to be lower) and 2-h (needed to be higher) glucose thresholds on the 75-g OGTT (16). As HAPO did not use a screening test, the 50-g GCT itself (having little empirical evidence [33]) was dropped. As a result, many of those with an isolated high fasting glucose that had previously been excluded from the OGTT were suddenly being diagnosed with GDM. The IADPSG criteria also require only one, rather than two, time points to be above the threshold, further increasing the importance of the fasting glucose threshold. Overall, 50% of HAPO women were diagnosed on the fasting result: a shift in the GDM glycemic profile. However, applying the IADPSG criteria to the HAPO results also revealed significant heterogeneity in the OGTT pattern, particularly between

ethnic groups, some of whom were considered hyperglycemic predominantly based upon the 1-h and/or 2-h post–glucose load test results (34).

However, HAPO tested women at 24–28 weeks, not in early pregnancy. A similar study involving 6,129 women but using only a fasting glucose test at a median of 9.5 weeks showed a similarly linear increase in pregnancy complications as glucose increased from <75 mg/dL (4.2 mmol/L) to 100–105 mg/dL (5.6–5.8 mmol/L) (35). The adverse pregnancy outcomes LGA/macrosomia and primary cesarean section increased from 7.9% to 19.4% and from 12.7% to 20.0%, respectively, across the glucose categories. GDM at 24–28 weeks using the 50-g GCT and 100-g OGTT increased from the lowest to the highest glucose category from 1% to 11.7%, respectively. Unlike HAPO, this was not a blinded study, and hence women were presumably treated. These data contributed to a growing shift in paradigm that women with higher glucose levels early in pregnancy, below overt diabetes, should be treated for their GDM.

Before the IADPSG recommendations for managing hyperglycemia in pregnancy, GDM was generally diagnosed early in pregnancy by applying existing GDM criteria used at 24–28 weeks. Overdiagnosis was avoided by limiting early OGTTs to those women with a prior history of GDM or, e.g., glycosuria. However, with the introduction of screening for ODIP among women with other type 2 diabetes risk factors, more women were found to have GDM using these criteria. The IADPSG acknowledged that there were limited trial data and initially recommended that an FPG $\geq$5.1 mmol/L (92 mg/dL) in early pregnancy also be used to diagnose GDM (16). However, within 5 years, data emerging from Italy and China (36) suggested many such women no longer fulfilled GDM when later retested. The Chinese study (37) found that at 24–28 weeks' gestation, GDM was only present in 37.0%, 52.7%, and 66.2%, respectively, of women with an FPG at the first antenatal visit of 5.10–5.59, 5.60–6.09, and 6.10–6.99 mmol/L. In response, the IADPSG recommended using an HbA$_{1c}$, and not a fasting glucose, to test for hyperglycemia in pregnancy (37). The situation is compounded by the potential for the "fetal steal phenomenon" (38) to have

lowered maternal glycemia, with the offspring already hyperinsulinemic and at risk for macrosomia. Furthermore, the HbA$_{1c}$ has now been shown to be an insensitive test for both hyperglycemia and adverse pregnancy outcomes (25), and two randomized controlled trials (RCTs) of treating women with HbA$_{1c}$ 5.7–6.4% (39, 40) showed no treatment benefit.

One major RCT has now been completed of early testing for GDM among 962 obese women with a subgroup analysis among those who had GDM diagnosed (early screening $n = 69$ [15.0%] vs. routine screening $n = 56$ [12.1%]) (41). Screening involved the two-step approach (50-g GCT followed by 100-g 3-h OGTT). Randomization was at mean 13.6–13.8 weeks' gestation. There was no significant difference in any pregnancy outcome, although insulin treatment was 3.70-fold (95% CI 1.04–13.17) more likely in the early-screen group. In fact, the primary composite outcome (macrosomia, primary cesarean delivery, gestational hypertension, preeclampsia, hyperbilirubinemia, shoulder dystocia, and neonatal hypoglycemia) was nonsignificantly higher in the early-screen group (56.9% vs. 50.8%, $P = 0.06$) with preeclampsia (13.6% vs. 9.5%, $P = 0.06$), in particular, nonsignificantly higher. Gestational age at delivery was lower (36.7 vs. 38.7 weeks, $P = 0.001$) among those with GDM in the early-treatment group, but the groups were too small to show a difference in less common, but more severe, outcomes. The early-screen group of course included treating the ~2.9% of women who would not have had GDM diagnosed at 24–28 weeks' gestation. Similarly, no significant difference in adverse pregnancy outcomes was found between women randomized to either lifestyle intervention ($n = 36$) or control ($n = 54$) in a Danish GDM prevention study post hoc analysis of participants with a fasting glucose 5.1–6.9 mmol/L and a 2-h capillary blood glucose <9.0 mmol/L (42).

The Treatment Of BOoking Gestational diabetes Mellitus (TOBOGM) Pilot and Main RCTs

Managing GDM is not without risk. While the iconic work of Freinkel and Pederson emphasized short- and long-term risks from fetal fuel oversupply (5), the "thrifty phenotype hypothesis" postulates that fetal undernutrition leads to future metabolic risks (15). Antenatal metformin therapy, insufficient gestational weight gain, and overmedication are all potentially associated with disturbances in fetal metabolism that might therefore lead to future obesity and dysglycemia (15, 43, 44). The TOBOGM RCT was commenced to address the equipoise between the potential for harm and there being no existing major RCTs showing benefits from treating GDM at the time of "booking" (i.e., early in pregnancy) (45, 46). There is good RCT evidence to show that GDM treatment at 24–28 weeks is of benefit (47, 48), although neither major trial used the IADPSG criteria.

The TOBOGM study is a multicenter RCT testing whether diagnosing and treating GDM from booking, rather than waiting for the OGTT at 24–28 weeks, reduces adverse pregnancy outcomes. Women at <20 weeks' gestation with GDM/diabetes risk factors are invited for an early OGTT. With this early OGTT, women are identified with "booking GDM" using the IADPSG 24–28 weeks criteria and randomized either to immediate referral for GDM management (and no

further OGTT) or to a repeat OGTT at 24–28 weeks' gestation. Clinicians are blinded to OGTT results. Antenatal and GDM care otherwise follow local/agreed guidelines. A pilot study (46) has been completed and the main TOBOGM RCT is currently underway (47). The pilot RCT randomized 11 women with "booking GDM" to early treatment and 10 women to a repeat OGTT at 24–28 weeks' gestation. A further 58 women served as decoys (i.e., women with normal glucose tolerance mingling in clinic with and labeled in the same way as the women randomized to untreated "booking GDM"). Important findings from the TOBOGM pilot study were, first, that GDM was still present in 89% of the women randomized to no early treatment and had developed in 20% of decoys. However, most important was that neonatal intensive care unit admission was highest in the treated group (36% vs. 0%, P = 0.043), largely due to SGA babies, while LGA babies were more common in the no-early-treatment group (0% vs. 33%, P = 0.030). This may indicate that early treatment (including gestational weight gain limitation) may have both benefits and harms, making completion of the

main TOBOGM RCT even more important. It certainly appears that lifestyle intervention (49) and weight management (50) have different impacts on GDM risk earlier and later in pregnancy and may require different management approaches early and later in pregnancy.

The main multicenter RCT is currently underway, requiring approximately 4,000 women to be recruited to identify 800 women with "booking GDM" with 400 randomized to early GDM treatment and 400 to the second OGTT at 24–28 weeks' gestation. A further 800 randomly selected women serve as decoys, with the remaining 2,400 for chart review only. Randomization is stratified by site. Women with ODIP and those with a fasting glucose 6.1–6.9 mmol/L are excluded from the RCT. The primary pregnancy outcome to detect the effects of maternal hyperglycemia is a composite of respiratory distress, phototherapy, birth trauma, birth <37 weeks, stillbirth/death, shoulder dystocia, and birth weight ≥4.5 kg. The primary neonatal outcome to detect any fetal undernutrition is neonatal lean body mass. The primary maternal outcome is preeclampsia. TOBOGM also stratifies its

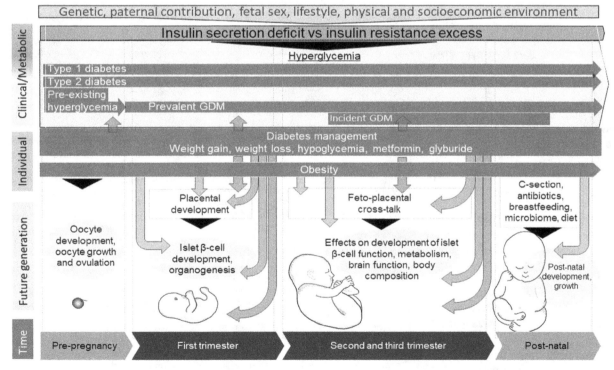

Figure 2—2021 adaptation of Freinkel model to include effects on the fetus beyond hyperglycemia. Blue = effects of maternal hyperglycemia; orange = effects of maternal obesity; dark pink = effects of maternal diabetes management including effects of weight change and pharmacotherapy. Light pink summarizes the wider effects of maternal genetics, any paternal contributions, fetal sex, maternal lifestyle, the physical (e.g., climate) and socioeconomic environment.

randomization within two glycemic bands: *1)* the HAPO 1.75 odds ratio band (FBG 5.1–5.2 mmol/L and/or 1-h blood glucose 10.0–10.5 mmol/L and/or 2-h blood glucose 8.5–8.9 mmol/L), and *2)* the HAPO 2.0 odds ratio band (FBG 5.3–6.9 mmol/L and/or 1-h blood glucose ≥10.6 mmol/L and/or 2-h blood glucose 9.0–11.0 mmol/L). The analyses will not only compare pregnancy outcomes between early-treated women and those who had the deferred OGTT but will repeat the comparisons within the two glycemic bands and between these bands and the decoys. Further analyses will be undertaken to identify the optimal OGTT time point thresholds.

What To Do While We Await the TOBOGM Results?

TOBOGM is the largest and most comprehensive RCT comparing treatment for women with early GDM and those with treatment deferred to the outcome of the OGTT at 24–28 weeks, and results will likely not be available for 2–3 years. In the meantime, the IADPSG recommendations provide no guidance for where to diagnose GDM <7.0 mmol/L and/or 2-h glucose <11.1 mmol/L (with confirmation). The American Diabetes Association recommends those with "prediabetes" be treated as if they have hyperglycemia (fasting ≥5.6 mmol/L and/or 2-h glucose ≥7.8 mmol/L), but there may be a risk of overtreatment early in pregnancy. HbA$_{1c}$ testing has been advised as an alternative, but there is no evidence of benefit. In terms of diagnosis, a 75-g OGTT is probably still the best test (with all its challenges). Previously, we have recommended using a threshold of 6.1–6.9 mmol/L to diagnose GDM early in pregnancy and this agrees with the recommendations by Zhu et al. (27, 37). A 2-h threshold of ≥8.5 mmol/L would identify those with significant postprandial hyperglycemia. All women without "early hyperglycemia in pregnancy" would then undertake the OGTT at 24–28 weeks.

Summary and Future Directions

There have been several paradigm shifts since Freinkel's iconic lecture of 1980. These include the growth in the importance and our understanding of type 2 diabetes in pregnancy, insights into the role of maternal obesity on fetal growth and metabolism, the realization that GDM is heterogenous with hyperglycemia often already present at conception, the introduction of oral antihyperglycemic agents in therapy, and the importance of the first trimester in the growth trajectory and metabolism of both the mother and offspring. Figure 2 brings each of these concepts into an adaptation of Fig. 1, also acknowledging the importance of the setting in which the pregnancy occurs.

Future work needs to consider the consequences of this new-found variation. This includes the potential for different screening strategies and diagnostic criteria early and later in pregnancy. Similarly, the use of metformin, weight management, glucose treatment thresholds, and lifestyle strategies may need to differ between women with GDM diagnosed early in pregnancy (who appear to have a more insulin-resistant pattern) and those diagnosed later. In view of these observed differences, it may be necessary to divide GDM into mild hyperglycemia already present at the beginning of pregnancy ("prevalent GDM") and that which arises de novo during pregnancy ("incident GDM"). Perhaps the move to subclassify GDM in this way should start now.

Acknowledgments. I am especially grateful to my mentors in epidemiology, Rhys Wlliams from Cardiff, Wales, and Paul Zimmett, Melbourne, Australia; my mentor in diabetes in pregnancy, the late David J. Scott; and my mentor in academic medicine, the late P. John Scott, who have between them guided me to broader and deeper insights into research. I am also grateful to my cultural mentors, all now passed, who gave me insights into indigenous communities: Betty Hunapo, Ngati Hine, Aotearoa/New Zealand; Buddy Te Whare, Ngati Maniapoto, Aotearoa/New Zealand; Rick Henderson, Goulburn Valley, Australia. I am grateful to all of the teams I work/have worked with in South Auckland and the Waikato in New Zealand, in Victoria and New South Wales in Australia, and the Addenbrookes/Rosie teams in Cambridge. Many thanks to the Vitamin D and Lifestyle Intervention for GDM Prevention (DALI) team for all of their insights—what a great group! Also thanks to my Swedish team members in Örebro, from whom I have learned a lot about obstetrics! I have to thank my colleagues in the Diabetic Pregnancy Study Group (DPSG) and Australasian Diabetes in Pregnancy Society (ADIPS) who have given such terrific insights into hyperglycemia in pregnancy over the years. I also wish to thank my good colleague Gernot Desoye, University of Graz, Graz, Austria, for critically reading the manuscript and important input into Fig. 2. Many thanks to Anand Hardikar, Western Sydney University, for the artwork and assistance with Fig. 2.

Funding. This work has been supported by multiple funders, particularly the Health Research Council in New Zealand, the European Commission, and the National Health and Medical Research Council of Australia.

Duality of Interest. No potential conflicts of interest relevant to this article were reported.

References

1. O'Sullivan JB, Mahan CM. Criteria for the oral glucose tolerance test in pregnancy. Diabetes 1964;13:278–285

2. Catalano PM, Tyzbir ED, Roman NM, Amini SB, Sims EAH. Longitudinal changes in insulin release and insulin resistance in nonobese pregnant women. Am J Obstet Gynecol 1991; 165:1667–1672

3. Pedersen J. Diabetes and pregnancy: blood sugar of newborn infants (PhD thesis). Copenhagen, Danish Science Press, 1952

4. Pedersen J. The Pregnant Diabetic and Her Newborn: Problems and Management. Baltimore, MD, William & Wilkins, 1967

5. Freinkel N. Banting Lecture 1980. Of pregnancy and progeny. Diabetes 1980;29:1023–1035

6. Gabbe SG. The gestational diabetes mellitus conferences. Three are history: focus on the fourth. Diabetes Care 1998;21(Suppl. 2):B1–B2

7. King H. Epidemiology of glucose intolerance and gestational diabetes in women of childbearing age. Diabetes Care 1998;21(Suppl. 2):B9–B13

8. Simmons D, Williams DR, Powell MJ. The Coventry Diabetes Study: prevalence of diabetes and impaired glucose tolerance in Europids and Asians. Q J Med 1991;81:1021–1030

9. Feig DS, Palda VA. Type 2 diabetes in pregnancy: a growing concern. Lancet 2002;359: 1690–1692

10. Albrecht SS, Kuklina EV, Bansil P, et al. Diabetes trends among delivery hospitalizations in the U.S., 1994-2004. Diabetes Care 2010;33: 768–773

11. Sina M, MacMillan F, Dune T, et al. Development of an integrated, district-wide approach to pre-pregnancy management for women with pre-existing diabetes in a multi-ethnic population. BMC Pregnancy Childbirth 2018;18:402

12. Feig DS, Donovan LE, Zinman B, et al.; MiTy Collaborative Group. Metformin in women with type 2 diabetes in pregnancy (MiTy): a multicentre, international, randomised, placebo-controlled trial. Lancet Diabetes Endocrinol 2020; 8:834–844

13. Simmons D, Thompson CF, Conroy C, Scott DJ. Use of insulin pumps in pregnancies complicated by type 2 diabetes and gestational diabetes in a multiethnic community. Diabetes Care 2001;24:2078–2082

14. Nielsen LR, Ekbom P, Damm P, et al. HbA$_{1c}$ levels are significantly lower in early and late pregnancy. Diabetes Care 2004;27:1200–1201

15. Hales CN, Barker DJ. Type 2 (non-insulin-dependent) diabetes mellitus: the thrifty phenotype hypothesis. Diabetologia 1992;35:595–601

16. Metzger BE, Gabbe SG, Persson B, et al.; International Association of Diabetes and Pregnancy Study Groups Consensus Panel. International Association of Diabetes and Pregnancy Study Groups recommendations on the diagnosis and classification of hyperglycaemia in pregnancy. Diabetes Care 2010;33:676–682

17. Colagiuri S, Falavigna M, Agarwal MM, et al. Strategies for implementing the WHO diagnostic criteria and classification of hyperglycaemia first detected in pregnancy. Diabetes Res Clin Pract 2014;103:364–372

18. HAPO Study Cooperative Research Group. Hyperglycemia and adverse pregnancy outcomes. N Engl J Med 2008;358:1991–2002

19. Immanuel J, Eagleton C, Baker J, Simmons D. Pregnancy outcomes among multi-ethnic women with hyperglycaemia during pregnancy in an urban New Zealand population and their association with postnatal HbA1c uptake. Aust N Z J Obstet Gynaecol 2021;61:69–77

20. Church D, Halsall D, Meek C, Parker RA, Murphy HR, Simmons D. Random blood glucose measurement at antenatal booking to screen for overt diabetes in pregnancy: a retrospective study. Diabetes Care 2011;34:2217–2219

21. Simmons D, Rudland VL, Wong V, et al. Options for screening for gestational diabetes mellitus during the SARS-CoV-2 pandemic. Aust N Z J Obstet Gynaecol 2020;60:660–666

22. Meek CL, Lindsay RS, Scott EM, et al. Approaches to screening for hyperglycaemia in pregnant women during and after the COVID-19 pandemic. Diabet Med 2021;38:e14380

23. Church D, Simmons D. More evidence of the problems of using HbA1c for diagnosing diabetes? The known knowns, the known unknowns and the unknown unknowns. J Int Med 2014;276:171–173

24. Hughes RC, Moore MP, Gullam JE, Mohamed K, Rowan J. An early pregnancy HbA1c ≥5.9% (41 mmol/mol) is optimal for detecting diabetes and identifies women at increased risk of adverse pregnancy outcomes. Diabetes Care 2014;37:2953–2959

25. Immanuel J, Simmons D, Desoye G, et al. Performance of early pregnancy HbA$_{1c}$ for predicting gestational diabetes mellitus and adverse pregnancy outcomes in obese European women. Diabetes Res Clin Pract 2020;168:108378

26. Harris MI. Gestational diabetes may represent discovery of preexisting glucose intolerance. Diabetes Care 1988;11:402–411

27. Immanuel J, Simmons D. Screening and treatment for early-onset gestational diabetes mellitus: a systematic review and meta-analysis. Curr Diab Rep 2017;17:115

28. Harreiter J, Simmons D, Desoye G, et al.; DALI Core Investigator group. IADPSG and WHO 2013 gestational diabetes mellitus criteria identify obese women with marked insulin resistance in early pregnancy. Diabetes Care 2016;39:e90–e92

29. Egan AM, Vellinga A, Harreiter J, et al.; DALI Core Investigator group. Epidemiology of gestational diabetes mellitus according to IADPSG/WHO 2013 criteria among obese pregnant women in Europe. Diabetologia 2017;60:1913–1921

30. Powe CE, Allard C, Battista MC, et al. Heterogeneous contribution of insulin sensitivity and secretion defects to gestational diabetes mellitus. Diabetes Care 2016;39:1052–1055

31. Immanuel J, Simmons D, Harreiter J, et al. Metabolic phenotypes of early gestational diabetes mellitus and their association with adverse pregnancy outcomes. Diabet Med 2020;38:e14413

32. Cutchie WA, Cheung NW, Simmons D. Comparison of international and New Zealand guidelines for the care of pregnant women with diabetes. Diabet Med 2006;23:460–468

33. Simmons D, Moses RG. Gestational diabetes mellitus: to screen or not to screen?: Is this really still a question? Diabetes Care 2013;36:2877–2878

34. Sacks DA, Hadden DR, Maresh M, et al.; HAPO Study Cooperative Research Group. Frequency of gestational diabetes mellitus at collaborating centers based on IADPSG consensus panel-recommended criteria: the Hyperglycemia and Adverse Pregnancy Outcome (HAPO) Study. Diabetes Care 2012;35:526–528

35. Riskin-Mashiah S, Younes G, Damti A, Auslender R. First-trimester fasting hyperglycemia and adverse pregnancy outcomes. Diabetes Care 2009;32:1639–1643

36. McIntyre HD, Sacks DA, Barbour LA, et al. Issues with the diagnosis and classification of hyperglycemia in early pregnancy. Diabetes Care 2016;39:53–54

37. Zhu WW, Yang HX, Wei YM, et al. Evaluation of the value of fasting plasma glucose in the first prenatal visit to diagnose gestational diabetes mellitus in China. Diabetes Care 2013;36:586–590

38. Desoye G, Nolan CJ. The fetal glucose steal: an underappreciated phenomenon in diabetic pregnancy. Diabetologia 2016;59:1089–1094

39. Osmundson SS, Norton ME, El-Sayed YY, Carter S, Faig JC, Kitzmiller JL. Early screening and treatment of women with prediabetes: a randomized controlled trial. Am J Perinatol 2016;33:172–179

40. Roeder HA, Moore TR, Wolfson T, Ramos GA. Treating prediabetes in the first trimester: a randomized controlled trial. Am J Obstet Gynecol 2017;216(Suppl.):S308

41. Harper LM, Jauk V, Longo S, Biggio JR, Szychowski JM, Tita AT. Early gestational diabetes screening in obese women: a randomized controlled trial. Am J Obstet Gynecol 2020;222:495.e1–495.e8

42. Vinter CA, Tanvig MH, Christensen MH, et al. Lifestyle intervention in Danish obese pregnant women with early gestational diabetes mellitus according to WHO 2013 criteria does not change pregnancy outcomes: results from the LiP (Lifestyle in Pregnancy) Study. Diabetes Care 2018;41:2079–2085

43. Catalano PM, Mele L, Landon MB, et al.; *Eunice Kennedy Shriver* National Institute of Child Health and Human Development Maternal-Fetal Medicine Units Network. Inadequate weight gain in overweight and obese pregnant women: what is the effect on fetal growth? Am J Obstet Gynecol 2014;211:137.e1–137.e7

44. Langer O, Levy J, Brustman L, Anyaegbunam A, Merkatz R, Divon M. Glycemic control in gestational diabetes mellitus—how tight is tight enough: small for gestational age versus large for gestational age? Am J Obstet Gynecol 1989;161:646–653

45. Simmons D, Hague WM, Teede HJ, et al. Hyperglycemia in early pregnancy: the Treatment of Booking Gestational diabetes Mellitus (TOBOGM) study. A randomised controlled trial. Med J Aust 2018;209:405–406

46. Simmons D, Nema J, Parton C, et al. The treatment of booking gestational diabetes mellitus (TOBOGM) pilot randomised controlled trial. BMC Pregnancy Childbirth 2018;18:151

47. Crowther CA, Hiller JE, Moss JR, McPhee AJ, Jeffries WS; Australian Carbohydrate Intolerance Study in Pregnant Women (ACHOIS) Trial Group. Effect of treatment of gestational diabetes mellitus on pregnancy outcomes. N Engl J Med 2005;352:2477–2486

48. Landon MB, Spong CY, Thom E, et al.; Eunice Kennedy Shriver National Institute of Child Health and Human Development Maternal-Fetal Medicine Units Network. A multicenter, randomized trial of treatment for mild gestational diabetes. N Engl J Med 2009;361:1339–1348

49. Song C, Li J, Leng J, Ma RC, Yang X. Lifestyle intervention can reduce the risk of gestational diabetes: a meta-analysis of randomized controlled trials. Obes Rev 2016;17:960–969

50. Hedderson MM, Gunderson EP, Ferrara A. Gestational weight gain and risk of gestational diabetes mellitus. Obstet Gynecol 2010;115:597–604

Cardiovascular Outcomes in Patients With Type 2 Diabetes and Obesity: Comparison of Gastric Bypass, Sleeve Gastrectomy, and Usual Care

Diabetes Care 2021;44:2552–2563 | https://doi.org/10.2337/dc20-3023

Ali Aminian,[1] Rickesha Wilson,[1] Alexander Zajichek,[2] Chao Tu,[2] Kathy E. Wolski,[3] Philip R. Schauer,[4] Michael W. Kattan,[2] Steven E. Nissen,[3] and Stacy A. Brethauer[5]

OBJECTIVE

To determine which one of the two most common metabolic surgical procedures is associated with greater reduction in risk of major adverse cardiovascular events (MACE) in patients with type 2 diabetes mellitus (T2DM) and obesity.

RESEARCH DESIGN AND METHODS

A total of 13,490 patients including 1,362 Roux-en-Y gastric bypass (RYGB), 693 sleeve gastrectomy (SG), and 11,435 matched nonsurgical patients with T2DM and obesity who received their care at the Cleveland Clinic (1998–2017) were analyzed, with follow-up through December 2018. With multivariable Cox regression analysis we estimated time to incident extended MACE, defined as first occurrence of coronary artery events, cerebrovascular events, heart failure, nephropathy, atrial fibrillation, and all-cause mortality.

RESULTS

The cumulative incidence of the primary end point at 5 years was 13.7% (95% CI 11.4–15.9) in the RYGB groups and 24.7% (95% CI 19.0–30.0) in the SG group, with an adjusted hazard ratio (HR) of 0.77 (95% CI 0.60–0.98, $P = 0.04$). Of the six individual end points, RYGB was associated with a significantly lower cumulative incidence of nephropathy at 5 years compared with SG (2.8% vs. 8.3%, respectively; HR 0.47 [95% CI 0.28–0.79], $P = 0.005$). Furthermore, RYGB was associated with a greater reduction in body weight, glycated hemoglobin, and use of medications to treat diabetes and cardiovascular diseases. Five years after RYGB, patients required more upper endoscopy (45.8% vs. 35.6%, $P < 0.001$) and abdominal surgical procedures (10.8% vs. 5.4%, $P = 0.001$) compared with SG.

CONCLUSIONS

In patients with obesity and T2DM, RYGB may be associated with greater weight loss, better diabetes control, and lower risk of MACE and nephropathy compared with SG.

[1]Bariatric and Metabolic Institute, Department of General Surgery, Cleveland Clinic, Cleveland, OH
[2]Department of Quantitative Health Sciences, Lerner Research Institute, Cleveland Clinic, Cleveland, OH
[3]Cleveland Clinic Coordinating Center for Clinical Research, Department of Cardiovascular Medicine, Cleveland Clinic, Cleveland, OH
[4]Pennington Biomedical Research Center, Baton Rouge, LA
[5]Department of Surgery, The Ohio State University Wexner Medical Center, Columbus, OH

Corresponding author: Ali Aminian, aminiaa@ccf.org

Received 13 December 2020 and accepted 29 July 2021

This article contains supplementary material online at https://doi.org/10.2337/figshare.15173139.

More than 10 small randomized clinical trials (RCTs) have shown that metabolic surgery is superior to usual medical therapy for diabetes control and modifying cardiometabolic risk factors in patients with type 2 diabetes mellitus (T2DM) and obesity (1–5). Furthermore, >30 large comparative cohort studies have consistently reported reduction in risk of mortality after metabolic surgery (6–9). The majority of these RCTs and large observational studies have only examined the favorable effects of Roux-en-Y gastric bypass (RYGB). Currently, sleeve gastrectomy (SG), a relatively new procedure, is the most commonly performed metabolic surgical procedure worldwide (10,11). However, long-term data on efficacy of SG for macro- and microvascular complications of T2DM and mortality are limited.

Guiding patients toward the most appropriate metabolic surgical procedure for treatment of chronic diseases of obesity, T2DM, and their adverse events is crucial for improving outcomes. The surgical risk, impact of each procedure on body weight and comorbidities, coexistence of other medical and mental conditions, and patient behavioral factors, values, and goals are important considerations in choosing the most appropriate metabolic surgical procedure (12,13). One factor that may help in decision-making would be understanding the differential impact of each surgical procedure on the risk of major adverse cardiovascular events (MACE) and mortality. This important consideration has not been studied yet.

RESEARCH DESIGN AND METHODS

This is a secondary analysis of a matched-cohort study that originally reported association of metabolic surgery with lower risk of MACE in adult patients with obesity and T2DM (6). The main aim of the current study is to determine which metabolic surgical procedure (RYGB vs. SG) is associated with greater risk reduction in development of MACE. In addition, since there are limited data on the effects of SG on cardiovascular health, the second aim of this study is to examine the association of each metabolic surgical procedure separately with risk of MACE and mortality.

A retrospective observational study on patients who received treatment within the Cleveland Clinic Health System between 1 January 1998 and 31 December 2017 with follow-up through 31 December 2018 was performed. The Cleveland Clinic's institutional review board approved the study as minimal risk research using data collected for routine clinical practice for which the requirement for informed consent was waived.

Details of the study protocol, enrollment criteria, construction of study cohorts, and statistical analysis have previously been published (6). The ICD-9, ICD-10, and Current Procedural Terminology (CPT) procedure codes that were used to extract data from the electronic health records (EHR) are summarized in Supplementary Tables 1 and 2.

Study Cohorts

A total of 2,287 adult patients with T2DM and BMI ≥30 kg/m² who underwent metabolic surgery and did not have a history of solid organ transplant, severe heart failure, or active cancer were identified. Among the 2,287 surgical patients of the original cohort, 1,362 RYGB and 693 SG cases are included in the current analysis. Patients who underwent adjustable gastric banding ($n = 109$), duodenal switch ($n = 5$), or conversion of primary SG and RYGB to other procedures ($n = 118$) were not included.

Enrollment criteria were implemented for identification of the nonsurgical patients who received usual care for T2DM and obesity. Each surgical patient was matched with a propensity score to five nonsurgical patients based on the index date, age at index date, sex, BMI at index date, location (Ohio vs. Florida), insulin use, and presence of diabetes end-organ complications (composite of coronary artery disease, heart failure, cerebrovascular disease, peripheral vascular disease, neuropathy, nephropathy, or requiring dialysis), resulting in 11,435 nonsurgical patients (6).

End Points

As described in the original study (6), the primary end point was the incidence of extended MACE, defined as first occurrence of any of six outcomes including all-cause mortality, coronary artery events (unstable angina, myocardial infarction, or coronary intervention/surgery), cerebrovascular events (ischemic stroke, hemorrhagic stroke, or carotid intervention/surgery), heart failure (diastolic and systolic), atrial fibrillation, and nephropathy (at least two measures of estimated glomerular filtration rate [eGFR] <60 mL/min), with the first occurrence after the index date recorded as the event date (see Supplementary Table 1 for definitions and codes). A secondary composite end point included three-component MACE (all-cause mortality, myocardial infarction, and ischemic stroke).

All patients were included in the assessment of the composite primary and secondary end points. However, the conditions or events that a patient had at baseline were omitted from the count toward the composite end points in follow-up. For example, in a patient with history of ischemic stroke before the index date, having a code for stroke after the index date was not considered an event for composite end points. However, development of myocardial infarction in this patient after the index date would count toward the composite end points (6).

Other secondary end points included the six individual components of the primary end point including coronary artery events, cerebrovascular events, heart failure, atrial fibrillation, nephropathy, and all-cause mortality. Death information was obtained from a combination of local EHR, Social Security, and state death indices. For assessment of individual secondary end points, patients who already had these conditions prior to the index date were eliminated from subsequent risk evaluation only for that specific outcome.

Other Outcomes

Weight, glycated hemoglobin (HbA_{1c}), and dates of prescription orders for diabetes and cardiovascular drugs were collected from the EHR for comparison of groups. Data on nutritional, endoscopic, radiologic, and surgical interventions until last follow-up were also compared between surgical procedures to serve as surrogates of surgical adverse events.

Statistical Analysis

Baseline data are expressed as median (interquartile range [IQR]) and number (%). Doubly robust estimation combining the propensity score and outcome regression was used to compare the outcomes between three study groups head-to-head.

Cause-specific event rates per 100 patient-years of follow-up starting from the index date were estimated for each outcome within each study group. Cumulative incidence estimates (Kaplan-Meier method) 5 years after the index date with 95% CIs for each outcome were calculated.

Fully adjusted Cox proportional hazards regression models were generated for two composite and six individual study outcomes. Regression analyses were performed for all of the factors used in the matching process as well as a larger range of potential confounding variables (all variables in Table 1). Therefore, any imbalances in the observed potential confounders that remained after the matching process were controlled for by the statistical analysis. The proportional hazards assumptions for the treatment variable were tested based on weighted residuals.

To address missing values, within each outcome data set, we imputed missing values at baseline (Table 1) with multiple imputation by chained equations (MICE) to create five imputed data sets. Predictive mean matching, logistic regression, and polytomous logistic regression were used for numeric, binary, and categorical variables, respectively. Imputation-corrected SEs of model estimates and contrasts were obtained with Rubin's formula (6, 14).

The Wald test was used for comparing mean changes in weight loss and HbA$_{1c}$, two-sample proportions test for comparing proportions of patients on diabetes and cardiovascular medications, and log-rank test for comparing interventions between the study groups at 5 years of follow-up.

A significance level of 0.05 for two-sided comparisons was considered statistically significant, and 95% CIs were reported where applicable. Because of the potential for a type 1 error due to multiple comparisons, findings should be interpreted as exploratory. All analysis was done in the R statistical programming language (version 3.5.0).

RESULTS

A total of 13,490 patients including 1,362 RYGB, 693 SG, and 11,435 matched nonsurgical patients were included in the analysis. The median BMI of RYGB, SG, and control group was 45.3, 44.7, and 42.6 kg/m^2, respectively. In total, 4.3% of

patients had a BMI between 30 and 34.9 kg/m^2.

The distribution of 37 baseline covariates was well balanced after matching among the RYGB, SG, and nonsurgical patient study groups (Table 1) including median HbA$_{1c}$ level (7.1% vs. 7.0% vs. 7.1%) and eGFR (91.3 vs. 90.4 vs. 91.9 mL/min) and percentage taking insulin (33.7% vs. 34.2% vs. 33.3%), cholesterol-lowering medications (52.6% vs. 51.5% vs. 52.5%), and renin-angiotensin system inhibitors (60.6% vs. 61% vs. 62.1%), respectively. Compared with RYGB patients, SG patients were older (54.6 vs. 51.2 years) and had higher rates of some comorbidities at baseline including heart failure (14.3% vs. 7.7%), history of myocardial infarction (3.3% vs. 1.9%), history of atrial fibrillation (9.1% vs. 5.2%), chronic obstructive pulmonary disease (11.1% vs. 8.4%), and nephropathy (9.8% vs. 6.9%). Conversely, the frequency of smoking (8.9% vs. 4.8%) and BMI $\geq$40 kg/m^2 (77.5% vs. 71.7%) was higher among patients receiving RYGB compared with SG. The median follow-up time for RYGB, SG, and nonsurgical patients was 4.0 years (IQR 1.3–7.0), 2.0 years (IQR 0.7–4.1), and 4.0 years (IQR 2.1–6.1), respectively.

Primary Composite End Point

The cumulative incidence of the primary end point at 5 years was 13.7% (95% CI 11.4–15.9) in the RYGB group and 24.7% (95% CI 19.0–30.0) in the SG group, with an adjusted hazard ratio (HR) of 0.77 (95% CI 0.60–0.98, P = 0.035) (Fig. 1A and Table 2). The cumulative incidence of the primary end point at 5 years was 30.4% (95% CI 29.4–31.5) in the nonsurgical group. Both metabolic surgical procedures were associated with a significantly lower cumulative incidence of the primary end point at 5 years compared with usual care: HR 0.53 (95% CI 0.46–0.61, P < 0.001) after RYGB and HR 0.69 (95% CI 0.56–0.85, P < 0.001) after SG (Fig. 1A and Table 2).

Secondary Composite End Point

The cumulative incidence of three-component MACE at 5 years was 6.4% (95% CI 4.8–8.0) in the RYGB group and 11.8% (95% CI 7.6–15.8) in the SG group, with an adjusted HR of 0.81 (95% CI 0.57–1.16, P = 0.258) (Fig. 1B and Table 2). The cumulative incidence

of three-component MACE at 5 years was 15.5% (95% CI 14.7–16.4) in the non-surgical group. Both metabolic surgical procedures were associated with significantly lower cumulative incidence of three-component MACE at 5 years in comparison with usual care: HR 0.53 (95% CI 0.43–0.65, P < 0.001) after RYGB and HR 0.65 (95% CI 0.48–0.88, P = 0.006) after SG (Fig. 1B and Table 2).

Secondary Individual End Points

RYGB was associated with a significantly lower cumulative incidence of nephropathy at 5 years compared with SG (2.8% vs. 8.3%, respectively) (HR 0.47 [95% CI 0.28–0.79, P = 0.005]). Although the 5-year cumulative incidences of the other five individual end points were lower after RYGB, the fully adjusted HRs were not significantly different in comparison of RYGB and SG (Fig. 2, Table 2, and Supplementary Table 3).

Compared with usual care, RYGB was associated with a significantly lower incidence of five out of six individual end points and SG was associated with a significantly lower incidence of three out of six individual end points. The incidence for these end points and adjusted HRs are reported in Table 2 and Supplementary Table 3. The proportional hazards assumption was satisfied for the primary and secondary composite outcomes and individual outcomes (see Supplementary Table 4 for P values testing the proportional hazards assumption).

Change in Status of Obesity, Diabetes, and Medications

Both metabolic surgical procedures were associated with a significant reduction in weight and HbA$_{1c}$ level in comparisons with the control group (P < 0.001 for all four comparisons at 5 years). Patients who underwent RYGB on average had 9.7%-points greater weight loss (95% CI 9.3–10.1, P < 0.001) and a 0.31% lower HbA$_{1c}$ level (95% CI 0.16–0.47, P < 0.001) at 5 years compared with SG patients (Fig. 3 and Supplementary Table 5).

Patients after RYGB and SG required significantly less diabetes and cardiovascular medication compared with those who received usual care. Furthermore, use of noninsulin diabetes medications, renin-angiotensin system blockers, lipid-lowering therapies, and aspirin was significantly lower after the

Table 1—Characteristics of patients at the index date

Baseline variable	RYGB (N = 1,362)	SG (N = 693)	Nonsurgical control (N = 11,435)
Demographic data			
Index year	2012 (2010, 2014)	2014 (2012, 2016)	2013 (2011, 2015)
Sex			
Female	908 (66.7)	439 (63.3)	7,339 (64.2)
Male	454 (33.3)	254 (36.7)	4,096 (35.8)
Age (years)	51.2 (43.1, 58.4)	54.6 (44.6, 62.8)	54.8 (46.2, 62.5)
BMI (kg/m^2)	45.3 (40.7, 51.5)	44.7 (39.3, 52.5)	42.6 (39.4, 47.2)
BMI category (kg/m^2)			
30–34.9	58 (4.3)	30 (4.3)	495 (4.3)
35–39.9	249 (18.3)	166 (24)	2,595 (22.7)
≥40	1,055 (77.5)	497 (71.7)	8,345 (73)
Weight (kg)	126.8 (112, 147)	125.6 (108.4, 149.4)	120.2 (106.8, 136.5)
Race			
White	1,066 (78.3)	492 (71)	7,994 (69.9)
Black	239 (17.5)	156 (22.5)	2,804 (24.5)
Other	23 (1.7)	27 (3.9)	234 (2)
Missing	34 (2.5)	18 (2.6)	403 (3.5)
Annual zip code income ($)	49,664 (39,730, 61,278)	50,925 (41,013, 63,445)	48,732 (36,951, 61,512)
Missing	29 (2.1)	34 (4.9)	125 (1.1)
Smoking status			
Never	724 (53.2)	383 (55.3)	5,615 (49.1)
Former	480 (35.2)	261 (37.7)	4,012 (35.1)
Current	121 (8.9)	33 (4.8)	1,607 (14.1)
Missing	37 (2.7)	16 (2.3)	201 (1.8)
Location			
Ohio	1,231 (90.4)	390 (56.3)	9,834 (86)
Florida	131 (9.6)	303 (43.7)	1,601 (14)
Medical history			
Hypertension	1,165 (85.5)	587 (84.7)	8,565 (74.9)
Dyslipidemia	1,042 (76.5)	483 (69.7)	7,457 (65.2)
Peripheral neuropathy	139 (10.2)	84 (12.1)	1,203 (10.5)
Heart failure	105 (7.7)	99 (14.3)	1,342 (11.7)
Coronary artery disease	129 (9.5)	81 (11.7)	1,104 (9.7)
COPD	114 (8.4)	77 (11.1)	1,188 (10.4)
Nephropathy	94 (6.9)	68 (9.8)	1,219 (10.7)
Atrial fibrillation	71 (5.2)	63 (9.1)	701 (6.1)
Peripheral arterial disease	66 (4.8)	47 (6.8)	755 (6.6)
Myocardial infarction	26 (1.9)	23 (3.3)	211 (1.8)
Cerebrovascular disease	18 (1.3)	19 (2.7)	358 (3.1)
Ischemic stroke	17 (1.2)	13 (1.9)	298 (2.6)
Dialysis	5 (0.4)	8 (1.2)	78 (0.7)
Clinical and laboratory data			
HbA$_{1c}$			
%	7.1 (6.3, 8.4)	7 (6.4, 8)	7.1 (6.4, 8.4)
mmol/mol	54 (45, 68)	53 (46, 64)	54 (46, 68)
Missing	88 (6.5)	50 (7.2)	1,288 (11.3)
Systolic blood pressure (mmHg)	136.7 (126, 147.3)	141.3 (130.8, 151.2)	130.2 (121, 142)
Missing	0 (0)	0 (0)	54 (0.5)
Diastolic blood pressure (mmHg)	72 (65.5, 79.7)	71.2 (65, 78)	78 (70, 84)
Missing	0 (0)	0 (0)	54 (0.5)
eGFR (mL/min)[a]	91.3 (74, 107.9)	90.4 (69.8, 111.5)	91.9 (72.5, 111.9)
Missing	0 (0)	1 (0.1)	432 (3.8)
HDL (mg/dL)	43 (36, 51)	45 (38, 51.5)	43 (36, 51)
Missing	378 (27.8)	346 (49.9)	3,512 (30.7)
LDL (mg/dL)	93 (72, 116)	91 (71, 116)	93 (72, 118)
Missing	121 (8.9)	56 (8.1)	2,947 (25.8)
Triglycerides (mg/dL)	150 (104, 216.5)	139 (96, 197.5)	146 (103, 208)
Missing	87 (6.4)	46 (6.6)	1,816 (15.9)
UACR (mg/g)	14 (6, 39.8)	14.2 (4.8, 39.8)	14 (5, 43)
Missing	532 (39.1)	353 (50.9)	4,224 (36.9)

Continued on p. 2556

Table 1—Continued

Baseline variable	RYGB (N = 1,362)	SG (N = 693)	Nonsurgical control (N = 11,435)
Medication history			
Noninsulin diabetes medication	1,139 (83.6)	553 (79.8)	9,253 (80.9)
0	223 (16.4)	140 (20.2)	2,182 (19.1)
1	628 (46.1)	351 (50.6)	5,218 (45.6)
2	362 (26.6)	148 (21.4)	2,929 (25.6)
3+	149 (10.9)	54 (7.8)	1,106 (9.7)
Insulin	459 (33.7)	237 (34.2)	3,806 (33.3)
Lipid-lowering medications	716 (52.6)	357 (51.5)	5,998 (52.5)
Renin-angiotensin system inhibitors[b]	825 (60.6)	423 (61)	7,102 (62.1)
Other antihypertensive medications	973 (71.4)	501 (72.3)	8,066 (70.5)
Aspirin	451 (33.1)	216 (31.2)	4,627 (40.5)
Warfarin	99 (7.3)	66 (9.5)	943 (8.2)

Data are n (%) or median (IQR). COPD, chronic obstructive pulmonary disease; UACR, urinary albumin-to-creatinine ratio. [a]eGFR was esti-mated using the MDRD study equation. [b]Including ACE inhibitors and angiotensin-receptor blockers.

RYGB compared with SG (Fig. 4 and Supplementary Table 6).

Adverse Events After Metabolic Surgery

The cumulative incidence of different interventions after RYGB and SG is shown in Fig. 5 and reported in Supplementary Table 7. More patients 5 years after RYGB required upper endoscopy (45.8% vs. 35.6%, $P < 0.001$) and abdominal surgical procedures (10.8% vs. 5.4%, $P = 0.001$) compared with patients after SG.

CONCLUSIONS

Findings of this study indicate that RYGB and SG were separately associated with a significant reduction in risk of MACE and all-cause mortality compared with usual care among patients with T2DM and a BMI ≥30 kg/m². Furthermore, during 5 years of follow-up, RYGB compared with SG was associated with a greater reduction in body weight, HbA$_{1c}$, use of medications to treat diabetes and cardiovascular diseases, and risk of six-component MACE. Among the individual components of MACE in this study, protective effects of RYGB versus SG were more prominent for risk of nephropathy than other end points. Nonetheless, more patients required endoscopic and abdominal surgical procedures after RYGB compared with SG.

In current practice, RYGB and SG account for >95% of metabolic surgical procedures performed in patients with T2DM (10,11). Despite the well-known metabolic effects of RYGB, SG has become a more popular procedure worldwide in the last several years, largely because of the relative ease of performing the procedure and fewer short- and long-term complications after SG (12,15–17). To date, there are only a few RCTs directly comparing long-term metabolic effects of RYGB with SG (3,18,19). These small trials were not primarily designed and adequately powered to specifically compare the impact of RYGB and SG on T2DM-related end

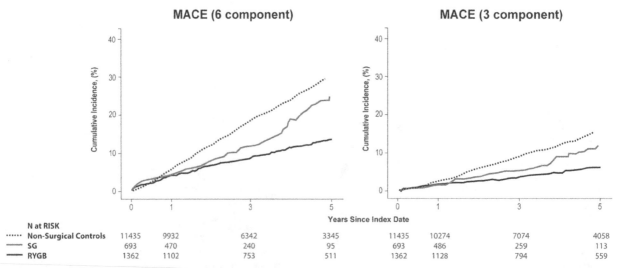

Figure 1—Five-year cumulative incidence estimates (Kaplan-Meier) for two composite end points. The primary end point was the incidence of extended MACE (composite of six outcomes), defined as first occurrence of coronary artery events, cerebrovascular events, heart failure, atrial fibrillation, nephropathy, and all-cause mortality, with the first occurrence after the index date recorded as the event date. The secondary composite end points included three-component MACE (all-cause mortality, myocardial infarction, and ischemic stroke), with the first occurrence after the index date recorded as the event date.

Table 2—Cumulative incidence estimates (%) and fully adjusted HRs from Cox models for each outcome stratified by treatment

| | Cumulative incidence at 5 years, % (95% CI) | | | | |
	RYGB	SG	Nonsurgical control	HR (95% CI)	P
Primary	13.7 (11.4–15.9)	24.7 (19.0–30.0)	30.4 (29.4–31.5)		
RYGB vs. SG				0.77 (0.60–0.98)	0.035
RYGB vs. control				0.53 (0.46–0.61)	<0.001
SG vs. control				0.69 (0.56–0.85)	<0.001
Secondary composite	6.4 (4.8–8.0)	11.8 (7.6–15.8)	15.5 (14.7–16.4)		
RYGB vs. SG				0.81 (0.57–1.16)	0.258
RYGB vs. control				0.53 (0.43–0.65)	<0.001
SG vs. control				0.65 (0.48–0.88)	0.006
All-cause mortality	3.9 (2.6–5.1)	4.5 (2.0–6.9)	10.1 (9.4–10.8)		
RYGB vs. SG				0.99 (0.60–1.66)	0.983
RYGB vs. control				0.51 (0.39–0.67)	<0.001
SG vs. control				0.52 (0.33–0.81)	0.004
Heart failure	2.9 (1.7–4.1)	5.3 (1.8–8.7)	10.7 (10.0–11.5)		
RYGB vs. SG				0.79 (0.45–1.39)	0.416
RYGB vs. control				0.32 (0.23–0.44)	<0.001
SG vs. control				0.40 (0.25–0.66)	<0.001
Coronary artery disease	2.7 (1.5–3.8)	7.1 (3.9–10.2)	7.1 (6.4–7.7)		
RYGB vs. SG				0.63 (0.38–1.05)	0.077
RYGB vs. control				0.56 (0.41–0.77)	<0.001
SG vs. control				0.89 (0.58–1.37)	0.606
Cerebrovascular disease	1.6 (0.7–2.5)	3.6 (0.9–6.2)	3.3 (2.8–3.7)		
RYGB vs. SG				0.70 (0.34–1.45)	0.340
RYGB vs. control				0.59 (0.38–0.92)	0.019
SG vs. control				0.85 (0.46–1.56)	0.593
Nephropathy	2.8 (1.6–4.0)	8.3 (4.1–12.3)	9.1 (8.3–9.9)		
RYGB vs. SG				0.47 (0.28–0.79)	0.005
RYGB vs. control				0.32 (0.23–0.45)	<0.001
SG vs. control				0.68 (0.45–1.05)	0.081
Atrial fibrillation	4.2 (2.9–5.6)	6.0 (2.5–9.4)	7.9 (7.3–8.6)		
RYGB vs. SG				1.30 (0.76–2.22)	0.340
RYGB vs. control				0.76 (0.57–1.00)	0.054
SG vs. control				0.58 (0.36–0.94)	0.027

HRs (95% CIs) and P values from adjusted Cox models comparing the relative instantaneous risk of each outcome among the study groups. When P value is <0.05, the "left" group is at a lower instantaneous risk of the outcome than the "right" group when the HR is <1. We included all baseline variables in Table 1 to adjust for potential confounding.

points. In the Surgical Treatment And Medications Potentially Eradicate Diabetes Efficiently (STAMPEDE) trial, 150 patients with T2DM were randomized to intensive medical therapy alone or intensive medical therapy plus RYGB or SG. Five years after enrollment, RYGB led to greater weight loss (~5 kg greater) compared with SG. However, the RCT did not show a difference in improvement of T2DM, hypertension, lipid profile, and quality of life indices in comparisons of RYGB with SG. At the end of the study, 45% of RYGB patients vs. 25% of SG patients were not taking any diabetes medications (P < 0.05) (3). In the SLEEVE versus byPASS (SLEEVE-PASS) RCT and the Swiss Multicenter Bypass or Sleeve Study (SM-BOSS), 101

(42%) and 54 (26%) enrolled patients with severe obesity had T2DM at baseline, respectively. After 5 years, both RCTs reported no significant differences between RYGB and SG in remission of diabetes, improvement of HbA_{1c}, and fasting glucose, although they were primarily designed to compare weight loss, and not T2DM-related end points, after two surgical procedures (18,19). There is only one RCT comparing RYGB and SG with T2DM remission at 1 year after surgery as the primary end point. In this trial on 109 patients who were randomly assigned to RYGB (n = 54) or SG (n = 55), RYGB was superior to SG for remission of T2DM at 1 year after surgery (relative risk 1.57 [95% CI 1.14–2.16], P = 0.005) (13).

In the current study, the greater and more sustained weight loss after RYGB compared with SG (10% difference in total weight loss at 5 years) could have meaningful physiologic effects. Similarly, in a recent retrospective observational cohort study from 41 health systems in the U.S. on nearly 5,000 patients, the average weight loss at 5 years was 71 lb (26% total body weight loss) after RYGB and 52 lb (19% total body weight loss) after SG (20). Although weight loss drives many of the metabolic improvements after bariatric surgery, the relative contribution of weight-independent mechanisms remains an area of active investigation. Current evidence suggests that RYGB may lead to greater weight-independent metabolic and neurohormonal

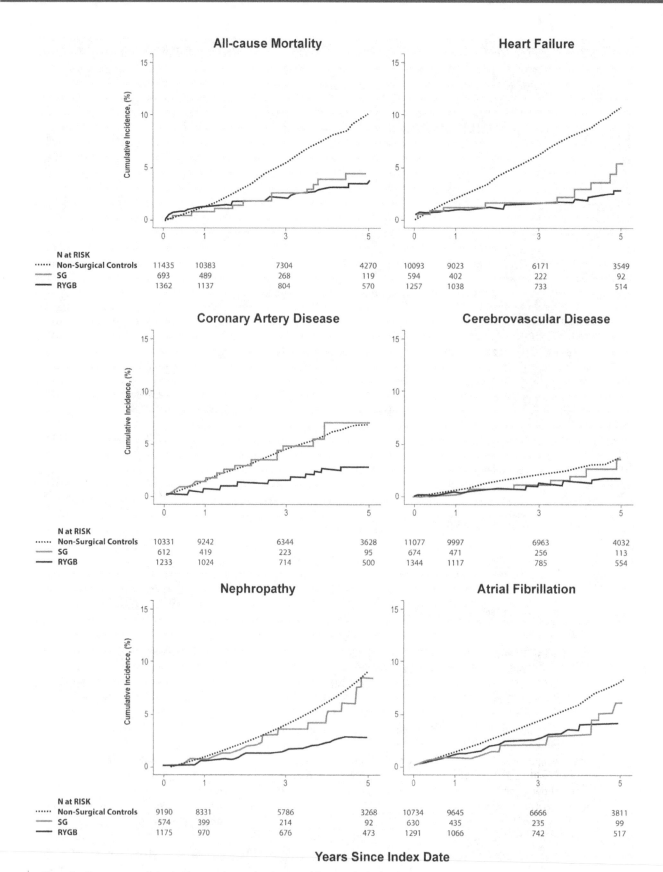

Figure 2—Five-year cumulative incidence estimates (Kaplan-Meier) for six individual end points. For each five individual outcomes (except all-cause mortality), any patient with a history of that outcome prior to the index date was eliminated from risk assessment only for that outcome.

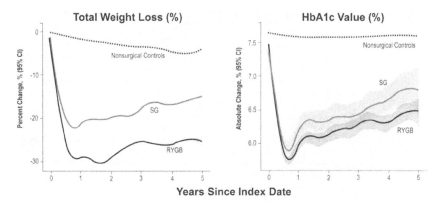

Figure 3—Mean trend curves of weight loss and HbA₁c over 5 years of follow-up. Figure displays smoothed mean trends of percent weight lost from baseline and absolute HbA₁c values (%) in three study groups during follow-up. Statistical comparisons between the study groups are reported in Supplementary Table 5.

benefits compared with SG (21,22). This constellation of favorable weight loss–dependent and weight-independent changes may explain better diabetes control, less medication use, and reduced risk of MACE after RYGB.

The combination of obesity, T2DM, and hypertension has a large negative impact on kidney integrity and function (23,24). Among the six individual secondary end points, RYGB was associated with 53% lower risk of nephropathy compared with SG. Although the exact explanation of this observation remains for future studies, this finding supports other evidence showing that the risk of nephropathy is extremely sensitive to weight changes and diabetes control (25–28). Despite no reduction in cardiovascular outcomes, findings of the Look AHEAD (Action for Health in Diabetes) randomized trial suggest that among patients with T2DM, intensive life modifications significantly decrease the risk of chronic kidney disease (26). Furthermore, in large clinical trials the impact of intensive glucose control has been more prominent on the risk of nephropathy than the risk of cardiovascular events (27,28). The relative contributions of weight loss, diabetes and blood pressure control, altered adipokine levels, decreased inflammation, and gut hormone signaling toward improving nephropathy risk and progression are yet to be elucidated (29–31). As shown in Table 2 and Fig. 2, we also observed some evidence of lower risk of coronary artery events favoring RYGB compared with SG (HR 0.63 [95% CI 0.38–1.05]), which did not reach conventional levels of statistical significance (*P* =

0.08). Both surgical groups had comparable effects for other secondary individual end points including all-cause mortality. Overall, there has been substantial evidence to support the improvement of cardiovascular risk after metabolic surgery. Because of the close association between diabetes and cardiovascular disease, it is also clear that greater metabolic improvements, particularly diabetes remission, lead to greater reduction in long-term cardiovascular risk (6–9).

The safety profile of metabolic surgery has remarkably improved in the last two decades (32–34). Consistent with prior studies (15–17,20), the current study showed fewer complications after SG compared with RYGB. The need for more reinterventions long-term after RYGB compared with SG has previously been documented and is primarily related to ulceration or stricture formation at the gastrojejunostomy and bowel obstructions. Although development of new gastroesophageal reflux disease or worsening of existing gastroesophageal reflux is a well-known adverse effect of SG (35), in the current study, similar to findings of prior studies (15–17), we found a lower rate of upper endoscopy in follow-up after SG compared with RYGB. Shorter operative time, lack of a gastrointestinal anastomosis, maintaining nutritional flow through an intact pylorus and small intestine, and unaltered gut absorption may contribute to a better safety profile of SG (12,15–17,20). In the field of metabolic surgery, gastrointestinal bypass procedures are generally associated with more weight loss and greater metabolic benefits but at a

cost of higher surgical and nutritional complications and reintervention rates (12,36,37). There also appears to be a dose-response relationship between the length of the intestinal bypass, particularly the biliopancreatic limb, and the magnitude and duration of metabolic improvement (38,39).

Several factors should be considered when the patient and medical team make a shared decision about the most appropriate metabolic surgical procedure (12). The current study shows that while both RYGB and SG are safe, effective, and durable operations, RYGB is associated with greater metabolic effects and greater reduction in risk of MACE and nephropathy. Overall, RYGB outperforms SG in achieving diabetes remission (40). Conversely, SG may be a better choice in patients with higher surgical risk, when there is limited intra-abdominal working space to perform more complex operations due to extreme obesity or complex abdominal wall hernias, in patients with certain small bowel diseases (e.g., Crohn disease, or history of multiple bowel resections), in solid organ transplant patients or in patients requiring psychotropic polypharmacy (because of possible lesser effect on absorption of medications), and in active smokers and patients dependent on chronic nonsteroidal antiinflammatory drugs (to avoid risk of anastomotic ulceration of RYGB) (12,41). Notably, the recommended nutritional surveillance in short- and long-term follow-up after RYGB and SG is similar (42).

This study has several limitations. First, the study cohorts were derived from the original study, where investigators comprehensively

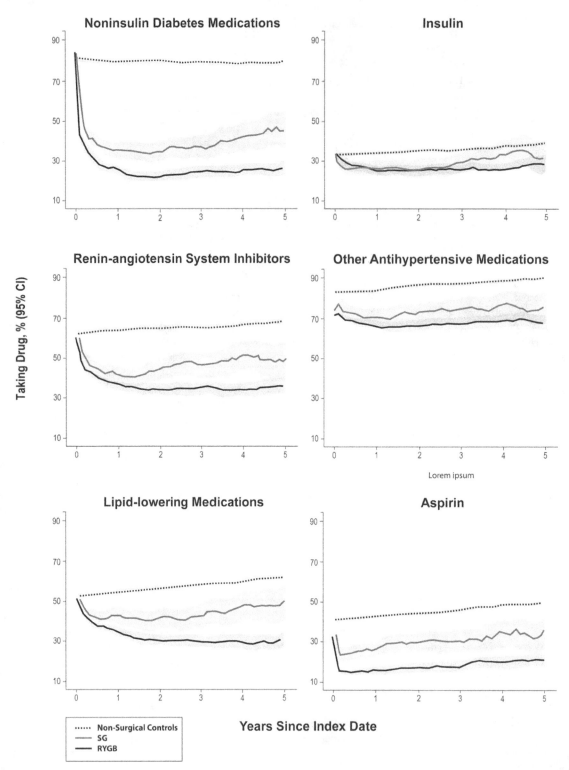

Figure 4—Proportions of patients taking diabetes and cardiovascular drugs over 5 years of follow-up. The proportion of patients on each drug was computed every one-tenth of a year starting at the index date through 5 years of follow-up. Displayed are the proportions over time with 95% point-wise CIs by surgical and nonsurgical patients. Statistical comparisons between the study groups are reported in Supplementary Table 6.

matched a surgical group with a nonsurgical group (6), which was not specifically designed to match and compare RYGB and SG subgroups. The propensity score matching was originally done to obtain a sample from a group of clinically valid comparators for the surgical patients— not to control for differences in every patient characteristic between RYGB and SG subgroups. The intention of the regression adjustment was to be the main method of actual statistical

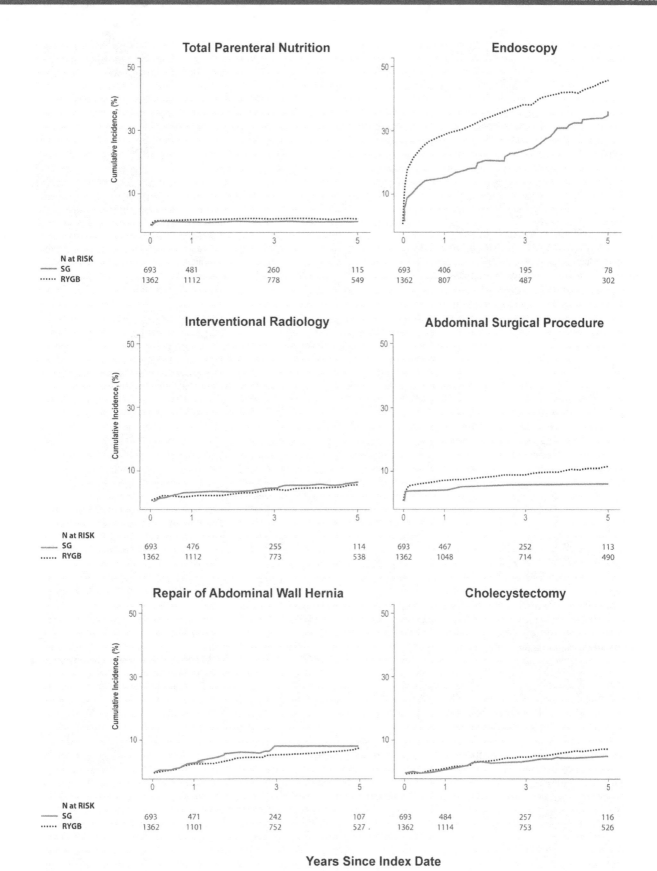

Figure 5—Five-year cumulative incidence estimates (Kaplan-Meier) for interventions after RYGB and SG. More patients after RYGB than after SG required upper endoscopy (45.8% vs. 35.6%, $P < 0.001$) and abdominal surgical procedures (10.8% vs. 5.4%, $P = 0.001$). Cumulative incidences and statistical comparisons are reported in Supplementary Table 7. Abdominal surgical procedure does not include repair of abdominal wall hernia or cholecystectomy.

adjustment for comparison of three study groups in order to control any imbalances that remained after the matching process. Nonetheless, residual measured or unmeasured confounders could have influenced findings of this retrospective observational study. Second, the SG group has a relatively smaller sample size and shorter follow-up time compared with other groups. Nonetheless, those were adequate to provide enough power to show differential impact of surgical procedures (favoring RYGB) on the primary composite end point of study. If this study could not show any difference in the primary end point between two surgical procedures, one valid argument would be lack of enough power due to smaller sample size and shorter follow-up time of the SG group than of the RYGB group. More studies with larger sample size, longer follow-up time, and higher number of events are needed to assess whether RYGB and SG have significantly different rates of "individual" cardiovascular end points beyond six-component MACE and nephropathy. In the current study, the HR for five of six individual cardiovascular end points favored RYGB compared with SG, although the upper 95% CI was <1 only for the nephropathy outcome. Particularly, the adjusted HR of coronary artery events for RYGB versus SG was 0.63 (95% CI 0.38–1.05), which did not reach conventional levels of statistical significance ($P = 0.08$). Third, coding errors, misclassification, and misdiagnosis can occur in EHR-driven data. Fourth, the causes of death could not be determined. Fifth, to analyze the status of diabetes and cardiovascular medications, prescription orders for medications were assessed, which does not necessarily equate to actual medication use. Sixth, surgical adverse events that did not lead to intervention were not analyzed. Indications and diagnoses associated with interventions were not collected. Seventh, a small percentage of nonsurgical patients received newer diabetes medications including glucagon-like peptide 1 receptor agonists and sodium–glucose cotransporter 2 inhibitors that could be associated with significant cardiovascular benefits (6).

Although cardiovascular and survival benefits of RYGB have been reported, the current study is among the first in the literature to show lower risk of MACE and mortality after SG compared with usual care. The findings of this large retrospective study also provide evidence suggesting that RYGB in patients with obesity and T2DM may be associated with greater weight loss, better diabetes control, and lower risk of six-component MACE and nephropathy compared with SG. However, given the nature of the study, these data should be considered hypothesis generating and not conclusive.

Acknowledgments. The authors acknowledge Alex Milinovich and Jian Jin from Department of Quantitative Health Sciences, Cleveland Clinic, for creation of the study database and data collection. The authors also acknowledge Dr. David E. Arterburn from Kaiser Permanente Washington Health Research Institute, Seattle, WA, for critical review of manuscript.

The individuals acknowledged above did not receive compensation for their role in the study.
Duality of Interest. A.A. reports receiving grants from Medtronic. P.R.S. reports receiving grants from Medtronic, Ethicon, and Pacira and receiving personal fees from Medtronic, GI Dynamics, W. L. Gore & Associates, Becton Dickinson Surgical, and Global Academy for Medical Education. M.W.K. reports receiving grants from Medtronic and Novo Nordisk. S.E.N. reports receiving a grant from Medtronic for the current study and receiving research support from Amgen, AbbVie, AstraZeneca, Cerenis Therapeutics, Eli Lilly, ESPERION Therapeutics, Novo Nordisk, The Medicines Company, Orexigen, Pfizer, and Takeda. S.A.B. reports receiving honoraria and consulting fees from Medtronic and GI Windows. No other potential conflicts of interest relevant to this article were reported.

S.E.N. reports consulting for a number of pharmaceutical companies without financial compensation (all honoraria, consulting fees, or any other payments from any for-profit entity are paid directly to charity, so income is not received and there is not any tax deduction).
Author Contributions. All authors contributed to study concept and design. A.A., R.W., A.Z., C.T., and M.W.K. contributed to acquisition and analysis of data. A.Z. and C.T. contributed to statistical analysis. All authors contributed to interpretation of data. A.A. and S.A.B. contributed to drafting of the manuscript. All authors contributed to critical revision of the manuscript. A.A., K.E.W., M.W.K., and S.E.N. provided administrative, technical, or material support. A.A. and S.E.N. provided supervision. A.A. is the guarantor of this work and, as such, had full access to all the data in the study and takes responsibility for the integrity of the data and the accuracy of the data analysis.

References

1. Ikramuddin S, Korner J, Lee WJ, et al. Lifestyle intervention and medical management with vs without Roux-en-Y gastric bypass and control of hemoglobin A1c, LDL cholesterol, and systolic blood pressure at 5 years in the Diabetes Surgery Study. JAMA 2018;319:266–278
2. Mingrone G, Panunzi S, De Gaetano A, et al. Bariatric-metabolic surgery versus conventional medical treatment in obese patients with type 2 diabetes: 5 year follow-up of an open-label, single-centre, randomised controlled trial. Lancet 2015;386:964–973
3. Schauer PR, Bhatt DL, Kirwan JP, et al.; STAMPEDE Investigators. Bariatric surgery versus intensive medical therapy for diabetes - 5-year outcomes. N Engl J Med 2017;376:641–651
4. Courcoulas AP, Gallagher JW, Neiberg RH, et al. Bariatric surgery vs lifestyle intervention for diabetes treatment: 5-year outcomes from a randomized trial. J Clin Endocrinol Metab 2020;105:866–876
5. Cummings DE, Arterburn DE, Westbrook EO, et al. Gastric bypass surgery vs intensive lifestyle and medical intervention for type 2 diabetes: the CROSSROADS randomised controlled trial. Diabetologia 2016;59:945–953
6. Aminian A, Zajichek A, Arterburn DE, et al. Association of metabolic surgery with major adverse cardiovascular outcomes in patients with type 2 diabetes and obesity. JAMA 2019;322:1271–1282
7. Fisher DP, Johnson E, Haneuse S, et al. Association between bariatric surgery and macrovascular disease outcomes in patients with type 2 diabetes and severe obesity. JAMA 2018;320:1570–1582
8. Aminian A, Nissen SE. Success (but unfinished) story of metabolic surgery. Diabetes Care 2020;43:1175–1177
9. Aminian A, Aleassa EM, Bhatt DL, et al. Bariatric surgery is associated with a lower rate of death after myocardial infarction and stroke: a nationwide study. Diabetes Obes Metab 2019;21:2058–2067
10. Angrisani L, Santonicola A, Iovino P, et al. IFSO worldwide survey 2016: primary, endoluminal, and revisional procedures. Obes Surg 2018;28:3783–3794
11. English WJ, DeMaria EJ, Hutter MM, et al. American Society for Metabolic and Bariatric Surgery 2018 estimate of metabolic and bariatric procedures performed in the United States. Surg Obes Relat Dis 2020;16:457–463
12. Aminian A. Bariatric procedure selection in patients with type 2 diabetes: choice between Roux-en-Y gastric bypass or sleeve gastrectomy. Surg Obes Relat Dis 2020;16:332–339
13. Hofsø D, Fatima F, Borgeraas H, et al. Gastric bypass versus sleeve gastrectomy in patients with type 2 diabetes (Oseberg): a single-centre, triple-blind, randomised controlled trial. Lancet Diabetes Endocrinol 2019;7:912–924
14. Rubin DB. Inference and missing data. Biometrika 1976;63:581–592
15. Lewis KH, Arterburn DE, Callaway K, et al. Risk of operative and nonoperative interventions up to 4 years after Roux-en-Y gastric bypass vs vertical sleeve gastrectomy in a nationwide US commercial insurance claims database. JAMA Netw Open 2019;2:e1917603
16. Li RA, Liu L, Arterburn D, et al. Five-year longitudinal cohort study of reinterventions after sleeve gastrectomy and Roux-en-Y gastric bypass. Ann Surg 2021;273:758–765

17. Courcoulas A, Coley RY, Clark JM, et al.; PCORnet Bariatric Study Collaborative. Interventions and operations 5 years after bariatric surgery in a cohort from the US National Patient-Centered Clinical Research Network Bariatric Study. JAMA Surg 2020;155:194–204

18. Salminen P, Helmiö M, Ovaska J, et al. Effect of laparoscopic sleeve gastrectomy vs laparoscopic Roux-en-Y gastric bypass on weight loss at 5 years among patients with morbid obesity: the SLEEVEPASS randomized clinical trial. JAMA 2018;319:241–254

19. Peterli R, Wölnerhanssen BK, Peters T, et al. Effect of laparoscopic sleeve gastrectomy vs laparoscopic Roux-en-Y gastric bypass on weight loss in patients with morbid obesity: the SM-BOSS randomized clinical trial. JAMA 2018;319:255–265

20. Arterburn D, Wellman R, Emiliano A, et al.; PCORnet Bariatric Study Collaborative. Comparative effectiveness and safety of bariatric procedures for weight loss: a PCORnet cohort study. Ann Intern Med 2018;169:741–750

21. Batterham RL, Cummings DE. Mechanisms of diabetes improvement following bariatric/metabolic surgery. Diabetes Care 2016;39:893–901

22. Chondronikola M, Harris LL, Klein S. Bariatric surgery and type 2 diabetes: are there weight loss-independent therapeutic effects of upper gastrointestinal bypass? J Intern Med 2016;280: 476–486

23. Hall JE, do Carmo JM, da Silva AA, Wang Z, Hall ME. Obesity, kidney dysfunction and hypertension: mechanistic links. Nat Rev Nephrol 2019;15:367–385

24. Hall ME, do Carmo JM, da Silva AA, Juncos LA, Wang Z, Hall JE. Obesity, hypertension, and chronic kidney disease. Int J Nephrol Renovasc Dis 2014;7:75–88

25. Cohen JB, Cohen DL. Cardiovascular and renal effects of weight reduction in obesity and the metabolic syndrome. Curr Hypertens Rep 2015;17:34

26. Look AHEAD Research Group. Effect of a long-term behavioural weight loss intervention on nephropathy in overweight or obese adults with type 2 diabetes: a secondary analysis of the Look AHEAD randomised clinical trial. Lancet Diabetes Endocrinol 2014;2:801–809

27. Patel A, MacMahon S, Chalmers J, et al.; ADVANCE Collaborative Group. Intensive blood glucose control and vascular outcomes in patients with type 2 diabetes. N Engl J Med 2008;358:2560–2572

28. UK Prospective Diabetes Study (UKPDS) Group. Intensive blood-glucose control with sulphonylureas or insulin compared with conventional treatment and risk of complications in patients with type 2 diabetes (UKPDS 33). Lancet 1998;352:837–853

29. Cohen RV, Pereira TV, Aboud CM, et al. Effect of gastric bypass vs best medical treatment on early-stage chronic kidney disease in patients with type 2 diabetes and obesity: a randomized clinical trial. JAMA Surg 2020;155:e200420

30. Young L, Nor Hanipah Z, Brethauer SA, Schauer PR, Aminian A. Long-term impact of bariatric surgery in diabetic nephropathy. Surg Endosc 2019;33:1654–1660

31. Scheurlen KM, Probst P, Kopf S, Nawroth PP, Billeter AT, Müller-Stich BP. Metabolic surgery improves renal injury independent of weight loss: a meta-analysis. Surg Obes Relat Dis 2019;15:1006–1020

32. Daigle CR, Brethauer SA, Tu C, et al. Which postoperative complications matter most after bariatric surgery? Prioritizing quality improvement efforts to improve national outcomes. Surg Obes Relat Dis 2018;14:652–657

33. Aminian A, Brethauer SA, Kirwan JP, Kashyap SR, Burguera B, Schauer PR. How safe is metabolic/diabetes surgery? Diabetes Obes Metab 2015;17:198–201

34. Sebastianelli L, Benois M, Vanbiervliet G, et al. Systematic endoscopy 5 years after sleeve gastrectomy results in a high rate of Barrett's esophagus: results of a multicenter study. Obes Surg 2019;29:1462–1469

36. Gu L, Huang X, Li S, et al. A meta-analysis of the medium- and long-term effects of laparoscopic sleeve gastrectomy and laparoscopic Roux-en-Y gastric bypass. BMC Surg 2020;20:30

37. Yang P, Chen B, Xiang S, Lin XF, Luo F, Li W. Long-term outcomes of laparoscopic sleeve gastrectomy versus Roux-en-Y gastric bypass for morbid obesity: results from a meta-analysis of randomized controlled trials. Surg Obes Relat Dis 2019;15:546–555

38. Patrício BG, Morais T, Guimarães M, et al. Gut hormone release after gastric bypass depends on the length of the biliopancreatic limb. Int J Obes 2019;43:1009–1018

39. Zorrilla-Nunez LF, Campbell A, Giambartolomei G, Lo Menzo E, Szomstein S, Rosenthal RJ. The importance of the biliopancreatic limb length in gastric bypass: A systematic review. Surg Obes Relat Dis 2019;15:43–49

40. Aminian A, Brethauer SA, Andalib A, et al. Individualized Metabolic Surgery score: procedure selection based on diabetes severity. Ann Surg 2017;266:650–657

41. Rosenthal RJ, Diaz AA, Arvidsson D, et al.; International Sleeve Gastrectomy Expert Panel. International Sleeve Gastrectomy Expert Panel Consensus Statement: best practice guidelines based on experience of >12,000 cases. Surg Obes Relat Dis 2012;8:8–19

42. O'Kane M, Parretti HM, Pinkney J, et al. British Obesity and Metabolic Surgery Society Guidelines on perioperative and postoperative biochemical monitoring and micronutrient replacement for patients undergoing bariatric surgery-2020 update. Obes Rev 2020;21:e13087

Thirty-Year Trends in Complications in U.S. Adults With Newly Diagnosed Type 2 Diabetes

Diabetes Care 2021;44:699–706 | https://doi.org/10.2337/dc20-2304

Michael Fang and Elizabeth Selvin

OBJECTIVE

To assess the prevalence of and trends in complications among U.S. adults with newly diagnosed diabetes.

RESEARCH DESIGN AND METHODS

We included 1,486 nonpregnant adults (aged ≥20 years) with newly diagnosed diabetes (diagnosed within the past 2 years) from the 1988–1994 and 1999–2018 National Health and Nutrition Examination Survey. We estimated trends in albuminuria (albumin-to-creatinine ratio ≥30 mg/g), reduced estimated glomerular filtration rate (eGFR <60 mL/min/1.73 m^2), retinopathy (any retinal microaneurysms or blot hemorrhages), and self-reported cardiovascular disease (history of congestive heart failure, heart attack, or stroke).

RESULTS

From 1988–1994 to 2011–2018, there was a significant decrease in the prevalence of albuminuria (38.9 to 18.7%, P for trend <0.001) but no change in the prevalence of reduced eGFR (7.5 to 9.9%, P for trend = 0.30), retinopathy (1988–1994 to 1999–2008 only; 13.2 to 12.1%, P for trend = 0.86), or self-reported cardiovascular disease (19.0 to 16.5%, P for trend = 0.64). There were improvements in glycemic, blood pressure, and lipid control in the population, and these partially explained the decline in albuminuria. Complications were more common at the time of diabetes diagnosis for adults who were older, lower income, less educated, and obese.

CONCLUSIONS

Over the past three decades, there have been encouraging reductions in albuminuria and risk factor control in adults with newly diagnosed diabetes. However, the overall burden of complications around the time of the diagnosis remains high.

Type 2 diabetes may be present in patients up to 12 years before its clinical diagnosis (1). During this latent period, hyperglycemia and cardiovascular risk factors are commonly present (2), contributing to a high burden of complications at the time of diagnosis (3).

Over the past three decades, there has been an increased focus on early diabetes detection in the U.S. (4), potentially reducing the time between disease onset and clinical diagnosis. In the late 1990s and early 2000s, expert groups increasingly emphasized regular diabetes screening for asymptomatic adults (5–9), contributing to a rise in testing, especially in high-risk populations (10,11). In 1997, the threshold for diagnosing diabetes was reduced from a fasting blood glucose of 140 mg/dL to

Department of Epidemiology and the Welch Center for Prevention, Epidemiology and Clinical Research, Johns Hopkins Bloomberg School of Public Health, Baltimore, MD

Corresponding author: Elizabeth Selvin, eselvin@jhu.edu

Received 14 September 2020 and accepted 28 November 2020

This article contains supplementary material online at https://doi.org/10.2337/figshare.13308467.

126 mg/dL (6), and a sharp increase in the diagnosis of diabetes followed (12). In 2009, glycated hemoglobin $\geq 6.5\%$ was first recommended for use in diagnosis (13).

The objective of our study was to assess the national prevalence of and trends in risk factors and microvascular and macrovascular complications among U.S. adults with newly diagnosed diabetes. To accomplish this, we analyzed three decades of data (1988–2018) from the National Health and Nutrition Examination Survey (NHANES).

RESEARCH DESIGN AND METHODS

Study Population

The NHANES is a nationally representative, cross-sectional survey designed to monitor the health of the U.S. population. During each survey cycle, a sample of participants is selected from the U.S. noninstitutionalized civilian population using a complex, stratified, multistage probability cluster sampling design. Data are collected from participants through in-home interviews and visits to a mobile examination center (14). The National Center for Health Statistics (NCHS) Institutional Review Board (Hyattsville, MD) approved study protocols, and all participants provided written informed consent. We analyzed data from the NHANES III (1988–1994) and the continuous NHANES (1999–2018).

All participants were asked whether they had ever been diagnosed with diabetes other than during pregnancy. Those reporting a diagnosis of diabetes were asked how old they were when they received their diagnosis. We calculated duration of diagnosed diabetes by subtracting participants' age of diabetes diagnosis from their age reported during the interview. We limited our analytic sample to nonpregnant adults aged ≥ 20 with newly diagnosed diabetes, defined as being diagnosed within the past 2 years ($n = 1,486$).

Risk Factor Treatment and Control

Hemoglobin A_{1c} (HbA_{1c}) was measured using high-performance liquid chromatography methods. To account for changes in laboratory methods over time, we calibrated HbA_{1c} using an equipercentile equating approach (15). We examined the proportion of participants with an HbA_{1c} <7.0% (<53 mmol/mol) (16). We defined receiving diabetes treatment as the self-reported current use of blood glucose-lowering pills or insulin.

Blood pressure was measured up to three times with a mercury sphygmomanometer, and the mean of all available readings was used in the analysis. We defined hypertension as having elevated mean blood pressure (mean systolic/diastolic blood pressure $\geq 140/90$ mmHg or $\geq 130/80$ mmHg) or the self-reported current use of antihypertensive medication (17,18). We defined receiving treatment as the self-reported current use of antihypertensive medication, and blood pressure control as having a mean blood pressure <140/90 mmHg or <130/80 mmHg.

Serum total cholesterol was measured enzymatically, and measurements from fasting and nonfasting participants were included in the analysis. We defined hyperlipidemia as having elevated lipids (total cholesterol ≥ 240 mg/dL or ≥ 200 mg/dL) or the self-reported current use of lipid-lowering medication (19). We defined receiving treatment as the self-reported current use of lipid-lowering medication and lipid control as total cholesterol <240 mg/dL or <200 mg/dL.

Microvascular Complications

Serum creatinine was measured using the Jaffe method. All creatinine measurements were recalibrated to standardized creatinine measurements using recommended equations that minimize the effects of laboratory drift (20). We determined the estimated glomerular filtration rate (eGFR) using the Chronic Kidney Disease Epidemiology Collaboration formula (21). We defined reduced eGFR as having an eGFR <60 mL/min/1.73 m^2. Urine albumin and creatinine concentrations were measured in a random urine sample using fluorescent immunoassay and a modified Jaffe method, respectively. We defined albuminuria as an albumin-to-creatinine ratio ≥ 30 mg/g. We defined any chronic kidney disease as having reduced eGFR, albuminuria, or both (22).

Medication use was assessed through pill bottle examination review. We evaluated use of ACE inhibitors or angiotensin II receptor blockers among those with chronic kidney disease.

Participants aged ≥ 40 had film photographs taken of one randomly selected eye in the NHANES III (1988–1994) and digital photographs taken of both eyes in the 2005–2008 NHANES. Retinopathy was assessed by graders using the Early Treatment Diabetic Retinopathy Study (ETDRS) protocol (23). We defined diabetic retinopathy as having any retinal microaneurysms or blot hemorrhages, with or without more severe lesions (24).

Participants aged ≥ 40 participated in a lower-extremity examination during the 1999–2004 cycles of the continuous NHANES. These participants received monofilament testing on three sites on each foot. We defined peripheral neuropathy as having one or more insensate areas. Blood pressure measurements were taken at participants' ankles and right arm. We computed the ankle-brachial pressure index by dividing systolic blood pressure measured at each ankle by the systolic blood pressure measured at the arm. We defined peripheral artery disease as having an ankle-brachial pressure index of <0.9 for either ankle (25). Participants reported whether they ever had an ulcer or sore on their legs or feet that lasted >4 weeks. We defined any lower-extremity disease as having peripheral neuropathy, peripheral artery disease, or a history of ulcers (26).

Cardiovascular Disease

Participants reported whether they had ever been diagnosed with congestive heart failure, stroke, or heart attack. We defined any cardiovascular disease as having at least one of these conditions.

Sociodemographic Measures and BMI

Participants self-reported their age, sex (male/female), race/ethnicity (non-Hispanic White, non-Hispanic Black, Mexican American, other), education (high school or less, some college, college graduate or above), family income (income-to-poverty ratio <130%, 130–349%, $\geq 350\%$), health insurance status (uninsured, any health insurance), access to a usual source of care (has access, no access), and smoking status (current, former, never). We calculated BMI as measured weight in kilograms divided by height in meters squared and classified participants into three weight status groups (normal, BMI <25 kg/m^2; overweight, BMI 25–29.9 kg/m^2; obese, BMI ≥ 30 kg/m^2).

Statistical Analyses

We calculated participant characteristics, the prevalence, treatment, and control of risk factors, and the prevalence of microvascular and cardiovascular disease over time. Because of the limited sample sizes in the individual 2-year survey cycles, we pooled survey years into three time intervals (1988–1994, 1999–2008, and 2009–2018) to improve the precision of our estimates (14). We assessed trends using logistic (binary outcomes), linear (mean of continuous outcomes), or quantile (median of continuous outcomes) regression models. Following NCHS guidelines to test for trends, we modeled the midpoint of each survey period as a continuous, linear predictor in the regression models (27). We examined the distribution of risk factors and compared changes over time using χ^2 tests. For complications that changed significantly over time, we used multivariable logistic regression models to explore how changes in social demographic characteristics, diabetes risk factors, and weight status might explain the observed trends. We examined risk factors for complications by combining data from 1988 to 2018 and estimating age-, sex-, and race/ethnicity-adjusted logistic regression models.

In sensitivity analyses, we repeated our trend analyses 1) adjusting for age, sex, and race/ethnicity using predictive margins (28); and 2) defining newly diagnosed diabetes as being diagnosed in ≤1 year, a common cut point used in surveillance research (29,30). Because the approach to assessing retinopathy changed over time, we also performed a sensitivity analysis using a randomly selected fundus photograph from one eye (rather than both eyes) for the NHANES 2005–2008 cycles. Following past studies (24), we used photographs from the right eye to classify participants with an even study identification number and the left eye for those with an odd number.

All analyses were conducted using Stata version 16.0 (StataCorp). The recommended sample weights were used, making our results representative of the civilian, noninstitutionalized U.S. adult population with newly diagnosed diabetes. A two-sided P value of <0.05 was considered statistically significant.

RESULTS

The age and sex distribution of U.S. adults with newly diagnosed diabetes did not change significantly from 1988 to 2018 (Table 1), whereas the proportion who were non-White, college educated, or had obesity increased substantially over the 30-year period.

The proportion of adults with good glycemic control (HbA_{1c} <7% [<53 mmol/mol]) increased substantially (59.8 to 73.7%, P for trend = 0.002) (Table 2 and Supplementary Fig. 1). While the proportion receiving any glucose-lowering treatment was unchanged, the proportion using any insulin declined from 12.8 to 7.5% (P for trend = 0.03).

Adults with newly diagnosed diabetes achieving blood pressure control increased during the 30-year period (Supplementary Fig. 1), as did the use of blood pressure-lowering medication (Table 2). The overall prevalence of hypertension increased when defined as ≥140/90 mmHg. When defined as ≥130/80 mmHg, the prevalence of hypertension was unchanged. An increasing proportion of adults with hypertension were treated and controlled to <140/90 mmHg (47.8 to 65.9%, P for trend = 0.02) and <130/80 mmHg (9.0 to 36.8%, P for trend <0.001), respectively.

The proportion with cholesterol control increased (Supplementary Fig. 1). The use of lipid-lowering medication rose significantly (Table 2), and the prevalence of hyperlipidemia was stable. An increasing share of those with hyperlipidemia were treated and controlled to total cholesterol <240 mg/dL (17.1 to 71.2%, P for trend <0.001) or <200 mg/dL (9.4 to 52.4%, P for trend <0.001), respectively.

The prevalence of any chronic kidney disease declined from 40.4 to 25.5% (P for trend = 0.003) (Table 3). These gains were driven by declines in albuminuria (38.9 to 18.7%, P for trend <0.001). In contrast, reduced eGFR remained stable over time (7.5 to 9.9%, P = 0.30). The use of ACE inhibitors/angiotensin II receptor blockers increased substantially among those with low eGFR or albuminuria (Supplementary Table 1).

The prevalence of retinopathy among U.S. adults aged ≥40 with newly diagnosed diabetes was unchanged from 1988 to 2008 (13.2 to 12.1%) (Table 3). Results were similar in sensitivity analyses using one fundus photograph to classify participants in the 2005–2008 NHANES (results not shown).

The prevalence of any self-reported cardiovascular disease was stable from 1988 to 2018 (19.0 to 16.5%) (Table 3).

The prevalence of lower-extremity diseases—peripheral neuropathy, peripheral arterial disease, or ulcers—in the 1999–2004 period was ~24%, 15%, 9%, and 6%, respectively (Supplementary Table 1). Limited data availability (1999–2004 only) precluded trend analyses of lower-extremity diseases.

We explored factors that might explain declines in the prevalence of albuminuria. Differences in albuminuria across time periods increased after adjusting for age, sex, and race/ethnicity but decreased after adjusting for education (Supplementary Table 2). Changes in HbA_{1c}, blood pressure, and total cholesterol partially accounted for the population-level improvements in albuminuria. Adjusting for weight status increased differences in albuminuria over time.

After adjusting for age, sex, and race/ethnicity, the prevalence of any complication for adults with newly diagnosed diabetes was higher among those who were older, lower income, less educated, current or former smokers, and obese (Table 4).

Trends in risk factors and complications were similar after adjusting for age, sex, and race/ethnicity (Supplementary Tables 3 and 4) and when defining newly diagnosed diabetes as being diagnosed within 1 year (Supplementary Tables 5 and 6).

CONCLUSIONS

From 1988 to 2018, there were marked improvements in the treatment and control of risk factors (HbA_{1c}, blood pressure, or cholesterol) and a substantial decline in the prevalence of albuminuria in U.S. adults with newly diagnosed type 2 diabetes. However, the burden of complications remained high. Approximately 26% had chronic kidney disease, 24% had lower-extremity disease, 12% had retinopathy, and 17% had a history of cardiovascular disease.

Our findings extend population research on the health status of adults with newly diagnosed type 2 diabetes. A prior U.S. population-based study using data from the National Health Interview Survey (NHIS) found that from 1997 to 2003 the prevalence of obesity rose among adults with newly diagnosed diabetes, while the prevalence of cardiovascular disease and hypertension was unchanged (31). However, data in the NHIS are entirely self-reported. When

Table 1—Characteristics of U.S. adults aged ≥20 years with newly diagnosed diabetes (diagnosed within the past 2 years), NHANES 1988–2018

	1988–1994 (Unweighted N = 312)	1999–2008 (Unweighted N = 518)	2009–2018 (Unweighted N = 656)	P for trend
Age, %				
20–44 years	30.1 (20.8–41.3)	27.8 (23.1–33.2)	21.4 (17.6–25.8)	0.12
45–64 years	44.9 (35.5–54.7)	47.6 (42.0–53.3)	52.3 (47.4–57.2)	0.24
≥65 years	25.0 (19.3–31.7)	24.5 (20.1–29.7)	26.3 (21.8–31.3)	0.67
Age, mean, years	54.3 (51.9–56.8)	54.0 (52.3–55.7)	55.3 (53.8–56.7)	0.51
Race/ethnicity, %				
Non-Hispanic White	71.1 (62.5–78.4)	60.1 (53.3–66.7)	59.1 (53.4–64.6)	0.01
Mexican American	5.4 (3.8–7.6)	8.3 (5.8–11.7)	9.8 (7.4–12.9)	0.003
Non-Hispanic Black	13.4 (9.8–18.0)	18.1 (14.2–22.8)	13.6 (10.6–17.4)	0.85
Non-Hispanic Asian*	—	—	5.0 (3.8–6.6)	—
Other†	10.2 (5.0–19.5)	13.5 (9.4–18.9)	12.4 (9.2–16.4)	—
Sex, %				0.57
Female	51.8 (41.6–61.8)	51.9 (46.3–57.5)	49.2 (43.5–55.0)	
Male	48.2 (38.2–58.4)	48.1 (42.5–53.7)	50.8 (45.0–56.5)	
Educational level, %				
High school or less	74.2 (64.8–81.8)	52.4 (45.8–58.8)	47.0 (41.4–52.7)	<0.001
Some college	13.1 (7.8–21.2)	30.8 (25.0–37.4)	31.3 (26.0–37.3)	0.001
College graduate	12.7 (7.3–21.2)	16.8 (13.1–21.3)	21.6 (16.8–27.5)	0.05
Poverty-to-income ratio, %				
<130%	26.7 (19.9–34.9)	27.2 (21.7–33.4)	23.5 (19.6–28.0)	0.37
130–350%	49.6 (39.7–59.6)	37.3 (31.2–43.9)	41.5 (36.5–46.8)	0.13
≥350%	23.7 (16.2–33.2)	35.5 (29.6–41.8)	34.9 (29.5–40.8)	0.02
Usual source of care, %				0.47
No usual care	6.2 (2.7–13.4)	2.8 (1.7–4.7)	4.0 (2.6–6.0)	
Any usual care	93.8 (86.6–97.3)	97.2 (95.3–98.3)	96.0 (94.0–97.4)	
Health insurance status, %				0.97
Uninsured	11.7 (6.5–20.2)	15.5 (11.7–20.3)	12.7 (10.1–16.0)	
Any insurance	88.3 (79.8–93.5)	84.5 (79.7–88.3)	87.3 (84.0–89.9)	
BMI categories, %‡				
Normal weight	17.6 (11.8–25.4)	10.9 (8.2–14.3)	8.1 (5.6–11.6)	0.01
Overweight	34.3 (27.0–42.5)	28.5 (23.4–34.2)	23.3 (19.2–27.9)	0.01
Obese	48.1 (39.8–56.5)	60.6 (53.9–66.9)	68.6 (63.1–73.7)	<0.001
BMI, mean, kg/m²	31.0 (30.0–32.0)	33.2 (32.2–34.2)	34.5 (33.5–35.6)	<0.001
Smoking, %				
Never smoker	37.1 (28.4–46.7)	50.2 (45.5–55.0)	47.3 (42.4–52.2)	0.09
Former smoker	39.7 (29.7–50.5)	26.6 (21.8–32.0)	34.5 (29.1–40.3)	0.47
Current smoker	23.2 (15.6–33.1)	23.2 (19.2–27.6)	18.2 (14.4–22.8)	0.29

Data are presented as percentages or means (with 95% CIs). *Representative information for non-Hispanic Asians only available in the 2011–2018 NHANES. †Trend not tested for "other" racial/ethnic group because of changing definition over survey years. ‡Normal weight defined as BMI <25 kg/m²; overweight defined as BMI ≥25 and <30 kg/m²; and obese defined as BMI ≥30 kg/m².

examining a broader range of objectively measured risk factors and comorbidities, we confirmed the increase in obesity but also found evidence of improvements in glycemic control and kidney health.

The reduction in albuminuria was likely related to major improvements in the detection of diabetes over the study period (4). This is consistent with research showing that the proportion of undiagnosed diabetes cases has decreased in the past two decades (2,32). Declines in albuminuria were especially pronounced from 1988–1994 to 1999–2008, corresponding to the reduction of the fasting blood glucose diagnostic threshold and increased emphasis on

diabetes screening (5–9). We also found that declines in HbA$_{1c}$, blood pressure, and total cholesterol explained some of the decrease in albuminuria. Results for HbA$_{1c}$ and blood pressure are consistent with landmark trials demonstrating the benefits of tight glycemic and blood pressure control (33,34), and findings for total cholesterol are congruent with research suggesting an association between dyslipidemia and kidney disease risk (35). Increasing educational attainment was another important contributor and suggests the fundamental importance of education in health. Growing awareness of the importance of albuminuria among clinicians, along with

rising use of renin-angiotensin system blockers, were likely important factors as well.

The high burden of complications suggests that timely detection of diabetes remains a challenge for some patients. In particular, we found that adults who were older, lower income, less educated, or obese had the highest prevalence of complications at the time of diagnosis. Approximately half of eligible U.S. adults receive recommended diabetes screenings, although uptake is significantly lower among certain high-risk groups, such as those who are low-income (11). More targeted screening programs for high-risk, underserved patients may thus

Table 2—Trends in the prevalence, treatment, and control of risk factors among U.S. adults with newly diagnosed diabetes (diagnosed within the past 2 years), NHANES 1988–2018

	1988–1994	1999–2008	2009–2018	P for trend
Glucose control				
HbA$_{1c}$, % points, median	6.3 (5.6–8.1)	6.2 (5.7–7.1)	6.2 (5.7–7.1)	0.24
HbA$_{1c}$, % points, mean	7.0 (6.6–7.3)	6.8 (6.5–7.1)	6.7 (6.5–6.8)	0.02
Treated, %				
Insulin or oral medication use	73.0 (65.1–79.6)	73.1 (67.6–78.1)	72.8 (67.3–77.6)	0.86
Oral medication use only	60.2 (51.8–68.0)	66.5 (60.8–71.9)	65.3 (59.3–70.8)	0.35
Any insulin use	12.8 (8.6–18.7)	6.6 (3.7–11.4)	7.5 (5.4–10.3)	0.03
HbA$_{1c}$ <7.0%-points (<53 mmol/mol), %	59.8 (50.0–69.0)	69.9 (63.0–76.0)	73.7 (68.9–78.1)	0.002
Blood pressure				
Systolic, mmHg median	130.0 (119.0–137.0)	126.7 (118.0–137.3)	124.0 (114.0–135.3)	0.02
Diastolic, mmHg, median	78.0 (73.0–85.0)	72.7 (64.0–82.0)	72.0 (64.7–79.0)	<0.001
Systolic, mmHg, mean	130.1 (127.4–132.8)	129.2 (127.0–131.4)	126.0 (124.2–127.7)	0.02
Diastolic, mmHg, mean	77.5 (75.9–79.2)	72.0 (69.9–74.1)	72.1 (70.8–73.5)	<0.001
Treated, %	39.5 (30.4–49.5)	51.5 (45.4–57.5)	55.2 (49.3–61.0)	0.01
Hypertension (≥140/90 mmHg or med use), %	48.9 (40.3–57.5)	59.5 (53.2–65.4)	61.2 (55.2–67.0)	0.03
Treated*	81.4 (69.3–89.5)	86.0 (79.8–90.5)	90.1 (86.1–93.1)	0.08
Treated and controlled (blood pressure <140/90 mmHg)*	47.8 (35.8–60.0)	58.9 (51.3–66.2)	65.9 (58.7–72.3)	0.02
Hypertension (≥130/80 mmHg or med use), %	71.4 (61.0–79.9)	71.1 (65.5–76.2)	71.1 (65.0–76.5)	0.97
Treated*	55.6 (43.9–66.6)	71.9 (64.9–78.0)	77.6 (72.0–82.4)	0.001
Treated and controlled (blood pressure <130/80 mmHg)*	9.0 (4.6–17.0)	28.5 (23.0–34.8)	36.8 (30.7–43.4)	<0.001
Lipids				
Total cholesterol, mg/dL, median	212.0 (187.0–246.0)	192.0 (166.0–218.0)	181.0 (153.0–208.0)	<0.001
Total cholesterol, mg/dL, mean	219.4 (210.0–228.8)	198.4 (192.5–204.2)	182.4 (178.3–186.6)	<0.001
Treated, %	14.1 (8.3–22.9)	35.2 (29.1–41.7)	43.8 (37.8–49.9)	<0.001
Hyperlipidemia (total cholesterol ≥240 mg/dL or med use), %	40.3 (30.2–51.3)	45.4 (39.5–51.4)	49.8 (44.3–55.4)	0.14
Treated†	32.4 (20.5–47.2)	71.1 (62.7–78.2)	86.1 (81.1–90.0)	<0.001
Treated and controlled (total cholesterol <240 mg/dL)†	17.1 (7.6–34.1)	45.0 (34.5–55.9)	71.2 (63.9–77.6)	<0.001
Hyperlipidemia (total cholesterol ≥200 mg/dL or med use), %	71.6 (65.3–77.1)	65.1 (59.7–70.2)	66.3 (61.3–70.9)	0.14
Treated†	18.5 (11.0–29.4)	51.5 (43.8–59.1)	65.4 (58.4–71.8)	<0.001
Treated and controlled (total cholesterol <200 mg/dL)†	9.4 (4.2–19.7)	29.9 (22.2–39.0)	52.4 (45.1–59.5)	<0.001
All three risk factors controlled				
HbA$_{1c}$ <7.0% (<53 mmol/mol) plus				
Blood pressure <130/80 mmHg, total cholesterol <200 mg/dL, %	9.4 (6.1–14.2)	18.1 (13.6–23.8)	33.0 (27.0–39.5)	<0.001
Blood pressure <140/90 mmHg, total cholesterol <240 mg/dL, %	31.6 (23.6–40.9)	47.8 (41.2–54.5)	56.2 (51.2–61.1)	<0.001

Data are presented as percentages or as means (with 95% CIs) or median (with interquartile range). *Computed for those with hypertension. †Computed for those with hyperlipidemia.

reduce complications at diagnosis. Our findings also indicate that more aggressive treatment of risk factors immediately after diagnosis may be needed. In particular, we found that control of hypertension or hyperlipidemia failed in up to 63% and 48% of adults with newly diagnosed diabetes, respectively, highlighting the need to prioritize blood pressure and lipid management.

We observed a nonsignificant increase in the prevalence of reduced eGFR from 1988–1994 to 1999–2008, followed by little change in 2009–2018. These trends are consistent with trends in the total population of adults with diabetes. In U.S. adults with diabetes, the prevalence of

reduced eGFR increased in 1988–1994 to 2003–2004 before subsequently leveling off in 2011–2012 (36). Prior studies speculate that rising blood pressure treatment and control may account for some of the increase in reduced eGFR in adults with diabetes due to their hemodynamic effects (37,38). Consistent with this suggestion, we found that trends in blood pressure-lowering medication use followed trends in reduced eGFR, rising from 1988–1994 to 1999–2008 and leveling off in 2009–2018.

We also did not observe any major improvements in the prevalence of retinopathy or cardiovascular disease in adults with newly diagnosed diabetes

over this 30-year period. However, these findings must be viewed in light of some methodological limitations. The NHANES III (1988–1994) used film photography to assess retinopathy, whereas the NHANES 2005–2008 used higher-quality digital photography. Detection of retinopathy may therefore have been more sensitive in the later survey years, potentially affecting the comparability of estimates across years (24). Likewise, we likely underestimate the true prevalence of cardiovascular disease, because this information is self-reported in NHANES. In particular, subclinical cardiovascular disease is common in older adults and those with diabetes (39). Trends will also reflect

Table 3—Trends in the prevalence of complications among U.S. adults with newly diagnosed diabetes (diagnosed within the past 2 years), NHANES 1988–2018

	1988–1994	1999–2008	2009–2018	P for trend
Any chronic kidney disease	40.4 (31.8–49.5)	28.0 (23.8–32.7)	25.5 (21.7–29.7)	0.003
Albuminuria (albumin-to-creatine ratio ≥30 mg/g)	38.9 (30.7–47.9)	21.0 (17.2–25.3)	18.7 (15.6–22.3)	<0.001
Reduced eGFR (<60 mL/min/1.73 m^2)	7.5 (4.4–12.5)	10.2 (7.4–13.9)	9.9 (7.3–13.3)	0.30
Retinopathy*	13.2 (6.7–24.3)	12.1 (6.8–20.4)	—	0.86
Any self-reported cardiovascular disease	19.0 (13.5–26.1)	14.8 (11.6–18.6)	16.5 (12.6–21.3)	0.64
History of congestive heart failure	6.9 (3.9–11.8)	6.4 (4.3–9.5)	5.1 (3.2–7.8)	0.35
History of stroke	6.8 (3.7–12.2)	6.4 (4.4–9.1)	6.4 (4.5–9.1)	0.95
History of heart attack	10.2 (6.1–16.4)	6.6 (4.8–9.1)	9.4 (6.3–13.7)	0.90

Data are presented as percentages (with 95% CIs). *Retinopathy was defined as ≥1 retinal microaneurysms or blot hemorrhages. Data were only available for adults aged ≥40 during the 1988–1994 and 2005–2008 NHANES survey cycles.

improvements in detection and survival; studies of the general population with diabetes have found steady declines in cardiovascular complications and all-cause and cardiovascular mortality (40–42).

Our study has several additional limitations. First, there may be misclassification of incident diabetes cases, because our definition relies on participants accurately reporting their diabetes status and age of diagnosis. However, prior research indicates that these measures are highly specific and reliable (43,44). Second,

because of sample size limitations, we may have lacked the power to detect small changes in complications over time. Third, retinopathy and lower-extremity disease assessments were only performed in those aged ≥40 years. Thus, we were not able to draw conclusions regarding these outcomes in younger individuals. Fourth, our study was cross-sectional, and we cannot determine the temporality of the observed associations.

Strengths of the study include the contemporary, nationally representative

sample of U.S. adults with newly diagnosed diabetes spanning 30 years. With the exception of cardiovascular disease, the assessment of risk factors and complications was based on objective, rigorous, and systematic measurement.

Over the past three decades, there were significant reductions in albuminuria and improvements in the treatment and control of HbA$_{1c}$, blood pressure, and cholesterol in adults with newly diagnosed type 2 diabetes. These results suggest that there have been improvements in diabetes

Table 4—Adjusted odds ratios (95% CIs) for the associations of risk factors with complications in U.S. adults with newly diagnosed diabetes (diagnosed within the past 2 years), NHANES 1988–2018*

	Any complication†	Any microvascular complication	Any self-reported cardiovascular disease
Age			
20–44 years (ref)	1	1	1
45–64 years	1.56 (0.93–2.62)	1.25 (0.69–2.26)	2.68 (1.02–7.03)
65 years	2.86 (1.66–4.94)	2.14 (1.21–3.79)	8.28 (3.41–20.15)
Race/ethnicity			
Non-Hispanic White (ref)	1	1	1
Mexican American	0.67 (0.45–1.01)	0.83 (0.56–1.23)	0.48 (0.25–0.91)
Non-Hispanic Black	0.90 (0.63–1.28)	0.88 (0.62–1.26)	1.09 (0.67–1.78)
Sex			
Female (ref)	1	1	1
Male	1.31 (0.90–1.91)	1.06 (0.73–1.54)	1.50 (0.94–2.40)
Income-to-poverty ratio			
≥350% (ref)	1	1	1
130–350%	1.98 (1.22–3.23)	1.58 (0.97–2.58)	1.82 (0.96–3.42)
<130%	1.81 (1.11–2.97)	1.49 (0.91–2.44)	2.04 (1.03–4.01)
Education level			
College graduate (ref)	1	1	1
Some college	1.63 (0.88–3.02)	1.14 (0.60–2.18)	2.13 (0.94–4.82)
≥ High school	2.31 (1.36–3.92)	1.68 (0.97–2.93)	2.43 (1.16–5.08)
Smoking status			
Never (ref)	1	1	1
Former	1.69 (1.09–2.61)	1.22 (0.78–1.93)	1.81 (1.07–3.08)
Current	1.80 (1.10–2.95)	1.48 (0.90–2.42)	2.46 (1.29–4.67)
Obese (BMI ≥30 kg/m^2)			
No (ref)	1	1	1
Yes	1.50 (1.04–2.18)	1.23 (0.85–1.77)	1.56 (0.99–2.45)

Ref, reference. *Odds ratios were adjusted for age, sex, and race/ethnicity. †Defined as any microvascular complication (chronic kidney disease, retinopathy, or lower-extremity disease) or any self-reported cardiovascular disease (history of congestive heart failure, heart attack, or stroke).

screening and that we are diagnosing cases earlier in the disease process. Nevertheless, the overall burden of complications and uncontrolled risk factors remains high. Targeted screening of high-risk populations and aggressive risk factor treatment immediately following diagnosis are important strategies for sustaining progress moving forward.

Funding. M.F. is supported by National Institutes of Health/National Heart, Lung, and Blood Institute grant T32 HL007024. E.S. is supported by National Institutes of Health/National Institute of Diabetes and Digestive and Kidney Diseases grant K24 DK106414.

The funders had no role in the design, analysis, interpretation, or writing of this study.

Duality of Interest. No potential conflicts of interest relevant to this article were reported.

Author Contributions. M.F. and E.S. designed the study. M.F. conducted the statistical analysis. M.F. drafted the manuscript. M.F. controlled the decision to publish. E.S. guided the statistical analysis. E.S. provided critical revisions to the manuscript. Both authors approved the final manuscript. The corresponding author, E.S., attests that all listed authors meet authorship criteria and that no others meeting the criteria have been omitted. M.F. is the guarantor of this work and, as such, had full access to all the data in the study and takes responsibility for the integrity of the data and the accuracy of the data analysis.

References

1. Harris MI, Klein R, Welborn TA, Knuiman MW. Onset of NIDDM occurs at least 4-7 yr before clinical diagnosis. Diabetes Care 1992;15:815–819
2. Selvin E, Wang D, Lee AK, Bergenstal RM, Coresh J. Identifying trends in undiagnosed diabetes in U.S. adults by using a confirmatory definition: a cross-sectional study. Ann Intern Med 2017;167:769–776
3. Engelgau MM, Narayan KM, Herman WH. Screening for type 2 diabetes. Diabetes Care 2000;23:1563–1580
4. Selvin E, Ali MK. Declines in the incidence of diabetes in the U.S.—real progress or artifact? Diabetes Care 2017;40:1139–1143
5. U.S. Preventive Services Task Force. Screening for type 2 diabetes mellitus in adults: recommendations and rationale. Ann Intern Med 2003; 138:212–214
6. Expert Committee on the Diagnosis and Classification of Diabetes Mellitus. Report of the Expert Committee on the Diagnosis and Classification of Diabetes Mellitus. Diabetes Care 1997; 20:1183–1197
7. Pearson TA, Blair SN, Daniels SR, et al.; American Heart Association Science Advisory and Coordinating Committee. AHA guidelines for primary prevention of cardiovascular disease and stroke: 2002 update: consensus panel guide to comprehensive risk reduction for adult patients without coronary or other atherosclerotic vascular diseases. Circulation 2002;106:388–391
8. Canadian Diabetes Association Clinical Practice Guidelines Expert Committee. Canadian Diabetes

Association 2003 Clinical Practice Guidelines for the Prevention and Management of Diabetes in Canada. Can J Diabetes 2003;27(Suppl. 2):S1–S152
9. World Health Organization. Screening for type 2 diabetes: report of a World Health Organization and International Diabetes Federation meeting. Geneva, Switzerland, World Health Organization, 2003
10. Cowie CC, Harris MI, Eberhardt MS. Frequency and determinants of screening for diabetes in the U.S. Diabetes Care 1994;17: 1158–1163
11. Bullard KM, Ali MK, Imperatore G, et al. Receipt of glucose testing and performance of two US diabetes screening guidelines, 2007–2012. PLoS One 2015;10:e0125249
12. Geiss LS, Wang J, Cheng YJ, et al. Prevalence and incidence trends for diagnosed diabetes among adults aged 20 to 79 years, United States, 1980-2012. JAMA 2014;312:1218–1226
13. International Expert Committee. International Expert Committee report on the role of the A1C assay in the diagnosis of diabetes. Diabetes Care 2009;32:1327–1334
14. Johnson CL, Paulose-Ram R, Ogden CL, et al. National Health and Nutrition Examination Survey: analytic guidelines, 1999-2010. Vital Health Stat 2 2013;1–24
15. Selvin E, Parrinello CM, Sacks DB, Coresh J. Trends in prevalence and control of diabetes in the United States, 1988-1994 and 1999-2010. Ann Intern Med 2014;160:517–525
16. American Diabetes Association. 6. Glycemic targets: *Standards of Medical Care in Diabetes—2020*. Diabetes Care 2020;43(Suppl. 1):S66–S76
17. American Diabetes Association. 10. Cardiovascular disease and risk management: *Standards of Medical Care in Diabetes—2020*. Diabetes Care 2020;43(Suppl. 1):S111–S134
18. Whelton PK, Carey RM, Aronow WS, et al. 2017 ACC/AHA/AAPA/ABC/ACPM/AGS/APhA/ASH/ASPC/NMA/PCNA guideline for the prevention, detection, evaluation, and management of high blood pressure in adults: a report of the American College of Cardiology/American Heart Association Task Force on Clinical Practice Guidelines [published correction appears in J Am Coll Cardiol 2018;71:2275–2279]. J Am Coll Cardiol 2018;71:e127–e248
19. National Cholesterol Education Program (NCEP) Expert Panel on Detection, Evaluation, and Treatment of High Blood Cholesterol in Adults (Adult Treatment Panel III). Third report of the National cholesterol Education Program (NCEP) Expert Panel on Detection, Evaluation, and Treatment of High Blood Cholesterol in Adults (Adult treatment Panel III) final report. Circulation 2002;106:3143–3421
20. Selvin E, Manzi J, Stevens LA, et al. Calibration of serum creatinine in the National Health and Nutrition Examination Surveys (NHANES) 1988-1994, 1999-2004. Am J Kidney Dis 2007; 50:918–926
21. Levey AS, Stevens LA, Schmid CH, et al.; CKD-EPI (Chronic Kidney Disease Epidemiology Collaboration). A new equation to estimate glomerular filtration rate [published correction appears in Ann Intern Med 2011;155:408]. Ann Intern Med 2009;150:604–612
22. Levey AS, Eckardt K-U, Tsukamoto Y, et al. Definition and classification of chronic kidney disease: a position statement from Kidney Disease:

Improving Global Outcomes (KDIGO). Kidney Int 2005;67:2089–2100
23. Early Treatment Diabetic Retinopathy Study Research Group. Grading diabetic retinopathy from stereoscopic color fundus photographs–an extension of the modified Airlie House classification. ETDRS report number 10. Early Treatment Diabetic Retinopathy Study Research Group. Ophthalmology 1991;98(Suppl.):786–806
24. Zhang X, Saaddine JB, Chou C-F, et al. Prevalence of diabetic retinopathy in the United States, 2005-2008. JAMA 2010;304:649–656
25. Gerhard-Herman MD, Gornik HL, Barrett C, et al. 2016 AHA/ACC guideline on the management of patients with lower extremity peripheral artery disease: executive summary: a report of the American College of Cardiology/American Heart Association Task Force on Clinical Practice Guidelines. J Am Coll Cardiol 2017;69:1465–1508
26. Gregg EW, Sorlie P, Paulose-Ram R, et al.; 1999-2000 National Health and Nutrition Examination Survey. Prevalence of lower-extremity disease in the US adult population $\geq$ =40 years of age with and without diabetes: 1999-2000 national health and nutrition examination survey. Diabetes Care 2004;27:1591–1597
27. Ingram DD, Malec DJ, Makuc DM, et al. National Center for Health Statistics guidelines for analysis of trends. Vital Health Stat 2 2018:1–71
28. Graubard BI, Korn EL. Predictive margins with survey data. Biometrics 1999;55:652–659
29. Centers for Disease Control and Prevention. National Diabetes Statistics Report, 2020: Estimates of Diabetes and Its Burden in the United States. 2020. Accessed 1 July 2020. Available from https://www.cdc.gov/diabetes/pdfs/data/statistics/national-diabetes-statistics-report.pdf
30. Benoit SR, Hora I, Albright AL, Gregg EW. New directions in incidence and prevalence of diagnosed diabetes in the USA. BMJ Open Diabetes Res Care 2019;7:e000657
31. Geiss LS, Pan L, Cadwell B, Gregg EW, Benjamin SM, Engelgau MM. Changes in incidence of diabetes in U.S. adults, 1997-2003. Am J Prev Med 2006;30:371–377
32. Menke A, Casagrande S, Geiss L, Cowie CC. Prevalence of and trends in diabetes among adults in the United States, 1988-2012. JAMA 2015;314:1021–1029
33. UK Prospective Diabetes Study (UKPDS) Group. Intensive blood-glucose control with sulphonylureas or insulin compared with conventional treatment and risk of complications in patients with type 2 diabetes (UKPDS 33) [published correction appears in Lancet 1999;354: 602]. Lancet 1998;352:837–853
34. UK Prospective Diabetes Study Group. Tight blood pressure control and risk of macrovascular and microvascular complications in type 2 diabetes: UKPDS 38 [published correction appears in BMJ 1999;318:29]. BMJ 1998;317:703–713
35. Muskiet MH, Tonneijck L, Smits MM, Kramer MH, Heerspink HJL, van Raalte DH. Pleiotropic effects of type 2 diabetes management strategies on renal risk factors. Lancet Diabetes Endocrinol 2015;3:367–381
36. Murphy D, McCulloch CE, Lin F, et al.; Centers for Disease Control and Prevention Chronic Kidney Disease Surveillance Team. Trends in prevalence of chronic kidney disease in the United States. Ann Intern Med 2016;165:473–481

37. Afkarian M, Zelnick LR, Hall YN, et al. Clinical manifestations of kidney disease among US adults with diabetes, 1988-2014. JAMA 2016; 316:602–610

38. de Boer IH, Rue TC, Hall YN, Heagerty PJ, Weiss NS, Himmelfarb J. Temporal trends in the prevalence of diabetic kidney disease in the United States. JAMA 2011;305:2532–2539

39. Kuller L, Borhani N, Furberg C, et al. Prevalence of subclinical atherosclerosis and cardiovascular disease and association with risk factors in the Cardiovascular Health Study. Am J Epidemiol 1994;139:1164–1179

40. Gregg EW, Li Y, Wang J, et al. Changes in diabetes-related complications in the United States, 1990-2010. N Engl J Med 2014;370: 1514–1523

41. Gregg EW, Cheng YJ, Srinivasan M, et al. Trends in cause-specific mortality among adults with and without diagnosed diabetes in the USA: an epidemiological analysis of linked national survey and vital statistics data. Lancet 2018;391: 2430–2440

42. Fox CS, Coady S, Sorlie PD, et al. Trends in cardiovascular complications of diabetes. JAMA 2004;292:2495–2499

43. Pastorino S, Richards M, Hardy R, et al.; National Survey of Health and Development Scientific and Data Collection Teams. Validation of self-reported diagnosis of diabetes in the 1946 British birth cohort. Prim Care Diabetes 2015;9:397–400

44. Schneider AL, Pankow JS, Heiss G, Selvin E. Validity and reliability of self-reported diabetes in the Atherosclerosis Risk in Communities Study. Am J Epidemiol 2012;176:738–743

Baseline Predictors of Glycemic Worsening in Youth and Adults With Impaired Glucose Tolerance or Recently Diagnosed Type 2 Diabetes in the Restoring Insulin Secretion (RISE) Study

Susan Sam,[1] Sharon L. Edelstein,[2]
Silva A. Arslanian,[3] Elena Barengolts,[1]
Thomas A. Buchanan,[4] Sonia Caprio,[5]
David A. Ehrmann,[1] Tamara S. Hannon,[6]
Ashley Hogan Tjaden,[2] Steven E. Kahn,[7]
Kieren J. Mather,[6] Mark Tripputi,[2]
Kristina M. Utzschneider,[7]
Anny H. Xiang,[8] and Kristen J. Nadeau,[9]
The RISE Consortium*

Diabetes Care 2021;44:1938–1947 | https://doi.org/10.2337/dc21-0027

OBJECTIVE

To identify predictors of glycemic worsening among youth and adults with impaired glucose tolerance (IGT) or recently diagnosed type 2 diabetes in the Restoring Insulin Secretion (RISE) Study.

RESEARCH DESIGN AND METHODS

A total of 91 youth (10–19 years) were randomized 1:1 to 12 months of metformin (MET) or 3 months of glargine, followed by 9 months of metformin (G-MET), and 267 adults were randomized to MET, G-MET, liraglutide plus MET (LIRA+MET), or placebo for 12 months. All participants underwent a baseline hyperglycemic clamp and a 3-h oral glucose tolerance test (OGTT) at baseline, month 6, month 12, and off treatment at month 15 and month 21. Cox models identified baseline predictors of glycemic worsening (HbA$_{1c}$ increase ≥0.5% from baseline).

RESULTS

Glycemic worsening occurred in 17.8% of youth versus 7.5% of adults at month 12 ($P = 0.008$) and in 36% of youth versus 20% of adults at month 21 ($P = 0.002$). In youth, glycemic worsening did not differ by treatment. In adults, month 12 glycemic worsening was less on LIRA+MET versus placebo (hazard ratio 0.21, 95% CI 0.05–0.96, $P = 0.044$). In both age-groups, lower baseline clamp-derived β-cell responses predicted month 12 and month 21 glycemic worsening ($P < 0.01$). Lower baseline OGTT-derived β-cell responses predicted month 21 worsening ($P < 0.05$). In youth, higher baseline HbA$_{1c}$ and 2-h glucose predicted month 12 and month 21 glycemic worsening, and higher fasting glucose predicted month 21 worsening ($P < 0.05$). In adults, lower clamp- and OGTT-derived insulin sensitivity predicted month 12 and month 21 worsening ($P < 0.05$).

CONCLUSIONS

Glycemic worsening was more common among youth than adults with IGT or recently diagnosed type 2 diabetes, predicted by lower baseline β-cell responses in both groups, hyperglycemia in youth, and insulin resistance in adults.

[1]University of Chicago, Chicago, IL
[2]George Washington University Biostatistics Center, Washington, DC
[3]University of Pittsburgh Medical Center-Children's Hospital of Pittsburgh, Pittsburgh, PA
[4]University of Southern California Keck School of Medicine, Los Angeles, CA
[5]Yale University, New Haven, CT
[6]Indiana University School of Medicine, Indianapolis, IN
[7]Veterans Affairs Puget Sound Health Care System and University of Washington, Seattle, WA
[8]Department of Research & Evaluation, Kaiser Permanente Southern California, Pasadena, CA
[9]University of Colorado Anschutz Medical Campus and Children's Hospital Colorado, Aurora, CO

Corresponding author: Sharon L. Edelstein, rise@bsc.gwu.edu

Received 6 January 2021 and accepted 31 March 2021

Clinical trial reg. nos. NCT01779362 and NCT01779375, clinicaltrials.gov

This article contains supplementary material online at https://doi.org/10.2337/figshare.14368220.

*A complete list of centers, RISE Consortium Investigators, and staff can be found in the supplementary material online.

This article is part of a special article collection available at https://care.diabetesjournals.org/collection/the-RISE-study-more-insights-into-T2D-in-youth-and-adults.

See accompanying articles, pp. 1934, 1948, and 1961.

Type 2 diabetes has become increasingly common in youth and adults as the prevalence of overweight and obesity increases. Progressive deterioration of islet β-cell function in individuals with prediabetes typically leads to type 2 diabetes (1). The rate of progression to type 2 diabetes and further loss of β-cell function once hyperglycemia is established varies widely among individuals with prediabetes. In an observational longitudinal study of 77,000 adults with prediabetes defined by HbA$_{1c}$, a small subset (5.2%) had a very high risk for development of type 2 diabetes within 2 years, while most (81.5%) were at lesser risk (2). Similarly, among obese youth with prediabetes based on HbA$_{1c}$, up to 8% developed type 2 diabetes after 12–22 months of follow-up (3). In youth with established type 2 diabetes monitored for a mean of 3.86 years in the Treatment Options for type 2 Diabetes in Adolescents and Youth (TODAY) study, insulin was required after oral treatments failed in 50% of participants, with a median time to treatment failure of 11.5 months, whereas other youth in TODAY maintained glycemic control on oral diabetes medications alone (4). Of note, youth in TODAY overall had a more rapid deterioration of β-cell function and glycemic control (4) than that previously reported in adults (5–8); however, no prior studies have directly compared youth and adults with type 2 diabetes longitudinally in the same study. Identification of factors that predispose to deterioration of β-cell function in youth and adults is essential to designing interventions to delay or prevent glycemic worsening in each age-group.

The Restoring Insulin Secretion (RISE) studies examined whether pharmacologic interventions could successfully restore or preserve β-cell function in youth and adults with impaired glucose intolerance (IGT) or recently diagnosed type 2 diabetes (9). As previously reported, none of the interventions resulted in sustained improvements in β-cell function after medication withdrawal in youth or adults (10,11). However, there was individual heterogeneity in responses both on and after withdrawal of therapy, ranging from normalization to rapid worsening of glycemia requiring study withdrawal; the latter was especially common among

youth (10,11). In this analysis, we aimed to compare glycemic worsening between youth and adult RISE participants with IGT or recently diagnosed type 2 diabetes and identify baseline characteristics that predict glycemic worsening in each group, while on treatment (month 12 [M12]) and 9 months after treatment withdrawal (month 21, [M21]).

RESEARCH DESIGN AND METHODS
Study Protocol
The RISE Pediatric and Adult Medication Studies were two of the three clinical trials performed as part of the RISE Consortium, funded by the National Institute of Diabetes and Digestive and Kidney Diseases (9). Both studies enrolled participants with IGT or recently diagnosed type 2 diabetes (12). The Pediatric Medication Study was a four-center, randomized, open-label clinical trial comparing 12-month interventions with insulin glargine for 3 months, followed by metformin (MET) for 9 months (G-MET) versus MET alone (9,10). The Adult Medication Study was a three-center, randomized, partially blinded clinical trial comparing 12-month interventions with 1) G-MET, 2) MET, 3) liraglutide plus MET (LIRA+MET), or 4) placebo. In the RISE Adult Medication Study, the placebo versus MET arms were double blinded. The rationale for and methods used in RISE were described previously in detail (9–11), and the study protocols can be found at https://rise.bsc.gwu.edu/web/rise/collaborators. Each center's Institutional Review Board (IRB) approved the protocol. Written informed consent was obtained from every adult participant, and parental or participant consent and child assent (when age-appropriate) were obtained before study procedures, consistent with the Declaration of Helsinki and each center's IRB guidelines.

Participants
A summary of the RISE Pediatric and Adult Medication Study participants and their rates of completion of oral glucose tolerance tests (OGTTs) during study visits are shown in the Consolidated Standards of Reporting Trials (CONSORT) diagram (Supplementary Figs. 1 and 2). The pediatric study randomized 91

youth aged 10–19 years with BMI ≥85th percentile for age and sex but <50 kg/m^2, with IGT (60%) or recently diagnosed (<6 months' duration) type 2 diabetes (40%), negative GAD and islet antigen 2 autoantibodies, and Tanner stage ≥2 (using breast development for females and testicular volume >3 mL for males) (9,10). Youth were also required to have a fasting glucose of ≥90 mg/dL (5 mmol/L) and an OGTT 2-h glucose ≥140 mg/dL (7.8 mmol/L), and if they were drug naive, HbA$_{1c}$ ≤8.0% (64 mmol/mol). Youth with type 2 diabetes already taking metformin had to have HbA$_{1c}$ ≤7.5% (58 mmol/mol) if on metformin for <3 months or HbA$_{1c}$ ≤7.0% (53 mmol/mol) if on metformin for 3–6 months (9,10). Eligible youth underwent baseline evaluations, followed by random 1:1 treatment assignment by study site, stratified by a baseline diagnosis of IGT versus type 2 diabetes (9,10). Eligibility criteria for adults included age 20–65 years and BMI ≥25 but <50 kg/m^2 (≥23 kg/m^2 for Asian Americans), with IGT or drug-naive physician-diagnosed type 2 diabetes <12 months' duration (9,11). Adults were required to have a fasting glucose 95–125 mg/dL (5.3–6.9 mmol/L), OGTT 2-h glucose ≥140 mg/dL (7.8 mmol/L), and HbA$_{1c}$ ≤7% (9,11). Eligible adults underwent baseline evaluations, followed by random 1:1:1:1 treatment assignment by study site, stratified by a baseline diagnosis of IGT versus type 2 diabetes (9,11).

Interventions
Complete details of the interventions were previously published (9–11), and the study timeline is shown in Supplementary Fig. 3. Youth and adult participants in the MET group both received 500 mg metformin that was titrated up to 1,000 mg twice daily over 4 weeks or to the maximal tolerated dose. The G-MET group in both youth and adults received 3 months of glargine insulin, titrated by study staff based on daily self-monitored fasting blood glucose. After 3 months, insulin glargine was stopped, and MET was initiated and titrated up to 1,000 mg twice daily (or the maximal tolerated dose) for the remainder of the 9-month intervention. For the adult LIRA+MET group, liraglutide was started first,

with weekly titration from 0.6 to 1.2 to a final dose of 1.8 mg daily as tolerated. After a tolerated liraglutide dose over the first 4 weeks was established, MET (unblinded) was added and titrated up to a goal of 1,000 mg twice daily (or the maximal tolerated dose) for the remainder of the intervention period (11). The adult placebo group received tablets that were identical in appearance to the metformin tablets and were titrated up in the same manner as the metformin and continued for 12 months.

The study medication for all participants in the Pediatric and Adult Medication Studies was withdrawn after 12 months of treatment (9–11). Study measurements in the present analysis included evaluations at baseline, M3, M6, M9, and M12 (on treatment) and M15, M18, and M21 (through 9 months after medication withdrawal). Measurements included in this analysis were baseline anthropometric measures, fasting and 2-h OGTT glucose, HbA_{1c}, and hyperglycemic clamp- and OGTT-derived measures of β-cell response and insulin sensitivity, as well as HbA_{1c} at M3, M6, M9, M12, M15, M18, and M21, and fasting and 2-h OGTT glucose at M6, M12, M15, and M21.

If protocol-specified HbA_{1c} safety thresholds were exceeded, outcome measures were promptly performed, if possible, and the participant was then withdrawn from the study and referred for additional clinical diabetes treatment. In addition to the IRB and the investigators, the study was regularly monitored by an independent National Institute of Diabetes and Digestive and Kidney Diseases-appointed Data and Safety Monitoring Board.

Procedures and Calculations
HbA_{1c} was measured at all quarterly visits. A two-step hyperglycemic clamp with target glucose concentrations of 200 mg/dL (11.1 mmol/L) and >450 mg/dL (>25 mmol/L), the latter paired with the insulin secretagogue arginine, was performed at baseline as previously described to assess pancreatic β-cell function (9,13–15). The hyperglycemic clamp simultaneously quantified insulin sensitivity (M/I) and three β-cell response measures: 1) acute (first-phase)

C-peptide and insulin responses to glucose ($ACPR_g$, AIR_g), 2) steady-state (second-phase) C-peptide (SSCP), and 3) acute C-peptide and insulin responses to arginine at maximal glycemic potentiation ($ACPR_{max}$ and AIR_{max}) achieved by glucose >450 mg/dL (16–19). M/I was calculated as the mean glucose infusion rate (M) at 100, 110, and 120 min of the clamp divided by the corresponding mean steady-state plasma insulin concentration. $ACPR_g$ and AIR_g were calculated as the mean incremental response above baseline for the first 10 min after the glucose bolus. Mean SSCP was calculated at 100, 110, and 120 min (16–19). $ACPR_{max}$ and AIR_{max} were calculated as the mean incremental response above concentrations before the arginine bolus.

A 3-h 75-g OGTT was performed at baseline to determine fasting and 2-h glucose, and fasting and 2-h insulin and C-peptide concentrations. From these, 1/fasting insulin (I/FI) was calculated to estimate insulin sensitivity, and OGTT-derived β-cell response measures were computed, including the C-peptide index (CPI, nmol/mmol; ΔC-$peptide_{30-0}$/$\Delta glucose_{30-0}$) and insulinogenic index (IGI, $\Delta insulin_{30-0}$/$\Delta glucose_{30-0}$) (14,20). The hyperglycemic clamp-derived insulin and C-peptide responses were adjusted for M/I, and OGTT-derived responses were adjusted for 1/FI.

Laboratory assessments were performed at the study's central biochemistry laboratory at the University of Washington (13,14). Glucose was measured using the glucose hexokinase method on a Roche c501 autoanalyzer (Roche Diagnostics, Indianapolis, IN). C-peptide and insulin were measured by a two-site immunoenzymometric assay performed on the Tosoh 2000 autoanalyzer (Tosoh Biosciences, South San Francisco, CA). Interassay coefficients of variation on quality control samples with low, medium, medium-high, and high concentrations were ≤2.0% for glucose, ≤4.3% for C-peptide, and ≤3.5% for insulin. HbA_{1c} was measured on a Tosoh G8 analyzer, under Level 1 NGSP certification. The interassay coefficients of variation, as measured on quality control samples with low and high HbA_{1c} levels, were 1.9% and 1.0%, respectively (9–11).

Statistics
Glycemic worsening was defined as an absolute increase in HbA_{1c} by ≥0.5% from baseline to M12 and from baseline to M21 (e.g., an increase from a baseline HbA_{1c} of 6.0% to 6.5% or from baseline of 7.7% to 8.2%, etc.). We additionally examined glycemic worsening defined as ≥5% and ≥10% relative increases from baseline HbA_{1c} to M12 and to M21 (e.g., a 5% relative increase from a baseline of 6.0% would be 6.3%, and a 10% relative increase from a baseline of 6% would be 6.6%). Cox proportional hazards models were used to identify baseline factors that were associated with time to glycemic worsening. Baseline characteristics used as predictors included age, sex, race/ethnicity, BMI, HbA_{1c}, fasting and 2-h OGTT glucose, and measures of β-cell response and insulin sensitivity from the OGTT and hyperglycemic clamp. Results from continuous variables in the Cox models are presented per 1 SD. Cox models were adjusted for treatment arm. β-Cell function measures were further adjusted for insulin sensitivity as assessed during the procedure, using M/I for hyperglycemic clamp-derived measures ($ACPR_g$, AIR_g, SSCP, $ACPR_{max}$, and AIR_{max}) and using 1/FI for OGTT-derived measures (CPI and IGI). When the analyses regarding β-cell responses were repeated without adjustment for insulin sensitivity, there was no significant impact on the results, so only the data that were adjusted are presented. Measures from the hyperglycemic clamp were log transformed before analyses to normalize the distributions. Additionally, progression from IGT to type 2 diabetes based on American Diabetes Association criteria for fasting and 2-h glucose concentrations (12) was evaluated at M06, M12, M15, and M21, and the impact of pharmacologic interventions on progression from IGT to type 2 diabetes was examined using Cox models.

RESULTS

Baseline demographic and metabolic characteristics of youth and adults and the primary outcome of the RISE studies have been reported (10,11) and are summarized in Supplementary Table 1. In brief, youth had a higher percentage of females, more racial/ethnic diversity, similar weight, and slightly but statistically higher BMI, and were markedly more insulin resistant than the adults. Furthermore, the proportion of youth with type 2 diabetes at baseline (40.7%) was higher than adults (26.2%) ($P = 0.0410$) (Supplementary Table 1). However, despite these differences, both groups had similar baseline HbA_{1c} and fasting and 2-h glucose concentrations (Supplementary Table 1).

Glycemic Worsening

At both M12 and M21, significantly more youth than adults developed glycemic worsening as defined by an absolute increase of $\geq 0.5\%$ in HbA_{1c} (M12: 17.8% vs. 7.5%, $P = 0.008$; M21 36.7% vs. 20%, respectively, $P = 0.002$) (Table 1, Fig. 1, top panel). Findings were similar even when analyses were restricted to the interventions common to youth and adults; i.e., MET and G-MET groups, both at M12 ($P = 0.011$) and M21 ($P = 0.005$, data not shown). Additionally, we evaluated the percentage of youth and adults who had a $\geq 5\%$ relative increase in HbA_{1c} from baseline to M12 and M21. Overall, 27.8% of youth and 22% of adults had a $\geq 5\%$ relative increase in HbA_{1c} at M12 ($P = 0.26$), as did 54.4% of youth and 42% of adults at M21 ($P = 0.041$) (Fig. 1, bottom panel). Using a $\geq 10\%$ relative increase in HbA_{1c}, we determined 14.4% of youth and 3.9% adults had such an increase in HbA_{1c} at M12 ($P < 0.001$), as did 31.3% of youth and 14.9% of adults at M21 ($P < 0.001$) (data not shown).

Predictors of Glycemic Worsening in Youth and Adults

In youth, treatment group did not affect glycemic worsening defined by an absolute increase of $\geq 0.5\%$ in HbA_{1c}, with glycemic worsening at M12 and M21 being associated with higher baseline HbA_{1c} ($P = 0.0241$ and $P = 0.008$, respectively) and higher baseline 2-h glucose ($P = 0.045$ and $P = 0.042$, respectively) (Table 2). Additionally, glycemic worsening at M21 in youth was associated with higher baseline fasting glucose ($P = 0.044$). In youth, glycemic worsening at M12 and M21 was also associated with lower baseline first-phase responses assessed by hyperglycemic clamp-derived $ACPR_g$ ($P = 0.006$ and $P < 0.001$, respectively) and AIR_g ($P = 0.014$ and $P < 0.001$, respectively) and lower baseline second-phase β-cell response by clamp-derived SSCP ($P = 0.004$ and $P = 0.001$, respectively). Glycemic worsening at M21 was also associated with lower baseline maximal β-cell response by clamp-derived $ACPR_{max}$ ($P = 0.015$) and AIR_{max} ($P = 0.007$). In youth, lower baseline OGTT-derived β-cell responses, including IGI ($P = 0.017$) and CPI $P = 0.006$), were associated with glycemic worsening at M21, and lower baseline CPI was also associated with glycemic worsening at M12 ($P = 0.031$).

Unlike youth, in adults, overall treatment group was borderline significant in predicting glycemic worsening defined by an absolute increase of $\geq 0.5\%$ in HbA_{1c} by M12 ($P = 0.089$) but not at M21 ($P = 0.233$) (Table 3). However,

treatment with LIRA+MET attenuated glycemic worsening at M12 compared with placebo (hazard ratio, 0.21; 95% CI 0.05–0.96, $P = 0.044$), although this beneficial effect was only borderline significant at M21 after withdrawal of LIRA+MET (hazard ratio 0.46, 95% CI 0.20–1.02, $P = 0.057$). Unlike youth, glycemic worsening in adults was not associated with baseline glycemic measures such as HbA_{1c} and fasting or 2-h glucose, but M12 and M21 glycemic worsening was associated with lower baseline insulin sensitivity by clamp-derived M/I ($P = 0.016$ and $P = 0.003$, respectively) and OGTT-derived 1/FI ($P = 0.010$ and $P = 0.029$, respectively). In addition, similar to youth, glycemic worsening in adults at M12 and M21 was associated with lower baseline clamp-derived first-phase responses, including $ACPR_g$ ($P = 0.010$ and $P = 0.011$) and AIR_g ($P = 0.001$ and $P = 0.007$). Like in youth, a lower baseline IGI on the OGTT was also associated with glycemic worsening at M21 in adults ($P = 0.034$).

Glycemic Worsening Based on Progression From IGT to Type 2 Diabetes

Among youth with IGT at baseline, 15.9% progressed to diabetes by M12 and 25% to diabetes by M21. In youth, treatment group did not affect progression from IGT to type 2 diabetes at M12 ($P = 0.28$) or M21 ($P = 0.40$) (Fig. 2A). Among adults with IGT at baseline, 21.2% progressed to diabetes by M12 and 39.1% by M21. In adults, treatment was borderline effective in reducing the progression from IGT to type 2 diabetes

Table 1—Glycemic worsening in youth and adults defined as an absolute increase of 0.5% in HbA_{1c} from baseline to M12 and M21

	M12				M21			
	No		Yes		No		Yes	
	n	%	n	%	n	%	n	%
Youth								
G-MET	35	79.5	9	20.5	30	68.2	14	31.8
MET	39	84.8	7	15.2	27	58.7	19	41.3
Total	74	82.2	16	**17.8***	57	63.3	33	**36.7†**
Adult								
G-MET	64	95.5	3	4.5	53	79.1	14	20.9
MET	57	91.9	5	8.1	51	82.3	11	17.7
LIRA+MET	61	96.8	2	3.2	54	85.7	9	14.3
Placebo	54	85.7	9	14.3	46	73.0	17	27.0
Total	236	92.5	19	**7.5**	204	80.0	51	**20.0**

Bold values are statistically significant comparing youth to adults. *$P = 0.008$ youth compared with adults at M12. †$P = 0.002$ youth compared with adults at M21.

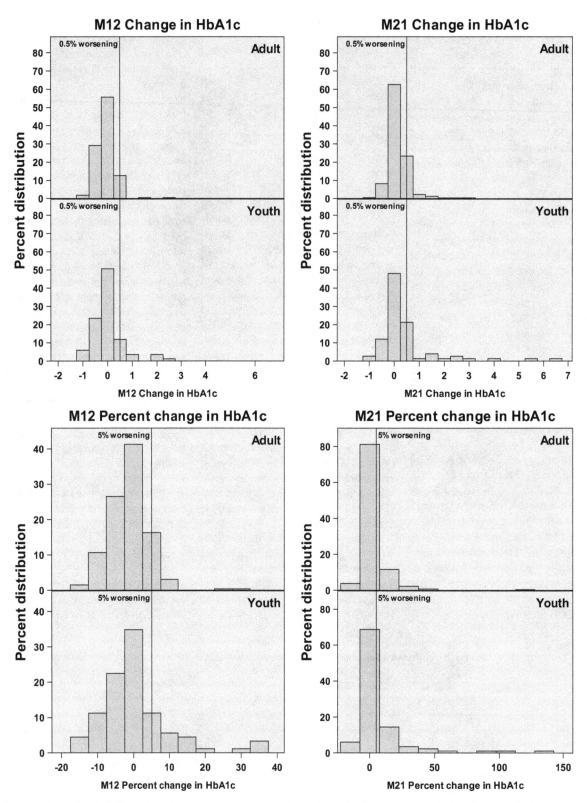

Figure 1—Change from baseline in glycemia at M12 (on treatment) and M21 (9 months after treatment withdrawal). Top panel: Glycemic worsening based on absolute increase in HbA_{1c} in adults and youth from baseline to M12 (left panel) and M21 (right panel). The vertical lines depict 0.5% worsening in absolute HbA_{1c}. On the left, there are no significant differences between adults and youth at M12. On the right, youth experienced greater glycemic worsening at M21 ($P = 0.041$). Bottom panel: Glycemic worsening based on the percentage (relative) increase in HbA_{1c} in adults and youth from baseline to M12 (left panel) and M21 (right panel). The vertical lines are shown at 5% worsening. Youth experienced greater glycemic worsening when defined as the percentage increase in HbA_{1c} at M12 ($P < 0.001$) and at M21 ($P < 0.001$).

Table 2—Cox regression models of predictors of glycemic worsening (an absolute increase of 0.5% in HbA$_{1c}$) in youth

	M12 hazard ratio†	Lower CI	Upper CI	P value	M21 hazard ratio†	Lower CI	Upper CI	P value
G-MET vs. MET	1.37	0.51	3.68	0.532	0.81	0.41	1.62	0.560
Sex (male vs. female)	1.52	0.54	4.31	0.432	0.94	0.41	2.13	0.878
Race/ethnicity								
White vs. other	0.35	0.08	1.56	0.170	0.54	0.22	1.32	0.177
Black vs. other	1.86	0.66	5.25	0.238	0.88	0.38	2.05	0.769
Hispanic vs. other	1.75	0.64	4.75	0.274	1.41	0.70	2.82	0.336
Baseline continuous measures								
Age (years)	0.98	0.59	1.63	0.932	0.99	0.70	1.41	0.956
BMI (kg/m^2)	1.14	0.68	1.92	0.614	1.14	0.79	1.64	0.496
HbA$_{1c}$ (%)	1.67	1.07	2.60	**0.024**	1.56	1.12	2.16	**0.008**
Fasting glucose (mg/dL)	1.43	0.93	2.19	0.100	1.33	1.01	1.77	**0.044**
2-h glucose (mg/dL)	1.49	1.01	2.20	**0.045**	1.33	1.01	1.75	**0.042**
Log M/I	0.83	0.50	1.38	0.472	0.93	0.65	1.34	0.704
Log ACPR$_g$	0.45	0.25	0.79	**0.006**	0.47	0.32	0.69	**<0.001**
Log AIR$_g$	0.57	0.36	0.89	**0.014**	0.61	0.45	0.81	**<0.001**
Log SSCP	0.45	0.26	0.78	**0.004**	0.54	0.37	0.78	**0.001**
Log ACPR$_{max}$	0.61	0.34	1.11	0.105	0.61	0.41	0.91	**0.015**
Log AIR$_{max}$	0.59	0.32	1.09	0.090	0.57	0.38	0.85	**0.007**
Log 1/FI	0.78	0.47	1.28	0.321	0.85	0.59	1.22	0.385
IGI	0.46	0.20	1.04	0.061	0.56	0.34	0.90	**0.017**
CPI	0.45	0.22	0.93	**0.031**	0.53	0.34	0.83	**0.006**

Bold P values are statistically significant (P < 0.05). All models included a term for the treatment arm. CI, 95% confidence interval. †Per 1 SD for continuous measures. Treatment arm is adjusted for insulin sensitivity by M/I, clamp-derived β-cell function responses are adjusted for treatment arm and insulin sensitivity by M/I, and all OGTT-derived β-cell function responses are adjusted for treatment arm and insulin sensitivity by 1/FI.

at M12 (P = 0.06 with the lowest rate in LIRA+MET) but not by M21 (P = 0.20) (Fig. 2B). The overall rate of progression from IGT to type 2 diabetes did not differ between youth and adults by M12 (P = 0.55) but was borderline significant by M21 (P = 0.089 with lower rates among youth). Limiting this comparison to include only adults randomized to MET or G-MET (to compare the interventions common to youth and adults) did not alter our findings (Fig. 2C).

In youth, progression to diabetes at M12 and M21 was associated with lower baseline maximal β-cell responses by clamp-derived ACPR$_{max}$ (P = 0.017 and P = 0.039, respectively, data not shown), at M12 by lower baseline AIR$_{max}$ (P = 0.004, data not shown), and at M21 by lower baseline first-phase response by clamp-derived AIRg (P = 0.039, data not shown). Similar to youth, in adults, lower baseline clamp-derived first-phase responses (AIRg and ACPRg) also predicted progression to diabetes at M12 (P = 0.001 and P = 0.010, respectively; data not shown) and M21 (P = 0.007 and P = 0.010, respectively; data not shown), as did lower baseline OGTT-derived IGI at M21

P = 0.034; data not shown). Different from youth, progression to type 2 diabetes at M12 and M21 in adults was associated with lower baseline insulin sensitivity by clamp-derived M/I (P = 0.016 and P = 0.003, respectively; data not shown) and by OGTT-derived 1/FI (P = 0.010 and P = 0.029, respectively; data not shown).

CONCLUSIONS

The current analysis of outcomes in the RISE study of youth and adults with IGT or recently diagnosed type 2 diabetes demonstrates that 1) short-term pharmacologic interventions did not reduce glycemic worsening or progression from IGT to type 2 diabetes in youth; 2) LIRA+MET was effective in reducing glycemic worsening while on therapy in adults, but this effectiveness did not persist 9 months after treatment withdrawal, consistent with our previous findings (10,14); 3) glycemic worsening was progressive in both groups, although greater in youth as 36% of youth versus 20% of adults (approaching 30% in adults randomized to placebo) developed glycemic worsening by the end of the 21-month study period, despite 12 months of active treatment

with pharmacologic agents; and 4) independent of pharmacologic intervention, β-cell dysfunction at baseline was a significant predictor of glycemic worsening in both youth and adults, both while they were on treatment and after treatment withdrawal, whereas while initial glycemia was predictive in youth, insulin sensitivity was predictive in adults.

By direct longitudinal comparison between youth and adults with a similar degree of dysglycemia at baseline, we clearly demonstrate for the first time that a greater fraction of youth with IGT or recently diagnosed type 2 diabetes had deterioration of glycemia compared with adults. Previous cross-sectional, observational, and randomized trials have suggested that youth have a more accelerated progression to type 2 diabetes and earlier development of diabetes complications compared with adults (8,10,11,21). The current study is also the first to directly compare youth and adults who were treated with a variety of medications, were monitored for nearly 2 years, and were studied in an identical manner across study sites using sensitive measures of insulin sensitivity and β-cell function. In both youth and adults, a lower baseline hyperglycemic

Table 3—Cox regression models of predictors of glycemic worsening (an absolute increase of 0.5% in HbA$_{1c}$) in adults

	M12 hazard ratio†	Lower CI	Upper CI	P value	M21 hazard ratio†	Lower CI	Upper CI	P value
Treatment group				0.089				0.233
G-MET vs. LIRA+MET	1.32	0.22	7.90	0.763	1.35	0.58	3.12	0.485
G-MET vs. MET	0.49	0.12	2.04	0.325	1.03	0.47	2.27	0.939
G-MET vs. placebo	0.27	0.07	1.01	0.051	0.61	0.30	1.25	0.179
LIRA+MET vs. MET	0.37	0.07	1.91	0.234	0.77	0.32	1.87	0.551
LIRA+MET vs. placebo	0.21	0.05	0.96	**0.044**	0.46	0.20	1.02	0.057
MET vs. placebo	0.56	0.19	1.67	0.296	0.60	0.28	1.27	0.181
Sex (male vs. female)	1.96	0.69	5.53	0.207	1.75	0.95	3.25	0.074
Race/ethnicity								
White vs. other	1.04	0.42	2.58	0.925	1.04	0.60	1.81	0.893
Black vs. other	0.75	0.27	2.09	0.581	0.95	0.52	1.73	0.870
Hispanic vs. other	1.68	0.48	5.88	0.418	0.89	0.32	2.51	0.831
Baseline continuous measures								
Age (years)	0.78	0.51	1.18	0.239	1.11	0.82	1.49	0.514
BMI (kg/m^2)	1.03	0.64	1.66	0.915	0.80	0.59	1.08	0.150
HbA$_{1c}$ (%)	1.05	0.66	1.65	0.842	0.94	0.70	1.27	0.695
Fasting glucose (mg/dL)	1.21	0.81	1.81	0.356	1.03	0.80	1.33	0.827
2-h glucose (mg/dL)	1.09	0.68	1.76	0.714	1.21	0.92	1.60	0.179
Log M/I	0.59	0.39	0.91	**0.016**	0.67	0.52	0.88	**0.0034**
Log ACPR$_g$	0.49	0.29	0.85	**0.010**	0.67	0.49	0.91	**0.011**
Log AIR$_g$	0.47	0.30	0.75	**0.001**	0.68	0.52	0.90	**0.007**
Log SSC-P	0.89	0.49	1.61	0.691	0.86	0.59	1.24	0.415
Log ACPR$_{max}$	0.94	0.59	1.48	0.778	0.90	0.68	1.20	0.476
Log AIR$_{max}$	0.82	0.51	1.33	0.426	0.79	0.59	1.05	0.108
Log 1/FI	0.57	0.37	0.87	**0.010**	0.75	0.57	0.97	**0.029**
IGI	0.49	0.22	1.08	0.078	0.65	0.43	0.97	**0.034**
CPI	0.60	0.31	1.15	0.122	0.72	0.51	1.02	0.062

Bold P values are statistically significant ($P < 0.05$). All models included a term for treatment arm. CI, 95% confidence interval. †Per 1 SD deviation for continuous measures. Treatment arm is adjusted for insulin sensitivity by M/I, clamp-derived β-cell function responses are adjusted for treatment arm and insulin sensitivity by M/I, and all OGTT-derived β-cell function responses are adjusted for treatment arm and Insulin sensitivity by 1/FI.

clamp-derived first-phase β-cell response to glucose was associated with a rise in HbA$_{1c}$ on treatment (M12) and after treatment withdrawal (M21), and lower OGTT-derived β-cell responses were similarly predictive after treatment withdrawal in both youth and adults. Lower baseline hyperglycemic clamp-derived second-phase and maximal C-peptide responses were also associated with glycemic worsening after treatment withdrawal in youth. Interestingly, baseline measures of glycemia in youth, such as fasting and OGTT 2-h glucose and HbA$_{1c}$, also predicted glycemic worsening after treatment withdrawal. In contrast to youth, in adults, reduced insulin sensitivity by hyperglycemic clamp and OGTT was a consistent additional predictor of glycemic worsening both on treatment and after treatment withdrawal. These data indicate potential differences in the pathophysiology of diabetes progression between youth and adults.

Our finding in youth with IGT and recently diagnosed type 2 diabetes

compliment and extend findings from the TODAY Study in youth with established type 2 diabetes (4,22). In TODAY, baseline OGTT-based β-cell dysfunction and dysglycemia predicted a greater probability of glycemic failure (defined as HbA$_{1c}$ ≥8% for 6 months); i.e., baseline proximity to a glycemic threshold predicted crossing that threshold during follow-up. In RISE, we focused on deterioration, defined as an increase in HbA$_{1c}$, rather than reaching a specific glycemic threshold. In RISE, baseline β-cell dysfunction and dysglycemia were the strongest predictors of glycemic worsening in youth; i.e., youth with the highest glucose levels and lowest β-cell function at baseline were deteriorating the fastest. This finding is consistent with a pattern of accelerating glycemia deterioration on a background of monotonous deterioration in β-cell-compensation (23). Further, RISE demonstrated that multiple β-cell responses (OGTT-based and first-phase, second-phase, and maximal glycemic potentiation responses during hyperglycemic

clamps) predicted glycemic worsening in youth. In contrast to the adults in RISE, neither TODAY (4,22) nor RISE found insulin sensitivity to be predictive of treatment failure or rising glycemia in youth. These findings point to β-cell dysfunction occurring on a background of severe insulin resistance as the key defect in youth that determines glycemic worsening, even at the earlier stage of IGT studied in RISE. Possible explanations for these age-related differences are that youth with IGT and type 2 diabetes are typically uniformly markedly insulin resistant due to multiple potential factors (the physiologic insulin resistance of puberty, lower physical activity, poor sleep, higher rates of racial/ethnic minorities, etc.), causing β-cell function to be the key differentiating factor in youth. In contrast, adults with IGT and type 2 diabetes may show more heterogeneity in their insulin sensitivity and β-cell responsiveness, allowing both to be predictors.

MET and G-MET did not reduce glycemic worsening in youth on treatment

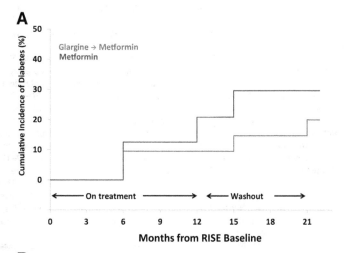

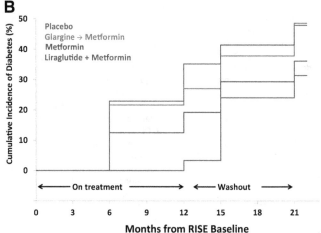

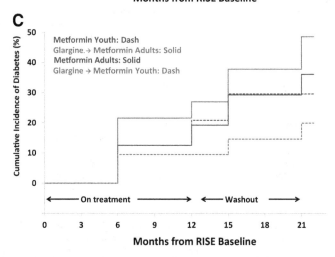

Figure 2—Life table estimate to progression from IGT to type 2 diabetes. *A*: Cumulative incidence of type 2 diabetes in youth over the duration of the study among youth with IGT at baseline. The progression to type 2 diabetes did not differ in youth between glargine, followed by metformin (G-MET) or metformin alone (MET) at M12 (*P* = 0.28) or M21 (*P* = 0.40). *B*: Cumulative incidence of type 2 diabetes in adults over the duration of the study among adults with IGT at baseline. The progression to type 2 diabetes was borderline significant between the four intervention arms at M12 (*P* = 0.06 for overall comparison) but not at M21 (*P* = 0.20 for overall comparison). *C*: Cumulative incidence of type 2 diabetes in youth and adults randomized to metformin (MET) alone vs. glargine, followed by metformin (G-MET), over the duration of the study, among youth and adults with IGT at baseline. The progression to type 2 diabetes did not differ between youth and adults in either intervention arm.

or after treatment withdrawal. In adults, only treatment with LIRA+MET was effective in reducing glycemic worsening while on therapy, but this beneficial effect did not persist after treatment withdrawal. This result is consistent with our earlier report of lack of durable benefit regarding β-cell function once LIRA+MET was discontinued for 3 months (11). Similarly, there are reports in the literature that the beneficial impact of glucagon-like peptide 1 agonists in reducing progression to type 2 diabetes in individuals with IGT is lost after withdrawal of therapy (24,25). Worsening of glycemia has also been reported upon withdrawal from liraglutide therapy in adults with type 2 diabetes of longer duration (26). In the Outcome Reduction With Initial Glargine Intervention (ORIGIN) study, insulin glargine was shown to reduce progression from IGT to type 2 diabetes in adults, although the effect was minimal (27). Similarly, a study from China demonstrated that intensive short-term glucose control with the use of multiple daily dose insulin injections or an insulin pump is associated with less progression of β-cell dysfunction in adults with newly diagnosed type 2 diabetes (28). In RISE, treatment with G-MET was not associated with a reduction in glycemic worsening in youth or adults with IGT or recently diagnosed type 2 diabetes while on treatment or after treatment withdrawal. Other reports in the literature are consistent with our observation that glargine does not prevent glycemic worsening (29). To date, thiazolidinediones have been the only pharmacologic class reported to durably prevent deterioration of β-cell function in adults (30–32) and in some youth (4,22).

Strengths of our study include the inclusion of both youth and adults of similar initial glycemia and inclusion of participants with IGT and recently diagnosed type 2 diabetes in protocols run in parallel at multiple sites using identical procedures and a central laboratory. Additional strengths include the use of measures of insulin sensitivity and β-cell responses by fasting, oral, and intravenous stimulation, inclusion of both glucose and arginine stimulation, as well as the racial/ethnic diversity among participants. The availability of longitudinal follow-up data both on treatment as well as after treatment withdrawal also contributes to the strength of our findings. Limitations include the lack of follow-up >21 months, baseline sex and racial/ethnic differences between youth and adults inherent to the affected populations, and the lack of a placebo and LIRA+MET group in youth.

In summary, in youth and adults with IGT or recently diagnosed type 2 diabetes, the incidence of glycemic worsening is high despite pharmacologic interventions, is worse in youth, and is predicted in both age-groups by baseline β-cell dysfunction with loss of the first-phase response. In adults, baseline insulin sensitivity is an additional predictor of glycemic worsening, whereas in youth, initial glycemia and β-cell dysfunction involving second-phase and maximal responses are also predictive. Although pharmacologic treatment in adults with LIRA+MET was not effective in reducing glycemic worsening after treatment withdrawal, it did decrease glycemic worsening while on therapy, arguing for long-term studies of β-cell function in youth receiving glucagon-like peptide 1 agonists. In addition, data on the impact of SGLT-2 inhibitors and of bariatric surgery on β-cell function are needed. Finally, our data also support the need for development of alternative approaches or therapies with a specific focus on preventing or improving insulin sensitivity and first-phase β-cell function in adults and all aspects of β-cell function in youth.

Acknowledgments. The RISE Consortium thanks the RISE Data and Safety Monitoring Board, Barbara Linder, the National Institute of Diabetes and Digestive and Kidney Diseases Program Official for RISE, and Ellen Leschek and Peter Savage, National Institute of Diabetes and Digestive and Kidney Diseases Scientific Officers for RISE, for their support and guidance. The Consortium is also grateful to the participants who, by volunteering, are furthering its ability to reduce the burden of diabetes. The authors dedicate this paper in memory of Bridget Pierpont, research associate from Yale University, for all she did to enrich their lives and further research in youth with diabetes.
Funding. RISE is supported by grants from the National Institutes of Health, National Institute of Diabetes and Digestive and Kidney Diseases (U01DK-094406, U01DK-094430, U01DK-094431, U01DK-094438, U01DK-094467, P30DK-017047, P30DK-020595, P30DK-045735, P30DK-097512) and the National Center for Advancing Translational Sciences (UL1TR-000430, UL1TR-001082, UL1TR-001108, UL1TR-001855, UL1TR-001857, UL1TR-001858, and UL1TR-001863), the Department of Veterans Affairs, and Kaiser Permanente Southern California. Additional financial and material support was received from the American Diabetes Association, Allergan Corporation, Apollo Endosurgery, Abbott Laboratories, and Novo Nordisk A/S.

The content of this publication is solely the responsibility of the authors and does not necessarily represent the official views of the National Institutes of Health.
Duality of Interest. S.A.A. is a paid consultant on advisory boards for Novo Nordisk, and a participant in a Novo Nordisk-sponsored clinical trial. S.E.K. is a paid consultant on advisory boards for Novo Nordisk and a steering committee for a Novo Nordisk-sponsored clinical trial. At the time of publication, K.J.M. was a full-time employee of Eli Lilly and Company. The data collection was performed before this employment, and the data analysis and preparation of the manuscript were independent of Eli Lilly and Company. No other potential conflicts of interest relevant to this article were reported.
Author Contributions. S.S., S.L.E., and K.J.N. wrote the first draft of the manuscript. S.S., S.L.E., K.J.N., S.A.A., E.B., T.A.B., S.C., D.A.E., T.S.H., A.H.T., S.E.K., K.J.M., M.T., K.M.U., and A.H.X. researched data, contributed to the discussion, and edited and approved the final version of the manuscript. S.L.E. is the guarantor of this work and performed all data analysis, and, as such, had full access to all the data in the study and takes responsibility for the integrity of the data and the accuracy of the data analysis.

References

1. Kahn SE, Hull RL, Utzschneider KM. Mechanisms linking obesity to insulin resistance and type 2 diabetes. Nature 2006;444:840–846
2. Glauber H, Vollmer WM, Nichols GA. A simple model for predicting two-year risk of diabetes development in individuals with prediabetes. Perm J 2018;22:17–050
3. Love-Osborne KA, Sheeder JL, Nadeau KJ, Zeitler P. Longitudinal follow up of dysglycemia in overweight and obese pediatric patients. Pediatr Diabetes 2018;19:199–204
4. Zeitler P, Hirst K, Pyle L, et al.; TODAY Study Group. A clinical trial to maintain glycemic control in youth with type 2 diabetes. N Engl J Med 2012;366:2247–2256
5. Turner RC, Cull CA, Frighi V; UK Prospective Diabetes Study (UKPDS) Group. Glycemic control with diet, sulfonylurea, metformin, or insulin in patients with type 2 diabetes mellitus: progressive requirement for multiple therapies (UKPDS 49). JAMA 1999;281:2005–2012
6. Brown JB, Conner C, Nichols GA. Secondary failure of metformin monotherapy in clinical practice. Diabetes Care 2010;33:501–506
7. Kahn SE, Haffner SM, Heise MA, et al.; ADOPT Study Group. Glycemic durability of rosiglitazone, metformin, or glyburide monotherapy. N Engl J Med 2006;355:2427–2443
8. Barrett T, Jalaludin MY, Turan S, Hafez M; Novo Nordisk Pediatric Type 2 Diabetes Global Expert Panel. Rapid progression of type 2 diabetes and related complications in children and young people—a literature review. Pediatr Diabetes 2020;21:158–172
9. RISE Consortium. Restoring Insulin Secretion (RISE): design of studies of β-cell preservation in prediabetes and early type 2 diabetes across the life span. Diabetes Care 2014;37:780–788
10. RISE Consortium. Impact of insulin and metformin versus metformin alone on β-cell function in youth with impaired glucose tolerance or recently diagnosed type 2 diabetes. Diabetes Care 2018;41:1717–1725
11. RISE Consortium. Lack of durable improvements in β-cell function following withdrawal of pharmacological interventions in adults with impaired glucose tolerance or recently diagnosed type 2 diabetes. Diabetes Care 2019;42: 1742–1751
12. American Diabetes Association. Diagnosis and classification of diabetes mellitus. Diabetes Care 2013;36 Suppl. 1(Suppl. 1):S67–S74
13. RISE Consortium. Metabolic contrasts between youth and adults with impaired glucose tolerance or recently diagnosed type 2 diabetes: I. Observations using the hyperglycemic clamp. Diabetes Care 2018;41:1696–1706
14. RISE Consortium. Metabolic contrasts between youth and adults with impaired glucose tolerance or recently diagnosed type 2 diabetes: II. Observations using the oral glucose tolerance test. Diabetes Care 2018;41:1707–1716
15. Hannon TS, Kahn SE, Utzschneider KM, et al.; RISE Consortium. Review of methods for measuring β-cell function: design considerations from the Restoring Insulin Secretion (RISE) Consortium. Diabetes Obes Metab 2018;20: 14–24
16. DeFronzo RA, Tobin JD, Andres R. Glucose clamp technique: a method for quantifying insulin secretion and resistance. Am J Physiol 1979;237:E214–E223
17. Elahi D. In praise of the hyperglycemic clamp. A method for assessment of β-cell sensitivity and insulin resistance. Diabetes Care 1996;19:278–286
18. Kahn SE, Prigeon RL, McCulloch DK, et al. Quantification of the relationship between insulin sensitivity and β-cell function in human subjects. Evidence for a hyperbolic function. Diabetes 1993;42:1663–1672
19. Ward WK, Bolgiano DC, McKnight B, Halter JB, Porte D Jr. Diminished B cell secretory capacity in patients with noninsulin-dependent diabetes mellitus. J Clin Invest 1984;74: 1318–1328
20. Solomon TP, Malin SK, Karstoft K, et al. Determining pancreatic β-cell compensation for changing insulin sensitivity using an oral glucose tolerance test. Am J Physiol Endocrinol Metab 2014;307:E822–E829
21. Hannon TS, Arslanian SA. The changing face of diabetes in youth: lessons learned from studies of type 2 diabetes. Ann N Y Acad Sci 2015;1353:113–137
22. TODAY Study Group. Effects of metformin, metformin plus rosiglitazone, and metformin plus lifestyle on insulin sensitivity and β-cell function in TODAY. Diabetes Care 2013;36:1749–1757
23. Xiang AH, Wang C, Peters RK, Trigo E, Kjos SL, Buchanan TA. Coordinate changes in plasma glucose and pancreatic β-cell function in Latino

women at high risk for type 2 diabetes. Diabetes 2006;55:1074–1079

24. le Roux CW, Astrup A, Fujioka K, et al.; SCALE Obesity Prediabetes NN8022-1839 Study Group. 3 years of liraglutide versus placebo for type 2 diabetes risk reduction and weight management in individuals with prediabetes: a randomised, double-blind trial. Lancet 2017;389:1399–1409

25. Retnakaran R, Kramer CK, Choi H, Swaminathan B, Zinman B. Liraglutide and the preservation of pancreatic β-cell function in early type 2 diabetes: the LIBRA trial. Diabetes Care 2014;37:3270–3278

26. Tran S, Kramer CK, Zinman B, Choi H, Retnakaran R. Effect of chronic liraglutide therapy and its withdrawal on time to postchallenge peak glucose in type 2 diabetes. Am J Physiol Endocrinol Metab 2018;314: E287–E295

27. Gerstein HC, Bosch J, Dagenais GR, et al.; ORIGIN Trial Investigators. Basal insulin and cardiovascular and other outcomes in dysglycemia. N Engl J Med 2012;367:319–328

28. Weng JL, Li Y, Xu W, et al. Effects of intensive insulin therapy on β-cell function and glycaemic control in patients with newly diagnosed type 2 diabetes: a multicentre randomised parallel-group trial. Lancet 2008;24:1753–1760

29. Retnakaran R, Choi H, Ye C, Kramer CK, Zinman B. Two-year trial of intermittent insulin therapy vs metformin for the preservation of β-cell function after initial short-term intensive insulin induction in early type 2 diabetes. Diabetes Obes Metab 2018;20: 1399–1407

30. DeFronzo RA, Tripathy D, Schwenke DC, et al.; ACT NOW Study. Pioglitazone for diabetes prevention in impaired glucose tolerance. N Engl J Med 2011;364:1104–1115

31. Knowler WC, Hamman RF, Edelstein SL, et al.; Diabetes Prevention Program Research Group. Prevention of type 2 diabetes with troglitazone in the Diabetes Prevention Program. Diabetes 2005;54: 1150–1156

32. Tripathy D, Schwenke DC, Banerji M, et al. Diabetes incidence and glucose tolerance after termination of pioglitazone therapy: results from ACT NOW. J Clin Endocrinol Metab 2016; 101:2056–2062

American Diabetes Association Framework for Glycemic Control in Older Adults: Implications for Risk of Hospitalization and Mortality

Mary R. Rooney,[1] Olive Tang,[1]
Justin B. Echouffo Tcheugui,[1,2]
Pamela L. Lutsey,[3] Morgan E. Grams,[1,4]
B. Gwen Windham,[5] and Elizabeth Selvin[1]

Diabetes Care 2021;44:1524–1531 | https://doi.org/10.2337/dc20-3045

OBJECTIVE

The 2021 American Diabetes Association (ADA) guidelines recommend different A1C targets in older adults that are based on comorbid health status. We assessed risk of mortality and hospitalizations in older adults with diabetes across glycemic control (A1C <7%, 7 to <8%, ≥8%) and ADA-defined health status (healthy, complex/intermediate, very complex/poor) categories.

RESEARCH DESIGN AND METHODS

Prospective cohort analysis of older adults aged 66–90 years with diagnosed diabetes in the Atherosclerosis Risk in Communities (ARIC) study.

RESULTS

Of the 1,841 participants (56% women, 29% Black), 32% were classified as healthy, 42% as complex/intermediate, and 27% as very complex/poor health. Over a median 6-year follow-up, there were 409 (22%) deaths and 4,130 hospitalizations (median [25th–75th percentile] 1 per person [0–3]). In the very complex/poor category, individuals with A1C ≥8% (vs. <7%) had higher mortality risk (hazard ratio 1.76 [95% CI 1.15–2.71]), even after adjustment for glucose-lowering medication use. Within the very complex/poor health category, individuals with A1C ≥8% (vs. <7%) had more hospitalizations (incidence rate ratio [IRR] 1.41 [95% CI 1.03–1.94]). In the complex/intermediate group, individuals with A1C ≥8% (vs. <7%) had more hospitalizations, even with adjustment for glucose-lowering medication use (IRR 1.64 [1.21–2.24]). Results were similar, but imprecise, when the analysis was restricted to insulin or sulfonylurea users (n = 663).

CONCLUSIONS

There were substantial differences in mortality and hospitalizations across ADA health status categories, but older adults with A1C <7% were not at elevated risk, regardless of health status. Our results support the 2021 ADA guidelines and indicate that <7% is a reasonable treatment goal in some older adults with diabetes.

The 2021 American Diabetes Association (ADA) guidelines provide a framework for treating older adults with diabetes (1). This framework recommends treatment

[1]Department of Epidemiology and Welch Center for Prevention, Epidemiology, and Clinical Research, Johns Hopkins University, Baltimore, MD
[2]Division of Endocrinology, Diabetes and Metabolism, Johns Hopkins University, Baltimore, MD
[3]Division of Epidemiology and Community Health, University of Minnesota, Minneapolis, MN
[4]Department of Medicine, Johns Hopkins University, Baltimore, MD
[5]Division of Geriatrics, Department of Medicine, University of Mississippi Medical Center, Jackson, MS

Corresponding author: Mary Rooney, mroone12@jhu.edu

Received 15 December 2020 and accepted 29 March 2021

This article contains supplementary material online at https://doi.org/10.2337/figshare.14365433.

goals for glycemic control that are based on older patients' comorbid health and functional status. The comorbidities are listed as arthritis, cancer, congestive heart failure, depression, emphysema, falls, hypertension, incontinence, stage 3 or worse chronic kidney disease (CKD), myocardial infarction, stroke, cognitive function, and activities of daily living dependencies, with three or more comorbidities reflecting a "high burden" (2).

The rationale for targeting differing A1C goals according to health status is driven by life expectancy and time-to-benefit principles, under the assumption that older adults with diabetes who have very complex or poor health status may be at highest risk for adverse effects of treatment and less likely to benefit from intensive glucose control. Yet, the prognosis of diabetes in older adults is poorly characterized (2,3). It is also unclear whether the health status categories set forth in the ADA guidelines provide discrimination for mortality risk (4).

We used data from the Atherosclerosis Risk in Communities (ARIC) study to assess the current ADA framework and treatment goals among older adults with diabetes. Specifically, we sought to 1) describe the characteristics of participants according to ADA comorbid health status categories and A1C treatment goals and 2) examine prospective associations of health status categories with mortality and total hospitalizations during 6 years of follow-up, overall, and according to A1C categories.

RESEARCH DESIGN AND METHODS

The ARIC study is a community-based cohort that began in 1987–1989 when participants were middle aged (5). Participants were recruited from four centers: Forsyth County, North Carolina; Jackson, Mississippi; Minneapolis, Minnesota; and Washington County, Maryland. Visit 5 occurred in 2011–2013 when all 6,538 participants were >65 years of age.

Approximately one in three ARIC participants had diagnosed diabetes at visit 5 (self-report physician diagnosis or use of glucose-lowering medication, n = 2,147). For our analysis, we excluded visit 5 participants who were missing A1C measurement (n =

60), were missing comorbidity status (n = 225), or did not contribute follow-up data after visit 5 (n = 2) (Supplementary Fig. 1). We also excluded participants who self-reported their race as neither Black nor White, and Black participants at the Maryland and Minnesota centers because of small numbers (n = 19). Our final analytic sample was 1,841 older adults with diagnosed diabetes.

Measurement of A1C and Ascertainment of Glucose-Lowering Medication Use

A1C was measured in whole blood using a Tosoh G7 automated high-performance liquid chromatography analyzer (Tosoh Bioscience), which was standardized to the Diabetes Control and Complications Trial (DCCT) assay. Participants were asked to bring medication bottles used in the prior 2 weeks. Medications were transcribed and coded. We categorized participants as using insulin or sulfonylurea (with or without other glucose-lowering medications), other glucose-lowering medications (noninsulin/sulfonylurea), or no glucose-lowering medication.

Measurement of Comorbidities

Prevalent comorbidities were assessed at visit 5 (2011–2013 unless specified otherwise), on the basis of a history of one or more ICD-9 codes identified through hospital surveillance between 1987 and 2011, or on the basis of claims identified through the Centers for Medicare & Medicaid Services (CMS) linkage between 1987 and 2011. Arthritis was based on CMS inpatient and outpatient claims, any hospitalization identified through ARIC standard surveillance procedures where arthritis was recorded (see Supplementary Table 1 for ICD-9 codes used) before visit 5 (2011–2013), or self-report of arthritis at visit 4 (1996–1998). Cancer was ascertained through linkage to cancer registries. Congestive heart failure (reduced or preserved ejection fraction), myocardial infarction, and stroke (ischemic or hemorrhagic) were based on self-report at ARIC visit 1 (1987–1989) or any adjudicated event before visit 5 (2011–2013) on the basis of previously published approaches (6–8). Depression was defined using a score of ≥9 on the validated Center

for Epidemiological Studies Depression 11-item questionnaire (9). Emphysema and chronic obstructive pulmonary disease (COPD) were self-reported at visit 5 and based on hospitalizations. History of falls was based on any prior fall-related hospitalization. Hypertension was defined as measured blood pressure ≥140/90 mmHg (mean of second and third measurement) or current hypertension medication use. Hypoglycemia was ascertained from hospitalizations and linkage to CMS claims (10,11). Incontinence was based on CMS claims and any hospitalization with incontinence recorded before visit 5. CKD was defined as an estimated glomerular filtration rate <60 mL/min/1.73 m^2 at visit 5 (stage 3+) on the basis of the Chronic Kidney Disease Epidemiology Collaboration equation using cystatin C and creatinine (12), an albumin-to-creatinine ratio of ≥30 mg/g at visit 5, prior CKD-related hospital admission by continuous active surveillance, or end-stage kidney disease event in the U.S. Renal Data System registry. Dementia was based on detailed neurocognitive testing and adjudication (13). Frailty was based on criteria previously described in ARIC on the basis of the presence of three or more of the following: low energy, low physical activity, low strength, slowed motor performance, and unintentional weight loss (14,15). Functional status was based on the Short Physical Performance Battery, with a score <7 indicating poor functional status and ≥7 indicating adequate functional status (16).

Outcomes

All-cause mortality was identified through semiannual follow-up telephone calls to participants or their proxies, state records, and linkage to the National Death Index. We also examined associations with number of hospitalizations. Hospitalization reports were identified from semiannual telephone contact with study participants or their proxies and from active surveillance of hospitalizations in community hospitals (17).

Statistical Analysis

Using the ADA framework, we categorized individuals with zero to two ADA comorbidities, no dementia, no frailty, and adequate functional status as healthy. We classified individuals with three or more comorbidities, no dementia or frailty, and adequate functional status as having complex or intermediate health status. Finally, we classified individuals with dementia, frailty, or poor functional status, irrespective of the number of ADA comorbidities, as having very complex or poor health status.

We described the proportion of individuals with each individual comorbidity and the proportion within each comorbid health status category (healthy, complex/intermediate, very complex/poor) overall and by A1C category (<7%, 7 to <8%, ≥8% [<53, 53 to <64, ≥64 mmol/mol]). We used Kaplan-Meier survival methods and multivariable Cox proportional hazards regression to examine associations of health status categories overall and according to A1C category with all-cause mortality. We estimated incidence rates for mortality and total hospitalizations by health status and A1C categories. We used negative binomial regression to quantify associations with number of hospitalizations with an offset for ln(person-time). We also examined the associations of individual comorbidities with mortality and hospitalizations. Follow-up for both outcomes was available through 31 December 2018. In model 1, we adjusted for age, sex, and race-center (Minnesota Whites, Maryland Whites, North Carolina Whites, North Carolina Blacks, Mississippi Blacks). In model 2, we adjusted for model 1 covariates plus glucose-lowering medication categories (insulin/sulfonylurea, noninsulin/sulfonylurea only, none). We tested whether the associations of A1C categories with mortality and hospitalizations differed according to health status by including a cross-product term in model 2. We conducted a sensitivity analysis where we restricted our analysis to insulin or sulfonylurea users. Additionally, we examined associations of comorbid health status within the A1C categories <6% (<42 mmol/mol) and ≥9% (≥75 mmol/mol) for mortality and total hospitalizations.

RESULTS

The 1,841 older participants with diabetes were, on average, 75.4 years (SD 5.1) old; 56% were women, and 29% self-reported Black race/ethnicity. In the study population, 36% were insulin or sulfonylurea users (with or without other glucose-lowering medications); 25% used only other glucose-lowering medications, while 39% used no glucose-lowering medication.

Overall, 32% were classified as healthy, 42% had complex/intermediate health status, and 27% had very complex/poor health (Table 1). The mean A1C was 6.6% (SD 1.1%) (49 mmol/mol [12 mmol/mol]). Across all health status categories, most individuals (~70%) had an A1C <7% (<53 mmol/mol). Compared with individuals categorized as healthy, those with very complex/poor health status were older, more likely to be using glucose-lowering medications, and had longer duration of diabetes. Overall, hypertension, arthritis, and CKD were the three most common comorbidities (Table 1). Only 3.1% of participants overall had a history of severe hypoglycemia. In the very complex/poor category, 7% had a history of severe hypoglycemia (5.9% in A1C <7% [<53 mmol/mol], 5.6% in A1C 7 to <8% [53 to <64 mmol/mol], and 10.6% in A1C ≥8% [≥64 mmol/mol]).

Over a median of 6 years follow-up, 409 (22%) deaths occurred. Regardless of health status, older adults with A1C <7% were not at significantly higher risk of mortality than those with A1C ≥7% (≥53 mmol/mol) (Fig. 1). Within the very complex/poor category, individuals with high A1C (≥8% [≥64 mmol/mol]) had higher mortality risk (hazard ratio [HR] 1.76 [95% CI 1.15–2.71]) than those with A1C <7% (<53 mmol/mol) (model 1, Table 2). This pattern remained even after adjusting for glucose-lowering medication use (model 2, Table 2). Within all health status categories, there were no statistically significant differences in mortality between individuals with A1C 7 to <8% (53 to <64 mmol/mol) compared with those with A1C <7% (<53 mmol/mol) (Table 2). The association between health status and mortality did not differ by A1C category (model 2 P for interaction = 0.74). Within all A1C categories, very complex/poor health was associated with greater mortality risk compared with individuals classified as healthy (Supplementary Table 2). When we examined mortality risk for individuals with A1C <6% (<42 mmol/mol) and those with A1C ≥9% (≥75 mmol/mol), our results were similar, but CIs were wider (Supplementary Table 2).

The majority (70%) of participants were hospitalized at least once over the study period, and the median number of hospitalizations per individual was one per person (25th–75th percentile 0–3). Within the very complex/poor category, individuals with high A1C (≥8% [≥64 mmol/mol]) had more hospitalizations (incidence rate ratio [IRR] 1.41 [95% CI 1.03–1.94]) than those with A1C <7% (model 1, Table 3). After further adjustment for glucose-lowering medication use, results were attenuated for the very complex/poor category (IRR 1.38 [0.99–1.91]) (Table 3). In the complex/intermediate category, individuals with an A1C 7 to <8% (53 to <64 mmol/mol) and ≥8% (≥64 mmol/mol) had more hospitalizations compared with those with an A1C <7% (<53 mmol/mol); the association for A1C 7 to <8% (53 to <64 mmol/mol) was attenuated with further adjustment for glucose-lowering medication use (Table 3). There were no statistically significant differences in total number of hospitalizations by A1C categories among those classified as healthy (Table 3). Total number of hospitalizations did not differ according to health status and A1C categories (model 2 P for interaction = 0.21). Regardless of A1C, very complex/poor health was associated with a higher incidence rate of total hospitalizations (Supplementary Table 2). This pattern was similar when we stratified A1C categories further to examine incidence of total hospitalizations for individuals with A1C <6% (<42 mmol/mol) and for individuals with A1C ≥9% (≥75 mmol/mol) (Supplementary Table 2).

Insulin or sulfonylurea use was more common among individuals with greater health status complexity (Supplementary Table 3). Insulin or sulfonylurea use was lower in the subset with an A1C <7% (<53 mmol/mol) than the overall population (insulin or sulfonylurea use in the very complex/poor category: 43% overall vs. 29% subset with A1C <7% [<53 mmol/mol]). Severe hypoglycemia was more common among insulin or sulfonylurea users at 6.6% (95% CI 4.9–8.8) compared with 1.1% (0.6–1.9) among individuals not taking insulin or sulfonylurea. Patterns of other glucose-lowering

Table 1—Baseline characteristics of older adults with diabetes according to health status: the ARIC study, 2011–2013

	Health status		
	Healthy	Complex/ intermediate	Very complex/ poor
n	582	766	493
Visit 5 age (years), mean (SD)	73.5 (4.2)	75.5 (4.9)	77.5 (5.5)
Women	305 (52.4)	411 (53.7)	312 (63.3)
Black	159 (27.3)	178 (23.2)	188 (38.1)
Number of medications,* mean (SD)	9.3 (4.7)	10.9 (4.9)	11.4 (5.0)
A1C			
<7%	433 (74.4)	547 (71.4)	337 (68.4)
7 to <8%	101 (17.4)	143 (18.7)	90 (18.3)
≥8%	48 (8.2)	76 (9.9)	66 (13.4)
Diabetes medication			
None	257 (44.2)	289 (37.7)	166 (33.7)
Noninsulin/sulfonylurea only	159 (27.3)	192 (25.1)	115 (23.3)
Insulin or sulfonylurea	166 (28.5)	285 (37.2)	212 (43.0)
Diabetes duration ≥10 years	196 (33.7)	341 (44.5)	284 (57.6)
Comorbidities			
Arthritis	238 (40.9)	618 (80.7)	414 (84.0)
Cancer	54 (9.3)	258 (33.7)	122 (24.7)
CKD†	124 (21.3)	534 (69.7)	354 (71.8)
Coronary heart disease	25 (4.3)	219 (28.6)	105 (21.3)
Depression	14 (2.4)	94 (12.3)	68 (13.8)
Emphysema or COPD	8 (1.4)	91 (11.9)	48 (9.7)
Heart failure	9 (1.5)	192 (25.1)	151 (30.6)
History of hospitalized fall	5 (0.9)	34 (4.4)	34 (6.9)
History of severe hypoglycemia	3 (0.5)	22 (2.9)	32 (6.5)
Hypertension	418 (71.8)	707 (92.3)	426 (86.4)
Incontinence	14 (2.4)	133 (17.4)	104 (21.1)
Stroke	9 (1.5)	40 (5.2)	49 (9.9)
Dementia‡	—	—	86 (17.4)
Frailty	—	—	191 (38.7)
Poor physical function	—	—	382 (77.5)

Data are n (%) unless otherwise indicated. *Inclusive of prescription and over-the-counter medications and dietary supplements. †CKD refers to stage 3+ (estimated glomerular filtration rate <60 mL/min/1.73 m^2) or albuminuria (albumin-to-creatinine ratio ≥30 mg/g). ‡By definition, "—" means that there are no participants in this category (i.e., dementia, frailty, or poor physical function were used to define the very complex/poor heath category).

medications (noninsulin/sulfonylureas) were similar across health categories overall and within the A1C <7% (<53 mmol/mol) subset (Supplementary Table 3). The associations across A1C and comorbid health status categories with mortality were similar (but less precise) when restricted to individuals treated with insulin/sulfonylurea (Supplementary Table 4).

Individuals with complex/intermediate (HR 2.00 [95% CI 1.48–2.70]) or very complex/poor health (4.30 [3.16–5.86]) had higher mortality risk than those classified as healthy after adjustment for age, sex, and race-center (Table 2 and Supplementary Fig. 2). Results were slightly attenuated with adjustment for glucose-lowering medication use but remained statistically significant. The individual comorbidities were generally associated with higher risk of mortality. Cancer, CKD, coronary heart disease, emphysema or COPD, heart failure, history of falls, history of hypoglycemia, dementia, frailty, and poor functional status were associated with elevated mortality risk. Arthritis, depression, hypertension, incontinence, and stroke were not significantly associated with mortality but had effect estimates consistent with the hypothesized direction of elevated mortality (Supplementary Fig. 3).

Those with complex/intermediate health (IRR 2.20 [95% CI 1.90–2.55]) or very complex/poor health (3.56 [3.01–4.21]) had higher total hospitalization rates than those classified as healthy with adjustment for age, sex, and race-center (Table 3). All the individual comorbidities were associated with a greater number of hospitalizations (Supplementary Fig. 4).

CONCLUSIONS

In this community-based population of adults aged 66–90 years with diabetes, individuals meeting more stringent A1C goals (<7% [<53 mmol/mol]) did not have higher 6-year risk of mortality or hospitalizations compared with individuals with elevated A1C in any of the health status categories. This pattern was consistent after adjustment for glucose-lowering medication use. There were substantial differences in mortality on the basis of the ADA health status categories; however, some of the individual components, such as arthritis, depression, hypertension, and incontinence, were not associated with mortality. All the individual comorbidities were associated with a greater number of hospitalizations. Our results suggest that certain patients may safely achieve lower A1C goals in older age, even in the presence of comorbidities, and suggest opportunities to improve ADA health status categorization.

There is controversy regarding the potential for "overtreatment" of older adults with diabetes; prior studies have raised concerns that overtreatment is common and may be doing harm (18–25). The term overtreatment implies that 1) the anticipated harms of glycemic control—typically hypoglycemia—exceed the benefits of glucose-lowering therapy (3) and 2) individuals with presumed limited life expectancy may not live to experience benefits of tighter glycemic management (26,27). Yet, a clear definition of what actually constitutes overtreatment is lacking. Objective measures for clinicians to operationalize the proposed ADA health status framework are also needed; it is unclear which comorbid conditions to consider in this approach (28). Confusion also arises from lack of adequate representation of older adults in clinical trials to inform guidelines on diabetes management (29). Our findings help to inform guidelines and suggest that certain components of the health status framework (e.g., dementia, functional status, frailty) may be of greater

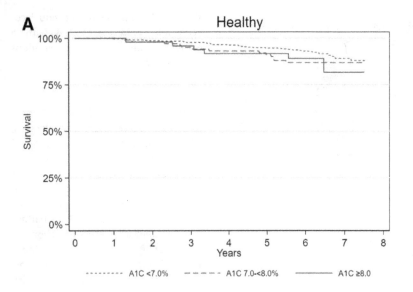

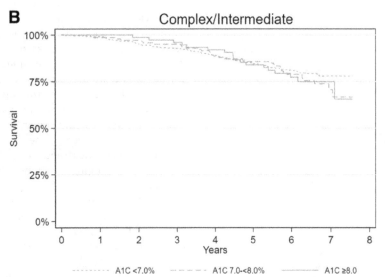

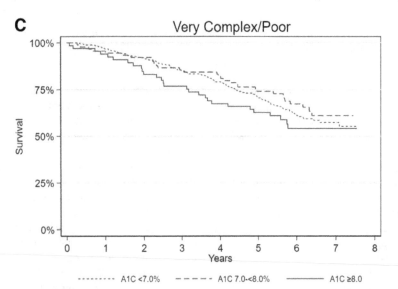

Figure 1—Kaplan-Meier curves of mortality in older adults with diabetes according to health status and A1C categories: the ARIC study, 2011–2018. *A*: Healthy. *B*: Complex/intermediate. *C*: Very complex/poor.

importance for the individualization of A1C goals. The presence of other comorbidities, such as arthritis or hypertension, should not carry as much influence for treatment decisions to relax A1C goals. Our findings highlight the need for research to inform evidence-based medicine for the management of diabetes in older adults.

Spotlighting the controversy regarding the benefits and risks of treatment intensification in older adults, the data safety and monitoring board for the Action to Control Cardiovascular Risk in Diabetes (ACCORD) trial recommended in 2003 (the trial was published in 2008 [30]) that recruitment of adults aged ≥80 years be stopped because of the greater number of participants experiencing severe hypoglycemia within the intensive control arm (31). However, in post hoc analyses, the risk of hypoglycemia in the intensive treatment arm was concentrated among participants who had high A1C but were not achieving the A1C goals (32–34). This finding is further supported by studies that have demonstrated that the highest rates of hypoglycemia are among those with poorly controlled diabetes (10,35). Longer diabetes duration in older age, which is correlated with poorer glycemic control, is also associated with greater risk for hypoglycemia (10,36) and mortality (37–39).

Older adults are particularly susceptible to hypoglycemia partly because of the higher prevalence of CKD (reducing clearance of glucose-lowering medications), cognitive impairment, depression (which can adversely affect diabetes self-care habits), and polypharmacy (40). Polypharmacy has a potential to increase risk of hypoglycemia and other adverse outcomes as a result of drug-drug interactions (3,41). Insulin and sulfonylureas are among the leading medications associated with hospitalizations in those aged >65 years (42). Therapy simplification may be appropriate if the insulin regimen is complex and hypoglycemia occurs (or recurs) (1). Shared decision making is an important tool for clinicians to decide with the patient whether to maintain, deintensify, or intensify glycemic goals (43).

Several observational studies have reported a high prevalence of potential overtreatment of older adults with diabetes (18–25). In a cross-sectional

Table 2—Mortality in older adults with diabetes according to comorbid health status overall and by A1C categories: the ARIC study, 2011–2018

	n	5-year cumulative mortality, % (95% CI)	Mortality rate per 1,000 person-years (95% CI)	HR (95% CI)† Model 1	HR (95% CI)† Model 2
Health status category*					
Healthy	582	6.3 (4.6–8.6)	16.2 (12.0–20.3)	1 (Ref)	1 (Ref)
Complex/intermediate	766	15.1 (12.8–17.9)	36.4 (30.8–42.0)	2.00 (1.48–2.70)	1.96 (1.45–2.66)
Very complex/poor	493	30.0 (26.1–34.3)	75.5 (64.7–86.2)	4.30 (3.16–5.86)	4.22 (3.10–5.76)
Health status and A1C categories					
Healthy					
A1C <7%	433	5.4 (3.6–8.0)	14.4 (9.9–18.9)	1 (Ref)	1 (Ref)
A1C 7 to <8%	101	9.1 (4.9–16.8)	21.5 (9.8–33.2)	1.32 (0.70–2.48)	1.24 (0.62–2.44)
A1C ≥8%	48	8.5 (3.3–21.1)	21.5 (4.3–38.7)	1.80 (0.74–4.39)	1.65 (0.64–4.26)
Complex/intermediate					
A1C <7%	547	15.2 (12.4–18.5)	34.5 (28.1–41.0)	1 (Ref)	1 (Ref)
A1C 7 to <8%	143	14.4 (9.5–21.4)	41.1 (27.3–55.0)	1.24 (0.84–1.82)	1.11 (0.73–1.71)
A1C ≥8%	76	16.2 (9.6–26.8)	41.3 (22.2–60.4)	1.35 (0.81–2.23)	1.18 (0.69–2.02)
Very complex/poor					
A1C <7%	337	29.5 (24.9–34.7)	75.1 (62.2–88.1)	1 (Ref)	1 (Ref)
A1C 7 to <8%	90	26.1 (18.2–36.7)	65.7 (42.6–88.9)	1.00 (0.67–1.48)	1.00 (0.66–1.52)
A1C ≥8%	66	37.8 (27.2–50.9)	92.4 (58.2–126.7)	1.76 (1.15–2.71)	1.73 (1.10–2.73)

Ref, reference. *Healthy: fewer than three ADA comorbidities, no dementia, no frailty, adequate physical function; complex/intermediate: three or more ADA comorbidities, no dementia, no frailty, adequate physical function; and very complex/poor: dementia or frailty or poor physical function. ADA comorbidities are arthritis, cancer, congestive heart failure, depression, emphysema, falls, hypertension, incontinence, CKD, myocardial infarction, and stroke. †Model 1: age, sex, race-center. Model 2: model 1 + glucose-lowering medication use (insulin/sulfonylurea, noninsulin/sulfonylurea only, none).

analysis of data from the 2001–2010 National Health and Nutrition Examination Survey (NHANES) cycles, 62% of older adults with diabetes had an A1C <7% (<53 mmol/mol) (18). Of the individuals with A1C <7% (<53 mmol/mol), 60% of those with poor/very complex health were being treated with insulin or sulfonylureas. This and several other observational studies have postulated that many older adults may be experiencing more harm (i.e., hypoglycemia) than benefit from intensive glycemic control (18–25). Unlike for randomized clinical trials, participants with diabetes in observational studies with well-controlled A1C (i.e., <7% [<53 mmol/mol]) will reflect a mix of intensively treated individuals on multiple medications and those who have "mild"

Table 3—Comorbidity categories with total count of hospitalizations overall and by A1C categories: the ARIC study, 2011–2018

	n	Total hospitalizations	Person-years	Incidence rate per 1,000 person-years	IRR (95% CI)† Model 1	IRR (95% CI)† Model 2
Health status category*						
Healthy	582	732	3,587	204.1	1 (Ref)	1 (Ref)
Complex/intermediate	766	1,859	4,473	415.6	2.20 (1.90–2.55)	2.12 (1.83–2.46)
Very complex/poor	493	1,539	2,477	621.3	3.56 (3.01–4.21)	3.41 (2.88–4.03)
Health status and A1C categories						
Healthy						
A1C <7%	433	546	2,704	201.9	1 (Ref)	1 (Ref)
A1C 7 to <8%	101	121	604	200.3	0.99 (0.71–1.39)	1.01 (0.71–1.44)
A1C ≥8%	48	65	279	233.0	1.16 (0.74–1.83)	1.17 (0.72–1.91)
Complex/intermediate						
A1C <7%	547	1,177	3,212	366.4	1 (Ref)	1 (Ref)
A1C 7 to <8%	143	393	826	475.8	1.32 (1.05–1.66)	1.24 (0.97–1.59)
A1C ≥8%	76	289	435	664.4	1.82 (1.36–2.44)	1.64 (1.21–2.24)
Very complex/poor						
A1C <7%	337	1,019	1,708	596.6	1 (Ref)	1 (Ref)
A1C 7 to <8%	90	276	469	588.5	0.98 (0.74–1.30)	0.94 (0.71–1.26)
A1C ≥8%	66	244	301	810.6	1.41 (1.03–1.94)	1.38 (0.99–1.91)

Ref, reference. *Healthy: fewer than three ADA comorbidities, no dementia, no frailty, adequate physical function; complex/intermediate: three or more ADA comorbidities, no dementia, no frailty, adequate physical function; very complex/poor: dementia or frailty or poor physical function. ADA comorbidities are arthritis, cancer, congestive heart failure, depression, emphysema, falls, hypertension, incontinence, CKD, myocardial infarction, stroke. †Model 1: age, sex, race-center. Model 2: model 1 + glucose-lowering medication use (insulin/sulfonylurea, noninsulin/sulfonylurea only, none).

disease and are on few medications. In an observational setting, the pathways by which patients achieve a well-controlled A1C will be diverse and typically unknown but would reflect real-world diabetes management practices. Indeed, older participants in our study with A1C <7% (<53 mmol/mol) were more likely to have a shorter duration of diabetes and to be taking fewer medications (any medications or for diabetes). It is not possible to know whether an older patient with diabetes with an achieved A1C <7% (<53 mmol/mol) is being overtreated per se.

Our study is not without limitations. First, the sample sizes were small in some subgroups, including in the A1C ≥8% (≥64 mmol/mol) group. However, we observed statistically significant higher risks of mortality and hospitalizations at higher A1C levels across all health status categories. Second, our analyses of combined comorbidities assume that each comorbidity had equal importance; this is unlikely to be the case. Nonetheless, our approach is consistent with how comorbidities are considered in the ADA guidelines. Third, we relied on hospital discharge codes and claims data to classify some comorbidities, which may have resulted in misclassification. For example, our definition of severe hypoglycemia (on the basis of hospitalization codes or claims) is a highly specific end point but likely underascertained (10,11). Finally, diabetes was defined on the basis of self-reported physician diagnosis or glucose-lowering medication use. This definition has been shown to be highly specific (44). Strengths of this analysis include the rigorous ascertainment of a wide array of comorbidities, information on diabetes duration, and standardized measurements conducted by trained personnel.

In summary, we found that among older adults with diabetes, there were substantial differences in mortality and hospitalizations on the basis of the ADA health status categories, but individuals meeting more stringent A1C goals (<7% [<53 mmol/mol]) were not at elevated risk, regardless of health status. Hospitalization and mortality risk were highest among individuals with high A1C (≥8% [≥64 mmol/mol]) across all

health status categories. Our results support the 2021 ADA Standards of Care and suggest that A1C <7% (<53 mmol/mol) is a reasonable treatment goal in some older adults with diabetes.

Acknowledgments. The authors thank the staff and participants of the ARIC study for their important contributions.
Funding. The ARIC study has been funded in whole or in part by federal funds from the National Heart, Lung, and Blood Institute, National Institutes of Health, Department of Health and Human Services, under contract numbers HHSN268201700001I, HHSN268201700002I, HHSN268201700003I, HHSN268201700005I, and HHSN268201700004I. Research reported in this publication was supported by National Heart, Lung, and Blood Institute grants T32-HL-007024 (M.R.R.) and K24-HL-152440 (E.S.) and National Institute of Diabetes and Digestive and Kidney Diseases grant R01-DK-089174 (E.S.).

The funding source had no role in the design or conduct of the study; collection, analysis, or interpretation of the data; or writing of the report.
Duality of Interest. No potential conflicts of interest relevant to this article were reported.
Author Contributions. M.R.R. conducted the analyses. M.R.R., O.T., J.B.E.T., P.L.L., M.E.G., B.G.W., and E.S. provided data interpretation and meaningful contributions to the revision of the manuscript. M.R.R., O.T., and E.S. designed the study. M.R.R. and E.S. drafted the manuscript. M.R.R. is the guarantor of this work and, as such, had full access to all the data in the study and takes responsibility for the integrity of the data and the accuracy of the data analysis.
Prior Presentation. Parts of this study were presented in abstract form at the 80th Scientific Sessions of the American Diabetes Association, 12–16 June 2020.

References

1. American Diabetes Association. 12. Older adults: *Standards of Care in Diabetes—2021.* Diabetes Care 2021;44(Suppl. 1):S168–S179
2. Kirkman MS, Briscoe VJ, Clark N, et al. Diabetes in older adults. Diabetes Care 2012;35:2650–2664
3. Schernthaner G, Schernthaner-Reiter MH. Diabetes in the older patient: heterogeneity requires individualisation of therapeutic strategies. Diabetologia 2018;61:1503–1516
4. Gagne JJ, Glynn RJ, Avorn J, Levin R, Schneeweiss S. A combined comorbidity score predicted mortality in elderly patients better than existing scores. J Clin Epidemiol 2011;64:749–759
5. The ARIC Investigators. The Atherosclerosis Risk in Communities (ARIC) study: design and objectives. Am J Epidemiol 1989;129:687–702
6. Rosamond WD, Chambless LE, Heiss G, et al. Twenty-two-year trends in incidence of myocardial infarction, coronary heart disease mortality, and case fatality in 4 US communities, 1987-2008. Circulation 2012;125:1848–1857

7. Loehr LR, Rosamond WD, Chang PP, Folsom AR, Chambless LE. Heart failure incidence and survival (from the Atherosclerosis Risk in Communities study). Am J Cardiol 2008;101:1016–1022
8. Rosamond WD, Folsom AR, Chambless LE, et al. Stroke incidence and survival among middle-aged adults: 9-year follow-up of the Atherosclerosis Risk in Communities (ARIC) cohort. Stroke 1999;30:736–743
9. Kohout FJ, Berkman LF, Evans DA, Cornoni-Huntley J. Two shorter forms of the CES-D (Center for Epidemiological Studies Depression) depression symptoms index. J Aging Health 1993;5:179–193
10. Lee AK, Lee CJ, Huang ES, Sharrett AR, Coresh J, Selvin E. Risk factors for severe hypoglycemia in Black and White adults with diabetes: the Atherosclerosis Risk in Communities (ARIC) study. Diabetes Care 2017;40:1661–1667
11. Ginde AA, Blanc PG, Lieberman RM, Camargo CA Jr. Validation of ICD-9-CM coding algorithm for improved identification of hypoglycemia visits. BMC Endocr Disord 2008;8:4
12. Inker LA, Schmid CH, Tighiouart H, et al.; CKD-EPI Investigators. Estimating glomerular filtration rate from serum creatinine and cystatin C. N Engl J Med 2012;367:20–29
13. Knopman DS, Gottesman RF, Sharrett AR, et al. Mild cognitive impairment and dementia prevalence: the Atherosclerosis Risk in Communities Neurocognitive Study (ARIC-NCS). Alzheimers Dement (Amst) 2016;2:1–11
14. Fried LP, Tangen CM, Walston J, et al.; Cardiovascular Health Study Collaborative Research Group. Frailty in older adults: evidence for a phenotype. J Gerontol A Biol Sci Med Sci 2001;56:M146–M156
15. Kucharska-Newton AM, Palta P, Burgard S, et al. Operationalizing frailty in the Atherosclerosis Risk in Communities study cohort. J Gerontol A Biol Sci Med Sci 2017;72:382–388
16. Windham BG, Harrison KL, Lirette ST, et al. Relationship between midlife cardiovascular health and late-life physical performance: the ARIC study. J Am Geriatr Soc 2017;65:1012–1018
17. White AD, Folsom AR, Chambless LE, et al. Community surveillance of coronary heart disease in the Atherosclerosis Risk in Communities (ARIC) study: methods and initial two years' experience. J Clin Epidemiol 1996;49:223–233
18. Lipska KJ, Ross JS, Miao Y, Shah ND, Lee SJ, Steinman MA. Potential overtreatment of diabetes mellitus in older adults with tight glycemic control. JAMA Intern Med 2015;175:356–362
19. Tseng CL, Soroka O, Maney M, Aron DC, Pogach LM. Assessing potential glycemic overtreatment in persons at hypoglycemic risk. JAMA Intern Med 2014;174:259–268
20. Arnold SV, Lipska KJ, Wang J, Seman L, Mehta SN, Kosiborod M. Use of intensive glycemic management in older adults with diabetes mellitus. J Am Geriatr Soc 2018;66:1190–1194
21. McCoy RG, Lipska KJ, Yao X, Ross JS, Montori VM, Shah ND. Intensive treatment and severe hypoglycemia among adults with type 2 diabetes. JAMA Intern Med 2016;176:969–978
22. Weiner JZ, Gopalan A, Mishra P, et al. Use and discontinuation of insulin treatment among

adults aged 75 to 79 years with type 2 diabetes. JAMA Intern Med 2019;179:1633–1641

23. Wojszel ZB, Kasiukiewicz A. A retrospective time trend study of diabetes overtreatment in geriatric patients. Diabetes Metab Syndr Obes 2019;12:2023–2032

24. Thorpe CT, Gellad WF, Good CB, et al. Tight glycemic control and use of hypoglycemic medications in older veterans with type 2 diabetes and comorbid dementia. Diabetes Care 2015;38:588–595

25. McCoy RG, Lipska KJ, Van Houten HK, Shah ND. Paradox of glycemic management: multi-morbidity, glycemic control, and high-risk medication use among adults with diabetes. BMJ Open Diabetes Res Care 2020;8:e001007

26. UK Prospective Diabetes Study (UKPDS) Group. Intensive blood-glucose control with sulphonylureas or insulin compared with conventional treatment and risk of complications in patients with type 2 diabetes (UKPDS 33). Lancet 1998;352:837–853

27. Holmes HM, Hayley DC, Alexander GC, Sachs GA. Reconsidering medication appropriateness for patients late in life. Arch Intern Med 2006;166:605–609

28. Tang O, Daya N, Matsushita K, et al. Performance of high-sensitivity cardiac troponin assays to reflect comorbidity burden and improve mortality risk stratification in older adults with diabetes. Diabetes Care 2020;43:1200–1208

29. Cruz-Jentoft AJ, Carpena-Ruiz M, Montero-Errasquín B, Sánchez-Castellano C, Sánchez-García E. Exclusion of older adults from ongoing clinical trials about type 2 diabetes mellitus. J Am Geriatr Soc 2013;61:734–738

30. Gerstein HC, Miller ME, Byington RP, et al.; Action to Control Cardiovascular Risk in Diabetes Study Group. Effects of intensive glucose lowering in type 2 diabetes. N Engl J Med 2008;358:2545–2559

31. Miller ME, Williamson JD, Gerstein HC, et al.; ACCORD Investigators. Effects of randomization to intensive glucose control on adverse events, cardiovascular disease, and mortality in older versus younger adults in the ACCORD Trial. Diabetes Care 2014;37:634–643

32. Zoungas S, Patel A, Chalmers J, et al.; ADVANCE Collaborative Group. Severe hypo-glycemia and risks of vascular events and death. N Engl J Med 2010;363:1410–1418

33. Miller ME, Bonds DE, Gerstein HC, et al.; ACCORD Investigators. The effects of baseline characteristics, glycaemia treatment approach, and glycated haemoglobin concentration on the risk of severe hypoglycaemia: post hoc epidemiological analysis of the ACCORD study. BMJ 2010;340:b5444

34. ORIGIN Trial Investigators. Predictors of nonsevere and severe hypoglycemia during glucose-lowering treatment with insulin glargine or standard drugs in the ORIGIN trial. Diabetes Care 2015;38:22–28

35. Lipska KJ, Warton EM, Huang ES, et al. HbA$_{1c}$ and risk of severe hypoglycemia in type 2 diabetes: the Diabetes and Aging Study. Diabetes Care 2013;36:3535–3542

36. Donnelly LA, Morris AD, Frier BM, et al.; DARTS/MEMO Collaboration. Frequency and predictors of hypoglycaemia in type 1 and insulin-treated type 2 diabetes: a population-based study. Diabet Med 2005;22:749–755

37. Ghouse J, Isaksen JL, Skov MW, et al. Effect of diabetes duration on the relationship between glycaemic control and risk of death in older adults with type 2 diabetes. Diabetes Obes Metab 2020;22:231–242

38. Tang O, Matsushita K, Coresh J, et al. Mortality implications of prediabetes and diabetes in older adults. Diabetes Care 2020;43:382–388

39. Huang ES, Laiteerapong N, Liu JY, John PM, Moffet HH, Karter AJ. Rates of complications and mortality in older patients with diabetes mellitus: the Diabetes and Aging Study. JAMA Intern Med 2014;174:251–258

40. Alagiakrishnan K, Mereu L. Approach to managing hypoglycemia in elderly patients with diabetes. Postgrad Med 2010;122:129–137

41. Lipska KJ, Krumholz H, Soones T, Lee SJ. Polypharmacy in the aging patient: a review of glycemic control in older adults with type 2 diabetes. JAMA 2016;315:1034–1045

42. Budnitz DS, Lovegrove MC, Shehab N, Richards CL. Emergency hospitalizations for adverse drug events in older Americans. N Engl J Med 2011;365:2002–2012

43. Rodriguez-Gutierrez R, Gionfriddo MR, Ospina NS, et al. Shared decision making in endocrinology: present and future directions. Lancet Diabetes Endocrinol 2016;4:706–716

44. Schneider AL, Pankow JS, Heiss G, Selvin E. Validity and reliability of self-reported diabetes in the Atherosclerosis Risk in Communities study. Am J Epidemiol 2012;176:738–743

Increased Hemoglobin A_{1c} Time in Range Reduces Adverse Health Outcomes in Older Adults With Diabetes

Julia C. Prentice,[1,2] David C. Mohr,[1,3] Libin Zhang,[1] Donglin Li,[1] Aaron Legler,[1] Richard E. Nelson,[4,5] and Paul R. Conlin[1,6]

Diabetes Care 2021;44:1750–1756 | https://doi.org/10.2337/dc21-0292

OBJECTIVE

Short- and long-term glycemic variability are risk factors for diabetes complications. However, there are no validated A1C target ranges or measures of A1C stability in older adults. We evaluated the association of a patient-specific A1C variability measure, A1C time in range (A1C TIR), on major adverse outcomes.

RESEARCH DESIGN AND METHODS

We conducted a retrospective observational study using administrative data from the Department of Veterans Affairs and Medicare from 2004 to 2016. Patients were ≥65 years old, had diabetes, and had at least four A1C tests during a 3-year baseline period. A1C TIR was the percentage of days during the baseline in which A1C was in an individualized target range (6.0–7.0% up to 8.0–9.0%) on the basis of clinical characteristics and predicted life expectancy. Increasing A1C TIR was divided into categories of 20% increments and linked to mortality and cardiovascular disease (CVD) (i.e., myocardial infarction, stroke).

RESULTS

The study included 402,043 veterans (mean [SD] age 76.9 [5.7] years, 98.8% male). During an average of 5.5 years of follow-up, A1C TIR had a graded relationship with mortality and CVD. Cox proportional hazards models showed that lower A1C TIR was associated with increased mortality (A1C TIR 0 to <20%: hazard ratio [HR] 1.22 [95% CI 1.20–1.25]) and CVD (A1C TIR 0 to <20%: HR 1.14 [95% CI 1.11–1.19]) compared with A1C TIR 80–100%. Competing risk models and shorter follow-up (e.g., 24 months) showed similar results.

CONCLUSIONS

In older adults with diabetes, maintaining A1C levels within individualized target ranges is associated with lower risk of mortality and CVD.

[1]VA Boston Healthcare System, Boston, MA
[2]Boston University School of Medicine, Boston, MA
[3]Boston University School of Public Health, Boston, MA
[4]VA Salt Lake City Healthcare System, Salt Lake City, UT
[5]University of Utah, Salt Lake City, UT
[6]Harvard Medical School, Boston, MA

Corresponding author: Julia C. Prentice, jprentic@bu.edu

Received 3 February 2021 and accepted 29 April 2021

This article contains supplementary material online at https://doi.org/10.2337/figshare.14515170.

Diabetes treatment often focuses on lowering A1C to prevent complications. Older patients with diabetes frequently have comorbidities and limited life expectancy, and this can affect the balance between benefits and harms of lower A1C levels. Many clinical practice guidelines (1–4) recommend higher A1C levels for older adults on the basis of patient-level factors such as life expectancy and treatment risks. However, A1C treatment goals that include only an upper limit (e.g., <8% or 64 mmol/mol) may place more weight on the risks of hyperglycemia and less on the risks of potential overtreatment, leading to a wide range of A1C levels considered acceptable.

Emerging evidence suggests that both short-term and long-term glycemic variability are linked to diabetes complications (5–16). Target ranges for day-to-day glucose measurements and thresholds for time in range (TIR) have been proposed to minimize risks of hypo- and hyperglycemia and microvascular complications (7). Many older adults with diabetes, and particularly those who are not treated with insulin, may derive limited benefits from periodic or continuous glucose monitoring (17–20), and their glucose control will be tracked by A1C levels. Long-term glycemic variability as measured by fluctuations in A1C over time also predicts diabetes complications, including micro- and macrovascular disease and mortality (8–16). Yet, there are no validated A1C target ranges that associate TIR with diabetes complications. Studies have focused on measures of A1C variability, such as SD or coefficient of variation, but have not linked A1C stability within specific ranges with adverse outcomes.

We developed a patient-level measure that captures A1C stability over time, termed A1C TIR, that is based on A1C target ranges adjusted to each patient's comorbidities, complications, and life expectancy. To demonstrate the usefulness of this measure as a predictor of adverse outcomes, we assessed the effects of A1C TIR on mortality and incident cardiovascular disease (CVD) in a large nationwide sample of Medicare-eligible veterans.

RESEARCH DESIGN AND METHODS

Study Population
The study was reviewed and approved by the institutional review board at the Department of Veterans Affairs (VA) Boston Healthcare System. We followed criteria by Miller et al. (21) to establish a diabetes diagnosis, which was based on at least one inpatient and/or two outpatient diagnosis codes and/or diabetes medications. Veterans aged ≥65 years who met these criteria were eligible for the study.

Study Timing
We used administrative and health care utilization data from VA and Medicare

from 2004 through 2016. Each patient had a 1-year clean period, a 3-year baseline period, and an outcome period that lasted until they experienced an outcome or the end of 2016, whichever came first. Since outcomes could take many years to develop, we followed patients for as many years as we had available data (through 2016).

The 1-year clean period was used to determine the presence of diabetes complications and to predict life expectancy before the baseline period. This information was used to set the individual's initial A1C target range during the baseline (see *Calculating A1C TIR* for more details).

To determine A1C TIR, we required that patients have at least four A1C tests during the 3-year baseline period, with tests no more than 1 year apart. VA performance metrics during the study period required annual A1C testing for patients with diabetes (22). Requiring four A1C tests during the 3-year baseline period identified patients who were more reliant on the VA for their health care, increasing the reliability of the A1C TIR because laboratory results were only available from VA data. Patients could enter the clean period from 2004 to 2011 and start the baseline period between 2005 and 2012, with follow-up through 2016 or when a participant experienced an outcome (Fig. 1).

The final sample size for the main analyses was 402,043 for mortality models after excluding patients with missing covariate data and those living outside the U.S. For incident myocardial infarction (MI) and stroke models, the sample size was 388,515 after excluding patients who had these diagnoses during the clean and baseline periods (Supplementary Appendix A).

Calculating A1C TIR
Patient-level A1C TIR was calculated as the percentage of days during the

3-year baseline period that a patient's A1C level was within an individualized target range. We used the VA/Department of Defense Diabetes Clinical Practice Guideline (2) to define individual A1C target ranges. This guideline proposes upper and lower bounds for A1C values and proposes different A1C target ranges on the basis of comorbidities, diabetes complications, and life expectancy.

To determine life expectancy, we predicted <5, 5–10, and ≥10 year mortality risk on the basis of 20 comorbidities or procedures, demographics, diabetes medications, biomarker and laboratory tests, and inpatient and outpatient health care utilization (23). The algorithm predicting life expectancy included several biomarkers that were recommended for annual screening (e.g., serum cholesterol, creatinine), so we used the 1-year clean period to minimize missing data on these biomarkers (24). To assess diabetes complications, we applied the Diabetes Complications Severity Index (DCSI) (25,26), with scores of 0–1, 2–3, or ≥4 considered to indicate absent/mild, moderate, or advanced diabetes complications, respectively. All predictors of life expectancy and diabetes complications were examined in the 1-year clean period to set the initial A1C target range. A1C target ranges were then updated annually to account for increasing age, new comorbidities, and development of diabetes complications.

To create the A1C TIR measure, we used linear interpolation and extrapolation between A1C levels and test dates to calculate monthly A1C values for the entire baseline period. We then computed A1C TIR as a percentage of time that A1C levels were within the target range (see Supplementary Appendix B for a detailed example). We tested A1C TIR for normality, graphically and statistically, and found that it was not normally distributed. Consequently, it was

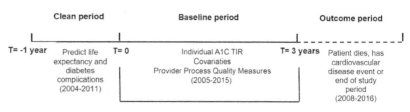

Figure 1—Study design. T, time.

divided into categories of 20% increments (i.e., 0 to <20%, 20 to <40%, 40 to <60%, 60 to <80%, 80–100%).

Covariates

Baseline covariates included demographics, measures of ability to obtain VA services, indicator variables for the calendar quarter in which a patient entered the outcome period to control for time trends, and VA medical center to control for facility variation. To examine whether A1C TIR was independent from A1C levels and other measures of glycemic variability, we included each individual's average A1C level and A1C SD throughout the baseline period. We also included the number of A1C tests during baseline since A1C TIR may be affected by the frequency of tests.

Comorbidities were taken from the Elixhauser comorbidity index (27) and were computed separately for each baseline year. Diabetes severity was based on the highest DCSI score (range 0–13) during baseline. We also modeled whether the individual was prescribed several categories of diabetes medications during baseline (e.g., insulin, metformin, sulfonylurea). Medication adherence was measured as a dichotomous indicator using the proportion of days covered by ≥80% for all prescribed diabetes medications.

Other laboratory and clinical measures included serum creatinine, albumin, urine albumin-to-creatinine ratio, BMI, blood lipids (HDL, LDL, triglycerides), and blood pressure. These measures were separated into three categories (i.e., low, normal, high) using clinical criteria, with a separate category if the measure was missing.

Clinical provider characteristics that may correlate with diabetes care were collected. These variables were computed at the clinician level for all other patients cared for by the same provider during the baseline period and included percentage of blood pressure readings >140/90 mmHg, percentage of LDL cholesterol levels >100 mg/dL, and percentage of A1C levels >9% (75 mmol/mol) (28). Also included were clinician type (physician, nurse practitioner, physician assistant, other) and whether the clinician was a primary care provider.

Outcomes

Outcomes included death and incident MI or stroke. The Medicare Vital Status

File, which determines the date of death from VA, Medicare, and Social Security Administration data, was used to determine all-cause mortality (29). We combined MI (24,30–32) and stroke (33) into a composite CVD outcome defined as the first occurrence of either event. MI included both ST elevation MI and non–ST elevation MI, and stroke included ischemic and hemorrhagic stroke.

Analyses

We estimated the effects of A1C TIR on the risks of mortality and CVD using separate Cox proportional hazards models for each outcome. Each model included patient A1C TIR as the main explanatory variable as well as all covariates. In the primary analyses, the outcome period extended through 2016 unless the individual experienced a censoring event. In the mortality model, individuals were censored upon death or at the end of 2016. In the CVD model, individuals were censored after experiencing MI or stroke, upon death, or at the end of the study period.

Several sensitivity analyses were conducted. We used separate models to predict mortality and CVD, but individuals are at risk for both outcomes at the same time, and this could lead to biased results (34–36). For the CVD outcome, we used Fine and Gray's competing risk Cox proportional hazards model using SAS 9.4 statistical software. We also tested whether results held with a shorter follow-up period limited to 24 months. Finally, we included A1C TIR as a continuous variable to test the robustness of the results. All other analyses were conducted using Stata 15 software (37).

RESULTS

Patients in the sample had a mean age 76.9 years and were predominantly White (86.3%) and male (98.8%); 26.4% had DCSI scores >5, and 24.4% were using insulin (Table 1). Fifty-two percent of the sample died, and 21% experienced a stroke or MI during an average outcome period of 5.5 years. Fifteen percent of the sample was followed for <2 years, and 47% were followed for ≥6 years.

Target A1C Levels To Determine TIR

Patients were assigned to different A1C target ranges on the basis of life

expectancy and diabetes complications, and these varied from 14% with an A1C target range of 6.0–7.0% (42–53 mmol/mol) to 17% with an A1C target range of 8.0–9.0% (64–75 mmol/mol) (Table 2).

A1C TIR and Clinical Outcomes

The average baseline A1C for the study sample was 7.0% (53 mmol/mol). Among the A1C TIR categories, mean A1C was lowest for the groups with A1C TIR 0 to <20% and 80–100%. A1C SD decreased with increasing A1C TIR (Supplementary Appendix C).

Sixty-eight percent of the sample was in the A1C TIR 0 to <20% or 20 to <40% category, with the remaining 32% having A1C TIR ≥40% during the baseline period (Table 3). There was a graded relationship between lower A1C TIR and higher mortality and CVD outcomes. In unadjusted analyses, patients with A1C TIR 0 to <20% had a 58.2% mortality rate during the outcome period compared with 31.3% with A1C TIR 80–100%. For CVD events, these clinical outcomes were 22.6% and 14.7%, respectively (data not shown).

In Cox proportional hazards models that controlled for covariates, including mean A1C level, A1C SD, and number of A1C tests, A1C TIR retained a significant relationship with mortality and CVD (Table 3). The risk of mortality increased with decreasing A1C TIR. Compared with A1C TIR 80–100%, the hazard ratio (HR) was 1.10 (95% CI 1.07–1.12) for A1C TIR 60 to <80%, 1.11 (95% CI 1.09–1.14) for A1C TIR 40 to <60%, 1.14 (95% CI 1.12–1.16) for A1C TIR 20 to <40%, and 1.22 (95% CI 1.20–1.25) for A1C TIR 0 to <20%.

Similar results emerged for the CVD outcome. Compared with A1C TIR 80–100%, the HR was 1.06 (95% CI 1.02–1.10) for A1C TIR 60 to <80%, 1.07 (95% CI 1.04–1.11) for A1C TIR 40 to <60%, 1.08 (95% CI 1.04–1.11) for A1C TIR 20 to <40%, and 1.14 (95% CI 1.11–1.19) for A1C TIR 0 to <20%.

Other covariates also had significant relationships with mortality and CVD. Older veterans, higher DCSI scores, insulin use, elevated urine albumin-to-creatinine ratio, and congestive heart failure had increased risk of both outcomes. Biguanide and thiazolidinedione use were associated with lower risk of both outcomes (Supplementary Appendix D).

Table 1—Selected descriptive demographic and comorbidity statistics at baseline (N = 402,043)

Parameter	Mean (SD) or n (%)
Demographics	
Age at the start of the outcome period (years)	
68–72	83,144 (20.7)
73–76	98,120 (24.4)
77–81	109,330 (27.2)
82–105	111,449 (27.7)
Sex	
Male	397,009 (98.8)
Female	5,034 (1.3)
Race/ethnicity	
White	346,909 (86.3)
Black	43,065 (10.7)
Hispanic	6,164 (1.5)
Asian	1,431 (0.4)
Other	4,474 (1.1)
Marital status	
Married	274,368 (68.2)
Divorced/separated	53,872 (13.4)
Widowed	54,560 (13.6)
Other	19,243 (4.8)
Years of follow-up	
Up to 2 years	58,800 (14.6)
2 to <4 years	75,091 (18.7)
4 to <6 years	75,365 (18.8)
6 to <8 years	70,310 (17.5)
≥8 years	122,477 (30.5)
Clinical characteristics	
A1C during baseline	
%	7.0 (1.0)
mmol/mol	53
A1C SD during baseline	0.56 (0.5)
Number of A1C tests	6.3 (2.4)
DCSI (highest score during the baseline period)	
0	29,173 (7.3)
1–2	103,321 (25.7)
3–5	163,691 (40.7)
6–8	87,483 (21.8)
≥9	18,375 (4.6)
Average BMI during the baseline period (kg/m^2)	
<18.5	647 (0.2)
18.5–24.9	51,442 (12.8)
25–29.9	152,662 (38.0)
30–39.9	162,025 (40.3)
≥40	17,962 (4.5)
Missing	17,305 (4.3)
Cardiovascular comorbidities	
Cardiac arrhythmias	169,215 (42.1)
Cardiovascular	277,401 (69.0)
Cerebrovascular	121,562 (30.2)
Congestive heart failure	120,914 (30.1)
Hypertension	385,495 (95.9)
Medications[a]	
Sulfonylureas	214,792 (53.4)
Biguanides	198,435 (49.4)
Insulin	98,086 (24.4)
Thiazolidinediones	63,362 (15.8)
α-Glucosidase inhibitors	7,694 (1.9)
Other medication[b]	6,569 (1.6)
Adherence	
Any diabetes medications with proportion of days covered ≥80%	228,430 (56.8)
Any diabetes medications with proportion of days covered <80%	173,613 (43.2)

A1C data are means (SD); otherwise, data are presented as n (%). [a]All medications taken by a patient; hence, the percentage represents prevalence within each medication category. [b]Other medications include amylin analog, bile acid sequestrants, dipeptidyl peptidase inhibitor, dopamine receptor agonist, glucagon-like peptide, meglitinides, and sodium–glucose cotransporter inhibitor.

Sensitivity Analyses

Sensitivity models further supported the relationship between A1C TIR and adverse outcomes (Supplementary Appendix E). In models that assessed a shorter outcome period (i.e., 24 months) lower A1C TIR was associated with a higher risk of mortality (A1C TIR 0 to <20%: HR 1.28 [95% CI 1.22–1.34]) and CVD events (A1C TIR 0 to <20%: HR 1.19 [95% CI 1.12–1.26]). Similarly, in a competing risk model that predicted CVD events with the competing risk of mortality, patients with higher A1C TIR had a lower risk of these outcomes (A1C TIR 0 to <20%: HR 1.11 [95% CI 1.08–1.14]). In models that included A1C TIR in linear form, there was a significant negative relationship between higher TIR and mortality and CVD outcomes (data not shown).

CONCLUSIONS

We show that in older adults with diabetes, maintaining stability of A1C levels within individualized target ranges over a 3-year period is associated with reduced risk of mortality and CVD outcomes. A1C TIR was based on comorbidities, complications, and life expectancy, and outcomes were measured over an average of 5.5 years and up to 9 years. The results were robust, with models that controlled for several relevant covariates, including mean A1C levels, A1C SD, and number of A1C tests.

These findings advance diabetes care in two important ways. First, A1C goal setting in older adults often balances reducing risks of acute hyperglycemia and microvascular complications with minimizing potential burdens and harms from hypoglycemia and polypharmacy. Clinical practice guidelines recognize these exigencies and propose treatment goals, often with higher A1C levels, that account for patients' unique characteristics and goals of care (1–4). However, A1C treatment goals that include only an upper limit may infer that a wide range of levels, including normal levels, may be acceptable. Our findings suggest that examining the time spent within specific A1C ranges with upper and lower bounds may have important implications. Patients with lower A1C TIR were more likely to experience mortality and CVD outcomes. Second, several studies have shown that increased short-term and long-term glycemic

Table 2—A1C target ranges for the study sample (N = 402,403)

| Life expectancy[a] | Diabetes complications | | |
	Absent or mild (DCSI = 0–1)	Moderate (DCSI = 2–3)	Advanced (DCSI ≥4)
>10 years			
A1C range, % (mmol/mol)	6.0–7.0 (42–53)	7.0–8.0 (53–64)	7.5–8.5 (58–69)
n (%)	56,124 (14.0)	73,968 (18.4)	82,764 (20.6)
5–10 years			
A1C range, % (mmol/mol)	7.0–8.0 (53–64)	7.5–8.5 (58–69)	7.5–8.5 (58–69)
n (%)	13,069 (3.3)	31,293 (7.8)	76,873 (19.1)
<5 years			
A1C range, % (mmol/mol)	8.0–9.0 (64–75)	8.0–9.0 (64–75)	8.0–9.0 (64–75)
n (%)	3,926 (1.0)	12,278 (3.1)	51,748 (12.9)

[a]Life expectancy was based on predicting the likelihood of mortality in <5 years, 5–10 years, and ≥10 years in the 3rd year of baseline.

variability are risk factors for diabetes complications (5,6,8–16). Measuring short-term glycemic variability requires frequent glucose testing with continuous glucose monitoring or conventional fingerstick methods. There are limited data on the benefits of daily glucose monitoring in older adults, although a recent study suggests that continuous glucose monitoring may identify patients with increased risk of all-cause and CVD mortality (18,19,38). Periodic A1C levels remain a mainstay for monitoring glucose control, and A1C TIR may be useful to risk stratify such patients.

Future studies may consider the influence of A1C TIR on other adverse events, such as hypoglycemia and microvascular complications, since increasing A1C variability is associated with each of these outcomes (39,40). One key question

is whether individuals who are consistently above their A1C target range will experience different risks for microvascular or macrovascular complications than individuals who are consistently below their A1C target range.

Strengths and Limitations

Our study has several strengths. We used a large nationwide sample of veterans with an extended follow-up period. The study design used a baseline period followed by an outcome period to minimize the possibility of reverse causation. The results were robust, and sensitivity analyses with a shorter outcome period corroborated the main results. Because it is unlikely that a randomized trial could be conducted to test the effects of A1C TIR on adverse

outcomes, observational studies are necessary to define such associations. We used data that are regularly included in electronic health records, so it is also possible to present A1C TIR as a measure of long-term glycemic stability to clinicians at the point of care.

Our study also has limitations. The study population was ≥65 years of age and predominantly male. Results may not generalize to females or younger individuals. Medicare data do not include laboratory test results, so we may be missing some A1C or other laboratory tests that were performed outside the VA. Diabetes complications tend to track with longer duration of disease, but we were unable to reliably determine duration of diabetes because this is not coded in administrative data. Our risk-adjusted A1C target ranges and

Table 3—HRs of A1C TIR predicting mortality and CVD

Cox proportional hazards model	HR	95% CI	P value
Mortality (n = 402,043)			
Individual A1C TIR (reference 80–100%, n = 36,642)			
60 to <80% (n = 41,042)	1.10	1.07–1.12	<0.001
40 to <60% (n = 51,609)	1.11	1.09–1.14	<0.001
20 to <40% (n = 76,801)	1.14	1.12–1.16	<0.001
0 to <20% (n = 195,949)	1.22	1.20–1.25	<0.001
A1C SD during baseline	1.14	1.13–1.16	<0.001
A1C average during baseline	1.04	1.03–1.05	<0.001
Myocardial infarction and stroke (n = 388,515)			
Individual A1C TIR (reference 80–100%, n = 36,309)			
60 to <80% (n = 40,181)	1.06	1.02–1.10	<0.001
40 to <60% (n = 50,015)	1.07	1.04–1.11	<0.001
20 to <40% (n = 73,980)	1.08	1.04–1.11	<0.001
0 to <20% (n = 188,030)	1.14	1.11–1.19	<0.001
A1C SD during baseline	1.03	1.01–1.05	<0.001
A1C average during baseline	1.12	1.11–1.13	<0.001

Model also includes all covariates listed in Supplementary Appendix D when predicting the outcomes.

the impact of greater A1C TIR on health outcomes derive from population data. Ultimately, risk assessments are best applied at the individual level. Treating older adults with diabetes should also consider individual circumstances beyond comorbidities and complications. Maintaining A1C stability over time may be affected by frailty or financial or social instability, and these are not always captured in coded health data.

This is an observation study. Unobserved factors, such as nutrition and self-management, may confound the apparent association among A1C TIR, mortality, and CVD outcomes, and we cannot affirm causality. While there are different clinical strategies for maintaining A1C stability, our results cannot assert that prospectively targeting A1C TIR as a treatment goal will reduce risks of adverse outcomes.

In summary, we show that in older adults with diabetes, maintaining A1C levels within specific and unique ranges over time is associated with a lower risk of mortality and CVD outcomes. These results support using both a personalized approach to A1C goal setting and A1C stability over time when treating older patients with diabetes.

Acknowledgments. The authors are indebted to Rebecca Lamkin at VA Boston Healthcare System for invaluable administrative support.
Funding. This work was supported by the U.S. Department of Veterans Affairs, Veterans Health Administration, Office of Research and Development, Health Services Research and Development (IIR 15-116), and the National Institutes of Health, National Institute of Diabetes and Digestive and Kidney Diseases (R01-DK-114098). Data were obtained with support from the VA Information Resource Center, VA/Centers for Medicare & Medicaid Services Data for Research Project (SDR 02-23).

The views expressed in this article are those of the authors and do not necessarily reflect the position or policy of the VA or the U.S. Government, Boston University, or University of Utah.
Duality of Interest. No potential conflicts of interest relevant to this article were reported.
Author Contributions. J.C.P., D.C.M., L.Z., D.L., and A.L. contributed to the statistical analyses. J.C.P., D.C.M., L.Z., D.L., A.L., R.E.N., and P.R.C. contributed to the interpretation of the data and drafting and critical revision of the manuscript. J.C.P. and P.R.C. contributed to the design of the study. L.Z., D.L., and A.L. contributed to the acquisition of data. J.C.P. is the guarantor of this work and, as such, had full access to all the data in the study and takes responsibility for the integrity of the data and the accuracy of the data analysis.

References

1. American Diabetes Association. 6. Glycemic targets. Diabetes Care 2017;40:S48–S56
2. U.S. Department of Veterans Affairs. VA/DOD Clinical Practice Guidelines: Management of Diabetes Mellitus in Primary Care. Accessed 17 April 2020. Available from https://www.healthquality.va.gov/guidelines/CD/diabetes/
3. LeRoith D, Biessels GJ, Braithwaite SS, et al. Treatment of diabetes in older adults: an Endocrine Society* clinical practice guideline. J Clin Endocrinol Metab 2019;104:1520–1574
4. Qaseem A, Wilt TJ, Kansagara D, Horwitch C, Barry MJ; Clinical Guidelines Committee of the American College of Physicians. Hemoglobin A1c targets for glycemic control with pharmacologic therapy for nonpregnant adults with type 2 diabetes mellitus: a guidance statement update from the American College of Physicians. Ann Intern Med 2018;168:569–576
5. Beck RW, Bergenstal RM, Riddlesworth TD, et al. Validation of time in range as an outcome measure for diabetes clinical trials. Diabetes Care 2019;42:400–405
6. Lu J, Ma X, Zhou J, et al. Association of time in range, as assessed by continuous glucose monitoring, with diabetic retinopathy in type 2 diabetes. Diabetes Care 2018;41:2370–2376
7. Battelino T, Danne T, Bergenstal RM, et al. Clinical targets for continuous glucose monitoring data interpretation: recommendations from the International Consensus on Time in Range. Diabetes Care 2019;42:1593–1603
8. Penno G, Solini A, Bonora E, et al.; Renal Insufficiency and Cardiovascular Events Study Group. HbA1c variability as an independent correlate of nephropathy, but not retinopathy, in patients with type 2 diabetes: the Renal Insufficiency and Cardiovascular Events (RIACE) Italian multicenter study. Diabetes Care 2013;36:2301–2310
9. Takao T, Matsuyama Y, Yanagisawa H, Kikuchi M, Kawazu S. Association between HbA1c variability and mortality in patients with type 2 diabetes. J Diabetes Complications 2014;28:494–499
10. Hirakawa Y, Arima H, Zoungas S, et al. Impact of visit-to-visit glycemic variability on the risks of macrovascular and microvascular events and all-cause mortality in type 2 diabetes: the ADVANCE trial. Diabetes Care 2014;37:2359–2365
11. Zoppini G, Verlato G, Targher G, Bonora E, Trombetta M, Muggeo M. Variability of body weight, pulse pressure and glycaemia strongly predict total mortality in elderly type 2 diabetic patients. The Verona Diabetes Study. Diabetes Metab Res Rev 2008;24:624–628
12. Prentice JC, Pizer SD, Conlin PR. Identifying the independent effect of HbA1c variability on adverse health outcomes in patients with type 2 diabetes. Diabet Med 2016;33:1640–1648
13. Forbes A, Murrells T, Mulnier H, Sinclair AJ. Mean HbA1c, HbA1c variability, and mortality in people with diabetes aged 70 years and older: a retrospective cohort study. Lancet Diabetes Endocrinol 2018;6:476–486
14. Critchley JA, Carey IM, Harris T, DeWilde S, Cook DG. Variability in glycated hemoglobin and risk of poor outcomes among people with type 2 diabetes in a large primary care cohort study. Diabetes Care 2019;42:2237–2246

15. Sheng CS, Tian J, Miao Y, et al. Prognostic significance of long-term HbA1c variability for all-cause mortality in the ACCORD trial. Diabetes Care 2020;43:1185–1190
16. Gorst C, Kwok CS, Aslam S, et al. Long-term glycemic variability and risk of adverse outcomes: a systematic review and meta-analysis. Diabetes Care 2015;38:2354–2369
17. Young LA, Buse JB, Weaver MA, et al.; Monitor Trial Group. Glucose self-monitoring in non-insulin-treated patients with type 2 diabetes in primary care settings: a randomized trial. JAMA Intern Med 2017;177:920–929
18. Malanda UL, Welschen LM, Riphagen II, Dekker JM, Nijpels G, Bot SD. Self-monitoring of blood glucose in patients with type 2 diabetes mellitus who are not using insulin. Cochrane Database Syst Rev 2012;1:CD005060
19. Vigersky RA, Fonda SJ, Chellappa M, Walker MS, Ehrhardt NM. Short- and long-term effects of real-time continuous glucose monitoring in patients with type 2 diabetes. Diabetes Care 2012;35:32–38
20. Park C, Le QA. The effectiveness of continuous glucose monitoring in patients with type 2 diabetes: a systemic review of literature and meta-analysis. Diabetes Technol Ther 2018;20:613–621
21. Miller DR, Safford MM, Pogach LM. Who has diabetes? Best estimates of diabetes prevalence in the Department of Veterans Affairs based on computerized patient data. Diabetes Care 2004;27:B10–B21
22. Kerr EA, Fleming B. Making performance indicators work: experiences of US Veterans Health Administration. BMJ 2007;335:971–973
23. Griffith KN, Prentice JC, Mohr DC, Conlin PR. Predicting 5- and 10-year mortality risk in older adults with diabetes. Diabetes Care 2020;43:1724–1731 PubMed
24. Prentice JC, Conlin PR, Gellad WF, Edelman D, Lee TA, Pizer SD. Capitalizing on prescribing pattern variation to compare medications for type 2 diabetes. Value Health 2014;17:854–862
25. Young BA, Lin E, Von Korff M, et al. Diabetes complications severity index and risk of mortality, hospitalization, and healthcare utilization. Am J Manag Care 2008;14:15–23
26. Glasheen WP, Renda A, Dong Y. Diabetes Complications Severity Index (DCSI)-update and ICD-10 translation. J Diabetes Complications 2017;31:1007–1013
27. Elixhauser A, Steiner C, Harris DR, Coffey RM. Comorbidity measures for use with administrative data. Med Care 1998;36:8–27
28. National Committee for Quality Assurance. *The State of Health Care Quality 2011: Continuous Improvement and the Expansion of Quality Measurement.* Washington, DC, National Committee for Quality Assurance, 2011
29. Arnold N, Maynard C, Hynes DM. VIReC Technical Report 2: VANDI Mortality Data Merge Project. Edward Hines, Jr. VA Hospital, Hines, IL: VA Information Resource Center, April 9, 2006.
30. Petersen LA, Wright S, Normand SL, Daley J. Positive predictive value of the diagnosis of acute myocardial infarction in an administrative database. J Gen Intern Med 1999;14:555–558
31. Kiyota Y, Schneeweiss S, Glynn RJ, Cannuscio CC, Avorn J, Solomon DH. Accuracy of Medicare claims-based diagnosis of acute myocardial infarction: estimating positive predictive value on

the basis of review of hospital records. Am Heart J 2004;148:99–104

32. Patel AB, Hude Q, Welsh RC, et al. Validity and utility of ICD-10 administrative health data for identifying ST- and non-ST-elevation myocardial infarction based on physician chart review. CMAJ Open 2015;3:E413–E418

33. Rothendler JA, Rose AJ, Reisman JI, Berlowitz DR, Kazis LE. Choices in the use of ICD-9 codes to identify stroke risk factors can affect the apparent population-level risk factor prevalence and distribution of CHADS2 scores. Am J Cardiovasc Dis 2012;2:184–191

34. Gooley TA, Leisenring W, Crowley J, Storer BE. Estimation of failure probabilities in the presence of competing risks: new representations of old estimators. Stat Med 1999;18:695–706

35. Southern DA, Faris PD, Brant R, et al.; APPROACH Investigators. Kaplan-Meier methods yielded misleading results in competing risk scenarios. J Clin Epidemiol 2006;59:1110–1114 PubMed

36. Kim HT. Cumulative incidence in competing risks data and competing risks regression analysis. Clin Cancer Res 2007;13:559–565

37. StataCorp. *Stata Statistical Software: Release 15*. College Station, TX, StataCorp LLC, 2017

38. Lu J, Wang C, Shen Y, et al. Time in range in relation to all-cause and cardiovascular mortality in patients with type 2 diabetes: a prospective cohort study. Diabetes Care 2021;44:549–555

39. Zhong VW, Juhaeri J, Cole SR, et al. HbA_{1C} variability and hypoglycemia hospitalization in adults with type 1 and type 2 diabetes: a nested case-control study. J Diabetes Complications 2018;32:203–209

40. Zhao MJY, Prentice JC, Mohr DC, Conlin PR. Association between hemoglobin A1c variability and hypoglycemia-related hospitalizations in veterans with diabetes mellitus. BMJ Open Diabetes Res Care 2021;9:e001797

Glycemic Control, Diabetic Complications, and Risk of Dementia in Patients With Diabetes: Results From a Large U.K. Cohort Study

Bang Zheng,[1] Bowen Su,[2] Geraint Price,[1] Ioanna Tzoulaki,[2] Sara Ahmadi-Abhari,[1] and Lefkos Middleton[1,3]

Diabetes Care 2021;44:1556–1563 | https://doi.org/10.2337/dc20-2850

OBJECTIVE

Type 2 diabetes is an established risk factor for dementia. However, the roles of glycemic control and diabetic complications in the development of dementia have been less well substantiated. This large-scale cohort study aims to examine associations of longitudinal HbA$_{1c}$ levels and diabetic complications with the risk of dementia incidence among patients with type 2 diabetes.

RESEARCH DESIGN AND METHODS

Data of eligible patients with diabetes, aged ≥50 years in the U.K. Clinical Practice Research Datalink from 1987 to 2018, were analyzed. Time-varying Cox regressions were used to estimate adjusted hazard ratios (HRs) and 95% CIs for dementia risk.

RESULTS

Among 457,902 patients with diabetes, 28,627 (6.3%) incident dementia cases were observed during a median of 6 years' follow-up. Patients with recorded hypoglycemic events or microvascular complications were at higher risk of dementia incidence compared with those without such complications (HR 1.30 [95% CI 1.22–1.39] and 1.10 [1.06–1.14], respectively). The HbA$_{1c}$ level, modeled as a time-varying exposure, was associated with increased dementia risk (HR 1.08 [95% CI 1.07–1.09] per 1% HbA$_{1c}$ increment) among 372,287 patients with diabetes with postdiagnosis HbA$_{1c}$ records. Similarly, a higher coefficient of variation of HbA$_{1c}$ during the initial 3 years of follow-up was associated with higher subsequent dementia risk (HR 1.03 [95% CI 1.01–1.04] per 1-SD increment).

CONCLUSIONS

Higher or unstable HbA$_{1c}$ levels and the presence of diabetic complications in patients with type 2 diabetes are associated with increased dementia risk. Effective management of glycemia might have a significant role in maintaining cognitive health among older adults with diabetes.

[1]Ageing Epidemiology Research Unit, School of Public Health, Imperial College London, London, U.K.
[2]Department of Epidemiology and Biostatistics, School of Public Health, Imperial College London, London, U.K.
[3]Public Health Directorate, Imperial College Healthcare NHS Trust, London, U.K.

Corresponding author: Lefkos Middleton, l.middleton@imperial.ac.uk

Received 21 November 2020 and accepted 23 April 2021

This article contains supplementary material online at https://doi.org/10.2337/figshare.14484852.

The number of older adults living with Alzheimer disease (AD) and other forms of late-onset dementia (LOD) is increasing exponentially, in parallel with increases in life expectancy and population ageing, across the globe (1,2). Type

2 diabetes is another highly prevalent chronic disease in late life and is a well-established risk factor for dementia (3). Three meta-analyses of previous cohort studies showed a 53–73% higher risk of LOD or AD in patients with diabetes compared with subjects without diabetes (4–6). Furthermore, several reports have linked type 2 diabetes with the presence of specific AD biomarkers, such as cerebrospinal fluid phosphorylated tau and total tau (7), reduced brain volume, and fluorodeoxyglucose uptake (7,8).

Most previous epidemiological studies mainly focused on defining the increased risk of dementia associated with diagnosis or presence of diabetes. However, the biological mechanisms underlying this relationship and the role of glycemic control and diabetic complications in dementia development are less well understood (9,10). Reports on plasma glucose or glycosylated hemoglobin A_{1c} (HbA_{1c}) levels and cognitive outcomes had contradictory results (11–14), probably limited by relatively small sample sizes, variable length of follow-up, or reverse causality bias. Of note, HbA_{1c} variability, an important indicator of long-term control of diabetes, has recently been found to be positively associated with micro- and macrovascular complications and mortality in patients with diabetes, independently of HbA_{1c} levels (15). The effect of HbA_{1c} variability on dementia risk is less clear.

With regard to diabetic complications, extensive evidence suggests that hypoglycemia, a common acute complication of diabetes treatment, is associated with adverse cognitive outcomes among older adults (16–18). In contrast, other prevalent diabetic complications resulting from microvascular lesions, such as diabetic retinopathy, nephropathy, and neuropathy, have drawn less attention with respect to dementia risk.

Our study aims to comprehensively evaluate the associations of longitudinal HbA_{1c} levels and their long-term variability, as well as of diabetic complications, with dementia incidence in a large cohort of older patients with type 2 diabetes, leveraging electronic health record (EHR) data from the U.K. Clinical Practice Research Datalink (CPRD) (19).

RESEARCH DESIGN AND METHODS

Data Sources

The U.K. CPRD GOLD database is a primary care database that includes ongoing longitudinal collection of fully coded EHRs of >17 million individuals who are (or were) registered with >700 participating general practitioner (GP) practices in the U.K. (19). The available data include symptomatology, clinical diagnosis, results of investigations, prescriptions, secondary care referrals, and vaccinations. CPRD was linked to secondary care data, such as the Hospital Episode Statistics (HES), mortality data from the Office for National Statistics (ONS), and regional data on measures of social deprivation. The demographic profiles of the patient population in CPRD are similar to those of the general population of the U.K. (19).

Study Population

Individual-level data between 1987 and 2018 were extracted for this study. Patients were included if they were aged ≥50 years at any point during their CPRD registration period and had a diagnosis of diabetes, based on relevant CPRD Medcode or a prescription of antidiabetes drugs (oral hypoglycemic agents or insulin) (Supplementary Table 1). In addition, eligible participants were required to have been registered in CPRD for at least 1 year prior to diabetes onset to ensure that the date of newly diagnosed diabetes was captured and to allow time for baseline information to be recorded. Patients with a diagnosis of type 1 diabetes or those who had a diagnosis of diabetes or initiation of treatment prior to 30 years of age were excluded. Patients were also excluded if they had a diagnosis of dementia before cohort entry. To account for reverse causality bias (i.e., that prodromal cognitive/functional impairment prior to dementia diagnosis could result in poorer management of diabetes), those who developed dementia or died during the first 2 years after cohort entry or the onset of diabetic complication were excluded from the analyses of diabetic complications and dementia risk; those who developed dementia or died during the first 2 years following the first post–diabetes diagnosis HbA_{1c} record after 50 years of age were excluded from the analyses of HbA_{1c} levels and dementia risk.

A total of 457,902 individuals fulfilled the inclusion and exclusion criteria and were included in the analysis on diabetic complications and dementia risk. Among these participants, 372,287 individuals had at least one HbA_{1c} record at ≥50 years of age and post–diabetes diagnosis and were included in the analysis of longitudinal HbA_{1c} levels and dementia risk.

Exposure Assessment

Episode of hypoglycemia, microvascular diabetic complications such as nephropathy, retinopathy, and neuropathy (including diabetic foot), and other complication events (such as coma, ulcer, and unspecified records of diabetic complications) were extracted using the corresponding CPRD Medcode (Supplementary Table 2). To comprehensively identify hypoglycemia episodes, we used codes of severe hypoglycemia, hospital-treated hypoglycemia, hypoglycemia without coma, and unspecified hypoglycemia (17). The date of onset of a specific type of complication was defined according to its first relevant health record. The date of onset of overall microvascular complications was defined as the earliest date of developing nephropathy, retinopathy, or neuropathy.

Longitudinal HbA_{1c} concentrations were recorded as test results and extracted using CPRD Medcode and Enttype code (Supplementary Table 3). The HbA_{1c} value, measured as a continuous variable, was also stratified into different clinically established categories (<6%, 6–7%, 7–8%, 8–9%, 9–10%, and ≥10%). For patients with at least three HbA_{1c} records during the first 3 years of follow-up, mean and coefficient of variation (CV; the ratio of the SD to the mean) of the 3-year HbA_{1c} measurements were estimated and assessed as additional exposure variables, reflecting the average level and variability of long-term HbA_{1c} concentrations.

In addition, information on the following covariates was extracted: age at cohort entry, sex, calendar year of cohort entry, region in U.K., index of multiple deprivation (IMD; a proxy of socioeconomic status linked to CPRD), BMI (latest record up to 10 years before cohort entry to reduce missing values), smoking status (latest record up to 5 years before cohort entry), duration of diabetes at cohort entry (based on the first clinical record of diabetes diagnosis), history of antidiabetes treatment, and history of major comorbidities, including chronic heart disease, stroke, hypertension, chronic kidney disease, chronic obstructive pulmonary disease, and cancer.

Outcome Ascertainment

The outcome event was dementia incidence. We did not distinguish by specific LOD type, as such granular level of data are variably registered in CPRD, and the precision of health data recording varies over time. Moreover, it is acknowledged that most cases of LOD involve mixed brain pathologies (20,21). Patients were considered to have dementia if they: *1*) had a dementia diagnosis based on Medcode in CPRD; *2*) had a dementia diagnosis based on ICD codes in linked HES or ONS databases; or *3*) had at least one dementia-specific drug prescription (donepezil, galantamine, rivastigmine, or memantine [22]) (Supplementary Table 4). Patients with dementia with diagnoses of unrelated etiologies, such as following HIV infection, Creutzfeldt-Jakob disease, or alcohol- and drug-induced, were excluded. Among the extracted subjects with dementia, 96% were based on diagnosis code, and 4% were based on dementia-specific drug prescription. The outcome event date was defined as the first dementia diagnosis date or the first prescription date of dementia-specific drugs, whichever occurred earlier.

Statistical Analysis

Distributions of baseline characteristics were summarized and compared between subcohort patients with baseline HbA_{1c} levels <7% (53 mmol/mol) and ≥7%. Time-varying Cox proportional hazards models, with age as the underlying time-scale, were used to estimate hazard ratios (HRs) and 95% CIs of dementia associated with diabetic complications or longitudinal HbA_{1c} levels in separate analyses. Exposures were treated as time-varying variables.

In analyses of diabetic complications, the presence of hypoglycemic episodes and microvascular complications in aggregate and by type (nephropathy, retinopathy, and neuropathy) in association

with dementia incidence were examined in separate Cox models. Patients who developed a relevant diabetic complication during follow-up contributed person-years to the no-complication group up until the complication diagnosis date and then contributed person-years to the complication group. Time of cohort entry for each patient was defined as date of diabetes onset, aged 50 or 1 January 1987, whichever was the latest. The end of follow-up was defined as date of dementia incidence, death, transfer-out date, last data collection date of GP practice, or 1 May 2018, whichever occurred first. The patient-level transfer-out date recorded in CPRD refers to the date the patient transferred out of the practice. The practice-level last data collection date refers to the date of the latest data upload from each GP practice (19). To examine independent effects of different types of microvascular complications, an additional analysis mutually adjusting for nephropathy, retinopathy, and neuropathy was conducted.

For the analysis of longitudinal HbA_{1c} level, given that glycemic levels change over time for each patient with diabetes, the time-varying Cox model was used to estimate the HR and 95% CI of dementia incidence per 1% increment (absolute value) of HbA_{1c} among patients with at least one HbA_{1c} record post–diabetes diagnosis after 50 years of age. In a separate Cox model, time-varying HbA_{1c} category (<6%, 6–7%, 7–8%, 8–9%, 9–10%, and ≥10%) was assessed as the exposure variable to explore the potential nonlinear relationship with dementia risk, with 6–7% as reference group. The beginning of follow-up for this cohort was defined as date of the first postdiagnosis HbA_{1c} record after 50 years of age (i.e., baseline HbA_{1c}). The end of follow-up was defined as above. To account for reverse causality bias, HbA_{1c} concentrations recorded within 2 years prior to dementia incidence or death were excluded.

For the analysis of long-term average level of HbA_{1c} and its variability, the 3-year mean and CV of HbA_{1c} were simultaneously entered into a conventional Cox model to estimate their independent associations with dementia incidence. Follow-up time for this analysis was calculated from 3 years after the baseline HbA_{1c} record (to avoid

concurrent bias), until the date of dementia incidence or censoring time. Patients who developed dementia or died during the first 2 years of follow-up were excluded. In addition, mean and CV of HbA_{1c} were both modeled as categorical variables (<6%, 6–7%, 7–8%, 8–9%, 9–10%, and ≥10% for mean value; quartiles for CV) in a separate Cox model.

To account for potential confounding factors, three sequential models with increasing levels of adjustment for covariates were created for all analyses: model 1 adjusted for age, sex, calendar year, and region; model 2 further adjusted for IMD (in quintile), smoking status (nonsmoker, current smoker, ex-smoker, or missing), BMI category (<25, 25–30, and ≥30 kg/m^2 or missing), and history of comorbidities; and model 3 additionally adjusted for diabetes-related factors, including duration of diabetes, presence of diabetic complications (only for HbA_{1c} analysis), baseline HbA_{1c} level (only for diabetic complications analysis), and prescription of antidiabetes drugs (no drug, only oral hypoglycemic drug, or insulin). Covariates were also modeled as time-varying variables and updated at complication diagnosis date or each HbA_{1c} record date during follow-up. Missing values in smoking status and BMI category during follow-up were imputed with last observation carried forward.

We further repeated the main analyses in males and females separately and tested the effect modification by sex. Several sensitivity analyses were conducted to assess the robustness of our findings: *1*) restricting to participants who were at least 60 years old at cohort entry; *2*) restricting to those who were at least 80 years old at the end of follow-up to account for the competing risk of premature death, in which the estimated HR reflects relative hazard of dementia conditional on patients surviving beyond 80 years of age; *3*) restricting to participants who entered cohort after 2004, as diabetes data quality was significantly improved in CPRD following the introduction of the Quality and Outcomes Framework indicators for diabetes, and to account for the change of clinical practice and guidelines of diabetes management over time (23); *4*) not excluding HbA_{1c} recorded within 2 years prior to dementia incidence or death in the analysis of longitudinal HbA_{1c}; *5*) excluding HbA_{1c} records within 5 years prior to dementia incidence or patients who developed dementia within the first 5 years of follow-up to further reduce reverse causality; 6) excluding possible outlier values in HbA_{1c} records (<4% or >12%); 7) adjusting the 3-year CV of HbA_{1c} for the possible influence of number of HbA_{1c} records (24) (adjusted CV = CV/[total records during 3-year follow-up/total records during 3-year follow-up − 1]$^{1/2}$) and also stratifying the analysis by the median number of HbA_{1c} records; 8) additionally adjusting for the average number of clinical visits per year during follow-up of each patient, since patients who visited a GP more frequently may have a systematically different profile or higher diagnosis rate; 9) additionally adjusting for the identifier of GP practices to account for the practice group variability; and 10) using a more stringent dementia ascertainment criterion that requires at least two dementia diagnosis records within or between data sources or at least one dementia diagnosis record plus one dementia-specific drug prescription (25).

The statistical analyses were performed using Stata (version 15; Stata Corp.). All statistical tests were two-sided, and the significance level was defined as $P < 0.05$.

Data and Resource Availability
This study is based on data from the CPRD obtained under license from the U.K. Medicines and Healthcare Products Regulatory Agency (protocol approved by the Independent Scientific Advisory Committee, number 19_065R). According to the U.K. Data Protection Act, information governance restrictions (to protect patient confidentiality) prevent data sharing via public deposition. Data extracts can be requested by applying to the CPRD (https://www.cprd.com).

RESULTS
Baseline Characteristics of Study Population
Of the 457,902 patients with type 2 diabetes, 52.1% were male; the mean baseline age was 64.5 (SD 10.8) years (Table 1). At cohort entry, 42.3% of patients had obesity (BMI $\geq$30 kg/m^2), and 19.0% were self-reported current smokers; 17.1% had been prescribed antidiabetes drugs, and the mean

baseline HbA_{1c} level was 7.4% (57 mmol/mol) (SD 2.1%). Prior to baseline, only 1,986 (0.4%) patients had hypoglycemic events, and 8,060 (1.8%) had microvascular complications (5,928 subjects with retinopathy, 2,275 with neuropathy, and 569 with nephropathy). During follow-up, 17,524 (3.8%) patients developed hypoglycemic episodes, and 103,188 (22.5%) patients developed microvascular complications (73,615 with retinopathy, 41,920 with neuropathy, and 8,660 with nephropathy).

Among the 372,287 patients included in analyses on longitudinal HbA_{1c}, 216,600 (58.2%) had HbA_{1c} levels <7% (53 mmol/mol) at baseline (Table 1). Compared with patients with HbA_{1c} <7%, those with HbA_{1c} $\geq$7% were slightly younger, entered the cohort earlier, presented with less comorbidities, and were more likely to be male, deprived, obese, and current smokers; they also had a longer duration of diabetes and higher proportion of antidiabetes drug use and diabetic complications before baseline ($P < 0.05$). Patients with post–diabetes diagnosis HbA_{1c} record were slightly more likely to have obesity, chronic heart disease, and hypertension at baseline than those without (Supplementary Table 5).

Diabetic Complications in Association With Dementia Risk
During a median of 6 years' follow-up (ranging from 0–31 years) of the 457,902 patients with diabetes, 28,627 (6.3%) incident dementia cases were recorded. After adjusting for a full set of covariates (model 3), there was evidence for an association between hypoglycemic events and a higher risk of dementia incidence (HR 1.30 [95% CI 1.22–1.39]) (Table 2). The HR estimates were 1.50 in model 1 and 1.44 in model 2 ($P < 0.05$).

Microvascular complications were also associated with a higher risk of dementia incidence in the fully adjusted model (HR 1.10 [95% CI 1.06–1.14]) as well as in models 1 and 2 (HR 1.22 and 1.21, respectively). Neuropathy and nephropathy had relatively stronger association with dementia incidence (HR 1.25 [95% CI 1.18–1.33] and 1.23 [1.13–1.33]; model 3) than retinopathy (HR 1.07 [95% CI 1.03–1.11]; model 3). The analysis mutually adjusting for neuropathy, nephropathy, and retinopathy revealed similar results; the HRs were 1.25

(95% CI 1.18–1.33), 1.24 (95% CI 1.14–1.35), and 1.06 (95% CI 1.02–1.10), respectively.

Longitudinal HbA_{1c} Level in Association With Dementia Risk
During a median of 6 years' follow-up (ranging from 0–30 years) of the 372,287 patients with diabetes with postdiagnosis HbA_{1c} data, 23,746 (6.4%) incident dementia cases were recorded. HbA_{1c} level was significantly associated with higher risk of dementia incidence, with an HR of 1.08 (95% CI 1.07–1.09) per 1% increment of HbA_{1c} in the fully adjusted model and 1.13 or 1.14 in models 1 and 2, respectively (Table 3). In a separate analysis in which time-varying HbA_{1c} was modeled as a categorical variable with 6–7% as reference group, patients with well-controlled HbA_{1c} (<6%) had lower risk of dementia incidence (HR 0.86 [95% CI 0.83–0.89]), while those with HbA_{1c} levels of 8–9%, 9–10%, and $\geq$10% had 15% (95% CI 9–21), 26% (95% CI 17–34), and 40% (95% CI 32–49) increased risk of dementia incidence, respectively (Fig. 1).

Long-Term Mean and Variability of HbA_{1c} in Association With Subsequent Dementia Risk
Consistent with the results of time-varying HbA_{1c} analysis, the mean value of 3-year HbA_{1c} measurements was significantly associated with higher risk of subsequent dementia incidence after controlling for HbA_{1c} variability, with an HR of 1.04 (95% CI 1.02–1.06) per 1% increment of HbA_{1c} in model 3 and 1.05 in models 1 and 2 (Table 3). Compared with patients who had a mean HbA_{1c} level at 6–7%, those with mean HbA_{1c} levels of 8–9%, 9–10%, and $\geq$10% had 9% (95% CI 3–16), 18% (95% CI 8–28), and 30% (95% CI 17–44) increased risk of dementia incidence (model 3), respectively.

The 3-year CV of HbA_{1c}, which reflects the long-term glycemic variability, was also independently associated with higher risk of dementia incidence. After controlling for the 3-year mean HbA_{1c} level, the HRs were 1.03 (95% CI 1.01–1.04) per 1-SD increment of CV in model 3 and 1.02 in models 1 and 2 (Table 3). Compared with patients in the lowest quartile (Q1) of CV, the Q2, Q3, and Q4 groups had 6% (95% CI 1–11), 12% (95% CI 6–18), and 13%

Table 1—Baseline characteristics of participants in diabetes cohort and HbA$_{1c}$ subcohort

Characteristics	Full diabetes cohort	HbA$_{1c}$ subcohort	Baseline HbA$_{1c}$ level <7%	Baseline HbA$_{1c}$ level ≥7%
Number of participants	457,902	372,287	216,600	155,687
Sex (male), %	52.1	53.3	51.8	55.3
Baseline age (mean), year	64.5	65.1	66.2	63.7
Ethnicity (White), %	87.5	87.5	88.6	85.9
Year of cohort entry (median)	2007	2007	2008	2005
IMD (most deprived), %	18.8	19.0	18.3	20.0
Obesity (BMI ≥30 kg/m^2), %	42.3	45.1	42.5	48.8
Current smoker, %	19.0	17.9	16.4	20.1
CHD, %	35.1	39.4	42.8	34.6
Stroke, %	6.8	7.6	8.1	6.9
Hypertension, %	85.0	92.0	92.4	91.5
CKD, %	5.9	6.6	8.3	4.2
COPD, %	3.8	4.2	4.5	3.7
Cancer, %	9.1	9.8	11.0	8.1
Duration of diabetes (mean), year	0.6	1.5	1.3	1.9
Ever use of antidiabetes drugs, %	17.1	31.1	20.0	46.5
Baseline HbA$_{1c}$ level (mean), %	7.4	7.3	—	—
Presence of hypoglycemic events, %	0.4	0.7	0.5	1.1
Presence of microvascular complications, %	1.8	4.2	2.9	6.0

In the diabetes cohort, ethnicity, IMD, BMI, smoking status, and baseline HbA$_{1c}$ had 69.9%, 6.7%, 11.4%, 18.5%, and 34.8% missing values, respectively. The statistics for these variables presented in this table are based on complete cases. CHD, chronic heart disease; CKD, chronic kidney disease; COPD, chronic obstructive pulmonary disease.

(95% CI 6–19) of increased risk of dementia incidence, respectively (Fig. 1).

The subgroup analyses by sex (Supplementary Table 6) showed a stronger association between hypoglycemia and dementia risk in men (HR 1.39) than in women (HR 1.23; $P_{interaction}$ = 0.002). Results of all sensitivity analyses were similar to those of the main analyses (Supplementary Table 7).

CONCLUSIONS

This is the largest cohort study to comprehensively evaluate the association between longitudinal diabetes control and subsequent dementia risk among patients with type 2 diabetes. Our results strengthen the previous evidence on the association between hypoglycemic events and increased risk of dementia incidence among patients with diabetes. Moreover, the presence of microvascular complications, as well as high and unstable HbA$_{1c}$ levels during follow-up, are also found to be independent risk factors for incident dementia.

Our results on hypoglycemic complications are in line with evidence from previous cohort studies. An EHR-based cohort study of 16,667 patients with type 2 diabetes showed that those with at least one severe hypoglycemic episode had higher risk of dementia than patients without such record (16). Another cohort study, using the earlier version of the U.K. CPRD (from 2003 to 2012) with 53,055 patients with type 2 diabetes, demonstrated that hypoglycemia was associated with a higher risk of subsequent dementia incidence (17). In contrast, as patients with dementia may have reduced functional ability to

Table 2—Associations between diabetic complications and risk of dementia among 457,902 patients with diabetes

Complications	Number of patients with complications	HR (95% CI) for dementia incidence Model 1	HR (95% CI) for dementia incidence Model 2	HR (95% CI) for dementia incidence Model 3
Hypoglycemic event	19,510	1.50 (1.42–1.59)	1.44 (1.37–1.53)	1.30 (1.22–1.39)
Microvascular complications	111,248	1.22 (1.18–1.26)	1.21 (1.17–1.24)	1.10 (1.06–1.14)
Retinopathy	79,543	1.19 (1.15–1.22)	1.17 (1.14–1.21)	1.07 (1.03–1.11)
Neuropathy	44,195	1.41 (1.34–1.48)	1.36 (1.30–1.44)	1.25 (1.18–1.33)
Nephropathy	9229	1.35 (1.25–1.45)	1.31 (1.21–1.41)	1.23 (1.13–1.33)

Results are based on time-varying Cox regressions, with no-complication group as the reference group. Model 1 adjusted for age, sex, calendar year, and region; model 2 further adjusted for IMD, smoking status, BMI category, and history of comorbidities (chronic heart disease, stroke, hypertension, chronic kidney disease, chronic obstructive pulmonary disease, and cancer); and model 3 additionally adjusted for duration of diabetes, prescriptions of antidiabetes drugs and baseline HbA$_{1c}$ level. $P < 0.05$ in all of the analyses in this table.

Table 3—Associations between longitudinal HbA$_{1c}$ levels of patients with diabetes and risk of dementia

HbA$_{1c}$ measures	HR (95% CI) for dementia incidence		
	Model 1	Model 2	Model 3
Time-varying HbA$_{1c}$ (per 1%)	1.13 (1.12–1.14)	1.14 (1.13–1.15)	1.08 (1.07–1.09)
Three-year mean HbA$_{1c}$ (per 1%)	1.05 (1.04–1.07)	1.05 (1.04–1.07)	1.04 (1.02–1.06)
Three-year CV of HbA$_{1c}$ (per 1 SD)	1.02 (1.00–1.04)	1.02 (1.00–1.04)	1.03 (1.01–1.04)

Results are based on time-varying Cox regressions (for time-varying HbA$_{1c}$) or conventional Cox regressions (for 3-year measures). Model 1 adjusted for age, sex, calendar year, and region; model 2 further adjusted for IMD, smoking status, BMI category, and history of comorbidities (chronic heart disease, stroke, hypertension, chronic kidney disease, chronic obstructive pulmonary disease, and cancer); and model 3 additionally adjusted for duration of diabetes, prescriptions of antidiabetes drugs and diabetic complications. In addition, for the analysis of 3-year HbA$_{1c}$ measures, the mean level and CV were mutually adjusted for in models 1 through 3, given that a moderate correlation was detected between these two variables. $P < 0.05$ in all of the analyses in this table.

achieve proper diabetes management, established dementia may in turn lead to frequent hypoglycemic episodes or other diabetic complications. A meta-analysis (18) of nine observational studies revealed a bidirectional association between hypoglycemic episode and dementia. Therefore, we have used a 2-year lag in the main analysis and 5-year lag in the sensitivity analyses to account for reverse causality bias. It has been postulated that hypoglycemia can disrupt the cerebral glucose metabolism and thus contribute to neuropathological changes (26). Previous experimental studies have shown that severe hypoglycemia could trigger apoptosis and neuronal loss (26). In this regard, hypoglycemia may not only serve as a reflection of poor management or progression of diabetes, but may also be directly implicated in the neurodegenerative process.

In terms of the relationship between microvascular diabetic complications and dementia risk, there has been one report on a predictive risk score of 10-year dementia risk for patients with type 2 diabetes (27). Among the 45

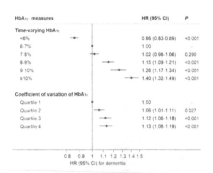

Figure 1—Associations of time-varying HbA$_{1c}$ and 3-year CV of HbA$_{1c}$ with the risk of dementia: results are based on fully adjusted time-varying Cox regression (for time-varying HbA$_{1c}$) or conventional Cox regression (for 3-year CV).

candidate predictors, the 8 strongest predictors were selected into the final prediction model, including microvascular disease (diabetic retinopathy/end-stage renal disease), diabetic foot, and acute hyper-/hypoglycemic events. Our findings further confirm the associations of overall and individual microvascular complications with risk of dementia incidence. It is likely that such complications merely represent peripheral markers of cerebral microvascular lesions (28) rather than contributing to the development of dementia through direct biological mechanisms. For instance, the retina is traditionally seen as an accessible extension of the central nervous system and may reflect possible cerebral pathology, such as cerebral small vessel disease, resulting from poor diabetes control and chronic hyperglycemia. In this context, our observed relatively weak association between retinopathy and dementia risk is intriguing. On one hand, our findings are in line with previous reports of weak direct evidence on associations between retinal microvascular changes and dementia incidence (29). For example, a report based on the Rotterdam Study found no association between retinopathy and dementia incidence (30). On the other hand, our effect estimate might have been attenuated due to underdiagnosis, as retinopathy may remain asymptomatic and undetected in the absence of routine ophthalmoscopic screening.

Our results of time-varying HbA$_{1c}$ levels and long-term average HbA$_{1c}$ levels confirm previous reports based on observational studies of much smaller sample sizes. A prospective cohort study monitored the glucose levels and dementia incidence of 2,067 older adults

for a median of 6.8 years (11). Among participants with diabetes at baseline, elevated average glucose levels were associated with a higher risk of dementia. A 9-year cohort study also demonstrated that elevated longitudinal glucose level was associated with worse cognitive performance among 717 older adults with diabetes (12). A previous cohort study in participants with and without diabetes found a J-shaped association between baseline HbA$_{1c}$ and incident dementia (31). In contrast, our results indicate a linear HbA$_{1c}$–dementia relationship among patients with diabetes, probably because we adjusted for hypoglycemic events or because the majority of patients in our sample had HbA$_{1c}$ levels >5.5% (37 mmol/mol). However, another cohort study of 2,246 older adults with type 2 diabetes showed that, for those with high or moderate HbA$_{1c}$ at baseline, a large reduction in HbA$_{1c}$ within the 1st year of follow-up was associated with higher incidence of dementia during follow-up (13). A pioneering large randomized controlled trial (32) tested the effects of intensive glycemic control treatment strategies (target HbA$_{1c}$ <6.0%) versus standard-care guidelines (HbA$_{1c}$ <7.0–7.9%) on cognitive outcomes in patients with type 2 diabetes. Although the intensive glycemic therapy group had larger total brain volume at 40 months and a slower rate of gray matter loss, no significant between-group difference in the rate of clinical cognitive decline was observed (32,33). Future adequately powered randomized controlled trials on long-term glycemic control and dementia prevention in patients with diabetes are further warranted.

Our findings also suggest that glycemic variability, an acknowledged indicator for diabetes control and predictor for mortality in older adults (15), is also independently associated with dementia risk. Currently, in the absence of an established "gold standard" measure, the CV has been recommended as a robust marker for glycemic variability (34). In accordance with our findings, a retrospective cohort study of 16,706 Chinese patients with type 2 diabetes suggested that CVs for fasting plasma glucose and HbA_{1c}, calculated during the 1st year of follow-up, were associated with increased risk of AD incidence (35). In this regard, a high and unstable glycemic level may contribute to dementia pathogenesis either through cerebrovascular lesions (28) and cerebral metabolic dysregulation (36) or as an indicator of the underlying "brain insulin resistance," shown to be associated with the AD pathological signature of brain amyloidosis, tau accumulation, and neurodegeneration (AT[N]) (10).

Studies based on EHRs are subject to potential sources of bias, which we have attempted to account for both in study design and through several sensitivity analyses. Firstly, selection bias is an acknowledged risk for studies based on real-world EHR data. In this study, this risk was mitigated by the use of a national database including data from virtually all patients registered in 8% of primary care/GP practices across the U.K. CPRD covers a wide range of urban and rural areas of diverse socioeconomic strata and has been shown to be well representative of the general population (19). Another possible limitation relates to the potential underreporting or misdiagnosis of dementia cases in EHR data sets. We maximized dementia case ascertainment by data linkage with HES and ONS databases (secondary diagnosis and cause of death). Moreover, assuming that the remaining misclassification in outcome events is independent of exposure variables, our estimates of association (i.e., HRs) are likely to have been biased toward the null rather than overestimated (37). To account for changes in dementia diagnostic criteria and the increasing diagnosis rate of dementia over time (38), we have adjusted for calendar year in all analyses and conducted a sensitivity analysis restricted to data collected after 2004, all of which produced consistent results. Future well-powered clinical studies, allowing for deep phenotyping and biomarker-based characterization of patients with dementia,

are warranted to elucidate the precise contribution of diabetes-related factors in the pathogenesis of AD and other LOD forms.

EHR-based studies are also vulnerable to information bias in exposure assessments. For example, although hospital admissions or emergency department attendances following severe hypoglycemia are typically recorded in GP practices through referral letters or hospital discharge notes, some instances may be missed. Another possible limitation is that measurement of HbA_{1c} may not be regularly conducted by GPs for each patient, which may potentially affect the calculation of the CV of HbA_{1c}. To overcome such limitations, a paradigm shift in data collection methods is warranted, as lack of real-time clinical data is a shared limitation of EHR-based and prospective cohort studies. Future real-time collection of clinical data using patient-administered portable and wearable devices and real-time reporting of adverse outcomes can improve disease management and data quality for research purposes. Furthermore, the possibility of residual confounding bias cannot be ruled out. For instance, there is little information on education level and on physical/social activities in CPRD, which are known risk factors for dementia (3,39). There were 7–19% missing values for IMD, BMI, and smoking status, but little difference was observed for effect estimates in models with and without adjustment for these covariates, suggesting that the effect of residual confounding is likely small. Finally, causality cannot be established from the results of our epidemiological analyses. Further mechanistic studies are required to elucidate the precise biological mechanisms underpinning the effect of poor diabetic control on dementia risk in older adults.

This CPRD-based study has several strengths, including the large sample size (457,902 patients with diabetes and 28,627 incident dementia cases), the long follow-up period of up to 30 years, and the broad age distribution of participants. We were also able to examine multiple indicators of diabetes control (HbA_{1c} level and its variability, hypoglycemia, and microvascular complications) in relation to dementia risk and have adjusted for a large set of potential confounding factors. In addition, we have

carefully accounted for reverse causality bias and conducted multiple sensitivity analyses to address issues such as data quality, change of clinical practice over time, and accuracy of dementia diagnosis, the results of which supported the robustness of our main findings.

In conclusion, this large-scale cohort study provides strong evidence that higher or unstable HbA_{1c} levels and the presence of diabetic complications in patients with type 2 diabetes are associated with higher dementia incidence. Given the lack of effective therapies for AD and other LOD forms and the long preclinical disease stage of progressively accumulating pathologies prior to clinical disease onset, the effective management of modifiable risk factors and conditions, such as type 2 diabetes (39,40), may have potential value in reducing the burden of cognitive and functional decline and dementia in the elderly population.

Funding. B.Z. was supported by the Imperial College London-China Scholarship Council scholarship.

Duality of Interest. No potential conflicts of interest relevant to this article were reported.

Author Contributions. B.Z. and L.M. contributed to study design. B.Z. carried out data analysis and drafted the first version of the manuscript. B.S. contributed to data analysis. B.Z., I.T., S.A.-A., and L.M. contributed to data interpretation. All authors critically reviewed and edited the manuscript. B.Z. is the guarantor of this work and, as such, had full access to all of the data in the study and takes responsibility for the integrity of the data and the accuracy of the data analysis.

Prior Presentation. Parts of this study were presented in abstract form at the 145th Annual Meeting of American Neurological Association, Virtual, on 9 October 2020.

References

1. Alzheimer's Association. 2020 Alzheimer's disease facts and figures. Alzheimers Dement 2020;16:391–460
2. Ahmadi-Abhari S, Guzman-Castillo M, Bandosz P, et al. Temporal trend in dementia incidence since 2002 and projections for prevalence in England and Wales to 2040: modelling study. BMJ 2017;358:j2856
3. Livingston G, Huntley J, Sommerlad A, et al. Dementia prevention, intervention, and care: 2020 report of the Lancet Commission. Lancet 2020;396:413–446
4. Gudala K, Bansal D, Schifano F, Bhansali A. Diabetes mellitus and risk of dementia: a meta-analysis of prospective observational studies. J Diabetes Investig 2013;4:640–650
5. Zhang J, Chen C, Hua S, et al. An updated meta-analysis of cohort studies: diabetes and risk

of Alzheimer's disease. Diabetes Res Clin Pract 2017;124:41–47

6. Chatterjee S, Peters SAE, Woodward M, et al. Type 2 diabetes as a risk factor for dementia in women compared with men: a pooled analysis of 2.3 million people comprising more than 100,000 cases of dementia. Diabetes Care 2016;39:300–307

7. Moran C, Beare R, Phan TG, Bruce DG, Callisaya ML; Alzheimer's Disease Neuroimaging Initiative (ADNI). Type 2 diabetes mellitus and biomarkers of neurodegeneration. Neurology 2015;85:1123–1130

8. Li W, Risacher SL, Huang E; Alzheimer's Disease Neuroimaging Initiative. Type 2 diabetes mellitus is associated with brain atrophy and hypometabolism in the ADNI cohort. Neurology 2016;87:595–600

9. Biessels GJ, Staekenborg S, Brunner E, Brayne C, Scheltens P. Risk of dementia in diabetes mellitus: a systematic review. Lancet Neurol 2006;5:64–74

10. Arnold SE, Arvanitakis Z, Macauley-Rambach SL, et al. Brain insulin resistance in type 2 diabetes and Alzheimer disease: concepts and conundrums. Nat Rev Neurol 2018;14:168–181

11. Crane PK, Walker R, Hubbard RA, et al. Glucose levels and risk of dementia. N Engl J Med 2013;369:540–548

12. Yaffe K, Falvey C, Hamilton N, et al. Diabetes, glucose control, and 9-year cognitive decline among older adults without dementia. Arch Neurol 2012;69:1170–1175

13. Lee ATC, Richards M, Chan WC, Chiu HFK, Lee RSY, Lam LCW. Higher dementia incidence in older adults with type 2 diabetes and large reduction in HbA1c. Age Ageing 2019;48:838–844

14. Mukai N, Ohara T, Hata J, et al. Alternative measures of hyperglycemia and risk of Alzheimer's disease in the community: the Hisayama study. J Clin Endocrinol Metab 2017;102:3002–3010

15. Gorst C, Kwok CS, Aslam S, et al. Long-term glycemic variability and risk of adverse outcomes: a systematic review and meta-analysis. Diabetes Care 2015;38:2354–2369

16. Whitmer RA, Karter AJ, Yaffe K, Quesenberry CP Jr, Selby JV. Hypoglycemic episodes and risk of dementia in older patients with type 2 diabetes mellitus. JAMA 2009;301:1565–1572

17. Mehta HB, Mehta V, Goodwin JS. Association of hypoglycemia with subsequent dementia in older patients with type 2 diabetes mellitus. J Gerontol A Biol Sci Med Sci 2017;72:1110–1116

18. Mattishent K, Loke YK. Bi-directional interaction between hypoglycaemia and cognitive impairment in elderly patients treated with glucose-lowering agents: a systematic review and meta-analysis. Diabetes Obes Metab 2016;18:135–141

19. Herrett E, Gallagher AM, Bhaskaran K, et al. Data resource profile: Clinical Practice Research Datalink (CPRD). Int J Epidemiol 2015;44:827–836

20. Schneider JA, Arvanitakis Z, Bang W, Bennett DA. Mixed brain pathologies account for most dementia cases in community-dwelling older persons. Neurology 2007;69:2197–2204

21. Toledo JB, Arnold SE, Raible K, et al. Contribution of cerebrovascular disease in autopsy confirmed neurodegenerative disease cases in the National Alzheimer's Coordinating Centre. Brain 2013;136:2697–2706

22. National Institute for Health and Care Excellence. Donepezil, galantamine, rivastigmine and memantine for the treatment of Alzheimer's disease. 2011. Accessed 29 March 2021. Available from https://www.nice.org.uk/guidance/ta217

23. Wilkinson S, Douglas I, Stirnadel-Farrant H, et al. Changing use of antidiabetic drugs in the UK: trends in prescribing 2000-2017. BMJ Open 2018;8:e022768

24. Kilpatrick ES, Rigby AS, Atkin SL. A1C variability and the risk of microvascular complications in type 1 diabetes: data from the Diabetes Control and Complications Trial. Diabetes Care 2008;31:2198–2202

25. Pujades-Rodriguez M, Assi V, Gonzalez-Izquierdo A, et al. The diagnosis, burden and prognosis of dementia: a record-linkage cohort study in England. PLoS One 2018;13:e0199026

26. Suh SW, Hamby AM, Swanson RA. Hypoglycemia, brain energetics, and hypoglycemic neuronal death. Glia 2007;55:1280–1286

27. Exalto LG, Biessels GJ, Karter AJ, et al. Risk score for prediction of 10 year dementia risk in individuals with type 2 diabetes: a cohort study. Lancet Diabetes Endocrinol 2013;1:183–190

28. Sonnen JA, Larson EB, Brickell K, et al. Different patterns of cerebral injury in dementia with or without diabetes. Arch Neurol 2009;66:315–322

29. Heringa SM, Bouvy WH, van den Berg E, Moll AC, Kappelle LJ, Biessels GJ. Associations between retinal microvascular changes and dementia, cognitive functioning, and brain imaging abnormalities: a systematic review. J Cereb Blood Flow Metab 2013;33:983–995

30. Schrijvers EM, Buitendijk GH, Ikram MK, et al. Retinopathy and risk of dementia: the Rotterdam Study. Neurology 2012;79:365–370

31. Rawlings AM, Sharrett AR, Albert MS, et al. The association of late-life diabetes status and hyperglycemia with incident mild cognitive impairment and dementia: the ARIC study. Diabetes Care 2019;42:1248–1254

32. Launer LJ, Miller ME, Williamson JD, et al.; ACCORD MIND investigators. Effects of intensive glucose lowering on brain structure and function in people with type 2 diabetes (ACCORD MIND): a randomised open-label substudy. Lancet Neurol 2011;10:969–977

33. Erus G, Battapady H, Zhang T, et al. Spatial patterns of structural brain changes in type 2 diabetic patients and their longitudinal progression with intensive control of blood glucose. Diabetes Care 2015;38:97–104

34. DeVries JH. Glucose variability: where it is important and how to measure it. Diabetes 2013;62:1405–1408

35. Li TC, Yang CP, Tseng ST, et al. Visit-to-visit variations in fasting plasma glucose and HbA1c associated with an increased risk of Alzheimer disease: Taiwan Diabetes Study. Diabetes Care 2017;40:1210–1217

36. Biessels GJ, Despa F. Cognitive decline and dementia in diabetes mellitus: mechanisms and clinical implications. Nat Rev Endocrinol 2018;14:591–604

37. Wang L, Hubbard RA, Walker RL, Lee EB, Larson EB, Crane PK. Assessing robustness of hazard ratio estimates to outcome misclassification in longitudinal panel studies with application to Alzheimer's disease. PLoS One 2017;12:e0190107

38. Donegan K, Fox N, Black N, Livingston G, Banerjee S, Burns A. Trends in diagnosis and treatment for people with dementia in the UK from 2005 to 2015: a longitudinal retrospective cohort study. Lancet Public Health 2017;2:e149–e156

39. Norton S, Matthews FE, Barnes DE, Yaffe K, Brayne C. Potential for primary prevention of Alzheimer's disease: an analysis of population-based data. Lancet Neurol 2014;13:788–794

40. Wheeler MJ, Dempsey PC, Grace MS, et al. Sedentary behavior as a risk factor for cognitive decline? A focus on the influence of glycemic control in brain health. Alzheimers Dement (NY) 2017;3:291–300

Practical Strategies to Help Reduce Added Sugars Consumption to Support Glycemic and Weight Management Goals

Hope Warshaw[1] and Steven V. Edelman[2,3]

Overconsumption of added sugars is a key contributor to the growing obesity, prediabetes, and type 2 diabetes pandemics. The nutrition therapy guidance of the American Diabetes Association recognizes that using low- and no-calorie sweeteners (LNCS) to reduce consumption of added sugars can reduce low–nutrient-density sources of calories and carbohydrate to beneficially affect glycemia, weight, and cardiometabolic health. This article provides information for primary care providers, diabetes care and education specialists, and other diabetes clinicians on the safety of LNCS and summarizes research evidence on the role of LNCS in glycemic and weight management. It also provides practical strategies for counseling individuals about how to integrate LNCS into their healthy eating pattern.

The increasing number of adults and children/adolescents who are overweight and obese in the United States is a national health concern. Numerous studies have shown that overweight and obesity are significant risk factors for several interrelated health conditions, including prediabetes, type 2 diabetes, cardiovascular and cerebrovascular disease, hypertension, stroke, and other significant health conditions of increasing concern (1,2), such as nonalcoholic steatohepatitis and nonalcoholic fatty liver disease (3). Excessive weight is a concern in individuals with type 1 or type 2 diabetes and is a leading risk factor for prediabetes (4) because it decreases insulin sensitivity, which creates additional challenges in achieving and maintaining management of glycemia and other cardiometabolic health metrics (5).

Given the growing pandemics of type 1 and type 2 diabetes, prediabetes, and obesity and their associated costs (6), it is imperative that primary care providers (PCPs), diabetes care and education specialists, and other diabetes clinicians provide people who have or are at risk for developing diabetes with practical strategies for weight management and healthier eating. For many people, the most challenging part of their diabetes care plan is knowing what to eat and adhering to a healthy eating plan over time (7). Some individuals can achieve some success by reducing consumption of added sugars by choosing foods and beverages sweetened with low- and no-calorie sweeteners (LNCS) and using their preferred type and forms of table-top LNCS to sweeten foods and beverages. LNCS, the term used throughout this publication, are also referred to as low-calorie sweeteners, nonnutritive sweeteners, sugar substitutes, and high-intensity sweeteners (8). As sweetening ingredients, LNCS add no or negligible calories to foods and beverages.

This article reviews evidence supporting the safety and efficacy of LNCS in glycemic and weight management. It also provides practical strategies for clinicians to help people with diabetes and prediabetes effectively use LNCS to replace full-calorie sources of added sugars to assist with weight management and glycemic goals.

Scope of the Problem

The National Center for Health Statistics reports that the prevalence of obesity was 42.4% in 2017–2018 (9). The prevalence of obesity among children and adolescents is estimated to be 18.5% (10).

Overconsumption of various sources of added sugars is one contributor to the growing obesity pandemic. Several recent meta-analyses confirm the strong relationship between the consumption of added sugars, including

---

[1]Hope Warshaw Associates, Asheville, NC; [2]University of California San Diego, San Diego, CA; [3]Taking Control of Your Diabetes, San Diego, CA

Corresponding author: Hope Warshaw, hope@hopewarshaw.com

https://doi.org/10.2337/cd20-0034

---

sugar-sweetened beverages (SSBs), and the onset of obesity and development of type 2 diabetes (11–19).

In a study by Schulze et al. (16), which followed >50,000 women for 8 years, investigators found that women who consumed more than one SSB per day had an 83% greater risk of developing type 2 diabetes than those who consumed less than one SSB per month. It has been speculated that high amounts of added sugars (particularly high-fructose corn syrup) are rapidly absorbed, and the excessive glycemic load may increase the risk of cardiovascular disease and type 2 diabetes independent of obesity (18). As recently reported by O'Connor et al. (20), higher intakes of added sugars from nonalcoholic beverages and full-calorie sweeteners added to tea, coffee, and cereal are associated with deleterious glycemia and inflammatory markers.

According to the 2015–2020 U.S. Dietary Guidelines Advisory Committee report, added sugars contribute, on average, 270 kcal/day, or ~13% of total daily calories. This amount is the equivalent of 17 teaspoons per day, which is two times the recommended intake (21). The estimated proportion of the U.S. population who met the guidance in the 2015–2020 Dietary Guidelines for Americans to consume <10% of energy from added sugars has increased from 30% in 2007–2010 to 37% in 2013–2016. Based on evidence explored by the 2020–2025 Dietary Guidelines Advisory Committee, the report recommends limiting added sugars to an even lower amount: ≤6% of total calories at most energy levels based on newer evidence about the negative health impacts of added sugars and to allow people to meet their nutrient needs from nutrient-dense foods (21). The report also states that added sugars could be reduced by consuming low- or no-sugar-added versions of foods and beverages that make positive nutrient contributions. This recommendation to further reduce added sugars aligns more closely with the added sugars recommendation of the World Health Organization (WHO), last issued in 2015 (22). At that time, the WHO strongly recommended that adults and children should reduce added sugars to <10%, with a conditional recommendation to further reduce added sugars to 5% of total calories.

Although consumption of SSBs has slowly declined during the past several years (23), they remain the single largest source of added sugars (47%) in the U.S. diet. Approximately 7% of added sugars from beverages are attributed to a variety of table-top sugars such as granulated sugar and honey that are added to coffee and tea (21). Additional sources of added sugars are found in snacks and sweets (31%), grains (8%), and condiments, gravies, spreads, and salad dressings (2%) (Figure 1) (21).

LNCS Available for Use in the U.S. Marketplace

Global regulatory authorities, including the U.S. Food and Drug Administration (FDA), Joint U.N. Food and Agriculture Organization/WHO Expert Committee on Food Additives, European Food Safety Authority, and Health Canada, have, over many years, determined the safety of LNCS using similar rigorous regulatory review protocols. The FDA regulates LNCS either through the Food Additive approval process or the Generally Recognized as Safe (GRAS) process (24–26). LNCS are deemed safe for their permitted uses and allowed for use by the general population, including people with diabetes, children, and pregnant and lactating women. One type of LNCS, aspartame, should be limited by individuals with a rare inherited metabolic disorder known as phenylketonuria because of its phenylalanine content.

As a result of increasing consumer demand for more natural products over the past decade, several plant-derived LNCS have entered the marketplace, including those derived from stevia and monk fruit. The dominant ingredients in the LNCS naturals category are derived from one or a combination of steviol glycosides. All are allowed on the U.S. marketplace as GRAS ingredients (27,28).

LNCS ingredients, either traditional or natural, are used in one of two ways: to replace added sugars in an array of commercially manufactured foods and beverages or as table-top sweetener substitutes for full-calorie sweeteners such as granulated sugar, honey, and brown sugar. Table 1 presents a list of added sugars used in foods and beverages.

When used as substitutes for added sugars, LNCS are most commonly used to sweeten coffee and other hot or cold beverages, hot or cold cereals, and yogurt and fruit; they are also used for cooking and baking. For these purposes, LNCS are available in various forms. Granulated LNCS are provided in individual packets for table-top use and in jars or pouches for use in beverages, baking, and cooking. "Squeeze and stir" liquid LNCS can be added to cold beverages and cereals without the need to dissolve. LNCS blends, with granulated sugar or granulated and brown sugar, can be used for an array of baking and cooking when the functional properties of sugar are needed but the benefit of fewer calories and carbohydrates per serving can be gained.

Evidence on Effectiveness of LNCS on Glycemic and Weight Management

Findings from Expert Consensus

Randomized controlled trials (RCTs) and meta-analyses/systematic reviews have demonstrated the impact of

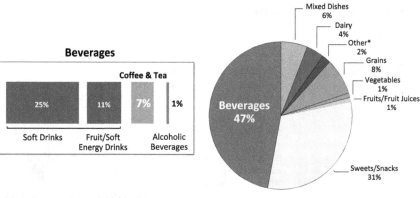

FIGURE 1 Sources of added sugars in the U.S. diet (21).

*Includes condiments, gravies, spreads, salad dressings

LNCS use on glucose metabolism (29–35) and weight management (36–39). A summary of findings from these studies is presented in Tables 2 and 3.

In 2018, an international panel of health care professionals, nutrition researchers, and food toxicologists evaluated the substantial body of evidence relevant to the associations between use of LNCS and weight and glycemic management (8). The following summarizes the panel's key findings, which are consistent with other recent international consensus statements (40,41):

- LNCS reduce calorie intake, can enhance adherence to nutrition recommendations, and assist in weight and glycemic management when substituted for added sugars in an individual's eating plan.
- LNCS do not adversely affect blood glucose levels (A1C or fasting or postprandial glucose) or insulin regulation in individuals with or without diabetes.
- There is a need to research and develop evidence-based strategies to communicate facts to consumers, health professionals, and policy makers.
- Experts agree that, with the reduction of added sugars being recommended globally to lower the risk and prevalence of obesity, LNCS are a strategy to consider.
- Efforts should be made to understand and, where possible, reconcile policy discrepancies between organizations and reduce regulatory hurdles that impede product development and reformulation designed to reduce sugars and calories.

Although water is considered by some to be an optimal beverage choice, a recent American Heart Association science advisory that was supported by the American Diabetes Association recognized that children with well-managed diabetes may be able to prevent excessive glucose excursions by substituting beverages with LNCS for SSBs when needed (42). The authors of this science advisory also determined that use of beverages with LNCS

may also be an effective replacement strategy for adults who are habitual consumers of SSBs. Carbonated soft drinks with LNCS were found in one study to assist adults in controlling calorie intake, weight loss, and weight maintenance (43).

Limitations of Observational Studies on LNCS

A common thread throughout all current recommendations on LNCS is recognition of the limitations inherent to using meta-analyses of observational study designs to assess the efficacy of LNCS in weight management (8,40,41,44). Unlike RCTs, which directly assess the effects of an identifiable intervention (e.g., use of LNCS) versus a comparator (i.e., control) intervention within a well-defined study population, observational studies cannot determine causal relationships between intervention and outcome. For example, whereas an observational study may show an association between use of LNCS and weight gain, it is not possible to determine whether individuals gained weight because they were consuming LNCS or whether they were consuming these products because they were overweight or were managing type 2 diabetes. Other limitations of these studies include small sample sizes, short study durations, and lack of participants' dietary history and information on other factors that can affect clinical outcomes.

TABLE 1 Added Sugars Commonly Used as Ingredients in Foods and Beverages

• Agave nectar	• Glucose	• Molasses
• Brown sugar	• High-fructose corn syrup	• Nectar
• Cane sugar	• Honey	• Powdered sugar
• Coconut sugar	• Invert sugar	• Raw sugar
• Corn sweetener	• Lactose	• Rice syrup
• Date sugar	• Malt syrup	• Sorghum
• Dextrose	• Maltose	• Sucrose
• Fructose	• Maple syrup	• Turbinado sugar

TABLE 2 Findings from Key Studies of the Effects of LNCS on Glycemic Management (Glucose Metabolism)

Glucose Metabolism Study	Study Design/Population	Findings
Jensen et al., 2020 (29)	• 8-year prospective trial • $n = 1,142$ adults with diabetes	• Eighty percent of participants reported regularly consuming LNCS soda (39%) or using LNCS to sweeten their beverages (41%). • No statistically significant associations of reported LNCS use consumption with fasting insulin or fasting glucose were observed.
Toora et al., 2018 (30)	• Single-arm, placebo-controlled trial • Healthy males/females • $n = 30$	• The mean glucose level 1 h after intake of glucose was 80.42 ± 8.97 mg/dL, and that of LNCS ranged from 74.42 ± 8.34 to 83.19 ± 5.62 mg/dL. • A statistically significant decrease ($P < 0.001$) compared with glucose intake was shown in the difference in blood glucose level between the two samples. • These findings showed a slight increase in the blood glucose level after the intake of LNCS; however, the increase was significantly less compared with the glucose consumption.
Nichol et al., 2018 (31)	• Systematic review of 29 RCTs • Normoglycemic adults and individuals with diabetes • $n = 741$	• LNCS consumption was not found to increase blood glucose level, and its concentration gradually declined over the course of observation after LNCS consumption. • The glycemic impact of LNCS consumption did not differ by type of LNCS but to some extent varied by participants' age, body weight, and diabetes status.
Grotz et al., 2017 (32)	• 12-week RCT • Normoglycemic males • $n = 47$	• A1C, glucose, insulin, and C-peptide levels remained within normal ranges throughout the study. • The findings support that sucralose has no effect on glycemic control. These results confirmed findings from an earlier study in type 2 diabetes (36) that showed no significant differences between sucralose and placebo groups in blood glucose control before, during, or after treatment or when analyzed over the 3-month study period.
Campos et al., 2015 (33)	• 12-week RCT • Healthy males/females • $n = 31$	• In subjects who were overweight or obese and had a high intake of sugar-sweetened beverages, replacement with LNCS beverages significantly decreased intrahepatocellular (IHCL) concentrations over a 12-week period. The decrease in hepatic fat was most significant in subjects with IHCL >60 mmol/L than in subjects with low IHCL concentrations.
Ma et al., 2009 (34)	• Single-blind, randomized order • Healthy males/females • $n = 10$	• No differences in blood glucose, plasma glucagon-like peptide 1, or serum 3-O-methylglucose concentrations between sucralose and control infusions were observed. • The findings showed that sucralose does not appear to modify the rate of glucose absorption or the glycemic or incretin response to intraduodenal glucose infusion when given acutely in healthy human subjects.
Grotz et al., 2003 (35)	• 17-week RCT • People with type 2 diabetes • $n = 136$	• No significant differences were observed between the sucralose and placebo groups in A1C, fasting plasma glucose, or fasting serum C-peptide changes from baseline. There were no clinically meaningful differences between the groups in any safety measure. • These findings demonstrated that, similar to cellulose, sucralose consumption for 3 months at doses of 7.5 mg/kg/day, which is approximately three times the estimated maximum intake, had no effect on glucose homeostasis in individuals with type 2 diabetes.

These limitations are compounded by reliance on meta-analyses/systematic reviews that are heavily weighted with observational studies (11,44–47). Many of these reports provide little or no information about the characteristics of included studies such as study designs, comparators assessed, effect sizes, and study quality (48).

Consideration of results from RCTs, reported individually or within well-designed meta-analyses, is the most appropriate approach for assessing the impact of LNCS relevant to glycemic control and weight management.

So, Why the Controversy About LNCS?

Despite the robust body of evidence supporting the benefits of use of LNCS in glycemic and weight management, these findings are often overshadowed by media headlines and stories based on unsubstantiated data or observational

TABLE 3 Findings from Key Studies of the Effects of LNCS on Weight Management

Weight Management Study	Study Design/Population	Findings
Laviada-Molina et al., 2020 (36)	• Systematic review of 20 RCTs • Normal-weight and overweight/obese children and adults • $n = 2,914$	• Participants consuming LNCS showed significant weight/BMI differences favoring LNCS compared with nonusers. • Participants with overweight/obesity showed significant favorable weight/BMI differences with LNCS. • These findings indicate that replacing added sugars with LNCS leads to weight reduction, an effect that is particularly evident in adults, subjects with overweight/obesity, and those following a specified or restricted eating plan.
Peters et al., 2016 (37)	• 1-year RCT (12 weeks weight loss, 9 months maintenance) • Overweight/obese adults • $n = 303$	• At 1 year, use of LNCS beverages was associated with greater weight loss than with water (-6.21 ± 7.65 vs. -2.45 ± 5.59 kg, $P < 0.001$). • Beverages with LNCS were superior to water for weight loss and weight maintenance in a population consisting of regular users of beverages with LNCS who either (based on study group) maintained or discontinued consumption of these beverages and consumed water during a 1-year structured weight loss program with 12 weeks for weight loss and 9 months of follow-up.
Piernas et al., 2013 (38)	• Subanalysis from Tate et al. (39) study (see below) • Overweight/obese adults • $n = 210$	• Micronutrient composition changed in both intervention groups (water and beverages containing LNCS). The water group showed increased grain intake at 3 months and a greater increase in fruit/vegetable intake at 6 months (both $P < 0.05$). The group drinking beverages with LNCS showed greater reductions in intake of desserts at 6 months ($P < 0.5$). • Participants in both intervention groups showed positive changes in energy intake and dietary patterns.
Tate et al., 2012 (39)	• 6-month RCT • Overweight/obese adults • $n = 318$	• Significant reduction in weight and waist circumference and improvement in systolic blood pressure were observed from 0 to 6 months. • No significant differences in weight loss were observed between participants who consumed beverages containing LNCS vs. water (-2.5 ± 0.45 vs. $-2.03 \pm 0.40\%$, respectively). • Replacement of caloric beverages with noncaloric beverages as a weight loss strategy resulted in average weight losses of 2–2.5%.

studies, which, as discussed earlier, are inherently flawed and inconclusive. For example, the recent study by Dalenberg et al. reported that "consumption of sucralose in the presence of a carbohydrate rapidly impairs glucose metabolism and results in longer-term decreases in brain but not perceptual, sensitivity to sweet taste, suggesting dysregulation of gut-brain control of glucose metabolism" (49). Adhering to established ethics for reporting medical research, the investigators appropriately listed the limitations of their study, which included:

• Small sample size: included only 13 people in the experimental group
• Short study duration: lasted only 2 weeks
• Nutrition data self-reported and collected only at baseline, allowing for the possibility that other

components of the diet and diet-related behavior could have affected the findings
• Questionable clinical significance: no group differences observed in glucose response

However, rather than provide an objective review of the study findings, the *Washington Post* instead published a uniformed article titled, "A common artificial sweetener might be making you fatter and sicker, a new study says: Sucralose in conjunction with carbohydrates may blunt the body's ability to metabolize sugar appropriately" (50). Although the article contained numerous references to observational studies "associating" use of LNCS to various adverse outcomes, it failed to report the limitations of the study that significantly diminished the credibility of its findings.

Sensationalized headlines have created unwarranted public alarm and confusion about the safety of LNCS over the course of many years. Conversely, a recent well-designed meta-analysis/systematic review by Laviada-Molina et al. (36), which demonstrated significant benefits of using LNCS in weight management, received no media coverage.

In short, meta-analyses and systematic reviews that include both RCTs and observational studies provide limited guidance. For example, a recent systematic review and meta-analysis by Azad et al. (50) reported no statistically or clinically relevant differences between subjects who consumed LNCS and those who regularly consumed sugar. Yet, the authors emphasized that many of the studies they included were of low quality and that the findings of the observational studies regarding the health effects of using LNCS should be interpreted with caution.

Importantly, the findings from Azad et al. (51) are in stark contrast to those reported in a meta-analysis by Rogers et al. (52), which included only RCTs in the analysis. In the study by Rogers et al., investigators concluded that the preponderance of evidence from all human RCTs indicates that LNCS do not increase energy intake or body weight and that the balance of evidence indicates that use of LNCS as a replacement for added sugars in children and adults leads to reduced body weight, and this reduction is also apparent when beverages containing LNCS are compared with water (52).

Practical Strategies to Reduce Consumption of Added Sugars

Motivations that Influence Use of LNCS

To our knowledge, no academic studies have been conducted to assess consumer motivations for using LNCS or preferences for specific LNCS. However, results from a 2020 survey of people who use LNCS (MarketLab, Philadelphia, PA; unpublished observations) provide some insights regarding consumer attitudes and behaviors. Conducted by an independent market research firm (MarketLab, unpublished observations), the survey included a national cohort of 919 respondents that was equally balanced in terms of sex, education, and income level.

As shown in Figure 2, the most commonly reported reasons for using LNCS were to reduce the intake of added sugars and to reduce overall calorie consumption. We hypothesize that "reduces calories" is a motivation for weight loss and management. When counseling individuals,

clinicians who deliver diabetes care should leverage the motivators for leading a healthier lifestyle and losing/managing weight to emphasize that reducing added sugars in both ready-to-eat and home-prepared foods and beverages can help people achieve the associated health benefits.

Importance of Taste in Successful Transition to Using LNCS

In the previously mentioned 2020 survey (MarketLab, unpublished observations), 514 users of LNCS were asked to identify the brand of LNCS they consistently use. As presented in Figure 3, survey respondents showed a stronger preference for Splenda (sucralose) compared with Equal and Sweet'N Low, the other traditional table-top sweeteners, as evidenced by a higher percentage of respondents who report consistent use of the brand. Splenda Naturals Stevia was consistently rated highest in the natural LNCS category.

These finding are important when counseling individuals because numerous studies have shown that the taste of food plays an important role in food choices, eating behaviors, and food intake (53–56) and that the more distant a recommended change is from the person's actual eating habits, the more difficult it is to gain sustained adherence to the recommended change (57,58). In a national survey of 2,967 U.S. adults (54), respondents were asked to rate the factors they felt were most influential in their food choices. On a 5-point Likert scale (from 1 = least to 5 = most), the mean score for importance of taste was 4.7, followed by cost (4.1), nutrition (3.9), convenience (3.8), and weight control (3.4). The investigators concluded that their results suggest that nutritional concerns per se are of less importance to most people than taste and cost. Therefore, product recommendations should focus on promoting healthy eating habits that are aligned with the consumer goals of having foods that are "tasty and inexpensive" (54).

Starting the Conversation

Although patients may generally understand the importance of limiting their intake of added sugars, many may not realize the quantity of added sugars they consume on a daily basis. As previously noted, U.S. adults consume, on average, 17 teaspoons of added sugars per day, which is nearly two times the recommended maximum daily intake. Therefore, a starting point for discussion could be to raise patients' awareness that their daily added sugars intake is likely much higher than they realize. The reason may be, in part, that they do not recognize that added sugars in foods

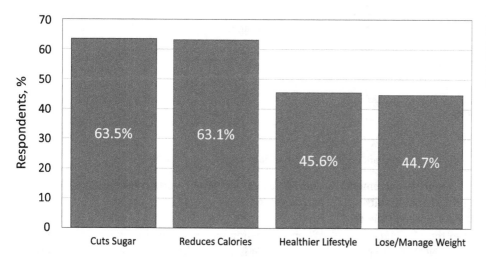

FIGURE 2 Most common reasons for using LNCS reported in a 2020 survey of 919 users of these products (MarketLab, unpublished observations).

and beverages are represented on food packaging nutrition labels by numerous ingredients and names, as listed in Table 1. It can be valuable to make this list a teaching tool to raise patients' awareness about the many sources of added sugars. With this knowledge in hand, encourage patients to read the ingredient lists on the foods and beverages they consider purchasing and to consider not buying those that contain large amounts of added sugars.

The next step might be to discuss the current recommendations for daily intake of added sugars. The current guidance from the 2015–2020 Dietary Guidelines for Americans (21), to limit intake of added sugars from all foods and beverages to <10% of total daily calories, translates to ≤9 teaspoons for men and ≤6 teaspoons for women. Table 4 illustrates how substituting LNCS for full-calorie sweeteners can help patients achieve these recommendations.

A

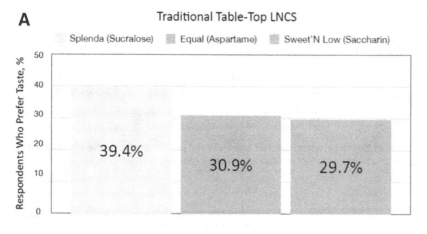

FIGURE 3 Consumer taste preferences for users of traditional (n = 514) (A) and natural (n = 512) (B) table-top sweeteners by brand name (MarketLab, unpublished observations).

B

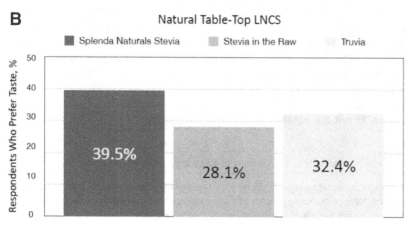

TABLE 4 Impact of Substituting LNCS for Added Sugars in Sweetened Beverages

Sweetened Beverage, 12 oz	Sweetened With Sugar		Sweetened With LNCS	
	Calories (Teaspoons of Sugar)	Carbohydrates, g	Calories, (Packets of LNCS)*	Carbohydrates, g
Iced tea	128 (8)	32	0 (4)	<1
Coffee	43 (3)	12	0 (1)	<1

*Per FDA guidance, all products with <5 calories per serving are listed as having 0 calories.

Successful weight loss and long-term weight management require making sustainable changes in eating habits and food choices. However, PCPs have limited time to spend offering nutrition guidance to their patients to reduce added sugars with the use of LNCS. To assist, Table 5 offers suggested open-ended questions that diabetes care clinicians can use to start a conversation with patients to assess their knowledge and, based on their readiness to change, help them set goals to reduce added sugars and consider the use of LNCS (both as table-top sweeteners and in products sweetened with LNCS). A crucial conceptual point to cover when encouraging patients to use LNCS to reduce added sugars is to avoid compensating for the reduction of calories with increased intake of calorie-containing foods and beverages.

When counseling patients, it is essential to provide guidance that is achievable and sustainable, empowering people with prediabetes and diabetes (type 1 or type 2) to adopt healthier food choices without compromising their taste preferences. It is also important to provide specific product recommendations when counseling individuals, particularly for people who have little or no previous experience using products made with LNCS (57,58). In their recent cross-sectional study of 91 people with type 2 diabetes, Jaworski et al. (59) reported that lack of knowledge about recommended

TABLE 5 Goals for Reducing Intake of Added Sugars

Goal: Assess total consumption of added sugars and types of foods and beverages.

Questions to ask:

1. List all of the beverages you drink (and the amounts) on a given day from the time you wake up until you go to sleep. (Follow-up: What do you add to hot and cold beverages such as coffee and tea?)

2. How many times a day (or week) do you eat sweets? (Follow-up: What types of sweets and in what amounts?)

3. Can you tell me what a few of the names are for added sugars on food and beverage ingredient labels? (Table 1 provides a list. Make this a handout and have a couple of representative products with nutrition facts and ingredient lists available to illustrate further.)

Goal: Assess knowledge and use of LNCS.

Questions to ask:

1. What are your thoughts about using LNCS (sugar substitutes) instead of sugar or other calorie-containing sweeteners? (If the response does not accurately reflect the science, attempt to offer accurate information.)

2. What are a few ways you could use LNCS to reduce the amount of sugars you eat and drink? (Use content in Table 4 to illustrate the calories and grams of carbohydrate saved when using LNCS rather than added sugars in beverages.) If the patient states that he or she does not use LNCS because they are not natural, you may note that there are now a variety of natural LNCS that may suit their product and taste preferences.

3. Tell me where you would find LNCS (sugar substitutes) in the supermarket?

4. What is the best way for you to find LNCS (sugar substitutes) that taste most like sugar?

Goal: Set a few small changes to reduce added sugars before the next appointment.

Question to ask:

1. What are two or three small changes you are willing and able to make to reduce the amount of added sugars you eat and drink?

Note: It is crucial to have patients write out or state their goals. PCPs should make a copy for or record their goals in their electronic health record. At the next appointment, ask about how successful they were with their goals. Having you spend a few minutes on this topic conveys an imperative to patients and sets expectations. Asking about their progress at the follow-up appointment increases this imperative.

TABLE 6 Most Common Brand-Name Table-Top LNCS

LNCS Ingredient	Brand Name
Aspartame	Equal NutraSweet
Saccharin	Sweet'N Low
Sucralose	Splenda
Steviol glycosides	Splenda Stevia Sweet Leaf Stevia in the Raw Truvia Whole Earth

products and their availability was the most common problem reported by study participants. For this reason, we suggest that diabetes care providers try the available table-top LNCS. The most commonly used table-top LNCS in the United States today are listed in Table 6.

Another important strategy is to present simple options for substituting LNCS for added sugars in common foods. Following are ideas to encourage switching from using added sugars to using LNCS:

- Use LNCS to sweeten hot or iced coffee or tea.
- Instead of SSBs, use a diet beverage or drink still or sparkling water instead. To increase the palatability of water, flavor it with a splash of fruit juice or a few squeezes of lemon or lime and then add an LNCS to sweeten. (Consider that some patients may find that drinking carbonated beverages is satisfying and quenches their desire for a sweet taste.)
- Use LNCS to sweeten fruit (e.g., grapefruit, strawberries, or other berries).
- Put LNCS in the sugar bowl instead of sugar.
- Use LNCS instead of sugar when making sweets, treats, and desserts.
- Use LNCS in homemade salad dressings, marinades, and sauces.

The impact of taste cannot be overemphasized. Diabetes care providers should consider the taste preference survey results when recommending LNCS options (Figure 3).

Summary

Individuals who are overweight or obese are at significant risk for developing prediabetes, coronary heart disease, hypertension, stroke, nonalcoholic steatohepatitis, and other health conditions (1–3). These risks are elevated among overweight or obese individuals with type 1 or type 2 diabetes, who are further challenged to maintain their glucose control because of decreased insulin sensitivity (5). Overconsumption of added sugars is a driver of overweight and obesity (21). Given the growing pandemics of diabetes and prediabetes, accompanied by the increasing prevalence of overweight and obesity (9), there is a clear need for effective strategies that promote healthier eating habits and alternatives to overconsumption of added sugars.

Based on evidence from recent RCTs (30–33,35,39,58), experts on LNCS have published consensus statements (8,40,41,59) that recognize the potential of LNCS to reduce calorie intake and assist in weight loss and weight management when consciously substituted for added sugars (30–33,35,58). Importantly, these benefits can be realized without adversely affecting blood glucose levels (A1C or fasting or postprandial blood glucose) or insulin regulation in individuals with diabetes (36,37,39).

Diabetes clinicians can play a significant role in assisting patients to reduce their intake of added sugars. In this article, we have outlined practical strategies clinicians can implement to help their patients obtain evidence-based information about LNCS. When encouraging lifestyle behavior modification to change food choices and eating habits, it is crucial to meet patients where they are, with an understanding of their current food choices, eating habits, food security, home and work situations, and other factors. In addition, if weight loss is being encouraged to prevent or delay prediabetes or type 2 diabetes, it is important to identify and leverage each patient's motivations for weight management. This strategy also provides an opportunity to dispel any myths and misinformation reported in the media and reinforces the message that LNCS are both safe and effective as a component of weight management efforts.

It is important to recognize the role of taste in choosing foods and to make specific product recommendations that consider taste as a key consumer factor. Therefore, clinicians should consider the preference data discussed earlier as a first option for patients. It is also important to present various options and forms of LNCS and to encourage experimentation with these alternatives.

Because most people require frequent, consistent nutrition counseling and support over time to make and adhere to behavioral lifestyle changes that assist with weight loss maintenance, it is suggested that clinicians refer people with or at high risk for prediabetes to a National Diabetes Prevention Program, Medicare Diabetes Prevention Program, or similar program (7,59). Additionally, diabetes self-management education and support and medical nutrition therapy should be provided at regular intervals through the course of patients' disease (60). These services are covered by Medicare and many private payors (7,59).

Perhaps most important is to establish an honest, collaborative, and person-centered relationship with patients to facilitate shared decision-making in setting practical, individualized, and achievable goals that address their preferences, circumstances, and capabilities.

FUNDING

Funding for the development of this manuscript was provided by Heartland Food Products Group.

DUALITY OF INTEREST

H.W. has received consulting and speaker fees from Heartland Food Products Group, Tate & Lyle, and several trade associations. No other potential conflicts of interest relevant to this article were reported.

AUTHOR CONTRIBUTIONS

H.W. and S.V.E. wrote, reviewed, and approved the manuscript for submission. H.W. is the guarantor of this work and, as such, takes responsibility for the integrity of the data and the accuracy of the content.

REFERENCES

1. Must A, Spadano J, Coakley EH, Field AE, Colditz G, Dietz WH. The disease burden associated with overweight and obesity. JAMA 1999;282:1523–1529

2. Allison DB, Fontaine KR, Manson JE, Stevens J, VanItallie TB. Annual deaths attributable to obesity in the United States. JAMA 1999;282:1530–1538

3. Sarwar R, Pierce N, Koppe S. Obesity and nonalcoholic fatty liver disease: current perspectives. Diabetes Metab Syndr Obes 2018;11:533–542

4. Naser KA, Gruber A, Thomson GA. The emerging pandemic of obesity and diabetes: are we doing enough to prevent a disaster? Int J Clin Pract 2006;60:1093–1097

5. Kahn BB, Flier JS. Obesity and insulin resistance. J Clin Invest 2000;106:473–481

6. Centers for Disease Control and Prevention. National Diabetes Statistics Report, 2020: Estimates of Diabetes and Its Burden in the United States. Available from https://www.cdc.gov/diabetes/pdfs/data/statistics/national-diabetes-statistics-report.pdf. Accessed 29 February 2020

7. American Diabetes Association. 5. Facilitating behavior change and well-being to improve health outcomes: *Standards of Medical Care in Diabetes—2020*. Diabetes Care 2020;43(Suppl. 1):S48–S65

8. Ashwell M, Gibson S, Bellisle F, et al. Expert consensus on low-calorie sweeteners: facts, research gaps and suggested actions. Nutr Res Rev 2020;33:145–154

9. Centers for Disease Control and Prevention, National Center for Health Statistics. Prevalence of obesity and severe obesity among adults: United States, 2017–2018. Available from https://www.cdc.gov/nchs/products/databriefs/db360.htm. Accessed 3 March 2020

10. Hales CM, Carroll MD, Fryar CD, Ogden CL. Prevalence of obesity among adults and youth: United States, 2015–2016: U.S. National Center for Health Statistics Data Brief, No. 28. Available from https://www.cdc.gov/nchs/data/databriefs/db288.pdf. Accessed 23 June 2020

11. Malik VS, Schulze MB, Hu FB. Intake of sugar-sweetened beverages and weight gain: a systematic review. Am J Clin Nutr 2006;84:274–288

12. Vartanian LR, Schwartz MB, Brownell KD. Effects of soft drink consumption on nutrition and health: a systematic review and meta-analysis. Am J Public Health 2007;97:667–675

13. Olsen NJ, Heitmann BL. Intake of calorically sweetened beverages and obesity. Obes Rev 2009;10:68–75

14. Malik VS, Willett WC, Hu FB. Global obesity: trends, risk factors and policy implications. Nat Rev Endocrinol 2013;9:13–27

15. Hu FB. Resolved: there is sufficient scientific evidence that decreasing sugar-sweetened beverage consumption will reduce the prevalence of obesity and obesity-related diseases. Obes Rev 2013;14:606–619

16. Schulze MB, Manson JE, Ludwig DS, et al. Sugar-sweetened beverages, weight gain, and incidence of type 2 diabetes in young and middle-aged women. JAMA 2004;292:927–934

17. Greenwood DC, Threapleton DE, Evans CEL, et al. Association between sugar-sweetened and artificially sweetened soft drinks and type 2 diabetes: systematic review and dose-response meta-analysis of prospective studies. Br J Nutr 2014;112:725–734

18. Malik VS, Popkin BM, Bray GA, Després JP, Willett WC, Hu FB. Sugar-sweetened beverages and risk of metabolic syndrome and type 2 diabetes: a meta-analysis. Diabetes Care 2010;33:2477–2483

19. Basu S, McKee M, Galea G, Stuckler D. Relationship of soft drink consumption to global overweight, obesity, and diabetes: a cross-national analysis of 75 countries. Am J Public Health 2013;103:2071–2077

20. O'Connor L, Imamura F, Brage S, Griffin SJ, Wareham NJ, Forouhi NG. Intakes and sources of dietary sugars and their association with metabolic and inflammatory markers. Clin Nutr 2018;37:1313–1322

21. Dietary Guidelines Advisory Committee. Scientific report of the 2015 Dietary Guidelines Advisory Committee: advisory report to the Secretary of Health and Human Services and the Secretary of Agriculture. Part D. Chapter 6: Cross-cutting topics of public health importance. Available from https://health.gov/our-work/food-nutrition/2015-2020-dietary-guidelines. Accessed 23 June 2020

22. World Health Organization. Guideline: sugars intake for adults and children. Available from https://www.who.int/publications/i/item/9789241549028. Accessed 23 June 2020

23. Welsh JA, Sharma AJ, Grellinger L, Vos MB. Consumption of added sugars is decreasing in the United States. Am J Clin Nutr 2011;94:726–734

24. Rulis AM, Levitt JA. FDA's food ingredient approval process: safety assurance based on scientific assessment. Regul Toxicol Pharmacol 2009;53:20–31

25. Roberts A. The safety and regulatory process for low calorie sweeteners in the United States. Physiol Behav 2016;164:439–444

26. World Health Organization. Joint FAO/WHO Expert Committee on Food Additives (JECFA). Available from https://www.who.int/foodsafety/areas_work/chemical-risks/jecfa/en. Accessed 4 April 2020

27. Perrier JD, Mihalov JJ, Carlson SJ. FDA regulatory approach to steviol glycosides. Food Chem Toxicol 2018;122:132–142

28. Samuel P, Ayoob KT, Magnuson BA, et al. Stevia leaf to stevia sweetener: exploring its science, benefits, and future potential. J Nutr 2018;148:1186S–1205S

29. Jensen PN, Howard BV, Best LG, et al. Associations of diet soda and non-caloric artificial sweetener use with markers of glucose and insulin homeostasis and incident diabetes: the Strong Heart Family Study. Eur J Clin Nutr 2020;74:322–327

30. Toora BD, Seema S, Manju M, Mishra S. Effect of artificial sweeteners on the blood glucose concentration. Journal of Medical Academics 2018;1:81–85

31. Nichol AD, Holle MJ, An R. Glycemic impact of non-nutritive sweeteners: a systematic review and meta-analysis of randomized controlled trials. Eur J Clin Nutr 2018;72:796–804

32. Grotz VL, Pi-Sunyer X, Porte D Jr, Roberts A, Richard Trout J. A 12-week randomized clinical trial investigating the potential for sucralose to affect glucose homeostasis. Regul Toxicol Pharmacol 2017;88:22–33

33. Campos V, Despland C, Brandejsky V, et al. Sugar- and artificially sweetened beverages and intrahepatic fat: a randomized controlled trial. Obes (Silver Spring) 2015;23:2335–2339

34. Ma J, Bellon M, Wishart JM, et al. Effect of the artificial sweetener, sucralose, on gastric emptying and incretin hormone release in healthy subjects. Am J Physiol Gastrointest Liver Physiol 2009;296:G735–G739

35. Grotz VL, Henry RR, McGill JB, et al. Lack of effect of sucralose on glucose homeostasis in subjects with type 2 diabetes. J Am Diet Assoc 2003;103:1607–1612

36. Laviada-Molina H, Molina-Segui F, Pérez-Gaxiola G, et al. Effects of nonnutritive sweeteners on body weight and BMI in diverse clinical contexts: systematic review and meta-analysis. Obes Rev 2020;21:e13020

37. Peters JC, Beck J, Cardel M, et al. The effects of water and non-nutritive sweetened beverages on weight loss and weight maintenance: a randomized clinical trial. Obesity (Silver Spring) 2016;24:297–304

38. Piernas C, Tate DF, Wang X, Popkin BM. Does diet-beverage intake affect dietary consumption patterns? Results from the Choose Healthy Options Consciously Everyday (CHOICE) randomized clinical trial. Am J Clin Nutr 2013;97:604–611

39. Tate DF, Turner-McGrievy G, Lyons E, et al. Replacing caloric beverages with water or diet beverages for weight loss in adults: main results of the Choose Healthy Options Consciously Everyday (CHOICE) randomized clinical trial. Am J Clin Nutr 2012;95:555–563

40. Serra-Majem L, Raposo A, Aranceta-Bartrina J, et al. Ibero-American consensus on low- and no-calorie sweeteners: safety, nutritional aspects and benefits in food and beverages. Nutrients 2018;10:818

41. Gibson S, Drewnowski A, Hill J, et al. Consensus statement on benefits of low-calorie sweeteners. Nutr Bull 2014;39:386–389

42. Johnson RK, Lichtenstein AH, Anderson CAM, et al. Low-calorie sweetened beverages and cardiometabolic health: a science advisory from the American Heart Association. Circulation 2018;138:e126–e140

43. Catenacci VA, Pan Z, Thomas JG, et al. Low/no calorie sweetened beverage consumption in the National Weight Control Registry. Obesity (Silver Spring) 2014;22:2244–2251

44. Sievenpiper JL, Khan TA, Ha V, Viguiliouk E, Auyeung R. The importance of study design in the assessment of nonnutritive sweeteners and cardiometabolic health. CMAJ 2017;189:E1424–E1425

45. Imamura F, O'Connor L, Ye Z, et al. Consumption of sugar sweetened beverages, artificially sweetened beverages, and fruit juice and incidence of type 2 diabetes: systematic review, meta-analysis, and estimation of population attributable fraction. Br J Sports Med 2016;50:496–504

46. Romo-Romo A, Aguilar-Salinas CA, Brito-Córdova GX, Gómez Díaz RA, Vilchis Valentín D, Almeda-Valdes P. Effects of the non-nutritive sweeteners on glucose metabolism and appetite regulating hormones: systematic review of observational prospective studies and clinical trials. PLoS One 2016;11:e0161264

47. Fowler SP, Williams K, Hazuda HP. Diet soda intake is associated with long-term increases in waist circumference in a biethnic cohort of older adults: the San Antonio Longitudinal Study of Aging. J Am Geriatr Soc 2015;63:708–715

48. Mosdøl A, Vist GE, Svendsen C, et al. Hypotheses and evidence related to intense sweeteners and effects on appetite and body weight changes: a scoping review of reviews. PLoS One 2018;13:e0199558

49. Dalenberg JR, Patel BP, Denis R, et al. Short-term consumption of sucralose with, but not without, carbohydrate impairs neural and metabolic sensitivity to sugar in humans. Cell Metab 2020;31:493–502.e7

50. Washington Post. A common artificial sweetener might be making you fatter and sicker, a new study says: sucralose in conjunction with carbohydrates may blunt the body's ability to metabolize sugar appropriately. Available from https://www.washingtonpost.com/business/2020/03/10/common-artificial-sweetener-might-be-making-you-fatter-sicker-new-study-says. Accessed 12 April 2020

51. Azad MB, Abou-Setta AM, Chauhan BF, et al. Nonnutritive sweeteners and cardiometabolic health: a systematic review and meta-analysis of randomized controlled trials and prospective cohort studies. CMAJ 2017;189:E929–E939

52. Rogers PJ, Hogenkamp PS, de Graaf C, et al. Does low-energy sweetener consumption affect energy intake and body weight? A systematic review, including meta-analyses, of the evidence from human and animal studies. Int J Obes 2016;40:381–394

53. Kourouniotis S, Keast RSJ, Riddell LJ, Lacy K, Thorpe MG, Cicerale S. The importance of taste on dietary choice, behaviour and intake in a group of young adults. Appetite 2016;103:1–7

54. Glanz K, Basil M, Maibach E, Goldberg J, Snyder D. Why Americans eat what they do: taste, nutrition, cost, convenience,

and weight control concerns as influences on food consumption. J Am Diet Assoc 1998;98:1118–1126

55. Ebrahim Z, Villiers A, Ahmed T. Factors influencing adherence to dietary guidelines: a qualitative study on the experiences of patients with type 2 diabetes attending a clinic in Cape Town. Journal of Endocrinology. Metabolism and Diabetes of South Africa 2014;19:76–84

56. Neumark-Sztainer D, Story M, Perry C, Casey MA. Factors influencing food choices of adolescents: findings from focus-group discussions with adolescents. J Am Diet Assoc 1999; 99:929–937

57. Jaworski M, Panczyk M, Cedro M, Kucharska A. Adherence to diet recommendations in diabetes mellitus: disease acceptance as a potential mediator. Patient Prefer Adherence 2018;12: 163–174

58. Ma J, Chang J, Checklin HL, et al. Effect of the artificial sweetener, sucralose, on small intestinal glucose absorption in healthy human subjects. Br J Nutr 2010;104:803–806

59. Evert AB, Dennison M, Gardner CD, et al. Nutrition therapy for adults with diabetes or prediabetes: a consensus report. Diabetes Care 2019;42:731–754

60. Powers MA, Bardsley JK, Cypress M, et al. Diabetes self-management education and support in adults with type 2 diabetes: a consensus report of the American Diabetes Association, the Association of Diabetes Care & Education Specialists, the Academy of Nutrition and Dietetics, the American Academy of Family Physicians, the American Academy of PAs, the American Association of Nurse Practitioners, and the American Pharmacists Association. Diabetes Educ 2020;46: 350–369

Rationale for the Use of Combination Injectable Therapy in Patients With Type 2 Diabetes Who Have High A1C (≥9%) and/or Long Duration (>8 Years): Executive Summary

Vivian A. Fonseca,[1] Minisha Sood,[2] and Rodolfo J. Galindo[3]

Recommended A1C targets for people with type 2 diabetes are between 6.5 and 8%; however, real-world data suggest that an increasing proportion of people with diabetes have suboptimal control, and ~15% have an A1C level >9%. People with A1C >9% are at increased risk for micro- and macrovascular complications and require treatment intensification to improve glycemic control as early as possible.

In a series of short videos now available on the *Clinical Diabetes* website, the authors discuss the pathophysiological changes that occur during the progression of type 2 diabetes, with particular focus on the key role of declining β-cell function. The authors review clinical characteristics—long diabetes duration and A1C ≥9%—that are indicative of diminishing β-cell function, and they discuss the clinical data that support the use of available treatment options for these individuals, consistent with current diabetes treatment guidelines.

This article is intended to briefly summarize those discussions. The videos described below are available in their entirety, along with short biographies of the authors, at https://diabetesjournals.org/clinical/pages/combination-injectable-therapy.

Video Summaries

Need for Glycemic Control in Individuals With A1C ≥9% (Video 1)

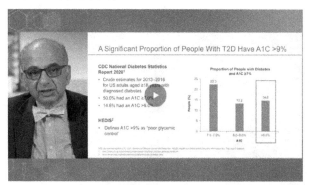

Video 1. Need for Glycemic Control in Individuals With A1C ≥9%. Available from https://bcove.video/3bda5FB.

Current treatment guidelines for people with type 2 diabetes from the American Diabetes Association, the American Association of Clinical Endocrinologists, the American College of Endocrinology, and the American College of Physicians recommend A1C targets within the range of 6.5–8% (1–3). However, public health reports suggest that a significant proportion of U.S. adults with diabetes have an A1C >9% (4), which is defined as "poor glycemic control" by the Healthcare Effectiveness Data and Information Set (5). Furthermore, A1C levels >9% can negatively affect reimbursement (e.g., through a decrease in the star ratings used to assess quality and performance) (6).

In this video, the authors discuss the deleterious health consequences for patients with high A1C levels, including data from the Diabetes & Aging Study, which demonstrated increased risk of microvascular events in individuals with A1C ≥9% (7). Data showing the relationship between the cumulative burden of microvascular disease and increased risk of cardiovascular disease (and the associated risk factors of hyperglycemia, hypertension, and dyslipidemia) in individuals with type 2 diabetes are also reviewed (8).

The UK Prospective Diabetes Study (9) showed that a 1% reduction in A1C was associated with a 37% reduction in the risk of microvascular complications. Although A1C targets differ among guidelines, all recommend individualization

[1]Tulane University Health Sciences Center, New Orleans, LA; [2]Fifth Avenue Endocrinology, New York, NY; [3]Emory University, Atlanta, GA

Corresponding author: Vivian A. Fonseca, vfonseca@tulane.edu

https://doi.org/10.2337/cd20-0121

©2021 by the American Diabetes Association. Readers may use this article as long as the work is properly cited, the use is educational and not for profit, and the work is not altered. More information is available at https://www.diabetesjournals.org/content/license.

of care and include caveats that targets should be relaxed in individuals at risk for hypoglycemia or with significant comorbidities and made more stringent for others, such as those with long life expectancy.

Role and Clinical Characteristics of Beta-Cell Dysfunction in the Progression of Type 2 Diabetes (Video 2)

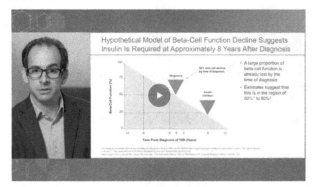

Video 2. Role and Clinical Characteristics of Beta-Cell Dysfunction in the Progression of Type 2 Diabetes. Available from https://bcove.video/306wFte.

The transition from impaired glucose tolerance to type 2 diabetes is associated with the progressive loss of β-cell mass and secretory capacity, which results in the inability to compensate for increased insulin resistance (10). In this video, the authors discuss the pathophysiological changes that occur during the progression of type 2 diabetes, with a particular focus on the key role of declining β-cell function. Estimates suggest that 50–80% of β-cell function is already lost at the time of type 2 diabetes diagnosis and that, ~8 years after diagnosis, β-cell function has declined to the point that insulin therapy may be needed (11).

The authors review clinical characteristics that are indicative of diminishing β-cell function. They discuss the results of the recent All New Diabetics in Scania cohort study (12), which suggest that nearly one-fifth of individuals with type 2 diabetes have severe insulin-deficient diabetes with characteristics such as younger age, lower BMI, and high A1C that are similar to those with type 1 diabetes; these individuals represent a higher proportion of the total type 2 diabetes population than is generally appreciated (12).

The authors review the complexities of determining whether β-cells are committed to failure and discuss the deleterious effect of glucotoxicity (i.e., high A1C) on β-cells, particularly when persistent (13). The authors also discuss the requirement for aggressive treatment in this setting to prevent not only complications, but also further deterioration of β-cell function. They advise that, ideally, clinicians should select agents

that do not act through a β-cell mechanism and do not overstimulate β-cells. The assessment of β-cell function as measured by C-peptide is discussed, and data from the Veterans Affairs Diabetes Trial cohort, which showed that C-peptide levels decrease with increasing duration of diabetes, are reviewed (14). However, the authors agree that C-peptide testing is often not practical in the primary care setting.

Increased awareness of patient characteristics may help practitioners to identify individuals who may be at risk for β-cell failure and for whom treatments that can facilitate β-cell rest should be considered. These characteristics include long duration of type 2 diabetes (>8 years), high A1C (≥9%) (15,16), and previous use of insulin secretagogue agents (17).

Clinical Implications of Beta-Cell Status on Therapeutic Selection (Video 3)

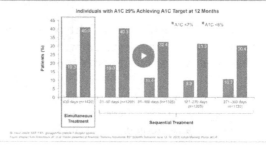

Video 3. Clinical Implications of Beta-Cell Status on Therapeutic Selection. Available from https://bcove.video/3bcEALW.

Several studies have shown that treatment with agents that stimulate β-cell function, including sulfonylureas and dipeptidyl peptidase 4 inhibitors, is associated with accelerated β-cell exhaustion and deterioration of glycemic control (18,19). In this video, the authors discuss treatments that do not stimulate β-cells.

The authors review evidence showing that early insulin therapy preserves β-cell function and can improve overall glycemic control (20). They also discuss glucagon-like peptide 1 receptor agonists (GLP-1 RAs), which are the recommended first injectable therapy for the majority of people with type 2 diabetes (1,2) because of their glycemic efficacy and lack of association with weight gain and hypoglycemia.

GLP-1 RAs suppress glucagon secretion and slow gastric emptying; however, agents within this class have differing mechanisms of action. Long-acting GLP-1 RAs act via glucose-dependent stimulation of insulin secretion and are hypothesized to increase secretory stress on β-cells; they also cause continuous stimulation of the GLP-1 receptor and consequent tachyphylaxis of the gastric emptying effect.

In contrast, short-acting GLP-1 RAs tend to exert their action primarily via a delay in gastric emptying and, because they have only intermittent receptor engagement, do not cause tachyphylaxis and are hypothesized to induce β-cell rest (21). The authors review results from a descriptive post hoc analysis, which showed that short-acting GLP-1 RA therapy reduced A1C, fasting plasma glucose, and postprandial glucose regardless of the level of β-cell function (22).

The rationale for combination therapy comprising a GLP-1 RA and basal insulin is based on the complementary effects of agents in these two drug classes. This combination has potent glucose-lowering actions and is associated with less weight gain and hypoglycemia than intensified insulin regimens (1). Real-world data have shown that, for the majority of individuals with A1C ≥9% and progression of type 2 diabetes despite oral therapy, neither a short-acting GLP-1 RA nor basal insulin was sufficient to reach glycemic targets when administered alone (23). Furthermore, the results of a retrospective cohort study of people with A1C ≥9% receiving oral antihyperglycemic agents who initiated both a GLP-1 RA and basal insulin in any order showed that those who initiated the two therapies on separate occasions were less likely to achieve glycemic control than those who initiated them on the same day or within 90 days of each other (24).

Two fixed-ratio combination (FRC) therapies comprising a basal insulin and a GLP-1 RA are currently available: iGlarLixi and IDegLira. iGlarLixi is an FRC of basal insulin glargine 100 units/mL and the short-acting GLP-1 RA lixisenatide 33 μg/mL that delivers doses from 15 to 60 units as a once-daily injection. IDegLira is an FRC of basal insulin degludec 100 units/mL and the long-acting GLP-1 RA liraglutide 3.6 mg/mL that delivers doses from 10 to 50 units, also as a once-daily injection.

Insulin/GLP-1 RA Fixed-Ratio Combination Therapy After Failure of Oral Antihyperglycemic Agents (Video 4)

LixiLan-O: High A1C (≥9%) Subgroup Analysis

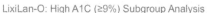
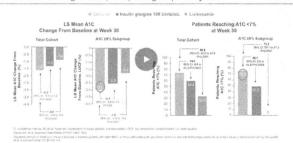

Video 4. Insulin/GLP-1 RA Fixed-Ratio Combination Therapy After Failure of Oral Antihyperglycemic Agents. Available from https://bcove.video/3sOEu3g.

In this video, the authors discuss the use of FRC therapies in individuals with type 2 diabetes and A1C inadequately controlled despite the use of oral antihyperglycemic therapy.

The efficacy and safety of the available FRC products in this patient population were investigated in open-label, randomized phase 3 studies: the LixiLan-O study for iGlarLixi (25) and the DUAL-I study for IDegLira (26). The LixiLan-O study was a 30-week, multicenter trial that compared treatment with iGlarLixi versus either insulin glargine or lixisenatide alone in adults who had received oral therapy for at least 3 months and who continued metformin therapy (25). DUAL-I was a 26-week study in adults who had received treatment with metformin with or without pioglitazone and compared daily injections of IDegLira, insulin degludec, or liraglutide (26). Reductions from baseline in A1C were greater with FRC therapies than with either of their components when used as single agents. Additionally, more people who received an FRC therapy achieved A1C targets (<7 and ≤6.5%). Mean body weight decreased with the FRC therapies, whereas it increased with basal insulin alone. Individuals who received FRC therapy reported fewer gastrointestinal adverse events than those who received a single-agent GLP-1 RA (25,26). Post hoc analyses demonstrated that the benefit of each FRC therapy over its individual components in reducing A1C is maintained in individuals with A1C ≥9% (27,28).

Insulin/GLP-1 RA Fixed-Ratio Combination Therapy After Failure of Previous GLP-1 RA Therapy (Video 5)

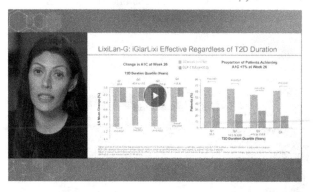

Video 5. Insulin/GLP-1 RA Fixed-Ratio Combination Therapy After Failure of Previous GLP-1 RA Therapy. Available from https://bcove.video/3uSzhJd.

In this video, the authors review the results of phase 3 randomized, open-label studies that assessed the efficacy and safety of FRC therapies in individuals with type 2 diabetes who had progressed despite their having received prior GLP-1 RA therapy. The 26-week LixiLan-G study enrolled adults on metformin and the maximum tolerated dose of a daily, twice-daily, or weekly GLP-1 RA, with or without pioglitazone and/or a sodium–glucose cotransporter 2 inhibitor and compared continuation of the GLP-1 RA with switching to iGlarLixi (29). In the DUAL III study, patients on a maximum-dose GLP-1 RA therapy (liraglutide once daily or exenatide twice daily) with oral agents (metformin alone or with pioglitazone and/or sulfonylurea therapy) were randomized to IDegLira once daily or to unchanged GLP-1 RA, continuing oral agents at pre-trial doses (30).

For both studies, the mean decrease in A1C from baseline was greater for the FRC than for stand-alone GLP-1 RA therapy, as was the proportion of individuals achieving target A1C levels. Weight change and gastro-intestinal adverse events appeared to be higher with FRC therapy than with a separate GLP-1 RA, but this was likely a consequence of switching from previous GLP-1 RA therapy. The results of a post hoc analysis of the LixiLan-G study according to C-peptide quartile showed that A1C reduction was significantly greater in the iGlarLixi arm than in the GLP-1 RA arm across all C-peptide quartiles, sug-gesting that the level of β-cell dysfunction has little, if any, impact on A1C outcomes achieved with iGlarLixi (31).

The authors also discussed the results of a propensity score–matched analysis (32) that compared outcomes from participants who received iGlarLixi in the LixiLan-L study (33) with those of participants who received basal-bolus insulin therapy in the GetGoal Duo-2 trial (34). The results of this analysis suggest that treatment intensification with iGlarLixi may be more efficacious and better tolerated than use of basal-bolus insulin (32).

Practical Tips for Using Fixed-Ratio Combination Therapies (Video 6)

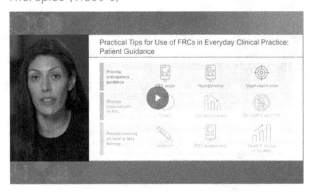

Video 6. Practical Tips for Using Fixed-Ratio Combination Therapies. Available from https://bcove.video/3qhUM2K.

The authors close their review by sharing their experience using FRC therapies, offering practical advice on patient selection, and providing points to consider before, and when initiating, an FRC therapy. Specifically, the authors focus on practical considerations for the initiation of FRCs in individuals with type 2 diabetes that is uncontrolled on two or more oral agents or on prior GLP-1 RA therapy, emphasizing that FRC therapies are particularly useful for patients with A1C ≥9% and a longer duration of type 2 diabetes. Changes to previous therapy and starting and maximum basal insulin doses are also discussed, as is the importance of anticipatory guidance on fasting plasma glucose, expectations of adverse events, and the provision of appropriate training. Finally, the authors provide practical tips for using an FRC therapy in individuals with type 2 diabetes who have renal insufficiency.

ACKNOWLEDGMENTS

The production of this video series and associated materials was funded by Sanofi US, Bridgewater, NJ. The authors received writing/editorial support in the preparation of the videos and executive summary from Helen Jones, PhD, CMPP, on behalf of Evidence Scientific Solutions in Philadelphia, PA. This assistance was also funded by Sanofi US.

REFERENCES

1. American Diabetes Association. 9. Pharmacologic approaches to glycemic treatment: *Standards of Medical Care in Diabetes—2021*. Diabetes Care 2021;44(Suppl. 1):S111–S124

2. Garber AJ, Handelsman Y, Grunberger G, et al. Consensus statement by the American Association of Clinical Endocrinol-ogists and American College of Endocrinology on the compre-hensive type 2 diabetes management algorithm: 2020 executive summary. Endocr Pract 2020;26:107–139

3. Qaseem A, Wilt TJ, Kansagara D, Horwitch C, Barry MJ; Clinical Guidelines Committee of the American College of Physicians. Hemoglobin A1c targets for glycemic control with pharmacologic therapy for nonpregnant adults with type 2 diabetes mellitus: a guidance statement update from the American College of Physicians. Ann Intern Med 2018;168:569–576

4. Centers for Disease Control and Prevention. National Diabetes Statistics Report, 2020: Estimates of Diabetes and Its Burden in the United States. Available from https://www.cdc.gov/diabetes/pdfs/data/statistics/national-diabetes-statistics-report.pdf. Accessed 12 October 2020

5. National Committee for Quality Assurance. Comprehensive diabetes care (CDC). Available from https://www.ncqa.org/hedis/measures/comprehensive-diabetes-care. Accessed 12 October 2020

6. Centers for Medicare & Medicaid Services. Medicare 2021 Part C & D star ratings technical notes. Available from https://www.cms.gov/files/document/2021technotes20201001.pdf-0. Accessed 4 January 2021

7. Laiteerapong N, Ham SA, Gao Y, et al. The legacy effect in type 2 diabetes: impact of early glycemic control on future complica-tions (the Diabetes & Aging Study). Diabetes Care 2019;42:416–426

8. Brownrigg JR, Hughes CO, Burleigh D, et al. Microvascular disease and risk of cardiovascular events among individuals with type 2 diabetes: a population-level cohort study. Lancet Diabetes Endocrinol 2016;4:588–597

9. Stratton IM, Adler AI, Neil HAW, et al. Association of glycaemia with macrovascular and microvascular complications of type 2 diabetes (UKPDS 35): prospective observational study. BMJ 2000; 321:405–412

10. Saisho Y. β-Cell dysfunction: its critical role in prevention and management of type 2 diabetes. World J Diabetes 2015;6:109–124

11. Lebovitz HE. Insulin secretagogues: old and new. Diabetes Rev (Alex) 1999;7:139–153

12. Ahlqvist E, Storm P, Käräjämäki A, et al. Novel subgroups of adult-onset diabetes and their association with outcomes: a data-driven cluster analysis of six variables. Lancet Diabetes Endocrinol 2018;6:361–369

13. Robertson RP, Harmon J, Tran PO, Tanaka Y, Takahashi H. Glucose toxicity in beta-cells: type 2 diabetes, good radicals gone bad, and the glutathione connection. Diabetes 2003;52:581–587

14. Duckworth WC, Abraira C, Moritz TE, et al.; Investigators of the VADT. The duration of diabetes affects the response to intensive glucose control in type 2 subjects: the VA Diabetes Trial. J Diabetes Complications 2011;25:355–361

15. Hou X, Liu J, Song J, et al. Relationship of hemoglobin A1c with β cell function and insulin resistance in newly diagnosed and drug naive type 2 diabetes patients. J Diabetes Res 2016;2016:8797316

16. Russo GT, Giorda CB, Cercone S, Nicolucci A; BetaDecline Study Group. Factors associated with beta-cell dysfunction in type 2 diabetes: the BETADECLINE study. PLoS One 2014;9:e109702

17. Russo GT, Giorda CB, Cercone S, De Cosmo S, Nicolucci A; BetaDecline Study Group. Beta cell stress in a 4-year follow-up of patients with type 2 diabetes: a longitudinal analysis of the BetaDecline study. Diabetes Metab Res Rev 2018;34:e3016

18. van Raalte DH, Verchere CB. Improving glycaemic control in type 2 diabetes: stimulate insulin secretion or provide beta-cell rest? Diabetes Obes Metab 2017;19:1205–1213

19. Biessels GJ, Verhagen C, Janssen J, et al. Effects of linagliptin versus glimepiride on cognitive performance in type 2 diabetes mellitus: the CAROLINA COGNITION sub-study (poster #583). Presented at the 55th Annual Meeting of the European Association for the Study of Diabetes in Barcelona, Spain, 16–20 September 2019

20. Kramer CK, Zinman B, Retnakaran R. Short-term intensive insulin therapy in type 2 diabetes mellitus: a systematic review and meta-analysis. Lancet Diabetes Endocrinol 2013;1:28–34

21. Miñambres I, Pérez A. Is there a justification for classifying GLP-1 receptor agonists as basal and prandial? Diabetol Metab Syndr 2017;9:6

22. Bonadonna RC, Blonde L, Antsiferov M, et al. Lixisenatide as add-on treatment among patients with different β-cell function levels as assessed by HOMA-β index. Diabetes Metab Res Rev 2017;33:e2897

23. Peng XV, Ayyagari R, Lubwama R, et al. Impact of simultaneous versus sequential initiation of basal insulin and glucagon-like peptide-1 receptor agonists on HbA1c in type 2

diabetes: a retrospective observational study. Diabetes Ther 2020;11:995–1005

24. Rosenstock J, Ampudia-Blasco FJ, Lubwama R, et al. Real-world evidence of the effectiveness on glycaemic control of early simultaneous versus later sequential initiation of basal insulin and glucagon-like peptide-1 receptor agonists. Diabetes Obes Metab 2020;22:2295–2304

25. Rosenstock J, Aronson R, Grunberger G, et al.; LixiLan-O Trial Investigators. Benefits of LixiLan, a titratable fixed-ratio combination of insulin glargine plus lixisenatide, versus insulin glargine and lixisenatide monocomponents in type 2 diabetes inadequately controlled on oral agents: the LixiLan-O randomized trial. Diabetes Care 2016;39:2026–2035

26. Gough SC, Bode B, Woo V, et al.; NN9068-3697 (DUAL-I) Trial Investigators. Efficacy and safety of a fixed-ratio combination of insulin degludec and liraglutide (IDegLira) compared with its components given alone: results of a phase 3, open-label, randomised, 26-week, treat-to-target trial in insulin-naive patients with type 2 diabetes. Lancet Diabetes Endocrinol 2014;2:885–893

27. Davies MJ, Russell-Jones D, Barber TM, et al. Glycaemic benefit of iGlarLixi in insulin-naive type 2 diabetes patients with high HbA1c or those with inadequate glycaemic control on two oral antihyperglycaemic drugs in the LixiLan-O randomized trial. Diabetes Obes Metab 2019;21:1967–1972

28. Sugimoto D, Frias J, Gouet D, et al. Effects of IDegLira (insulin degludec/liraglutide) in patients with poorly controlled type 2 diabetes (T2D) with A1C >9%: analyses from the DUAL program [Abstract]. Diabetes 2018;67(Suppl. 1);1092-P

29. Blonde L, Rosenstock J, Del Prato S, et al. Switching to iGlarLixi versus continuing daily or weekly GLP-1 RA in type 2 diabetes inadequately controlled by GLP-1 RA and oral anti-hyperglycemic therapy: the LixiLan-G randomized clinical trial. Diabetes Care 2019;42:2108–2116

30. Linjawi S, Bode BW, Chaykin LB, et al. The efficacy of IDegLira (insulin degludec/liraglutide combination) in adults with type 2 diabetes inadequately controlled with a GLP-1 receptor agonist and oral therapy: DUAL III randomized clinical trial. Diabetes Ther 2017;8:101–114

31. Del Prato S, Frias JP, Blonde L, et al. Impact of disease duration and β-cell reserve on the efficacy of switching to iGlarLixi in adults with type 2 diabetes on glucagon-like peptide-1 receptor agonist therapy: exploratory analyses from the LixiLan-G trial. Diabetes Obes Metab 2020;22:1567–1576

32. Tabák AG, Anderson J, Aschner P, et al. Efficacy and safety of iGlarLixi, fixed-ratio combination of insulin glargine and lixisenatide, compared with basal-bolus regimen in patients with type 2 diabetes: propensity score matched analysis. Diabetes Ther 2020;11:305–318

33. Aroda VR, Rosenstock J, Wysham C, et al.; LixiLan-L Trial Investigators. Efficacy and safety of LixiLan, a titratable fixed-ratio combination of insulin glargine plus lixisenatide in type 2 diabetes inadequately controlled on basal insulin and metformin: the LixiLan-L randomized trial. Diabetes Care 2016;39:1972–1980

34. Rosenstock J, Guerci B, Hanefeld M, et al.; GetGoal Duo-2 Trial Investigators. Prandial options to advance basal insulin glargine therapy: testing lixisenatide plus basal insulin versus insulin glulisine either as basal-plus or basal-bolus in type 2 diabetes: the GetGoal Duo-2 trial. Diabetes Care 2016;39:1318–1328

Ultra-Rapid-Acting Insulins: How Fast Is Really Needed?

Eva Y. Wong[1] and Lisa Kroon[2]

OBJECTIVE. To review the new ultra-rapid-acting insulin analogs and describe the benefits and limitations compared with other bolus insulins.

SUMMARY. The options for bolus insulins, which are usually taken at mealtime or for correction of hyperglycemia, are expanding, with recent approvals of faster-acting insulin aspart and insulin lispro-aabc. These new-generation insulins contain additives that enhance absorption and accelerate onset of action. Clinical studies demonstrate that, although these insulins are faster acting, their efficacy for A1C lowering and safety in terms of hypoglycemia risk are similar to those of other available bolus insulin options such as rapid-acting insulin analogs. However, their use resulted in significant reductions in 1- and 2-hour postprandial glucose levels.

CONCLUSION. Novel ultra-rapid-acting insulins provide additional bolus insulin options, and their quick onset of action provides additional dosing flexibility for people with diabetes. Given their comparable efficacy and safety compared to other quick-acting insulins, health care providers should engage in shared decision-making with patients and their caregivers regarding possible use of ultra-rapid-acting insulin, taking into account their preferences, individualized considerations, and insurance formulary coverage. These new insulin formulations may be a suitable option for people with diabetes who are not able to achieve postprandial glycemic targets with other bolus insulins.

In the United States, there are 34.2 million children and adults (10.5% of the population) with diabetes. Approximately one in five people with diabetes have not been diagnosed (1). Because of autoimmune destruction of insulin-producing pancreatic β-cells, insulin is required for people with type 1 diabetes. Among those with type 2 diabetes, some patients may eventually need insulin therapy because of the progressive course of the disease and eventual β-cell failure (2). The prevalence of type 2 diabetes and diabetes-related complications is expected to increase continually based on increases in risk factors, including overweight and obesity, physical inactivity, and tobacco use, as well as common coexisting conditions such as hypertension and dyslipidemia (3).

In 1923, Iletin, a short-acting regular insulin derived from porcine pancreas, became the first type of insulin commercially available for diabetes management (4). Sixty years later, in 1983, recombinant human insulin produced by genetically altered bacteria was approved for the U.S. market (5). This recombinant formulation eliminated the risk of allergic reactions from earlier insulins derived from animal sources such as the bovine or porcine pancreas (5).

Further advancements in insulin therapy followed, with the approval of rapid-acting insulin analogs that better mimic the bolus secretion of physiological insulin (Figure 1). The first rapid-acting analog formulation, insulin lispro (Humalog), was approved in 1996, followed by insulin aspart (Novolog) in 2002, and insulin glulisine (Apidra) in 2004 (6). Most recently, a new class of insulins that have an even faster onset, referred to as "ultra-rapid-acting" insulins, have been introduced, with faster-acting insulin aspart (faster aspart; sold under the brand name Fiasp) approved in 2017 (7) and insulin lispro-aabc (URLi; sold under the brand name Lyumjev) approved in 2020 (8). With these new additions, clinicians have several bolus insulin options, with short-, rapid-, or ultra-rapid-acting time-action profiles, to assist patients with diabetes in managing postprandial glucose levels and making hyperglycemia corrections.

Ultra-Rapid-Acting Insulins

Faster Aspart

Insulin aspart is an analog of human insulin created by the replacement of amino acid proline (Pro) with aspartic acid (Asp) in the 28-amino-acid residues in the C-terminus of the β-chain (9). The substitution of ProB28 to

[1]Department of Pharmacy Practice, Marshall B. Ketchum University College of Pharmacy, Fullerton, CA; [2]Department of Clinical Pharmacy, University of California, San Francisco School of Pharmacy, San Francisco, CA

Corresponding author: Eva Y. Wong, ewong@ketchum.edu

https://doi.org/10.2337/cd20-0119

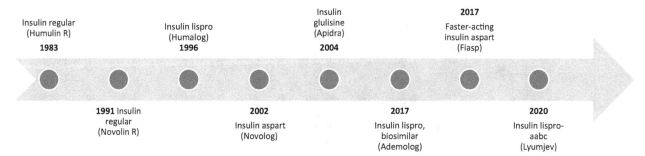

FIGURE 1 Timeline of U.S. Food and Drug Administration approval of bolus insulins (6).

AspB28 decreases the affinity of the insulin molecule to self-associate into hexamer formations. This change in the insulin structure results in a rapid onset of insulin activity compared with human insulin (10).

Faster aspart is similar to conventional insulin aspart (IAsp) except that it is formulated with niacinamide (vitamin B3) for faster absorption and a naturally occurring amino acid (L-arginine) to improve stability (11). These additives enable it to appear in the bloodstream in 2.5 minutes compared with 5.2 minutes with IAsp (12). Time to maximum insulin concentration is achieved 63 minutes after administration of faster aspart, which is 7.3 minutes earlier than with IAsp (12). Compared with that of IAsp, the pharmacodynamic profile of faster aspart includes a faster onset of action, occurring within 20–30 minutes, which is ~5 minutes earlier; a faster time to peak effect, occurring in 1.5–2.2 hours, which is ~10 minutes earlier; and a comparable duration of action (5 vs. 3–5 hours) (12). Faster aspart was initially approved in 2017 for the treatment of adults with diabetes, but in 2020, its indication was expanded to include children ≥2 years of age with diabetes (13).

In patients with type 1 diabetes, the results from the onset 1 clinical trial demonstrated that faster aspart was not inferior to IAsp in A1C reduction in the mealtime (administered 0–2 minutes before meals) and postmeal (administered 20 minutes after the start of meals) treatment groups ($P < 0.0001$) (Table 1) (14). One- and two-hour postprandial glucose (PPG) increments were statistically significantly lower in favor of faster aspart given at mealtimes ($P < 0.0001$ and $P = 0.0089$, respectively) (14). The initial study period was 26 weeks, which was extended an additional 26 weeks to determine whether faster aspart can maintain improved A1C glycemic control in the longer term. The full 52-week trial results were consistent with the initial 26-week findings in that patients treated with mealtime

faster aspart achieved similar improvements in A1C in comparison with IAsp ($P = 0.0424$). Improvements were seen at the 1-hour PPG increment end point (−16.7 mg/dL [95% CI −28.5 to −5.0], $P = 0.0054$); however, there was no statistically significant difference in 2-hour PPG reduction (−7.2 mg/dL [95% CI −21.5 to 7.13], $P = $ NS) (15). The results of the onset 1 trial favored faster aspart given at mealtime in comparison with postmeal timing, with varying degrees of 1- and 2-hour PPG A1C reduction, but similar long-term A1C reduction in patients with type 1 diabetes.

Faster aspart was tested in patients with type 2 diabetes in the onset 2 clinical trial, and results were similar to those in the onset 1 trial, demonstrating noninferiority for A1C reduction compared with IAsp ($P < 0.0001$). Additionally, the improvement in 1-hour PPG increment was statistically significant (−10.63 mg/dL [95% CI −19.56 to −1.69], $P = 0.0198$); however, the 2-hour PPG increment did not reach statistical significance (−6.57 mg/dL [95% CI −14.54 to 1.41], $P = 0.1063$) (16). Overall, the results from the onset 1 and onset 2 clinical trials demonstrated noninferiority in A1C reduction, with greater 1- and 2-hour PPG reductions with faster aspart compared with IAsp; however, the 2-hour PPG reductions were not sustained in the extended 52-week onset 1 trial or the onset 2 trial. Accordingly, the results demonstrating glycemic efficacy similar to IAsp and potential for further lowering of PPG support the consideration of faster aspart as an alternative bolus insulin for patients with type 1 or type 2 diabetes.

URLi

Insulin lispro is an analog of human insulin created by two amino acid changes of proline (Pro) and lysine (Lys) in the 28- and 29-amino-acid residues in the C-terminus of the β-chain (9). There is an inversion of ProB28 to LysB28 and LysB29 to ProB29, which reduces the tendency for hexamer formations (9). As in other

TABLE 1 Summary of Ultra-Rapid-Acting Insulin Randomized Controlled Trials (14,15,16,20,21)

Trial	Patient Demographics	Intervention(s)	A1C Outcome (ETD, %)	PPG Outcome (ETD, mg/dL)
onset 1 (26 weeks)	• T1D; n = 1,143 • Duration of diabetes: 20.9 ± 12.9 vs. 19.5 ± 12.1 vs. 19.3 ± 11.8 years • Baseline A1C: 7.6 ± 0.7 vs. 7.6 ± 0.7 vs. 7.6 ± 0.7% • Baseline FPG: 151.4 ± 55.8 vs. 145.6 ± 57.6 vs. 141.8 ± 50.2 mg/dL	Faster aspart mealtime (0–2 minutes before meals) vs. faster aspart postmeal (20 minutes after meals) vs. IAsp mealtime (0–2 minutes before meals)	Faster aspart mealtime vs. IAsp: −0.15% (95% CI −0.23 to −0.07), P <0.0001, noninferiority confirmed Faster aspart postmeal vs. IAsp: 0.04% (95% CI −0.04 to 0.12), P <0.0001, noninferiority confirmed	1-hour PPG: Faster aspart mealtime vs IAsp: −25.44 (95% CI −36.12 to −14.76), P <0.0001 in favor of faster aspart mealtime Faster aspart postmeal vs. IAsp: 12.38 (95% CI 1.65–23.11), P = 0.0238 in favor of IAsp 2-hour PPG: Faster aspart mealtime vs. IAsp: −16.73 (95% CI −29.26 to −4.20), P = 0.0089 in favor of faster aspart mealtime 2-hour PPG: Faster aspart postmeal vs. IAsp: 1.08 (95% CI −11.49 to 13.66), P = NS
onset 1 (52 weeks; initial 26 weeks plus an additional 26 weeks)	• T1D; n = 761 • Duration of diabetes: 20.9 ± 12.9 vs. 19.8 ± 11.8 years • Baseline A1C: 7.6 ± 0.7 vs. 7.6 ± 0.7% • Baseline FPG: 151.4 ± 55.8 vs. 141.8 ± 50.2 mg/dL	Faster aspart mealtime (0–2 minutes before meals) vs. IAsp mealtime (0–2 minutes before meals)	Faster aspart mealtime vs. IAsp: −0.10% (95% CI −0.19 to −0.00), P = 0.0424, noninferiority confirmed	1-hour PPG: Faster aspart mealtime vs. IAsp: −16.7 (95% CI −28.5 to −5.0), P = 0.0054 in favor of faster aspart mealtime 2-hour PPG: Faster aspart mealtime vs. IAsp: −7.2 (95% CI −21.5 to 7.13), P = NS
onset 2 (26 weeks)	• T2D; n = 689 • Duration of diabetes: 13.2 ± 6.7 vs. 12.3 ± 6.3 years • Baseline A1C: 8.0 ± 0.7 vs. 7.9 ± 0.7% • Baseline FPG: 121.7 ± 32.7 vs. 122.7 ± 35.1 mg/dL	Faster aspart mealtime (0–2 minutes before meals) vs. IAsp mealtime (0–2 minutes before meals)	Faster aspart mealtime vs. IAsp: −0.02% (95% CI −0.15 to 0.10), P <0.0001, noninferiority confirmed	1-hour PPG: Faster aspart mealtime vs. IAsp: −10.63 (95% CI −19.56 to −1.69), P = 0.0198 in favor of faster aspart mealtime 2-hour PPG: Faster aspart mealtime vs. IAsp: −6.57 (95% CI −14.54 to 1.41), P = NS

»*Continued from p. 417*

TABLE 1 Summary of Ultra-Rapid-Acting Insulin Randomized Controlled Trials [14,15,16,20,21]

Trial	Patient Demographics	Intervention(s)	A1C Outcome (ETD, %)	PPG Outcome (ETD, mg/dL)
PRONTO-T1D (26 weeks)	• T1D; n = 1,222 • Duration of diabetes: 18.8 ± 12.3 vs. 18.8 ± 11.7 vs. 19.1 ± 12.0 years • Baseline A1C: 7.34 ± 0.65 vs. 7.36 ± 0.64 vs. 7.33 ± 0.67% • Baseline FPG: NR	URLi mealtime (0–2 minutes before meals) vs. URLi postmeal (20 minutes after meals) vs. lispro mealtime (0–2 minutes before meals)	URLi mealtime vs. lispro: −0.08% (95% CI −0.16 to 0.00), P = 0.06, noninferiority confirmed URLi postmeal vs. lispro: 0.13% (95% CI 0.04–0.22), P = 0.003, noninferiority confirmed	1-hour PPG: URLi mealtime vs. lispro: −27.9 (95% CI −35.3 to −20.5), P <0.001 in favor of URLi mealtime URLi postmeal vs. lispro: 13.1 (95% CI 5.0–21.4), P <0.05 in favor of lispro URLi postmeal vs. URLi mealtime: 41.0 (95% CI 32.9-39.1), P <0.001 in favor of URLi mealtime 2-hour PPG: URLi mealtime vs. lispro: −31.1 (95% CI −41.0 to −21.2), P <0.001 in favor of URLi mealtime URLi postmeal vs. lispro: 13.1 (95% CI −17.6 to 4.3), P = NS URLi postmeal vs. URLi mealtime: 24.5 (95% CI 13.5–35.5), P <0.001 in favor of URLi mealtime
PRONTO-T2D (26 weeks)	• T2D; n = 673 • Duration of diabetes: 16.4 ± 7.8 vs. 6.6 ± 7.9 years • Baseline A1C: 7.27 ± 0.68 vs. 7.31 ± 0.72% • Baseline FPG: NR	URLi mealtime (0–2 minutes before meals) vs. lispro mealtime (0–2 minutes before meals)	URLi mealtime vs. lispro: 0.06% (95% CI −0.05 to 0.16), P = NR, noninferiority confirmed	1-hour PPG: URLi mealtime vs. lispro: −11.9 (95% CI −18.2 to −5.4), P <0.001 in favor of URLi mealtime 2-hour PPG: URLi mealtime vs. lispro: −17.3 (95% CI −25.4 to −9.4), P <0.001 in favor of URLi mealtime

ETD, estimated treatment difference; FPG, fasting plasma glucose; NR, not reported; NS, not significant; T1D, type 1 diabetes; T2D, type 2 diabetes.

rapid-acting insulin analogs, this change in the insulin structure results in a faster onset of action (9).

URLi is an ultra-rapid-acting insulin formulated with treprostinil and citrate to improve the absorption of insulin lispro (17). Treprostinil is a prostacyclin analog that improves absorption via local vasodilation, and citrate allows for faster absorption via local vascular permeability (17). In a pharmacokinetic and pharmacodynamic study, URLi appears in the bloodstream ~1 minute after injection; its time to maximum concentration is 57 minutes after administration, which is 14 minutes faster in patients with type 1 diabetes and 11 minutes faster in patients with type 2 diabetes than convention insulin lispro (18). In comparison with insulin lispro, URLi's time to measurable effect is 20.1 minutes (vs. 31 minutes) in patients with type 1 diabetes and 32 minutes (vs. 45 minutes) in patients with type 2 diabetes. Its peak effect is 2–2.9 hours (vs. 2.4–2.8 hours), and its duration of action is 5 hours (vs. 5.5–6.6 hours) in patients with type 1 diabetes and 6.4 hours (vs. 6.7 hours) in patients with type 2 diabetes (19). At this time, URLi is approved only for adults with type 1 or type 2 diabetes.

The PRONTO-T1D and PRONTO-T2D clinical trials demonstrated that mealtime (administered 0–2 minutes before meals) and postmeal (administered 20 minutes after the start of meals) URLi levels were noninferior to conventional insulin lispro in the primary outcome of A1C for patients with type 1 or type 2 diabetes (20,21). In patients with type 1 diabetes, URLi achieved a similar end-of-treatment A1C change whether given at mealtime (−0.08% [95% CI −0.16 to 0.00], $P = 0.06$) or postmeal (0.13% [95% CI 0.04–0.22], $P = 0.003$). Improvements in 1-hour PPG (−27.9 mg/dL [95% CI −35.3 to −20.5], $P < 0.001$) and 2-hour PPG (−31.1 mg/dL [95% CI −41.0 to −21.2], $P < 0.001$) favored URLi given at mealtime (18). In patients with type 2 diabetes, URLi achieved similar end-of-treatment A1C change (0.06% [95% CI −0.05 to 0.16]), confirming noninferiority, and demonstrated statistical significance in reducing 1-hour PPG (−11.9 mg/dL [95% CI −18.2 to −5.4], $P < 0.001$) and 2-hour PPG (−17.3 mg/dL [95% CI −25.4 to −9.4], $P < 0.001$) excursions in patients with type 2 diabetes (21).

Place for Ultra-Rapid-Acting Insulins in Diabetes Treatment

The new generation of ultra-rapid-acting insulins, including faster aspart and URLi, offers additional bolus insulin options for patients with type 1 or type 2 diabetes. Advantages to these faster-acting agents include

potential glycemic benefits in patients whose PPG is not at target, use in infusion pumps (only faster aspart is approved for such use at this time [22]), and their availability in convenient pen delivery devices.

These ultra-rapid-acting insulins provide a quick onset of action by achieving faster insulin absorption and faster times to maximum insulin concentration than other bolus insulins such as conventional short- and rapid-acting insulins. With faster aspart, the onset of action occurs 5 minutes earlier than with IAsp (23). URLi begins to act 10.9 minutes faster in patients with type 1 diabetes (24) and 13 minutes faster in patients with type 2 diabetes than conventional insulin lispro (19). With their faster onsets of action, these faster-acting bolus insulins provide patients the extra flexibility associated with injecting the medication just before or after meals. Their durations of action are similar to those of rapid-acting insulins, and, generally, there is no need to adjust basal insulin dosing when switching to the newer formulations. The onset 1 (26 weeks) and PRONTO-T1D trials demonstrated that faster aspart and URLi could be delivered either at mealtime (0–2 minutes before meals) or postmeal (20 minutes after meal), although mealtime administration provided statistically significant greater reductions in 1- and 2-hour PPG.

Compared with conventional rapid-acting analogs in phase 3, randomized, controlled trials, these newer faster-acting agents were confirmed to be noninferior in A1C reduction from baseline and achieved mixed results in reductions of 1- and 2-hour PPG (Table 1). Faster aspart demonstrated statistically significant greater reductions in both 1- and 2-hour PPG in the onset 1 (26 weeks) trial. Although there was a statistically significant reduction in 1-hour PPG compared with IAsp in the onset 1 (extended to 52 weeks) and onset 2 trials, the reductions in 2-hour PPG were not maintained and were not statistically significant in these trials. Alternatively, URLi demonstrated greater reductions in both 1- and 2-hour PPG in comparison with conventional lispro that were statistically significant in the PRONTO-T1D and PRONTO-T2D trials.

The results from these clinical studies suggest potential additional benefits in PPG control and may be useful in patients whose PPG targets have not been reached with other bolus insulin agents. These findings are especially relevant as more and more patients on insulin therapy self-monitor their glucose levels using continuous glucose monitoring (CGM) devices and tracking the metric of time in range.

These faster-acting agents are available in pen delivery devices, which are easier to use than traditional insulin vials and syringes. Both faster aspart and URLi are available in the standard U-100 (100 units/mL) concentration, but URLi also comes in a U-200 (200 units/mL) concentration for patients with higher bolus insulin dosage requirements. URLi U-100 is available in the Junior Kwikpen, which delivers 0.5-unit increments; the URLi U-100 KwikPen, URLi U-100 Tempo Pen, URLi U-200 Kwikpen, and faster aspart U-100 FlexTouch pen all deliver 1-unit increments (7,8).

Patients with diabetes who are using insulin infusion pumps may use either regular insulin or one of the rapid-acting insulin options. In clinical practice, ultra-rapid-acting insulins are also used in insulin pumps for the convenience and flexibility afforded by their quick action times. Based on the results of the onset 5 trial, the U.S. Food and Drug Administration approved faster aspart use in insulin pumps in October 2019 (22). With the recent approval of URLi, more studies are warranted to evaluate its efficacy and safety when used in insulin pumps.

Limitations and Additional Considerations

Additional considerations when evaluating the option of using a faster-acting insulin include the patient's age and pregnancy status, the ease of acquisition and cost of the medication, and the medication's long-term clinical and safety outcomes. Although faster aspart is approved for use in both children and adult patients (7), URLi is only approved for use in adult patients at this time; it has not yet been studied in children, and therefore its safety and efficacy in children with type 1 or type 2 diabetes are unknown (8).

Insulin therapy is the preferred treatment for managing hyperglycemia in women with gestational diabetes and in those with type 1 or type 2 diabetes during pregnancy, if pharmacotherapy is clinically indicated (25). The American College of Obstetricians and Gynecologists and The Endocrine Society recommend the use of insulin aspart and insulin lispro over regular insulin in patients with diabetes during pregnancy (26,27). However, these clinical guidelines were published before ultra-rapid-acting insulins became available. It is unknown whether faster aspart or URLi cross the placenta, and, because of methodological limitations, studies completed to date could not determine whether there are medication-related risks for major birth defects or miscarriage with these agents (7,8). Glycemic control in patients with diabetes is vital to maternal and fetal health and mitigates the risk for complications, including diabetic ketoacidosis, preterm delivery, preeclampsia, delivery complications, macrosomia, and major birth defects. Based on the limited data available, ultra-rapid-acting insulins cannot be recommended as a bolus option during pregnancy at this time, and rapid-acting insulins would be safer options.

Medication acquisition and costs should be considered when initiating or adjusting therapy. The costs of the ultra-rapid-acting insulin analogs are similar to those of rapid-acting insulin analogs (Table 2). For patients who have medication acquisition issues or for whom cost is a primary concern (e.g., those who self-pay for health care or are under-or uninsured), clinicians may consider prescribing more affordable bolus insulins such as regular human insulin, including the Walmart-branded ReliOn Novolin regular insulin (28) or the biosimilar insulin lispro analog Admelog (29). For patients with commercial or government insurance, the drug formulary should be reviewed first to select the plan's preferred bolus insulin agent.

With the steeply rising costs of insulins, many professional diabetes associations and patient advocacy groups, as well as the federal government, have pressured insulin manufacturers to reduce their insulin prices. Some manufacturers have reduced copayment programs (e.g., $35/month out of pocket), but not all people with diabetes are eligible (e.g., Medicare patients) (30). Fortunately, several Medicare Part D plans are now offering maximum copayments of $35 or less as of January 2021 (25).

Although ultra-rapid-acting insulins appear more quickly in the bloodstream and have a quicker time to first measurable effect, these characteristics have not been found to translate into clinically significant improvements in long-term glycemic control and safety outcomes. The clinical trials demonstrated that the efficacy of ultra-rapid-acting insulins in overall glycemic control as measured by A1C is comparable to that of their rapid-acting insulin counterparts. Secondary outcomes assessing medication safety found no significant treatment differences between the treatment groups in rates and incidences of severe, documented hypoglycemia. Ultimately, based on comparable efficacy and safety, all mealtime insulins may be considered viable options for bolus dosing in patients with type 1 or type 2 diabetes, depending on clinician judgment, glycemic response, and patient preference.

TABLE 2 Bolus Insulins Available in the United States (28,29,31,32)

Generic Name	Trade Name	Form	Concentration	Onset, minutes	Peak, minutes	Duration, hours	Cost (WAC) (29)
Ultra-rapid-acting insulins							
Faster aspart	Fiasp	Analog	U-100	16–20	63	5–7	$289.36/one 10-mL vial
							$558.83/five 3-mL FlexPens
							$537.47/five 3-mL Penfill cartridges
URLi	Lyumjev	Analog	U-100				$274.70/one 10-mL vial
							$530.40/five 3-mL KwikPens
			U-200	15–17	57	4.6–7.3	$424.32/two 3-mL KwikPens
Rapid-acting insulins							
Insulin aspart	Novolog	Analog	U-100	10–20	30–90	3–5	$289.36/one 10-mL vial
							$537.45/five 3-mL Penfill cartridges
							$558.83/five 3-mL FlexPens
Insulin glulisine	Apidra	Analog	U-100	10–20	30–90	3–5	$283.95/one 10-mL vial
							$548.52/five 3-mL SoloStar pens
Insulin lispro	Humalog	Analog	U-100	10–20	30–90	3–5	$137.35/one 10-mL vial
							$265.20/five 3-mL KwikPens or KwikPen Juniors
			U-200	15	30–90	3–5	$424.32/two 3-mL KwikPens
Insulin lispro, biosimilar	Admelog	Analog	U-100	15	30–90	3–5	$130.76/one 10-mL vial
							$39.23/one 3-mL vial
							$252.47/five 3-mL SoloStar pens
Insulin, inhaled	Afrezza	Human	U-100	12	35–55	1.5–4.5	$353.91/90 4-unit cartridges
							$707.82/90 8-unit cartridges
							$1,061.74/90 12-unit cartridges
Short-acting insulins							
Insulin, regular	Humulin R	Human	U-100	30–60	120–240	5–8	$148.70/one 10-mL vial
							$44.61/one 3-mL vial
	Novolin R	Human	U-100	30	80–120	Up to 8	$137.70/one 10-mL vial
							$25/one 10-mL vial (ReliOn) (29)

WAC, wholesale acquisition cost.

In collaboration with patients and caregivers, other important factors (e.g., patients' preferences, vision impairment, hearing impairment, and hand dexterity) should also be taken into consideration when starting or switching to a particular bolus insulin and delivery device.

Conclusion

The availability of ultra-fast-acting insulins provides additional bolus insulin alternatives for patients with type 1 or type 2 diabetes. Although this new generation, including faster aspart and URLi, allow for a quicker rate of absorption and onset of action, the array of available bolus insulins all provide similar A1C-lowering effects and similar rates of severe, confirmed hypoglycemia in patients with diabetes. When initiating or switching to a new bolus insulin, health care providers can select from the bolus insulin options and should keep in mind patient-specific considerations and patients' insurance coverage. An ultra-rapid-acting insulin may be a good choice for patients with diabetes who are not reaching PPG targets with other bolus agents.

DUALITY OF INTEREST

No potential conflicts of interest relevant to this article were reported.

AUTHOR CONTRIBUTIONS

Both authors conceptualized, wrote, reviewed, and edited the manuscript. Both authors are guarantors of this work and, as such, had full access to all of the data reported and take responsibility for the integrity and accuracy of the article.

REFERENCES

1. Centers for Disease Control and Prevention. *National Diabetes Statistics Report, 2020*. Available from https://www.cdc.gov/diabetes/pdfs/data/statistics/national-diabetes-statistics-report.pdf. Accessed 7 July 2020

2. American Diabetes Association. 2. Pharmacologic approaches to glycemic treatment: *Standards of Medical Care in Diabetes—2020*. Diabetes Care 2020;43(Suppl. 1):S98–S110

3. Centers for Disease Control and Prevention, U.S. Diabetes Surveillance System. Diagnosed diabetes. Available from https://gis.cdc.gov/grasp/diabetes/diabetesatlas.html. Accessed 7 July 2020

4. White JR Jr. A brief history of the development of diabetes medications. Diabetes Spectr 2014;27:82–86

5. American Diabetes Association. Timeline. Available from https://www.diabetes.org/resources/timeline. Accessed 7 July 2020

6. U.S. Food and Drug Administration. Drugs@FDA: FDA-approved drugs. Available from https://www.accessdata.fda.gov/scripts/cder/daf. Accessed 7 July 2020

7. Novo Nordisk. Fiasp [package insert]. Plainsboro, NJ, Novo Nordisk, 2019

8. Eli Lilly and Company. Lyumjev [package insert]. Indianapolis, IN, Eli Lilly and Company, 2020

9. Williams DA. *Foye's Principles of Medicinal Chemistry*. 7th ed. Philadelphia, PA, Lippincott Williams & Wilkins, 2012

10. Mudaliar SR, Lindberg FA, Joyce M, et al. Insulin aspart (B28 asp-insulin): a fast-acting analog of human insulin: absorption kinetics and action profile compared with regular human insulin in healthy nondiabetic subjects. Diabetes Care 1999;22:1501–1506

11. Kildegaard J, Buckley ST, Nielsen RH, et al. Elucidating the mechanism of absorption of fast-acting insulin aspart: the role of niacinamide. Pharm Res 2019;36:49

12. Heise T, Hövelmann U, Brøndsted L, Adrian CL, Nosek L, Haahr H. Faster-acting insulin aspart: earlier onset of appearance and greater early pharmacokinetic and pharmacodynamic effects than insulin aspart. Diabetes Obes Metab 2015;17:682–688

13. Melillo G. FDA approves Fiasp for children with diabetes. Available from https://www.ajmc.com/newsroom/fda-approves-fiasp-for-children-with-diabetes. Accessed 8 July 2020

14. Russell-Jones D, Bode BW, De Block C, et al. Fast-acting insulin aspart improves glycemic control in basal-bolus treatment for type 1 diabetes: results of a 26-week multicenter, active-controlled, treat-to-target, randomized, parallel-group trial (onset 1). Diabetes Care 2017;40:943–950

15. Mathieu C, Bode BW, Franek E, et al. Efficacy and safety of fast-acting insulin aspart in comparison with insulin aspart in type 1 diabetes (onset 1): a 52-week, randomized, treat-to-target, phase III trial. Diabetes Obes Metab 2018;20:1148–1155

16. Bowering K, Case C, Harvey J, et al. Faster aspart versus insulin aspart as part of a basal-bolus regimen in inadequately controlled type 2 diabetes: the onset 2 trial. Diabetes Care 2017;40:951–957

17. Pratt E, Leohr J, Heilmann C, Johnson J, Landschulz W. Treprostinil causes local vasodilation, is well tolerated, and results in faster absorption of insulin lispro [Abstract]. Diabetes 2017;66(Suppl. 1):A253

18. Michael MD, Zhang C, Siesky AM, et al. Exploration of the mechanism of accelerated absorption for a novel insulin lispro formulation [Abstract]. Diabetes 2017;66(Suppl. 1):A250

19. Leohr J, Dellva MA, Coutant DE, et al. Pharmacokinetics and glucodynamics of ultra rapid lispro (URLi) versus Humalog (lispro) in patients with type 2 diabetes mellitus: a phase I randomised, crossover study. Clin Pharmacokinet 2020;59:1601–1610

20. Klaff L, Cao D, Dellva MA, et al. Ultra rapid lispro improves postprandial glucose control compared with lispro in patients with type 1 diabetes: results from the 26-week PRONTO-T1D study. Diabetes Obes Metab 2020;22:1799–1807

21. Blevins T, Zhang Q, Frias JP, Jinnouchi H; PRONTO-T2D Investigators. Randomized double-blind clinical trial comparing ultra rapid lispro with lispro in a basal-bolus regimen in patients with type 2 diabetes: PRONTO-T2D. Diabetes Care 2020;43:2991–2998

22. Klonoff DC, Evans ML, Lane W, et al. A randomized, multicentre trial evaluating the efficacy and safety of fast-acting insulin aspart in continuous subcutaneous insulin infusion in adults with type 1 diabetes (onset 5). Diabetes Obes Metab 2019;21:961–967

23. Heise T, Linnebjerg H, Coutant D, et al. Ultra rapid lispro lowers postprandial glucose and more closely matches normal physiological glucose response compared to other rapid insulin analogues: a phase 1 randomized, crossover study. Diabetes Obes Metab 2020;22:1789–1798

24. Linnebjerg H, Zhang Q, LaBell E, et al. Pharmacokinetics and glucodynamics of ultra rapid lispro (URLi) versus Humalog (lispro) in younger adults and elderly patients with type 1 diabetes mellitus: a randomised controlled trial. Clin Pharmacokinet 2020;59:1589–1599

25. American Diabetes Association. 14. Management of diabetes in pregnancy: *Standards of Medical Care in Diabetes—2021*. Diabetes Care 2021;44(Suppl. 1):S200–S210

26. American College of Obstetricians and Gynecologists (ACOG) Committee on Practice Bulletins—Obstetrics. ACOG Practice Bulletin No. 190: gestational diabetes mellitus. Obstet Gynecol 2018;131:e49–e64

27. Blumer I, Hadar E, Hadden DR, et al. Diabetes and pregnancy: an Endocrine Society clinical practice guideline. J Clin Endocrinol Metab 2013;98:4227–4249

28. Fennell D. ReliOn insulin for $25 a vial at Walmart. Available from http://www.diabetesselfmanagement.com/blog/relion-insulin-for-25-a-vial-at-walmart. Accessed 6 October 2020

29. Micromedex. RED BOOK Online. Available from https://www.micromedexsolutions.com. Accessed 9 July 2020

30. Hayes TO, Farmer J. Insulin cost and pricing trends. Available from https://www.americanactionforum.org/research/insulin-cost-and-pricing-trends. Accessed 6 October 2020

31. American Diabetes Association. Consumer guide 2017: medications. Available from http://main.diabetes.org/dforg/pdfs/2017/2017-cg-medications.pdf. Accessed 20 June 2020

32. Sanofi. Admelog [package insert]. Bridgewater, NJ, Sanofi, 2019

Prevalence of and Characteristics Associated With Overbasalization Among Patients With Type 2 Diabetes Using Basal Insulin: A Cross-Sectional Study

Kevin Cowart,[1,2] Wendy H. Updike,[1,3] and Rashmi Pathak[4]

This article describes a cross-sectional analysis of 655 patients to determine the prevalence of and patient-specific characteristics associated with overbasalization in patients with type 2 diabetes. Overbasalization was defined as uncontrolled A1C (>8%) plus a basal insulin dose >0.5 units/kg/day. The period prevalence of overbasalization was found to be 38.1, 42.7, and 42% for those with an A1C >8, ≥9, and ≥10%, respectively. Those with an A1C ≥9% had the greatest likelihood of experiencing overbasalization. These results suggest that overbasalization may play a role in patients not achieving optimal glycemic control in type 2 diabetes.

Overbasalization is defined as the titration of basal insulin beyond an appropriate dose in an attempt to achieve glycemic targets (1). Current clinical practice guidelines suggest treatment intensification to address postprandial hyperglycemia when a patient's A1C target is not being achieved at a basal insulin dose >0.5 units/kg/day (2,3). However, the strength of this recommendation is based on expert opinion because few studies have investigated the maximum effective dose of basal insulin at which treatment intensification is indicated (4). Overbasalization is not well studied as a barrier to achieving glycemic targets. The aim of this study was to identify the prevalence of and patient-specific characteristics associated with overbasalization in patients with type 2 diabetes.

Research Design and Methods

This was a cross-sectional study conducted at the University of South Florida Department of Family Medicine between 1 January 2015 and 31 December 2018.

Inclusion criteria were age 18–80 years, diagnosis of type 2 diabetes for at least 12 months, and at least one clinic visit with a medical provider. The first clinic visit within the study time frame at which a prescription for a basal insulin (glargine U-100, glargine U-300, detemir, degludec U-100, degludec U-200, regular U-500, or NPH insulin) was generated was defined as the index date. The basal insulin dose must have been included on the prescription for inclusion in the study.

The most recent A1C prior to 90 days of the index date was used for the analysis. If an A1C was not available within this time frame, the subject was excluded. Prisoners, pregnant women, and individuals prescribed prandial insulin, a noninsulin injectable (glucagon-like peptide-1 [GLP-1] receptor agonist or pramlintide), or a fixed ratio combination of a basal insulin and a GLP-1 receptor agonist were excluded.

Baseline demographics were analyzed using descriptive statistics. Overbasalization was defined as an A1C >8% plus a basal insulin dose >0.5 units/kg/day. The period prevalence of overbasalization was calculated by determining the number of patients with uncontrolled type 2 diabetes (A1C >8%), and who had a basal insulin dose >0.5 units/kg/day, as compared with patients with the same A1C but without a basal insulin dose >0.5 units/kg/day. The period prevalence was also calculated for those with an A1C of ≥9 and ≥10%.

Univariate logistic regression analysis was performed to determine the significance of several baseline patient characteristics (age, BMI, sex, A1C, race/ethnicity, and type of basal insulin) with the dependent variable (overbasalization). Variables found to be significant in

[1]Department of Pharmacotherapeutics & Clinical Research, Taneja College of Pharmacy, University of South Florida, Tampa, FL; [2]Department of Internal Medicine, Morsani College of Medicine, University of South Florida, Tampa, FL; [3]Department of Family Medicine, Morsani College of Medicine, University of South Florida, Tampa, FL; [4]College of Public Health, University of South Florida, Tampa, FL

Corresponding author: Kevin Cowart, kcowart2@usf.edu

https://doi.org/10.2337/cd20-0080

the univariate analysis were then included in a backward-elimination multivariate regression model. The concentrated insulin products (regular U-500, glargine U-300, and degludec U-200) were excluded from the multivariate regression model to minimize confounding by indication because they may be indicated for people with a basal insulin dose >0.5 units/kg/day. Statistical significance was defined as $\alpha < 0.05$ for all analyses. The analysis was conducted using SAS, v. 9.4 (SAS Institute, Cary, NC). This study was certified exempt by the University of South Florida's institutional review board.

Results

A total of 655 patients (mean age 57 ± 13.4 years) were included in this analysis. The mean BMI was 32.4 kg/m^2 (SD ± 8.7), and 48% of the subjects were male. The majority of patients (57.3%) were White, followed by 24.4% being Black or African American. The mean A1C was 8.4% (SD ± 2.2) and the mean dose of basal insulin was 0.4 units/kg/day (SD ± 0.4). The majority of patients were prescribed insulin glargine U-100 (63.2%), followed by insulin detemir U-100 (21.4%). The period prevalence of overbasalization in this population was found to be 38.1, 42.7, and 42% for those with an A1C >8, ≥9, and ≥10%, respectively. Mean BMI did not differ clinically between these groups (A1C >8%: 32.1 kg/m^2 [SD ± 8.8]; A1C ≥9%: 31.5 kg/m^2 [SD ± 8.4]; A1C ≥10%: 31.5 kg/m^2 [SD ± 8.1]).

In the univariate regression analysis, the following patient characteristics were independently associated with overbasalization: age 35–54 years (odds ratio [OR] 1.89, 95% CI 1.24–2.88), age 65–80 years (OR 0.44, 95% CI 0.27–0.73), A1C ≥9% (OR 13.97, 95% CI 8.43–23.14), A1C ≥10% (OR 6.04, 95% CI 3.93–9.29), and prescription for insulin glargine U-100 (OR 0.62, 95% CI 0.41–0.93). In the multivariate analysis, only A1C ≥9% remained significant; thus, all other variables were eliminated from the model.

Discussion

This is the first report to our knowledge describing the prevalence of overbasalization in a primary care setting among patients with type 2 diabetes. Just under half of the population sampled in this cross-sectional study experienced overbasalization. It is worth mentioning that, regardless of the degree to which A1C was elevated, the prevalence of overbasalization remained similar (~40%). This finding suggests that a large number of patients with type 2 diabetes who are using basal insulin without

prandial insulin or a GLP-1 receptor agonist may benefit clinically from treatment intensification. Because the degree of fasting versus postprandial hyperglycemia varies by level of A1C and the prevalence of overbasalization was similar across varying A1C levels, it cannot be determined from this study whether individuals not meeting glycemic targets need additional basal insulin or postprandial coverage. Therefore, these preliminary findings are hypothesis-generating and support the need for additional investigation into the optimal dose of basal insulin at which to initiate postprandial coverage.

Several patient-specific characteristics were found to be independently associated with overbasalization, although when adjusted for potential confounders, an A1C ≥9% was the strongest predictor of overbasalization. These findings suggest that overbasalization may play a role in patients with type 2 diabetes not achieving optimal glycemic control, although this hypothesis requires additional investigation in a larger sample. Additionally, studies are needed to determine the association of hypoglycemia with overbasalization because that was not measured as a variable in this study and is an expected adverse outcome associated with overbasalization.

Limitations to this analysis include the limited independent variables that were measured to predict the dependent variable. Furthermore, oral antidiabetic medication use and length of time basal insulin was prescribed were not captured, and both may affect treatment decisions. Additionally, we did not exclude patients using steroids, which may transiently increase insulin requirements. Future work should also evaluate the following characteristics to define overbasalization: postmeal blood glucose >180 mg/dL, A1C not at goal despite attaining fasting blood glucose targets, or a bedtime-morning blood glucose differential ≥50 mg/dL (1). There may also be patients seen in clinical practice whose basal insulin dose is much larger than their prandial insulin dose (i.e., >50% of their total daily insulin dose) who may also be overbasalized (5–8), although such patients were not accounted for in the present analysis because prandial insulin use was an exclusion criterion. An additional consideration in light of high basal insulin doses in patients with suboptimal glycemic control is the potential for poor insulin injection technique. Given the retrospective nature and limited variables available for collection in the electronic medical record, we could not assess this, although it should be considered in future prospective evaluations. Additional limitations include the observational design (lack of temporality) and low external validity because analyzed data were from one academic family medicine practice. However, the study's strengths include its large sample size and an adjusted analysis for potential confounders affecting the dependent variable.

In conclusion, our findings are hypothesis-generating but suggest that overbasalization may play a role in patients with type 2 diabetes not achieving optimal glycemic control. The results highlight the need for additional investigation into therapeutic strategies that ascribe to a physiologic approach in the management of patients with type 2 diabetes using basal insulin. These strategies may involve continuous glucose monitoring or having shorter intervals between routine clinic visits to appropriately titrate basal insulin without delay in treatment intensification when warranted in those not meeting glycemic goals.

ACKNOWLEDGMENTS

The authors thank the following individuals who were Doctor of Pharmacy (PharmD) candidates at the time of publication for their assistance with data collection: C. Cayanan, T. Phan, J. Rummage, Y. Saba, N. Wesson, and S. Zambito.

DUALITY OF INTEREST

No potential conflicts of interest relevant to this article were reported.

AUTHOR CONTRIBUTIONS

K.C. contributed to the conception, study design, and statistical analysis and wrote the first draft of the manuscript. W.H.U. contributed to the acquisition and interpretation of the data and provided critical revisions to the manuscript for important intellectual content. R.P. contributed to the statistical analysis. K.C. is the guarantor of this work and, as such, had full access to all the data in the project and takes responsibility for the integrity of the data and the accuracy of the data analysis.

REFERENCES

1. Cowart K. Overbasalization: addressing hesitancy in treatment intensification beyond basal insulin. Clin Diabetes 2020;38:304–310

2. American Diabetes Association. 9. Pharmacologic approaches to glycemic treatment: *Standards of Medical Care in Diabetes—2020*. Diabetes Care 2020;43(Suppl. 1):S98–S110

3. Garber AJ, Handelsman Y, Grunberger G, et al. Consensus statement by the American Association of Clinical Endocrinologists and American College of Endocrinology on the comprehensive type 2 diabetes management algorithm: 2020 executive summary. Endocr Pract 2020;26:107–139

4. Umpierrez GE, Skolnik N, Dex T, Traylor L, Chao J, Shaefer C. When basal insulin is not enough: a dose-response relationship between insulin glargine 100 units/mL and glycaemic control. Diabetes Obes Metab 2019;21:1305–1310

5. LaSalle JR, Berria R. Insulin therapy in type 2 diabetes mellitus: a practical approach for primary care physicians and other health care professionals. J Am Osteopath Assoc 2013;113:152–162

6. Shubrook JH. Insulin for type 2 diabetes: how and when to get started. J Fam Pract 2014;63:76–81

7. Patel D, Triplitt C, Trujillo J. Appropriate titration of basal insulin in type 2 diabetes and the potential role of the pharmacist. Adv Ther 2019;36:1031–1051

8. Johnson EL, Frias JP, Trujillo JM. Anticipatory guidance in type 2 diabetes to improve disease management: next steps after basal insulin. Postgrad Med 2018;130:365–374

Optimizing Management of Type 2 Diabetes and Its Complications in Patients With Heart Failure

Christie A. Schumacher,[1] Elizabeth K. Van Dril,[2] Kayce M. Shealy,[3] and Jennifer D. Goldman[4]

Diabetes is an independent risk factor for heart failure (HF), with current trends indicating that nearly half of patients with type 2 diabetes will develop this complication. The presence of diabetes also worsens the prognosis of those with HF; people with both conditions have nearly double the mortality rate of those with HF who do not have diabetes (1–3). Additional risk factors for the development of HF in people with diabetes include increasing age, longer duration of disease, insulin use, ischemic heart disease, peripheral artery disease, nephropathy, poor glycemic management, hypertension, obesity, and higher levels of N-terminal pro b-type natriuretic peptide (2,4,5). Recently, HF, including diabetic cardiomyopathy, has become a more well-recognized complication of diabetes, with a prevalence rivaling that of established cardiovascular disease (CVD). Clinical interest in the management of type 2 diabetes in the presence of HF has grown with the publication of cardiovascular outcomes trials (CVOTs) for sodium–glucose cotransporter 2 (SGLT2) inhibitors demonstrating HF-related benefits and other trials showing heightened risk with the use of certain other antihyperglycemic therapies.

To understand the interrelatedness of diabetes and HF, it is important to understand the pathophysiology of HF in people with diabetes. Structural heart disease via cardiac ischemia and infarction, also known as ischemic cardiomyopathy, is a documented complication of hyperglycemia. Yet, ischemic events are not a requirement for the development of HF in people with diabetes. The presence of systolic or diastolic dysfunction in people with diabetes, in the absence of common causes such as coronary artery disease, hypertension, or valvular heart disease, is termed "diabetic cardiomyopathy" (5). The development of diabetic cardiomyopathy is multifactorial, with insulin resistance, changes in cellular metabolism, and hyperglycemia-induced advanced glycation end products triggering a cascade of deleterious effects that contribute to hypertrophy, fibrosis, autonomic dysfunction, and ultimately impaired ventricular contraction and relaxation (Figure 1) (5–10). These mechanisms lead to the development of HF and should be taken into consideration when selecting pharmacologic therapy for type 2 diabetes.

Recent guidelines for the management of type 2 diabetes focus on patients' comorbidities to determine the most appropriate add-on therapy. In its *Standards of Medical Care in Diabetes—2020,* the American Diabetes Association (ADA) stratifies specific comorbidities that include atherosclerotic CVD, chronic kidney disease (CKD), and HF (11). Metformin, in conjunction with lifestyle modifications that improve glycemic management, continues to be the preferred first-line therapy for the management of type 2 diabetes regardless of comorbidities. For patients with HF, SGLT2 inhibitors demonstrate the strongest evidence for clinical benefit related to HF morbidity and mortality and are recommended regardless of the patient's baseline A1C. A glucagon-like peptide 1 (GLP-1) receptor agonist with established cardiovascular benefit can be considered in this population if SGLT2 inhibitor use is contraindicated or not tolerated or can be added to SGLT2 inhibitor therapy, if needed. Other agents with demonstrated cardiovascular safety may be considered if additional or alternative therapy is needed to further reduce the patient's A1C. These include select dipeptidyl peptidase-4 (DPP-4) inhibitors (i.e., sitagliptin and linagliptin), select basal insulins (i.e., degludec and glargine 100 units/mL), and sulfonylureas with a lower risk of hypoglycemia (i.e., glipizide and glimepiride).

This review describes the co-management of diabetes and HF, provides a review of the preferred medication classes for the treatment of people with both of these diseases, and discusses recent clinical trial data for newer antihyperglycemic agents. It also offers practical considerations for clinicians who treat people with both diabetes

[1]Chicago College of Pharmacy, Midwestern University, Downers Grove, IL; [2]College of Pharmacy, University of Illinois at Chicago, Chicago, IL; [3]School of Pharmacy, Presbyterian College Clinton, SC; [4]MCPHS University, Boston, MA

Corresponding author: Christie A. Schumacher, cschum@midwestern.edu

https://doi.org/10.2337/cd20-0008

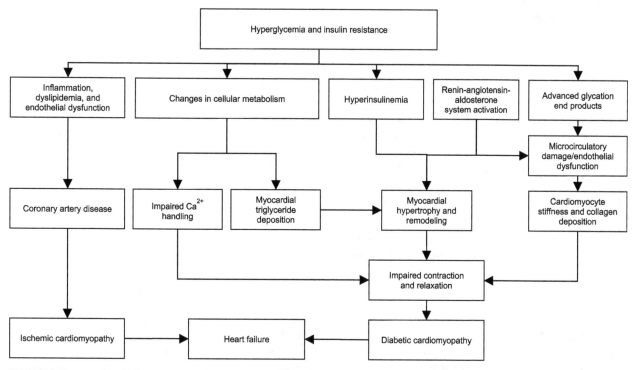

FIGURE 1 Proposed pathophysiology for HF in people with diabetes (5–10).

and HF. For a more extensive review of all of the drugs used for the treatment of type 2 diabetes, readers are referred to the ADA's Standards of Care (11).

Antihyperglycemic Therapy in People With Type 2 Diabetes and HF

The following noninsulin therapies are highlighted in the ADA's Standards of Care as options for the management of type 2 diabetes in people with HF. Below, we discuss hypothesized mechanisms of benefit or harm in people with HF and review relevant recent clinical trial data.

Metformin

Metformin is the preferred initial therapy in the management of patients with type 2 diabetes, including those with HF, because it is affordable, efficacious, and generally well tolerated (11). Metformin exerts its blood glucose–lowering effects by decreasing hepatic glucose production and intestinal absorption of glucose and increasing peripheral glucose uptake and utilization, thereby improving insulin sensitivity.

Despite initial concerns of lactic acidosis, metformin is considered safe in patients with stable HF and can safely be used in patients with an estimated glomerular filtration rate >30 mL/min/1.73 m^2 (12,13). A systematic review of nine cohort studies involving nearly 34,000 patients

demonstrated that patients with concomitant diabetes and HF who were receiving metformin had a 31% lower risk of all-cause mortality (14). A recent population-based retrospective cohort study further supported this finding, demonstrating a lower risk of hospitalization for HF (HHF) in patients treated with metformin when compared with those who have never been treated with metformin, with an overall risk reduction of 65% in the unmatched cohort and 43% in the matched cohort (15). These two studies and others have demonstrated the cost-effectiveness and safety of metformin in patients with diabetes and HF (14–16).

Caution should be used if there is a decline in cardiac output and subsequent decrease in renal perfusion from acute decompensated HF because the risk of lactic acidosis is greatest in hypoxic states. Metformin should be held or discontinued in such situations and can be reinitiated if patients' renal function recovers and they are hemodynamically stable.

SGLT2 Inhibitors

The significant reduction in HHF seen with SGLT2 inhibitors in clinical trials has established them as second-line therapy after metformin for patients with established atherosclerotic CVD, and they should be considered before a GLP-1 receptor agonist with cardiovascular benefit in patients with CKD or HF independent of baseline

TABLE 1 Summary of SGLT2 Inhibitor CVOTs in Patients With Type 2 Diabetes (17–19)

	EMPA-REG Outcome (Empagliflozin)	CANVAS Program (Canagliflozin)	DECLARE-TIMI 58 (Dapagliflozin)
Study size, n	7,020	10,142	17,160
Median follow-up, years	3.1	2.4	4.2
Patient population	A1C 7.0-9.0% without therapy or 7.0-10.0% on therapy; established CVD	A1C 7.0-10.5%; age ≥50 years with at least two CVD risk factors or age ≥30 years with a history of symptomatic CVD	A1C 6.5-12.0%; men age ≥55 years and women age ≥60 years with at least one CVD risk factor or established CVD
Primary end point(s), HR (95% CI)	3-point MACE*: 0.86 (0.74-0.99)	3-point MACE*: 0.86 (0.75-0.97)	3-point MACE*: 0.93 (0.84-1.03); cardiovascular death + HHF: 0.83 (0.73-0.95)
HF-related secondary end point, HR (95% CI)	HHF: 0.65 (0.50-0.85)	HHF: 0.67 (0.52-0.87)	HHF: 0.73 (0.61-0.88)

*3-point MACE included cardiovascular death, nonfatal myocardial infarction, and nonfatal stroke. CANVAS, Canagliflozin Cardiovascular Assessment Study; DECLARE-TIMI 58, Dapagliflozin Effect on Cardiovascular Events; EMPA-REG Outcome, BI 10773 (Empagliflozin) Cardiovascular Outcome Event Trial in Type 2 Diabetes Mellitus Patients; HR, hazard ratio.

A1C or individualized A1C target (11). SGLT2 inhibitors promote glucose homeostasis through an insulin-independent mechanism at the proximal tubule of the kidney. SGLT2 facilitates ~90% of renal glucose reabsorption, thereby increasing urinary glucose excretion and ultimately lowering blood glucose levels. In addition, inhibition of SGLT2 increases the fractional excretion of sodium, resulting in a moderate diuretic effect.

Three CVOTs evaluating SGLT2 inhibitors have demonstrated significant reductions in the risk for HHF in patients with type 2 diabetes (35% with empagliflozin, 33% with canagliflozin, and 27% with dapagliflozin) (Table 1) (17–19). These results were consistent regardless of whether patients had a history of HF or established CVD at baseline, and they have been further confirmed in real-world analyses (20–22). In the DAPA-HF (Dapagliflozin and Prevention of Adverse Outcomes in Heart Failure) trial, dapagliflozin was shown to decrease both the risk for worsening HF and death from cardiovascular causes in patients with HF with and without diabetes (23). These results appear to be independent of blood glucose, body weight, and blood pressure reductions, a finding that has led investigators to propose potential mechanisms for cardiac benefit. The three most commonly discussed proposed mechanisms are 1) the diuretic hypothesis, 2) the "thrifty substrate" hypothesis, and 3) the sodium hypothesis (24,25).

The diuretic hypothesis is derived from the natriuretic and osmotic effect of inhibition of glucose-coupled sodium reabsorption in the proximal tubule. The increase in sodium excretion drives plasma volume contraction, which may hemodynamically reduce the preload and ventricle filling pressure, leading to a decrease in myocardial oxygen demand, myocardial stretch, and ventricular wall tension (25). In addition, the increase in osmotic diuresis has been shown to decrease both systolic and diastolic blood pressure, which may be the result of persistent volume depletion. Clinical data regarding the diuretic effect are controversial because the plasma volume contraction has been shown to level off at ~12 weeks of treatment (26). In addition, diuretics have not demonstrated morbidity and mortality benefit in patients with HF, leading researchers to believe the benefit extends beyond natriuresis (27).

The thrifty substrate hypothesis is derived from the observation that SGLT2 inhibitors produce an increase in mean plasma ketone levels, notably β-hydroxybutyrate (BHB) (28). The lower glucose levels from SGLT2 inhibitors decrease the insulin response leading to lipolysis and ketogenesis, and it has been suggested that SGLT2 inhibitors directly stimulate glucagon secretion from pancreatic α-cells, which in turn stimulates hepatic ketogenesis. Research has suggested that BHB is a "super fuel" that is used preferentially by cardiomyocytes over fatty acids and glucose and is more energy efficient, improving cardiac contractility. BHB oxidation increases cardiac efficiency and decreases oxygen consumption compared with fatty acids and glucose, leading to a cardioprotective state. In addition, BHB has been shown to have antioxidative, anti-inflammatory, and antiarrhythmic properties, which may also provide cardiac benefit (24,25,29).

The sodium hypothesis is related to the direct effects of SGLT2 inhibitors on cardiac ion homeostasis. Failing cardiac myocytes demonstrate an increase in activity of the sarcolemmal sodium-hydrogen exchanger, leading to an efflux of calcium from the mitochondria, which further results in a decline in cellular function and a decrease in antioxidant capacity (25). SGLT2 inhibitors may directly bind to the sodium-hydrogen exchanger, decreasing their activity in myocardial cells, leading to a decrease in intracellular sodium, an influx in calcium, and restored myocardial calcium handling. This process is thought to improve mitochondrial energetics, prevent oxidative stress, and subsequently decrease the incidence of ventricular arrhythmias and sudden cardiac death. More detail regarding these hypotheses can be found in a recent publication by Bertero et al. (25).

Despite the cardioprotective benefits demonstrated by SGLT2 inhibitors in recent clinical trials, some precautions exist for their use. Genitourinary tract infections are of concern after initial premarketing studies showed an increased risk; however, real-world data recently demonstrated that the risk may not be as high as previously described (30). Patients should be counseled on good hygiene on initiation of therapy to reduce the risk of this undesirable side effect.

Although SGLT2 inhibitors increase the production of ketones, which may be a mechanism for their cardiovascular benefit, this increase may result in the accumulation of ketones, and patients may experience the rare side effect of euglycemic diabetic ketoacidosis (euDKA). It would be prudent to alert patients to possible precipitating factors for euDKA such as dehydration, discontinued or reduced insulin doses, surgery, and infections (28). Patients should also be educated on possible symptoms of euDKA such as abdominal pain, shortness of breath, fatigue, nausea, and vomiting and should seek immediate medical attention if they experience these symptoms.

The effects of SGLT2 inhibitors on systemic and renal hemodynamics have raised concerns regarding their safety with concomitant use of diuretics or renin-angiotensin-aldosterone system (RAAS) inhibitors, given their duplicative ability to reduce intravascular volume and intraglomerular pressure. The U.S. Food and Drug Administration (FDA) has strengthened its warning about the risk for acute kidney injury with SGLT2 inhibitors in combination with diuretics and RAAS inhibitors; however, these agents all play a valuable role in the management of patients with HF (31).

To reduce the risk of acute kidney injury, caution should be used when starting or increasing the dose of an SGLT2 inhibitor at the same time as an RAAS inhibitor to minimize hemodynamic changes at the kidney.

Additionally, clinicians should reevaluate the need for traditional diuretic therapies, specifically thiazide diuretics, given their mechanism for sodium-wasting at the distal convoluted tubule. Clinical judgement should be used when determining whether to decrease the dose of a loop diuretic when initiating an SGLT2 inhibitor, taking into consideration kidney function, functional class, and volume status.

Another clinical concern may be the risk for hyperkalemia with concomitant use of ACE inhibitors, angiotensin receptor blockers (ARBs), angiotensin receptor-neprilysin (ARN) inhibitors, or aldosterone antagonists as guideline-directed medical therapy for HF (32,33). Despite initial concerns for hyperkalemia from the increased sodium load to the distal tubule, subsequent studies have shown that these agents pose no higher risk for this adverse effect compared with placebo and that these medications can be used together safely (34,35).

GLP-1 Receptor Agonists

The ADA Standards of Care recommends an SGLT2 inhibitor after metformin for patients with type 2 diabetes and comorbid HF (11). A GLP-1 receptor agonist with proven cardiovascular benefit is preferred in this population if SGLT2 inhibitor use is contraindicated or is not tolerated by the patient or can be added to SGLT2 inhibitor therapy if further blood glucose lowering is needed. GLP-1 receptor agonists decrease glucagon secretion, increase glucose-dependent insulin secretion, delay gastric emptying, decrease food intake, and preserve β-cell function.

Seven CVOTs have been published investigating the cardiovascular safety of GLP-1 receptor agonists, including oral semaglutide (Table 2). Like other CVOTs, these trials included a primary composite outcome of major adverse cardiovascular events (MACE), which most often included cardiovascular death, nonfatal myocardial infarction, and nonfatal stroke (36–42). All agents demonstrated at least noninferiority compared with placebo regarding the composite MACE outcome, and four agents (albiglutide, dulaglutide, liraglutide, and semaglutide) demonstrated a reduction in cardiovascular events (37,38,40–42).

Each of the CVOTs with GLP-1 receptor agonists included HHF as a secondary or exploratory outcome. There was no significant difference compared with placebo for any agent with regard to HHF, indicating that these agents are likely safe in patients with HF (36–42). In addition, a subanalysis of patients enrolled in the HARMONY Outcomes (A Long Term, Randomized, Double-Blind, Placebo-Controlled Study to Determine the Effect of

TABLE 2 Summary of GLP-1 Receptor Agonist CVOTs in Patients With Type 2 Diabetes (36–42)

	ELIXA (Lixisenatide)	LEADER (Liraglutide)	SUSTAIN-6 (Semaglutide)	EXSCEL (Exenatide ER)	HARMONY Outcomes (Albiglutide)	REWIND (Dulaglutide)	PIONEER-6 (Oral Semaglutide)
Study size, n	6,068	9,340	3,297	14,752	9,463	9,901	3,183
Median follow-up, years	2.1	3.8	2.1	3.2	1.6	5.4	1.3
Patient population	A1C 5.5–11.0%; age ≥30 years with ACS within 180 days of screening	A1C ≥7.0%; age ≥60 years with at least one CVD risk factor or age ≥50 years with established CVD, CKD stage ≥3, or chronic heart failure (NYHA class II or III)	A1C ≥7.0%; age ≥60 years with at least one CVD risk factor, or age ≥50 years with established CVD, CKD stage ≥3, or chronic heart failure (NYHA class II or III)	A1C 6.5–10.0%; no specifications for established CVD or CVD risk factors; per investigators, "designed so that 70% of patients had a history of a CV event"	A1C ≥7.0%; age ≥40 years with established coronary artery disease, cerebrovascular disease, or peripheral arterial disease	A1C ≤9.5%; age ≥60 years with at least two CVD risk factors or age ≥55 years with subclinical vascular or renal disease or age ≥50 years with established CVD	A1C ≥7.0%; age ≥60 years with at least one CVD risk factor or age ≥50 years with established CVD, CKD stage ≥3, or chronic heart failure (NYHA class II or III)
Primary end point(s),* HR (95% CI)	4-point MACE: 1.02 (0.89–1.17)	3-point MACE: 0.87 (0.78–0.97)	3-point MACE: 0.74 (0.58–0.95)	3-point MACE: 0.91 (0.83–1.00)	3-point MACE: 0.78 (0.68–0.90)	3-point MACE: 0.88 (0.79–0.99)	3-point MACE: 0.79 (0.57–1.11)
HF-related secondary end points, HR (95% CI)	HHF: 0.96 (0.75–1.23)	HHF: 0.87 (0.73–1.05)	HHF: 1.11 (0.77–1.61)	HHF: 0.94 (0.78–1.13)	Cardiovascular death + HHF: 0.85 (0.70–1.04)	HHF: 0.93 (0.77–1.12)	HHF: 0.86 (0.48–1.55)

*3-point MACE included cardiovascular death, nonfatal myocardial infarction, and nonfatal stroke; 4-point MACE also included hospitalization for unstable angina. ACS, acute coronary syndrome; ELIXA, Evaluation of Lixisenatide in Acute Coronary Syndrome; ER, extended release; EXSCEL, Exenatide Study of Cardiovascular Event Lowering; HR, hazard ratio; LEADER, Liraglutide Effect and Action in Diabetes: Evaluation of Cardiovascular Outcome Results; PIONEER-6, A Trial Investigating the Cardiovascular Safety of Oral Semaglutide in Subjects With Type 2 Diabetes; REWIND, Researching Cardiovascular Events With a Weekly Incretin in Diabetes; SUSTAIN-6, Trial to Evaluate Cardiovascular and Other Long-Term Outcomes With Semaglutide in Subjects With Type 2 Diabetes.

Albiglutide, When Added to Standard Blood Glucose Lowering Therapies, on Major Cardiovascular Events in Patients With Type 2 Diabetes Mellitus) trial demonstrated that patients with a history of HF were less likely to experience the primary composite outcome compared with those with no such history when treated with the commercially unavailable albiglutide (40).

Liraglutide has also been evaluated for its impact on clinical stability in high-risk patients within the first 180 days after an admission for HF (43). Approximately 60% of the 300 patients enrolled in the study had a history of type 2 diabetes, 63% had New York Heart Association (NYHA) Class III HF, and liraglutide was titrated to the maximum dose of 1.8 mg per day. There was no difference in clinical stability based on death, hospitalization, and N-terminal pro b-type natriuretic peptide levels. An additional trial evaluating the use of liraglutide in patients with chronic HF with and without diabetes found that liraglutide did not affect left ventricular function; however, it was associated with an increase in heart rate and adverse cardiovascular events, warranting further evaluation of GLP-1 receptor agonists in this population (44).

Weight loss is an additional potential benefit of GLP-1 receptor agonist use in patients with HF. Obesity has been considered a risk factor for developing HF and type 2 diabetes, and strategies to safely reduce weight are encouraged as part of the management plan for both conditions (5,32). Dulaglutide, liraglutide, and semaglutide have demonstrated the strongest cardiovascular benefit in their CVOTs, and although they have shown no impact on the risk of HHF, their overall efficacy and weight loss benefit may still provide benefit to patients with both diabetes and HF (37,38,41). These agents should be considered after metformin and an SGLT2 inhibitor in patients with type 2 diabetes and HF as long no contraindications are present.

DPP-4 Inhibitors

The ADA recommends using a DPP-4 inhibitor, with the exception of saxagliptin, as an alternative to an SGLT2 inhibitor or GLP-1 receptor agonist or as additional antihyperglycemic therapy after an SGLT2 inhibitor, given their neutral effect on MACE. Conversely, a combined statement from the American Heart Association and the Heart Failure Society of America noted the lack of patients with HF at baseline in the DPP-4 inhibitor CVOTs and acknowledged concerning signals with DPP-4 inhibitors in mechanistic trials (5). The statement concluded that the risk-benefit profile for most DPP-4 inhibitors does not justify their use in patients with type 2 diabetes and comorbid HF or those at risk for HF. DPP-4 inhibitors act by inhibiting the degradation of endogenous GLP-1 and therefore modestly increasing the effects of the incretin system to augment pancreatic insulin secretion.

The four CVOTs evaluating DPP-4 inhibitors established that these agents are noninferior compared with placebo for the FDA-mandated primary MACE outcome (Table 3) (45–49). Despite demonstrating safety with regard to the MACE end point, there was an unexpected 27% relative increase in the risk of HHF with the use of saxagliptin in the

TABLE 3 Summary of DPP-4 Inhibitor CVOTs in Patients With Type 2 Diabetes (45–49)

	SAVOR-TIMI 53 (Saxagliptin)	EXAMINE (Alogliptin)	TECOS (Sitagliptin)	CARMELINA (Linagliptin)
Study size, n	16,492	5,380	14,671	6,979
Median follow-up, years	2.1	1.5	3.0	2.2
Patient population	A1C 6.5-12.0%; men age ≥55 years and women age ≥60 years with at least one CVD risk factor or men and women age ≥40 years with established CVD	A1C 6.5-11.0%; hospitalization for ACS within 15-90 days of randomization	A1C 6.5-8.0%; age ≥50 years with established CVD	A1C 6.5-10.0%; age >18 years with high risk of cardiovascular events
Primary end point,* HR (95% CI)	3-point MACE: 1.00 (0.89-1.12)	3-point MACE: 0.96 (≤1.16)	4-point MACE: 0.98 (0.88-1.09)	3-point MACE: 1.02 (0.89-1.17)
HF-related secondary end points, HR (95% CI)	HHF: 1.27 (1.07-1.51)	HHF: 1.19 (0.90-1.58)†; HHF for patients with no history of HF at baseline: 1.76 (1.07-2.90)†	HHF: 1.00 (0.83-1.20)	HHF: 0.90 (0.74-1.08)

*3-point MACE included cardiovascular death, nonfatal myocardial infarction, and nonfatal stroke; 4-point MACE also included hospitalization for unstable angina. †Based on a post hoc analysis from the EXAMINE trial. ACS, acute coronary syndrome; HR, hazard ratio.

SAVOR-TIMI 53 (Saxagliptin Assessment of Vascular Outcomes Recorded in Patients with Diabetes Mellitus–Thrombolysis in Myocardial Infarction) trial (45). The EXAMINE (Examination of Cardiovascular Outcomes With Alogliptin Versus Standard of Care) trial evaluating alogliptin did not initially measure rates of HHF; however, a post hoc analysis identified a 76% relative risk increase for HHF in patients with recent acute coronary syndrome and no history of HF at baseline, which constituted the majority of the study population (46,49). In contrast, TECOS (Trial Evaluating Cardiovascular Outcomes with Sitagliptin) and CARMELINA (Cardio-vascular and Renal Microvascular Outcome Study With Linagliptin in Patients With Type 2 Diabetes Mellitus) evaluating sitagliptin and linagliptin, respectively, dem-onstrated no increased risk of HHF with these agents compared with placebo (47,48). Signals for increased HHF seen with saxagliptin and alogliptin prompted the FDA to issue a safety alert, mandate that warnings be included in the labeling for these agents, specifically for patients who already have CVD or CKD, and recommend their discontinuation in patients who develop HF (50).

Since then, two meta-analyses evaluating DPP-4 inhibi-tion compared with placebo showed no statistically significant increase in risk for HHF; however, one meta-analysis evaluated 236 trials and found a 22 and 81% increase in relative risk for HHF with these agents when compared with GLP-1 receptor agonists and SGLT2 in-hibitors, respectively (51,52). Additional meta-analyses have demonstrated a 13–24% increase in HF-related end points with the use of all DPP-4 inhibitors, with no significant heterogeneity among drugs within the class (53–55).

The proposed mechanism for increased risk of HHF in patients with diabetes is partially derived from the effect of DPP-4 inhibition on plasma concentrations of stromal cell–derived factor 1 (SDF-1) (56). DPP-4 is responsible for the degradation of several substrates, including SDF-1, which has been linked to cardiac fibrosis, central nervous system activation with subsequent increases in myocar-dial cyclic adenosine monophosphate (AMP), and distal tubular natriuresis. Endogenous GLP-1 is also associated with an increase in cyclic AMP in cardiomyocytes; however, unlike the GLP-1 receptor agonists, DPP-4 inhibitors are not associated with a clinically significant chronotropic effect.

These proposed deleterious effects of DPP-4 inhibitors may be attenuated by a natriuretic effect, which would offset cardiac loading conditions; however, because the DPP-4 inhibitors exert their natriuretic effect through

potentiation of SDF-1 at the distal tubule, they do not exhibit a natriuretic effect significant enough to reduce cardiac filling pressures. This process is in contrast to the SGLT2 inhibitors and GLP-1 receptor agonists, which are proposed to exert their natriuretic effect at the proximal tubule, the major site of sodium reabsorption, and therefore may assist in decreasing cardiac filling pressures.

In light of these postulated mechanisms for the increased HHF risk in patients using DPP-4 inhibitors, further re-search is required to confirm their safety in patients with HF. Although the initial signal for increased risk for HHF was isolated to saxagliptin with potential concern with the use of alogliptin, the proposed mechanisms for this in-creased risk and inconsistent findings from multiple meta-analyses may be enough evidence to give pause to using this drug class in patients at high risk for or with established HF (45,46,49).

Thiazolidinediones

Thiazolidinediones (TZDs) are generally not recom-mended in patients with HF because of their potential to cause fluid retention (11). These agents are selective agonists for the peroxisome proliferator–activated receptor-γ (PPAR-γ). Activation of PPAR-γ receptors increases the production of gene products responsible for glucose and lipid metabolism, thereby improving insulin sensitivity. PPAR-γ is found in the cells within the renal tubule, and therefore stimulation increases sodium reabsorption (57). Rosiglitazone was shown to increase the risk of HF causing hospitalization or death by twofold in the RECORD (Rosiglitazone Evaluated for Cardio-vascular Outcomes in Oral Agent Combination Therapy for Type 2 Diabetes) trial, and a 42-trial meta-analysis found that rosiglitazone increased the risk for cardio-vascular death (58,59). The PROactive (Prospective Pioglitazone Clinical Trial in Macrovascular Events) trial demonstrated that pioglitazone was associated with a reduction in risk of MACE; however, pioglitazone was associated with an increase in the rate of HHF, and the incidence of edema was 26.4% compared with 15.1% in the placebo group (60,61). Additional trials cite a sig-nificant increase in edema and risk of HHF and related events with TZDs compared with other therapies used in the management of people with diabetes (62–65).

If TZDs are used in patients with NYHA Class I or II HF, it should be noted that these patients are more resistant to loop diuretics, and edema will resolve with discontinu-ation of TZD therapy. In addition, patients using these agents should be educated on careful monitoring for fluid retention and daily weight monitoring. The increase in the risk of HHF and edema in people with diabetes and HF makes this class of medications an undesirable choice in this population, and drugs in this class should be avoided (11).

Sulfonylureas

The ADA supports sulfonylureas as a treatment option for patients with type 2 diabetes and HF who cannot afford an SGLT2 inhibitor, a GLP-1 receptor agonist, or a DPP-4 inhibitor. Drugs in this class stimulate insulin secretion from the pancreatic β-cells and have fallen out of favor because of their inability to reduce cardiovascular risk and concern about β-cell burnout. CAROLINA (Cardiovascular Outcome Study of Linagliptin Versus Glimepiride in Patients With Type 2 Diabetes) evaluated the cardiovascular safety of the sulfonylurea glimepiride in comparison with the DPP-4 inhibitor linagliptin (66). The study found no difference between the two agents in the primary outcome, which was time to first occurrence of the composite MACE outcome. In addition, there was no difference in the risk of HHF between the two groups (3.7 vs. 3.1% with linagliptin and glimepiride, respectively). Although these agents do not confer any additional cardiovascular benefit, they also have not been shown to cause cardiovascular harm and remain a viable option for patients with type 2 diabetes and HF.

Other Considerations for the Co-Management of Type 2 Diabetes and HF

β-Blockers in Patients With HF and Diabetes

Historically, clinicians have been reluctant to use β-blockers in patients with diabetes because of concerns regarding hypoglycemia unawareness, worsening glycemic control, and insulin sensitivity. Because β-blockers are a first-line therapy along with ACE inhibitors, ARBs, and ARN inhibitors in patients with HF, their use is critical in patients with diabetes and concomitant HF.

Three mortality-reducing β-blockers are currently recommended for the treatment of patients with HF with reduced ejection fraction: carvedilol, metoprolol succinate, and bisoprolol (32). Metoprolol succinate and bisoprolol are β-1–selective agents and have been shown to significantly decrease insulin sensitivity in patients with hypertension, and many of the negative perceptions regarding β-blocker use are from clinical trials studying nonspecific first-generation β-blockers (e.g., propranolol) and second-generation β-1–selective agents (67).

Carvedilol, a nonselective third-generation β-blocker with additional vasodilatory activity produced by additional α-1 adrenergic receptor blockade, has been recommended as the preferred agent in the past for patients with diabetes who need additional blood pressure lowering (68). Beneficial effects were demonstrated in multiple studies comparing carvedilol to metoprolol, in which carvedilol increased insulin sensitivity compared with metoprolol and stabilized glycemic management (69,70). Unless patients have concomitant severe restrictive lung disease, a low baseline blood pressure, or another indication that would make carvedilol less favorable, carvedilol is the preferred β-blocker in patients with HF and diabetes.

Another concern with β-blocker use is the theoretical increased risk of masking common signs and symptoms of hypoglycemia, such as weakness, shakiness, and palpitations. In HF, the mortality-reducing benefits were found at the maximum doses of these agents, so the fear of hypoglycemia unawareness cannot deter clinicians from titrating to mortality-reducing doses. It is important for clinicians to counsel patients to look for signs such as sweating or agitation, which may not be affected by the antiadrenergic effects of β-blockers (32,67).

Fluid Restriction and Diuretic Management

Increasing fluid intake has been shown to have a beneficial effect on renal function in patients with or at risk for CKD, making it a desirable recommendation for patients with diabetes (71). In patients with HF and diabetes, a careful fluid intake balance must be maintained to ensure adequate hydration benefits on the kidney and prevent congestive symptoms of HF. Many clinicians continue to follow a tight fluid restriction recommendation in patients with HF, educating patients to consume no more than 1.5–2 L of liquid per day. However, recent HF guidelines have relinquished fluid restriction recommendations for all except those with stage D HF, especially in patients with hyponatremia. More general fluid restriction in all patients with HF regardless of symptoms or other considerations does not appear to result in significant benefit (32,72).

Patients should be counseled on signs and symptoms of fluid retention, such as edema, abdominal fullness, shortness of breath, paroxysmal nocturnal dyspnea, and orthopnea. Daily weight monitoring should be recommended, and patients should be instructed to contact their provider if they gain 2 lb or more in 1 day or 3–5 lb in 1 week.

Certain HF symptoms should be monitored more closely in patients taking GLP-1 receptor agonists because they have the potential to cause weight loss and early satiety, especially upon initiation. These effects may mask weight gain from fluid overload and early satiety from fluid collection around the abdomen in patients with worsening HF. A more thorough examination for edema and heart and lung sounds may be required in patients with symptomatic HF who are started on GLP-1 receptor agonists.

Management of Diabetes Complications in Patients With HF

Inappropriate management of the complications of diabetes in the setting of HF may have a detrimental effect on morbidity and mortality in this patient population, as well as increase the cost of care. For example, when considering pharmacologic options for the treatment of peripheral neuropathy resulting from longstanding hyperglycemia, clinicians should avoid the use of pregabalin. Although the manufacturer's labeling specifically notes that clinicians should use caution in the setting of NYHA class III or IV HF because of the risk for peripheral edema, there are case reports of acute decompensation with pregabalin in patients with stable, NYHA class I through III HF, which further support avoiding this agent in patients with diabetes and HF (73–75).

Furthermore, it is paramount to take measures to prevent acute infections or optimize therapy for inflammatory conditions that occur as a result of or in conjunction with suboptimal glycemic management to limit the use of glucocorticoids in this population. These therapies not only acutely worsen hyperglycemia, but also promote sodium and water retention to further increase the risk for HF exacerbation. The same can be said for the use of nonsteroidal anti-inflammatory drugs (NSAIDs). The increased risk for volume expansion with NSAIDs' inherent ability to cause sodium and water retention is further compounded by their tendency to impair renal function in the presence of RAAS inhibitors and diuretics. As a result, NSAIDs may diminish the effects of diuretics used for maintaining euvolemia in patients with HF. It is imperative to be mindful of the use of these agents given their multimodal detrimental effects in patients with diabetes and HF.

The management of other comorbidities that commonly occur alongside diabetes and HF may require careful consideration of the risks versus benefits of certain therapies in this population, and publications exist to promote awareness of treatments to avoid in HF (76).

Future Directions and Conclusion

The management of diabetes in the setting of HF requires a comprehensive approach to optimize clinical outcomes for both conditions. Data from the published CVOTs provide some insight into the potential benefits of SGLT2 inhibitor therapy in patients with diabetes. The DAPA-HF trial, the anticipated Empagliflozin Outcome Trial in Patients with Chronic Heart Failure (EMPEROR)-Reduced, and additional follow-up studies examining their use in patients with HF with reduced ejection fraction regardless of diabetes status will provide more conclusive evidence (23,77). Additionally, multiple ongoing studies evaluating SGLT2 inhibitors will elucidate the role of these agents in patients with HF with preserved and midrange ejection fraction and may provide evidence that these therapies offer clinical benefits to this patient population (78,79).

The abundance of both cardiovascular safety and efficacy evidence for SGLT2 inhibitors make them a preferred choice for patients with HF regardless of glycemic control. Despite the aforementioned ongoing trials to establish the role of SGLT2 inhibitors in patients with HF, practitioners should not wait for the results of these studies to implement SGLT2 inhibitors and replicate their benefit in patients with diabetes and HF in clinical practice. In addition, it is equally imperative to ensure that patients do not receive medications, including those for diabetes and related complications, that may worsen or exacerbate HF. The optimal care of patients with diabetes and HF is an evolving area of clinical practice. Clinicians should be mindful of the interrelatedness of these comorbidities as they develop individualized management plans for their patients who have both conditions.

DUALITY OF INTEREST

C.A.S. serves as a consultant for Becton Dickinson. K.M.S serves on a speakers bureau for Novo Nordisk. J.D.G. serves on speakers bureaus for Novo Nordisk, Sanofi, and Xeris and as a consultant for Becton Dickinson. No other potential conflicts of interest relevant to this article were reported.

AUTHOR CONTRIBUTIONS

C.A.S., K.M.S., and E.K.V.D. researched and identified literature for the publication and wrote the manuscript, and E.K.V.D. formatted the manuscript. J.D.G. reviewed and edited the manuscript. C.A.S. is the guarantor of this work and, as such, had full access to all of the references used and takes responsibility for the integrity and accuracy of the manuscript.

REFERENCES

1. Kannel WB, Hjortland M, Castelli WP. Role of diabetes in congestive heart failure: the Framingham study. Am J Cardiol 1974;34:29–34

2. Nichols GA, Gullion CM, Koro CE, Ephross SA, Brown JB. The incidence of congestive heart failure in type 2 diabetes: an update. Diabetes Care 2004;27:1879–1884

3. Ohkuma T, Komorita Y, Peters SAE, Woodward M. Diabetes as a risk factor for heart failure in women and men: a systematic review and meta-analysis of 47 cohorts including 12 million individuals. Diabetologia 2019;62:1550–1560

4. Bertoni AG, Hundley WG, Massing MW, Bonds DE, Burke GL, Goff DC Jr. Heart failure prevalence, incidence, and mortality in the elderly with diabetes. Diabetes Care 2004;27:699–703

5. Dunlay SM, Givertz MM, Aguilar D, et al.; American Heart Association Heart Failure and Transplantation Committee of the Council on Clinical Cardiology; Council on Cardiovascular and Stroke Nursing; and the Heart Failure Society of America. Type 2 diabetes mellitus and heart failure: a scientific statement from the American Heart Association and the Heart Failure Society of America: this statement does not represent an update of the 2017 ACC/AHA/HFSA heart failure guideline update. Circulation 2019; 140:e294–e324

6. Levelt E, Mahmod M, Piechnik SK, et al. Relationship between left ventricular structural and metabolic remodeling in type 2 diabetes. Diabetes 2016;65:44–52

7. Shimizu I, Minamino T, Toko H, et al. Excessive cardiac insulin signaling exacerbates systolic dysfunction induced by pressure overload in rodents. J Clin Invest 2010;120:1506–1514

8. Levelt E, Rodgers CT, Clarke WT, et al. Cardiac energetics, oxygenation, and perfusion during increased workload in patients with type 2 diabetes mellitus. Eur Heart J 2016;37:3461–3469

9. Falcão-Pires I, Hamdani N, Borbély A, et al. Diabetes mellitus worsens diastolic left ventricular dysfunction in aortic stenosis through altered myocardial structure and cardiomyocyte stiffness. Circulation 2011;124:1151–1159

10. Basta G, Schmidt AM, De Caterina R. Advanced glycation end products and vascular inflammation: implications for accelerated atherosclerosis in diabetes. Cardiovasc Res 2004; 63:582–592

11. American Diabetes Association. 9. Pharmacologic approaches to glycemic treatment: *Standards of Medical Care in Diabetes—2020*. Diabetes Care 2020;43(Suppl. 1): S98–S110

12. Aguilar D, Chan W, Bozkurt B, Ramasubbu K, Deswal A. Metformin use and mortality in ambulatory patients with diabetes and heart failure. Circ Heart Fail 2011;4:53–58

13. Andersson C, Olesen JB, Hansen PR, et al. Metformin treatment is associated with a low risk of mortality in diabetic patients with heart failure: a retrospective nationwide cohort study. Diabetologia 2010;53:2546–2553

14. Eurich DT, Weir DL, Majumdar SR, et al. Comparative safety and effectiveness of metformin in patients with diabetes mellitus and heart failure: systematic review of observational studies involving 34,000 patients. Circ Heart Fail 2013;6:395–402

15. Tseng CH. Metformin use is associated with a lower risk of hospitalization for heart failure in patients with type 2 diabetes mellitus: a retrospective cohort analysis. J Am Heart Assoc 2019; 8:e011640

16. Crowley MJ, Diamantidis CJ, McDuffie JR, et al. Clinical outcomes of metformin use in populations with chronic kidney disease, congestive heart failure, or chronic liver disease: a systematic review. Ann Intern Med 2017;166:191–200

17. Zinman B, Wanner C, Lachin JM, et al.; EMPA-REG OUTCOME Investigators. Empagliflozin, cardiovascular outcomes, and mortality in type 2 diabetes. N Engl J Med 2015;373:2117–2128

18. Neal B, Perkovic V, Mahaffey KW, et al.; CANVAS Program Collaborative Group. Canagliflozin and cardiovascular and renal events in type 2 diabetes. N Engl J Med 2017;377:644–657

19. Wiviott SD, Raz I, Bonaca MP, et al.; DECLARE–TIMI 58 Investigators. Dapagliflozin and cardiovascular outcomes in type 2 diabetes. N Engl J Med 2019;380:347–357

20. Kosiborod M, Cavender MA, Fu AZ, et al.; CVD-REAL Investigators and Study Group. Lower risk of heart failure and death in patients initiated on sodium-glucose cotransporter-2 inhibitors versus other glucose-lowering drugs: the CVD-REAL study (Comparative Effectiveness of Cardiovascular Outcomes in New Users of Sodium–Glucose Cotransporter-2 Inhibitors). Circulation 2017;136:249–259

21. Kosiborod M, Lam CSP, Kohsaka S, et al.; CVD-REAL Investigators and Study Group. Cardiovascular events associated with SGLT-2 inhibitors versus other glucose-lowering drugs: the CVD-REAL 2 study. J Am Coll Cardiol 2018;71:2628–2639

22. Patorno E, Pawar A, Franklin JM, et al. Empagliflozin and the risk of heart failure hospitalization in routine clinical care. Circulation 2019;139:2822–2830

23. McMurray JJV, Solomon SD, Inzucchi SE, et al.; DAPA-HF Trial Committees and Investigators. Dapagliflozin in patients with heart failure and reduced ejection fraction. N Engl J Med 2019;381:1995–2008

24. Mudaliar S, Alloju S, Henry RR. Can a shift in fuel energetics explain the beneficial cardiorenal outcomes in the EMPA-REG OUTCOME study? A unifying hypothesis. Diabetes Care 2016;39: 1115–1122

25. Bertero E, Prates Roma L, Ameri P, Maack C. Cardiac effects of SGLT2 inhibitors: the sodium hypothesis. Cardiovasc Res 2018;114:12–18

26. Sha S, Polidori D, Heise T, et al. Effect of the sodium glucose co-transporter 2 inhibitor canagliflozin on plasma volume in patients with type 2 diabetes mellitus. Diabetes Obes Metab 2014; 16:1087–1095

27. Casu G, Merella P. Diuretic therapy in heart failure: current approaches. Eur Cardiol 2015;10:42–47

28. Rosenstock J, Ferrannini E. Euglycemic diabetic ketoacidosis: a predictable, detectable, and preventable safety concern with SGLT2 inhibitors. Diabetes Care 2015;38:1638–1642

29. Prattichizzo F, De Nigris V, Micheloni S, La Sala L, Ceriello A. Increases in circulating levels of ketone bodies and cardiovascular protection with SGLT2 inhibitors: is low-grade inflammation the neglected component? Diabetes Obes Metab 2018;20: 2515–2522

30. Dave CV, Schneeweiss S, Kim D, Fralick M, Tong A, Patorno E. Sodium-glucose cotransporter-2 inhibitors and the risk for severe urinary tract infections: a population-based cohort study. Ann Intern Med 2019;171:248–256

31. U.S. Food and Drug Administration. FDA drug safety communication: FDA strengthens kidney warnings for diabetes medicines canagliflozin (Invokana, Invokamet) and dapagliflozin (Farxiga, Xigduo XR). Available from https://www.fda.gov/drugs/drug-safety-and-availability/fda-drug-safety-communication-fda-strengthens-kidney-warnings-diabetes-medicines-canagliflozin. Accessed 19 January 2020

32. Yancy CW, Jessup M, Bozkurt B, et al.; American College of Cardiology Foundation; American Heart Association Task Force on Practice Guidelines. 2013 ACCF/AHA guideline for the management of heart failure: a report of the American College of Cardiology Foundation/American Heart Association Task Force on Practice Guidelines. J Am Coll Cardiol 2013;62: e147–e239

33. Yancy CW, Jessup M, Bozkurt B, et al. 2017 ACC/AHA/HFSA focused update of the 2013 ACCF/AHA guideline for the management of heart failure: Report of the American College of Cardiology/American Heart Association Task Force on Clinical Practice Guidelines and the Heart Failure Society of America. Circulation 2017;136:e137–e161

34. Wanner C, Lachin JM, Inzucchi SE, et al.; EMPA-REG OUTCOME Investigators. Empagliflozin and clinical outcomes in patients with type 2 diabetes mellitus, established cardiovascular disease, and chronic kidney disease. Circulation 2018;137: 119–129

35. Tang H, Zhang X, Zhang J, et al. Elevated serum magnesium associated with SGLT2 inhibitor use in type 2 diabetes patients: a meta-analysis of randomised controlled trials. Diabetologia 2016; 59:2546–2551

36. Pfeffer MA, Claggett B, Diaz R, et al.; ELIXA Investigators. Lixisenatide in patients with type 2 diabetes and acute coronary syndrome. N Engl J Med 2015;373:2247–2257

37. Marso SP, Daniels GH, Brown-Frandsen K, et al.; LEADER Steering Committee; LEADER Trial Investigators. Liraglutide and cardiovascular outcomes in type 2 diabetes. N Engl J Med 2016; 375:311–322

38. Marso SP, Bain SC, Consoli A, et al.; SUSTAIN-6 Investigators. Semaglutide and cardiovascular outcomes in patients with type 2 diabetes. N Engl J Med 2016;375:1834–1844

39. Holman RR, Bethel MA, Mentz RJ, et al.; EXSCEL Study Group. Effects of once-weekly exenatide on cardiovascular outcomes in type 2 diabetes. N Engl J Med 2017;377: 1228–1239

40. Hernandez AF, Green JB, Janmohamed S, et al.; Harmony Outcomes committees and investigators. Albiglutide and cardiovascular outcomes in patients with type 2 diabetes and cardiovascular disease (Harmony Outcomes): a double-blind, randomised placebo-controlled trial. Lancet 2018;392: 1519–1529

41. Gerstein HC, Colhoun HM, Dagenais GR, et al.; REWIND Investigators. Dulaglutide and cardiovascular outcomes in type 2 diabetes (REWIND): a double-blind, randomised placebo-controlled trial. Lancet 2019;394:121–130

42. Husain M, Birkenfeld AL, Donsmark M, et al.; PIONEER 6 Investigators. Oral semaglutide and cardiovascular outcomes in patients with type 2 diabetes. N Engl J Med 2019;381:841–851

43. Margulies KB, Hernandez AF, Redfield MM, et al.; NHLBI Heart Failure Clinical Research Network. Effects of liraglutide on clinical stability among patients with advanced heart failure and reduced ejection fraction: a randomized clinical trial. JAMA 2016; 316:500–508

44. Jorsal A, Kistorp C, Holmager P, et al. Effect of liraglutide, a glucagon-like peptide-1 analogue, on left ventricular function in stable chronic heart failure patients with and without diabetes (LIVE): a multicentre, double-blind, randomised, placebo-controlled trial. Eur J Heart Fail 2017;19:69–77

45. Scirica BM, Bhatt DL, Braunwald E, et al.; SAVOR-TIMI 53 Steering Committee and Investigators. Saxagliptin and cardiovascular outcomes in patients with type 2 diabetes mellitus. N Engl J Med 2013;369:1317–1326

46. White WB, Cannon CP, Heller SR, et al.; EXAMINE Investigators. Alogliptin after acute coronary syndrome in patients with type 2 diabetes. N Engl J Med 2013;369:1327–1335

47. Green JB, Bethel MA, Armstrong PW, et al.; TECOS Study Group. Effect of sitagliptin on cardiovascular outcomes in type 2 diabetes. N Engl J Med 2015;373:232–242

48. Rosenstock J, Perkovic V, Johansen OE, et al.; CARMELINA Investigators. Effect of linagliptin vs placebo on major cardiovascular events in adults with type 2 diabetes and high cardiovascular and renal risk: the CARMELINA randomized clinical trial. JAMA 2019;321:69–79

49. Zannad F, Cannon CP, Cushman WC, et al.; EXAMINE Investigators. Heart failure and mortality outcomes in patients with type 2 diabetes taking alogliptin versus placebo in EXAMINE: a multicentre, randomised, double-blind trial. Lancet 2015;385: 2067–2076

50. U.S. Food and Drug Administration. FDA drug safety communication: FDA adds warnings about heart failure risk to labels of type 2 diabetes medicines containing saxagliptin and alogliptin. Available from https://www.fda.gov/Drugs/DrugSafety/ucm486096.htm. Accessed 19 January 2020

51. Kankanala SR, Syed R, Gong Q, Ren B, Rao X, Zhong J. Cardiovascular safety of dipeptidyl peptidase-4 inhibitors: recent evidence on heart failure. Am J Transl Res 2016;8: 2450–2458

52. Zheng SL, Roddick AJ, Aghar-Jaffar R, et al. Association between use of sodium-glucose cotransporter 2 inhibitors, glucagon-like peptide 1 agonists, and dipeptidyl peptidase 4 inhibitors with all-cause mortality in patients with type 2 diabetes: a systematic review and meta-analysis. JAMA 2018;319: 1580–1591

53. Verma S, Goldenberg RM, Bhatt DL, et al. Dipeptidyl peptidase-4 inhibitors and the risk of heart failure: a systematic review and meta-analysis. CMAJ Open 2017;5:E152–E177

54. Monami M, Dicembrini I, Mannucci E. Dipeptidyl peptidase-4 inhibitors and heart failure: a meta-analysis of randomized clinical trials. Nutr Metab Cardiovasc Dis 2014;24:689–697

55. Clifton P. Do dipeptidyl peptidase IV (DPP-IV) inhibitors cause heart failure? Clin Ther 2014;36:2072–2079

56. Packer M. Worsening heart failure during the use of DPP-4 inhibitors: pathophysiological mechanisms, clinical risks, and potential influence of concomitant antidiabetic medications. JACC Heart Fail 2018;6:445–451

57. Staels B. Fluid retention mediated by renal PPARgamma. Cell Metab 2005;2:77–78

58. Home PD, Pocock SJ, Beck-Nielsen H, et al.; RECORD Study Team. Rosiglitazone evaluated for cardiovascular outcomes in oral agent combination therapy for type 2 diabetes (RECORD): a multicentre, randomised, open-label trial. Lancet 2009;373: 2125–2135

59. Nissen SE, Wolski K. Effect of rosiglitazone on the risk of myocardial infarction and death from cardiovascular causes. N Engl J Med 2007;356:2457–2471

60. Dormandy JA, Charbonnel B, Eckland DJ, et al.; PROactive Investigators. Secondary prevention of macrovascular events in patients with type 2 diabetes in the PROactive Study (PROspective pioglitAzone Clinical Trial In macroVascular Events): a randomised controlled trial. Lancet 2005;366: 1279–1289

61. Dormandy J, Bhattacharya M, van Troostenburg de Bruyn AR; PROactive investigators. Safety and tolerability of pioglitazone in high-risk patients with type 2 diabetes: an overview of data from PROactive. Drug Saf 2009;32:187–202

62. Berlie HD, Kalus JS, Jaber LA. Thiazolidinediones and the risk of edema: a meta-analysis. Diabetes Res Clin Pract 2007;76: 279–289

63. Hernandez AV, Usmani A, Rajamanickam A, Moheet A. Thiazolidinediones and risk of heart failure in patients with or at high risk of type 2 diabetes mellitus: a meta-analysis and meta-regression analysis of placebo-controlled randomized clinical trials. Am J Cardiovasc Drugs 2011;11:115–128

64. Lincoff AM, Wolski K, Nicholls SJ, Nissen SE. Pioglitazone and risk of cardiovascular events in patients with type 2 diabetes mellitus: a meta-analysis of randomized trials. JAMA 2007;298: 1180–1188

65. Lago RM, Singh PP, Nesto RW. Congestive heart failure and cardiovascular death in patients with prediabetes and type 2 diabetes given thiazolidinediones: a meta-analysis of randomised clinical trials. Lancet 2007;370:1129–1136

66. Rosenstock J, Kahn SE, Johansen OE, et al.; CAROLINA Investigators. Effect of linagliptin vs glimepiride on major adverse cardiovascular outcomes in patients with type 2 diabetes: the CAROLINA randomized clinical trial. JAMA 2019;322:1155–1166

67. McGill JB. Reexamining misconceptions about β-blockers in patients with diabetes. Clin Diabetes 2009;27:36–46

68. Torre JJ, Bloomgarden ZT, Dickey RA, et al.; AACE Hypertension Task Force. American Association of Clinical Endocrinologists medical guidelines for clinical practice for the diagnosis and treatment of hypertension. Endocr Pract 2006;12:193–222

69. Jacob S, Rett K, Wicklmayr M, Agrawal B, Augustin HJ, Dietze GJ. Differential effect of chronic treatment with two beta-blocking agents on insulin sensitivity: the carvedilol-metoprolol study. J Hypertens 1996;14:489–494

70. Bakris GL, Fonseca V, Katholi RE, et al.; GEMINI Investigators. Metabolic effects of carvedilol vs metoprolol in patients with type 2 diabetes mellitus and hypertension: a randomized controlled trial. JAMA 2004;292:2227–2236

71. Clark WF, Sontrop JM, Huang SH, Moist L, Bouby N, Bankir L. Hydration and chronic kidney disease progression: a critical review of the evidence. Am J Nephrol 2016;43:281–292

72. Travers B, O'Loughlin C, Murphy NF, et al. Fluid restriction in the management of decompensated heart failure: no impact on time to clinical stability. J Card Fail 2007;13:128–132

73. Lyrica (pregabalin) [package insert]. New York, NY, Pfizer, 2019

74. Fong T, Lee AJ. Pregabalin-associated heart failure decompensation in a patient with a history of stage I heart failure. Ann Pharmacother 2014;48:1077–1081

75. Page RL 2nd, Cantu M, Lindenfeld J, Hergott LJ, Lowes BD. Possible heart failure exacerbation associated with pregabalin: case discussion and literature review. J Cardiovasc Med (Hagerstown) 2008;9:922–925

76. Page RL 2nd, O'Bryant CL, Cheng D, et al.; American Heart Association Clinical Pharmacology and Heart Failure and Transplantation Committees of the Council on Clinical Cardiology; Council on Cardiovascular Surgery and Anesthesia; Council on Cardiovascular and Stroke Nursing; and Council on Quality of Care and Outcomes Research. Drugs that may cause or exacerbate heart failure: a scientific statement from the American Heart Association. Circulation 2016;134:e32–e69

77. Boehringer Ingelheim. Empagliflozin outcome trial in patients with chronic heart failure with reduced ejection fraction (EMPEROR-Reduced). Available from https://clinicaltrials.gov/ct2/show/NCT03057977. Accessed 19 January 2020

78. Boehringer Ingelheim. Empagliflozin outcome trial in patients with chronic heart failure with preserved ejection fraction (EMPEROR-Preserved). Available from https://clinicaltrials.gov/ct2/show/NCT03057951. Accessed 19 January 2020

79. AstraZeneca. Dapagliflozin evaluation to improve the lives of patients with preserved ejection fraction heart failure (DELIVER). Available from https://clinicaltrials.gov/ct2/show/NCT03619213. Accessed 19 January 2020

Flash Continuous Glucose Monitoring: A Summary Review of Recent Real-World Evidence

Clifford J. Bailey[1] and James R. Gavin III[2]

Optimizing glycemic control remains a shared challenge for clinicians and their patients with diabetes. Flash continuous glucose monitoring (CGM) provides immediate information about an individual's current and projected glucose level, allowing users to respond promptly to mitigate or prevent pending hypoglycemia or hyperglycemia. Large randomized controlled trials (RCTs) have demonstrated the glycemic benefits of flash CGM use in both type 1 and type 2 diabetes. However, whereas RCTs are mostly focused on the efficacy of this technology in defined circumstances, real-world studies can assess its effectiveness in wider clinical settings. This review assesses the most recent real-world studies demonstrating the effectiveness of flash CGM use to improve clinical outcomes and health care resource utilization in populations with diabetes.

During the past 5 years, increasing numbers of people with type 1 or type 2 diabetes have integrated continuous glucose monitoring (CGM) into their diabetes self-management regimens. Unlike traditional blood glucose meters, CGM systems provide immediate information about the concentration and the direction and rate of change of interstitial glucose. This information enables patients to intervene promptly to prevent or reduce acute hypoglycemia or hyperglycemia.

Flash CGM is among the most recent CGM technologies. Currently, the FreeStyle Libre 14-day system (Abbott Diabetes Care) and FreeStyle Libre 2 are the only flash CGM systems available, and these systems are being adopted rapidly. Large randomized controlled trials (RCTs) have confirmed the glycemic benefits of flash CGM use in people with type 1 diabetes (1,2) and those with type 2 diabetes (3–6). However, because RCTs are mostly focused on measures of efficacy in defined circumstances, real-world studies can usefully assess the effectiveness of flash CGM in wider clinical settings.

Although adoption of flash CGM continues to expand within endocrinology and diabetes specialty practices, primary care providers may be less familiar with this technology and how it can benefit patients with diabetes. This review assesses recent real-world studies demonstrating the impact of flash CGM use on clinical outcomes and health care resource utilization in both type 1 and type 2 diabetes populations.

Rationale for Intensive Interventions to Improve Glycemic Control

The International Diabetes Federation estimated the global prevalence of diabetes in 2019 to be 9.3% (463 million people), and this proportion is expected to rise to 10.2% (578 million people) by 2030 (7), with associated annual costs of ~$2.25 trillion (7). This figure includes $1.5 trillion in direct costs and $730 billion in indirect costs (e.g., absenteeism and societal costs) resulting from uncontrolled diabetes (7).

Therefore, preventing or reducing the severity of acute and long-term diabetes complications through patient-centered care remains a primary goal of diabetes management, and maintaining optimal glycemic control is central to achieving this goal (8,9). Although improvements in glycemic control should always be a priority, it is also important to strike a balance among the clinical benefits of new diabetes technologies, the initial and ongoing costs associated with their use, and the long-term gains for health and well-being.

Lowering A1C Levels Reduces Health Care Costs

Many studies have demonstrated that lower A1C levels result in lower health care resource utilization and associated costs (10–14). In a recent U.K. analysis using the IMS Core Diabetes Model, the per-person cost reductions

[1]Life and Health Sciences, Aston University, Birmingham, U.K.; [2]Emory University School of Medicine, Atlanta, GA

Corresponding author: Clifford J. Bailey, c.j.bailey@aston.ac.uk

https://doi.org/10.2337/cd20-0076

TABLE 1 Cost Reductions per Person for an A1C Reduction From Baseline by 0.4% (4.4 mmol/mol) in U.K. Adults With Diabetes (12)

Baseline A1C	5 Years	10 Years	15 Years	20 Years	25 Years
Adults with type 1 diabetes					
<7.5%	£66 ($87)	£271 ($359)	£719 ($953)	£1,379 ($1,828)	£2,057 ($2,726)
7.5–8.0%	£89 ($118)	£358 ($474)	£901 ($1,194)	£1,713 ($,2270)	£2,621 ($3,473)
>8.0–9.0%	£103 ($137)	£494 ($655)	£1,224 ($1,622)	£2,138 ($2,833)	£2,831 ($3,752)
>9.0%	£184 ($244)	£808 ($1,071)	£1,880 ($2,491)	£3,147 ($4,171)	£4,136 ($5,481)
Adults with type 2 diabetes					
<7.5%	£83 ($110)	£317 ($420)	£682 ($904)	£1,280 ($1,429)	£1,280 ($1,696)
7.5–8.0%	£132 ($175)	£449 ($595)	£995 ($1,319)	£1,510 ($2,001)	£1,678 ($2,224))
>8.0–9.0%	£138 ($183)	£607 ($804)	£1,366 ($1,820)	£1,999 ($2,649)	£2,223 ($2,946)
>9.0%	£105 ($139)	£662 ($877)	£1,274 ($1,688)	£1,591 ($2,108)	£1,559 ($2,065)

Costs are based on a 1.32 USD ($) to GBP (£) calculation.

that could be achieved over time were calculated based on a 0.4% (4.4 mmol/mol) reduction from baseline A1C (12). As shown in Table 1, the cost savings are most notable for individuals with the highest baseline A1C levels.

Reducing the Incidence and Severity of Hypoglycemia Reduces Health Care Costs

The global HAT (Hypoglycemia Assessment Tool) study, a 6-month retrospective and 4-week prospective investigation of 27,585 insulin-treated patients (type 1 diabetes, $n = 8,022$; type 2 diabetes, $n = 19,563$) in 24 countries noted the costs of inadequate glycemic control (15). During the prospective period, 83% of patients with type 1 diabetes and 46.5% of those with type 2 diabetes reported hypoglycemia, resulting in increased blood glucose monitoring, a marked increase in contact with health care providers, and increased hospitalizations. Significant indirect costs were incurred during the prospective period, with lost work time averaging 2.0 days for patients with type 1 diabetes and 1.8 days for those with type 2 diabetes. Other studies have had similar findings (15). Importantly, any level of hypoglycemia confers substantial indirect costs on employers as well as on individuals with diabetes because of increased work days lost (16–18).

Glycemic and Economic Benefits of Flash CGM Use in Real-World Studies

Although well-designed RCTs provide high levels of evidence, there is growing recognition for the complementary relationship between RCTs and real-world

prospective and retrospective observational studies. An increasing number of payers and regulators now request that pharmaceutical and medical device companies provide real-world evidence alongside RCT findings when evaluating the safety and effectiveness of new drugs and medical devices (19–22).

Large RCTs have clearly established that use of flash CGM improves glycemic control, reduces hypoglycemia, and achieves higher treatment satisfaction scores among individuals with type 1 diabetes (1,2) or type 2 diabetes (4,5) who are treated with intensive insulin therapy. Now real-world studies are investigating the use of flash CGM within different clinical settings and diverse diabetes populations.

Recent Study Results

As presented in Table 2, results from recently published prospective, observational studies closely align with glycemic benefits reported in earlier RCTs and also demonstrate the value of flash CGM use on cost outcomes and quality of life (QoL) measures (23–31). While these studies confirm significant reductions in A1C (23–25,32) and hypoglycemia (23,24) within large populations with type 1 or type 2 diabetes, they also provide strong evidence linking metabolic outcomes of flash CGM use to reductions in health care resource utilization. For example, one prospective, observational study assessed the impact of flash CGM in an unselected real-world cohort of 1,913 adults with type 1 diabetes (23). Over the 12-month study period, admissions for severe hypoglycemia and/or diabetic ketoacidosis (DKA) decreased from 3.3 to 2.2%

TABLE 2 Summary of Recently Published Real-World, Prospective, Observational Studies

Published Report	Design/Intervention	Outcome Measures	Findings
Charleer et al., 2020 (23)	• 12-month, prospective, observational, multicenter, cohort study (Belgium) • 1,913 adults with type 1 diabetes • Use of flash CGM	• Hospitalization with DKA and/or severe hypoglycemia • Hypoglycemia • Absenteeism • QoL	• Hospitalizations decreased from 3.3 to 2.2% ($P = 0.031$). • Severe hypoglycemic events decreased from 14.6 to 7.8% ($P < 0.0001$). • Hypoglycemic comas decreased from 2.7 to 1.1% ($P = 0.001$). • Fewer people were absent from work (2.9 vs. 5.8%). • Questionnaire-derived measures of treatment satisfaction improved.
Fokkert et al., 2019 (24)	• 12-month, prospective nationwide registry (the Netherlands) • 1,365 adults with type 1 diabetes (77%), type 2 diabetes (16%), or other diabetes (7%) • Use of flash CGM	• A1C • Hypoglycemia • Diabetes-related hospitalizations • Absenteeism • QoL	• A1C decreased from 64.1 to 60.1 mmol/mol (difference of −4 [95% CI −6 to 3] mmol/mol; $P < 0.001$). • In participants with a baseline A1C >70 mmol/mol, the A1C decrease was −9 (95% CI −12 to 5) mmol/mol. • The proportion of participants who reported hypoglycemia decreased from 93.5 to 91.0% ($P < 0.05$). • The diabetes-related hospital admission rate (per year) decreased from 13.7 to 4.7% ($P < 0.05$). • Absenteeism (per 6 months) decreased from 18.5 to 7.7% ($P < 0.05$). • Questionnaire-derived measures of QoL improved.
Kröger et al., 2020 (32)	• European pragmatic, parallel retrospective, noninterventional chart review study • 363 adults with type 2 diabetes • Use of flash CGM over 3–6 months	• A1C	• Mean (± SD) A1C levels were reduced by 9.6 ± 8.8 mmol/mol (0.9 ± 0.8%, $P < 0.0001$) in Austria, 8.9 ± 12.5 mmol/mol (0.8% ± 1.1%, $P < 0.0001$) in France, and 10.1 ± 12.2 mmol/mol (0.9% ± 1.1%, $P < 0.0001$) in Germany compared with levels recorded up to 90 days before starting use of the device. • No significant differences were detected for age, sex, BMI, or duration of insulin use.
Tyndall et al., 2019 (25)	• 8-month, prospective observational study (United Kingdom) • 900 adults with type 1 diabetes • Use of flash CGM • SMBG comparator group ($n = 518$)	• A1C • Hypoglycemia • Hospitalization • QoL	• A1C levels decreased by 0.6% ($P < 0.001$) among participants with a baseline A1C ≥7.5%; there was no change in the comparator group. • The percentage of participants who achieved an A1C <7.5% increased from 34.2 to 50.9% ($P < 0.001$). • More symptomatic (OR 1.9, $P < 0.001$) and asymptomatic (OR 1.4, $P < 0.001$) hypoglycemia was reported with flash CGM. • Hospitalizations for DKA were reduced ($P = 0.043$) with flash CGM. • Participants experienced less regimen-related and emotional distress, but more patients had elevated anxiety and depression with flash CGM use.
Paris et al., 2018 (26)	• 12-month, observational study (Belgium) • 120 adults with type 1 diabetes • Use of flash CGM	• A1C • Scanning frequency • Hypoglycemia	• A1C levels decreased from 8.51 to 8.16% ($P < 0.0001$) among participants with baseline A1C >7.5%. • Number of daily scans was negatively correlated with decreased A1C. • Number of hypoglycemic events (<70 mg/dL) increased from 16.9 to 22.9 events per month ($P < 0.05$). • No severe hypoglycemic events were reported. • Less fear of hypoglycemia was reported.

TABLE 2 Summary of Recently Published Real-World, Prospective, Observational Studies (continued)

Published Report	Design/Intervention	Outcome Measures	Findings
Messaaoui et al., 2019 (27)	• 12-month, prospective, observational study (Belgium) • 335 children/adolescents (10.9–16.3 years of age) with type 1 diabetes • Use of flash CGM	• Hypoglycemia • Hypoglycemia change • Use of SMBG • A1C • Acceptance • Adverse events	• Proportion of flash CGM continuers who experienced a severe hypoglycemic event decreased by 86% ($P = 0.037$); no change was seen in the SMBG group. • SMBG use decreased during use of flash CGM from 4.3 to 0 tests per day; SMBG use did not change in the SMBG group. • No significant changes in A1C occurred with either flash CGM or SMBG monitoring. • A total of 278 participants (83.2%) switched from SMBG to flash CGM, 234 participants were still using their device at end of the follow-up period, and 44 (15.8%) reverted to SMBG after a median use of 5.3 months. • Discontinuers reported more frequent occurrence of adverse events than continuers, including premature loss of sensor (31.8 vs. 12.4%), skin reactions (18.2 vs. 2.6%), and local pain (6.8 vs. 0%) (all $P < 0.001$). • Discontinuation of flash CGM was associated with longer duration of diabetes and higher baseline A1C level.
Pintus et al., 2019 (28)	• 12-month, prospective study (UK) • 52 children (4 months to 17 years of age) with type 1 diabetes • Use of flash CGM with education/support from health care professionals	• A1C • QoL	• Improvements were seen in A1C post-flash CGM compared with values at 12 ($P < 0.04$), 6 ($P < 0.04$), and 3 months ($P = 0.012$) pre-flash CGM use. • Questionnaire-derived measures of QoL improved ($P = 0.014$), diabetes symptoms decreased ($P = 0.018$), and treatment barriers were reduced ($P = 0.035$).
Al Hayek et al., 2019 (29)	• 12-week, prospective study (Saudi Arabia) • 33 adolescents/young adults (14–21 years of age) with type 1 diabetes • Use of flash CGM	• Well-being	• Questionnaire-derived measures of well-being improved: mean ($\pm$ SD) DTSQ score increased from 14.4 $\pm$ 6.5 to 32.1 $\pm$ 1.8 ($P < 0.001$), and percentage score for the WHO-5 Well-Being Index increased from 45.1% at baseline to 93.6% ($P < 0.001$).

DTSQ, Diabetes Treatment Satisfaction Questionnaire; OR, odds ratio.

($P = 0.031$), and fewer individuals reported severe hypoglycemic events (7.8 vs. 14.6%, $P < 0.0001$) or experienced hypoglycemic coma (1.1 vs. 2.7%, $P = 0.001$). Although measures of general and diabetes-specific QoL were relatively high at baseline and remained stable throughout the study, treatment satisfaction was increased by study end. Moreover, fewer subjects were absent from work (2.9 vs. 5.8%, $P < 0.0001$), a metric that is often not reported in RCTs and provides an informative indicator of economic benefit.

Similarly, an analysis of a Dutch registry assessed the impact of flash CGM use among 1,365 individuals with diabetes (77% with type 1 diabetes, 16% with type 2 diabetes, and 7% with other types of diabetes) (24). After 12 months of flash CGM use, A1C decreased from 8.0 to 7.4%, with the greatest reductions occurring among participants with a baseline A1C >8.6%. The percentage

of patients experiencing any hypoglycemic event decreased from 93.5 to 91.0% ($P < 0.05$), and the number of diabetes-related hospital admissions decreased from 144 before baseline to 22 at 12 months ($P < 0.001$). Additionally, flash CGM users reported reduced diabetes burden with the SF-12 (12-item Short Form, v. 2) survey, EQ-5D-3 L (EuroQol 5-Dimension, three-level version) instrument, and DVN-PROM (Diabetes Vereniging Nederland Patient-Reported Outcomes Measure) questionnaire. The majority of study participants reported fewer hypoglycemic events (77%), less severe hypoglycemia (78%), more frequent insulin dose adjustments (80%), better understanding of their glucose fluctuations (95%), and less worry about their diabetes among housemates and family members (62%). Moreover, 81.7% felt no inhibitions about measuring their glucose in the presence of strangers, which was consistent with an increased frequency of sensor scanning. Also, in addition to the cost savings associated with reduced hospitalizations, there were fewer absences from work (7.8 vs. 18.55%, P <0.001).

While findings from these real-world studies further support the metabolic benefits associated with flash CGM use reported in RCTs, the reductions in hospitalizations (23–25,33) and in absenteeism (23,24) also demonstrate the immediate and substantial economic benefits of flash CGM use within populations with type 1 or type 2 diabetes. The improvements observed in treatment satisfaction (23,29), levels of hypoglycemia fear (26,29), sense of well-being (29), and other health-related measures (23–25,28,29) additionally support patient-reported outcomes described in RCTs (1,5).

Additional Emerging Real-World Evidence

As use of flash CGM technology continues to grow, large national and commercial database studies are being investigated to discern the impact of flash CGM on both A1C and acute diabetes-related events (Table 3). Two recent analyses showed significant reductions in all-cause hospitalizations and diabetes-related events among adults with either type 1 or type 2 diabetes who acquired flash CGM.

Analysis of a French national reimbursement claims database identified 74,158 adults with diabetes (type 1: $n = 33,203$, type 2: $n = 40,955$) who initiated flash CGM during the last 6 months of 2017 (34). Over the next 12 months, yearly hospitalization rates for DKA and acute hyperglycemia were reduced by 52% among patients with type 1 diabetes and by 47% for those with type 2 diabetes. The reduced rates were most evident for people with very low or very high adherence to self-monitoring of blood glucose (SMBG).

Significant reductions in acute diabetes-related adverse events (ADEs) and all-cause hospitalizations (ACH) were noted among 1,244 adults with type 2 diabetes treated with rapid- or short-acting insulin who acquired flash CGM (35). At 6 months post-acquisition, ADE rates decreased from 0.158 to 0.077 events/patient-year (hazard ratio [HR] 0.49 [95% CI 0.34–0.69], P <0.001). Hospitalizations also decreased from 0.345 to 0.247 events/patient-year (HR 0.72 [95% CI 0.58–0.88], P = 0.002). These findings equate to numbers needed to treat of 12 and 10 for 1 year to avoid one ADE or 1 ACH, respectively.

Strong evidence for the clinical and economic benefits associated with use of flash CGM has also emerged from studies of individuals treated less intensively with insulin

or noninsulin therapy (30,31,33). In addition to significant reductions in ADEs and hospitalization rates (33), there were substantial and sustained reductions in A1C among adults with type 2 diabetes treated with long-acting insulin or noninsulin therapies (30). For those not treated with insulin, the reductions in A1C were similar to what would be expected from adding insulin glargine (36). Further studies (34,37) have established that there is no correlation between previous frequency of daily blood glucose monitoring and ADEs.

These findings challenge the view that CGM should be made available only to patients who are treated with intensive insulin therapy and who have a documented history of frequent blood glucose monitoring. This perception may have reduced the coverage of CGM offered by some commercial and public insurers. For example, the Centers for Medicare & Medicaid Services currently limit coverage to patients who administer three or more insulin injections per day (or use an insulin pump) and perform four or more glucose tests per day.

Summary

Many individuals with diabetes experience poor glycemic control (38,39), which puts them at increased risk for acute adverse glycemic events (40,41) and the long-term development of microvascular and macrovascular disease (42–44). In addition to its clinical consequences, uncontrolled diabetes is driving an inordinate economic burden on private payers and national health care systems (7).

Numerous studies have shown that optimizing A1C levels and reducing the incidence of severe hypoglycemia and DKA can significantly lower health care costs (10–14,45–47). However, achieving optimal diabetes control necessitates expanded adoption of diabetes medications and technologies that are effective, safe, and feasible in real-world clinical settings.

Flash CGM provides immediate information about an individual's current and projected glucose level using rate-of-change arrows, which allows users to respond promptly to mitigate or prevent pending hypoglycemia or hyperglycemia. Findings from large RCTs and prospective, observational studies have shown that use of flash CGM is associated with improved overall glycemic control (23–26,28), reductions in hypoglycemia (23–25), fewer diabetes-related hospitalizations (23–25,33), decreased absenteeism (23,24), and improvements in treatment satisfaction (23,29) and measures of well-being (23,25,28,29). These outcomes indicate both clinical and economic benefits, and use of flash CGM can enable these

TABLE 3 Summary of Emerging Real-World Evidence

Published Reports	Design/Intervention	Outcome Measures	Findings
A1C reductions			
Miller et al., 2020 (30)	• 6- and 12-month retrospective, observational analyses using medical/pharmacy claims database and Quest laboratory A1C values (United States) • 6- and 12-month: 774 and 207 adults, respectively, with type 2 diabetes treated with long-acting insulin or premixed insulin (*n* = 277 and 87, respectively) or noninsulin therapy (*n* = 497 and 120, respectively) • Acquisition of flash CGM	• A1C	• A1C decreased by −0.8% (*P* <0.0001) in the 6-month cohort: long-acting insulin by −0.6% (*P* <0.0001), noninsulin by −0.9% (*P* <0.0001). • A1C decreased by −0.6% (*P* <0.0001) in the 12-month cohort: long-acting insulin by −0.5% (*P* = 0.0014), noninsulin by −0.7% (*P* <0.0001).
Wright et al., 2020 (31)	• 12-month, retrospective, observational study using IBM Explorys, a U.S. EHR database • 1,183 adults with type 2 diabetes using long-acting insulin or premixed insulin (*n* = 378) or noninsulin (*n* = 805) therapy • 12-month, retrospective, observational study using IBM Explorys, a U.S. EHR database	• A1C	• A1C decreased by −1.38% (from 10.16 to 8.78%, *P* <0.0001) at 6 months post–flash CGM acquisition. • Greatest reductions of A1C were seen in participants with highest baseline A1C levels.
Eeg-Olofsson et al., 2020 (48)	• 12-month, retrospective, observational study using Swedish National Diabetes Register • 538 adults with type 1 or type 2 diabetes • Flash CGM use	• A1C	• A1C decreased by −0.52% (*P* <0.0001) at 12 months.
Reductions in events/hospitalizations			
Hirsch et al., 2020 (37)	• 12-month, retrospective, observational study using IBM MarketScan Commercial Claims and Medicare Supplemental databases • 12,521 adults with type 1 or type 2 diabetes • Acquisition of flash CGM	• Acute ADEs for hypoglycemia or hyperglycemia	• ADE decreased from 0.245 to 0.132 events/patient-year (HR: 0.54 [95% CI 0.49-0.59], *P* <0.001). • Similar reductions in ADE were seen in participants with a history of performing four or more or less than four glucose tests per day.
Bergenstal et al., 2020 (35)	• 12-month, retrospective, observational study using IBM MarketScan Commercial Claims and Medicare Supplemental databases • 1,244 adults with type 2 diabetes • Acquisition of flash CGM	• Acute ADEs for hypoglycemia or hyperglycemia • ACH	• ADEs decreased from 0.158 to 0.077 events/patient-year (HR: 0.49 [95% CI 0.34-0.69], *P* <0.001). • ACH decreased from 0.345 to 0.247 events/patient-year (HR: 0.72 [95% CI 0.58-0.88], *P* = 0.002).
Miller et al., 2020 (33)	• 12-month, retrospective, observational study using IBM MarketScan Commercial Claims and Medicare Supplemental databases • 7,167 adults with type 2 diabetes treated with long-acting insulin or noninsulin therapy • Acquisition of flash CGM	• Acute ADEs • Hospitalization or outpatient emergency for hypoglycemia or hyperglycemia	• ADEs decreased at 6 months post-acquisition of flash CGM from 0.071 to 0.052 events/patient-year (HR: 0.70 [95% CI 0.57-0.85], *P* <0.001). • Hospitalizations decreased from 0.180 to 0.161 events/patient-year (HR: 0.87 [95% CI 0.78-0.98], *P* = 0.025).
Roussel et al., 2020 (34)	• 12-month, retrospective, observational study using the French nationwide reimbursement claims database • 33,203 individuals with type 1 diabetes and 40,955 individuals with type 2 diabetes • Flash CGM use for 12 months	• Hospitalizations for DKA	• DKA hospitalizations decreased by 52% in participants with type 1 diabetes and by 47% in those with type 2 diabetes.

EHR, electronic health record; IBM, International Business Machines.

outcomes regardless of therapy and previous blood glucose monitoring frequency (30,31,33,34,37).

Given the growing global prevalence of diabetes and its associated costs, there is an opportunity to take advantage of flash CGM to facilitate improvements in metabolic control and patient QoL while reducing the projected costs of diabetes care.

ACKNOWLEDGMENTS

The authors thank Christopher G. Parkin, CGParkin Communications, Inc., for his thoughtful assistance in developing this manuscript.

FUNDING

Funding for the development of this manuscript was provided by Abbott Diabetes Care.

DUALITY OF INTEREST

C.J.B. has served on advisory boards for Abbott Diabetes Care, Boehringer Ingelheim, Lexicon, Novo Nordisk, and Sanofi. J.R.G. has served on advisory boards and/or speaker bureaus for Abbott Diabetes Care.

AUTHOR CONTRIBUTIONS

C.J.B. and J.R.G. wrote, reviewed, and approved the manuscript for submission. C.J.B. is the guarantor of this work and takes responsibility for the integrity of the data and the accuracy of the content.

REFERENCES

1. Bolinder J, Antuna R, Geelhoed-Duijvestijn P, Kröger J, Weitgasser R. Novel glucose-sensing technology and hypoglycaemia in type 1 diabetes: a multicentre, non-masked, randomised controlled trial. Lancet 2016;388: 2254–2263

2. Oskarsson P, Antuna R, Geelhoed-Duijvestijn P, Kröger J, Weitgasser R, Bolinder J. Impact of flash glucose monitoring on hypoglycaemia in adults with type 1 diabetes managed with multiple daily injection therapy: a pre-specified subgroup analysis of the IMPACT randomised controlled trial. Diabetologia 2018;61:539–550

3. Evans M, Welsh Z, Ells S, Seibold A. The impact of flash glucose monitoring on glycaemic control as measured by HbA1c: a meta-analysis of clinical trials and real-world observational studies. Diabetes Ther 2020;11:83–95

4. Haak T, Hanaire H, Ajjan R, Hermanns N, Riveline JP, Rayman G. Use of flash glucose-sensing technology for 12 months as a replacement for blood glucose monitoring in insulin-treated type 2 diabetes. Diabetes Ther 2017;8:573–586

5. Haak T, Hanaire H, Ajjan R, Hermanns N, Riveline JP, Rayman G. Flash glucose-sensing technology as a replacement for blood glucose monitoring for the management of insulin-treated type 2 diabetes: a multicenter, open-label randomized controlled trial. Diabetes Ther 2017; 8:55–73

6. Yaron M, Roitman E, Aharon-Hananel G, et al. Effect of flash glucose monitoring technology on glycemic control and treatment satisfaction in patients with type 2 diabetes. Diabetes Care 2019;42:1178–1184

7. Bommer C, Sagalova V, Heesemann E, et al. Global economic burden of diabetes in adults: projections from 2015 to 2030. Diabetes Care 2018;41:963–970

8. Davies MJ, D'Alessio DA, Fradkin J, et al. Management of hyperglycaemia in type 2 diabetes, 2018. A consensus report by the American Diabetes Association (ADA) and the European Association for the Study of Diabetes (EASD). Diabetologia 2018; 61:2461–2498

9. National Institute for Health and Care Excellence. Type 1 diabetes in adults: diagnosis and management. Available from https://www.nice.org.uk/guidance/ng17. Accessed 1 July 2019

10. Fitch K, Pyenson BS, Iwasaki K. Medical claim cost impact of improved diabetes control for medicare and commercially insured patients with type 2 diabetes. J Manag Care Pharm 2013;19: 609–620, 620a–620d

11. Bansal M, Shah M, Reilly B, Willman S, Gill M, Kaufman FR. Impact of reducing glycated hemoglobin on healthcare costs among a population with uncontrolled diabetes. Appl Health Econ Health Policy 2018;16:675–684

12. Baxter M, Hudson R, Mahon J, et al. Estimating the impact of better management of glycaemic control in adults with type 1 and type 2 diabetes on the number of clinical complications and the associated financial benefit. Diabet Med 2016;33:1575–1581

13. Gilmer TP, O'Connor PJ, Rush WA, et al. Predictors of health care costs in adults with diabetes. Diabetes Care 2005;28:59–64

14. Juarez D, Goo R, Tokumaru S, Sentell T, Davis J, Mau M. Association between sustained glycated hemoglobin control and healthcare costs. Am J Pharm Benefits 2013;5:59–64

15. Aronson R, Galstyan G, Goldfracht M, Al Sifri S, Elliott L, Khunti K. Direct and indirect health economic impact of hypoglycaemia in a global population of patients with insulin-treated diabetes. Diabetes Res Clin Pract 2018;138:35–43

16. Pawaskar M, Iglay K, Witt EA, Engel SS, Rajpathak S. Impact of the severity of hypoglycemia on health-related quality of life, productivity, resource use, and costs among US patients with type 2 diabetes. J Diabetes Complications 2018;32:451–457

17. Brod M, Christensen T, Thomsen TL, Bushnell DM. The impact of non-severe hypoglycemic events on work productivity and diabetes management. Value Health 2011;14:665–671

18. Giorda CB, Rossi MC, Ozzello O, et al.; HYPOS-1 Study Group of AMD. Healthcare resource use, direct and indirect costs of hypoglycemia in type 1 and type 2 diabetes, and nationwide projections: results of the HYPOS-1 study. Nutr Metab Cardiovasc Dis 2017;27:209–216

19. Khosla S, White R, Medina J, et al. Real world evidence (RWE): a disruptive innovation or the quiet evolution of medical evidence generation? F1000 Res 2018;7:111

20. U.S. Food and Drug Administration. Use of real-world evidence to support regulatory decision-making for medical devices. Available from https://www.fda.gov/media/99447/download. Accessed 30 March 2019

21. Resnic FS, Matheny ME. Medical devices in the real world. N Engl J Med 2018;378:595–597

22. Katkade VB, Sanders KN, Zou KH. Real world data: an opportunity to supplement existing evidence for the use of long-established medicines in health care decision making. J Multidiscip Healthc 2018;11:295–304

23. Charleer S, De Block C, Van Huffel L, et al. Quality of life and glucose control after 1 year of nationwide reimbursement of intermittently scanned continuous glucose monitoring in adults living with type 1 diabetes (FUTURE): a prospective observational real-world cohort study. Diabetes Care 2020;43:389–397

24. Fokkert M, van Dijk P, Edens M, et al. Improved well-being and decreased disease burden after 1-year use of flash glucose monitoring (FLARE-NL4). BMJ Open Diabetes Res Care 2019;7: e000809

25. Tyndall V, Stimson RH, Zammitt NN, et al. Marked improvement in HbA$_{1c}$ following commencement of flash glucose monitoring in people with type 1 diabetes. Diabetologia 2019;62: 1349–1356

26. Paris I, Henry C, Pirard F, Gérard A-C, Colin IM. The new FreeStyle Libre flash glucose monitoring system improves the glycaemic control in a cohort of people with type 1 diabetes followed in real-life conditions over a period of one year. Endocrinol Diabetes Metab 2018;1:e00023

27. Messaaoui A, Tenoutasse S, Crenier L. Flash glucose monitoring accepted in daily life of children and adolescents with type 1 diabetes and reduction of severe hypoglycemia in real-life use. Diabetes Technol Ther 2019;21:329–335

28. Pintus D, Ng SM. FreeStyle Libre flash glucose monitoring improves patient quality of life measures in children with type 1 diabetes mellitus (T1DM) with appropriate provision of education and support by healthcare professionals. Diabetes Metab Syndr 2019;13:2923–2926

29. Al Hayek AA, Al Dawish MA. The potential impact of the FreeStyle Libre flash glucose monitoring system on mental well-being and treatment satisfaction in patients with type 1 diabetes: a prospective study. Diabetes Ther 2019;10:1239–1248

30. Miller E, Brandner L, Wright E. HbA1c reduction after initiation of the FreeStyle Libre system in type 2 diabetes patients on long-acting insulin or non-insulin therapy [Abstract]. Diabetes 2020; 69(Suppl. 1):84-LB

31. Wright E, Kerr MSD, Reyes I, Nabutovsky Y, Miller E. HbA1c reduction associated with a FreeStyle Libre system in people with type 2 diabetes not on bolus insulin therapy [Abstract]. Diabetes 2020;69(Suppl. 1):78-LB-P

32. Kröger J, Fasching P, Hanaire H. Three European retrospective real-world chart review studies to determine the effectiveness of flash glucose monitoring on HbA1c in adults with type 2 diabetes. Diabetes Ther 2020;11:279–291

33. Miller E, Kerr MSD, Roberts GJ, Souto D, Nabutovsky Y, Wright E. FreeStyle Libre system use associated with reduction in acute diabetes events and all-cause hospitalizations in patients with type 2 diabetes without bolus insulin [Abstract]. Diabetes 2020; 69(Suppl. 1):85-LB

34. Roussel R, Bruno Guerci B, Vicaut E, et al. Dramatic drop in ketoacidosis rate after FreeStyle Libre system initiation in type 1

and type 2 diabetes in France, especially in people with low self-monitoring of blood glucose (SMBG): a nationwide study [Abstract]. Diabetes 2020;69(Suppl. 1):68-OR

35. Bergenstal RM, Kerr MSD, Gregory J, et al. FreeStyle Libre system use is associated with reduction in inpatient and outpatient emergency acute diabetes events and all-cause hospitalizations in patients with type 2 diabetes [Abstract]. Diabetes 2020;69(Suppl. 1):69-OR

36. Sanofi. Lantus [prescribing information]. Available from https://products.sanofi.us/Lantus/Lantus.html#section-15.1. Accessed 25 June 2020

37. Hirsch IB, Kerr MSD, Roberts GJ, et al. Utilization of continuous glucose monitors is associated with reduction in inpatient and outpatient emergency acute diabetes events regardless of prior blood test strip usage [Abstract]. Diabetes 2020;69(Suppl. 1): 875-P

38. Carls G, Huynh J, Tuttle E, Yee J, Edelman SV. Achievement of glycated hemoglobin goals in the US remains unchanged through 2014. Diabetes Ther 2017;8:863–873

39. Brath H, Paldánius PM, Bader G, Kolaczynski WM, Nilsson PM. Differences in glycemic control across world regions: a post-hoc analysis in patients with type 2 diabetes mellitus on dual antidiabetes drug therapy. Nutr Diabetes 2016;6:e217

40. Monnier L, Colette C, Wojtusciszyn A, et al. Toward defining the threshold between low and high glucose variability in diabetes. Diabetes Care 2017;40:832–838

41. Qu Y, Jacober SJ, Zhang Q, Wolka LL, DeVries JH. Rate of hypoglycemia in insulin-treated patients with type 2 diabetes can be predicted from glycemic variability data. Diabetes Technol Ther 2012;14:1008–1012

42. Diabetes Control and Complications Trial Research Group. The relationship of glycemic exposure (HbA1c) to the risk of development and progression of retinopathy in the Diabetes Control and Complications Trial. Diabetes 1995;44:968–983

43. Lind M, Pivodic A, Svensson A-M, Ólafsdóttir AF, Wedel H, Ludvigsson J. HbA$_{1c}$ level as a risk factor for retinopathy and nephropathy in children and adults with type 1 diabetes: Swedish population based cohort study. BMJ 2019;366:l4894

44. Sherwani SI, Khan HA, Ekhzaimy A, Masood A, Sakharkar MK. Significance of HbA1c test in diagnosis and prognosis of diabetic patients. Biomark Insights 2016;11:95–104

45. Liu J, Wang R, Ganz ML, Paprocki Y, Schneider D, Weatherall J. The burden of severe hypoglycemia in type 1 diabetes. Curr Med Res Opin 2018;34:171–177

46. Liu J, Wang R, Ganz ML, Paprocki Y, Schneider D, Weatherall J. The burden of severe hypoglycemia in type 2 diabetes. Curr Med Res Opin 2018;34:179–186

47. Agency for Healthcare Research and Quality. Healthcare Cost and Utilization Project (HCUP). Available from https://www.ahrq.gov/research/data/hcup/index.html. Accessed 1 February 2020

48. Eeg-Olofsson K, Svensson A-M, Franzén S, Ismail HA, Levrat-Guillen F. Sustainable HbA1c decrease at 12 months for adults with type 1 and type 2 diabetes using the FreeStyle Libre system: a study within the National Diabetes Register in Sweden [Abstract]. Diabetes 2020;69(Suppl. 1):74-LB-P

Use of Flash Continuous Glucose Monitoring Is Associated With A1C Reduction in People With Type 2 Diabetes Treated With Basal Insulin or Noninsulin Therapy

Eugene E. Wright Jr.,[1] Matthew S.D. Kerr,[2] Ignacio J. Reyes,[2] Yelena Nabutovsky,[2] and Eden Miller[3]

[1]Charlotte Area Health Education Center, Charlotte, NC; [2]Abbott, Sylmar, CA; [3]Diabetes Nation, Sisters, OR

BACKGROUND | Glycemic control is suboptimal in many individuals with type 2 diabetes. Although use of flash continuous glucose monitoring (CGM) has demonstrated A1C reductions in patients with type 2 diabetes treated with a multiple daily injection or insulin pump therapy regimen, the glycemic benefit of this technology in patients with type 2 diabetes using nonintensive treatment regimens has not been well studied.

METHODS | This retrospective, observational study used the IBM Explorys database to assess changes in A1C after flash CGM prescription in a large population with suboptimally controlled type 2 diabetes treated with nonintensive therapy. Inclusion criteria were diagnosis of type 2 diabetes, age <65 years, treatment with basal insulin or noninsulin therapy, naive to any CGM, baseline A1C ≥8%, and a prescription for the FreeStyle Libre flash CGM system during the period between October 2017 and February 2020. Patients served as their own control subject.

RESULTS | A total of 1,034 adults with type 2 diabetes (mean age 51.6 ± 9.2 years, 50.9% male, baseline A1C $10.1 \pm 1.7\%$) were assessed. More patients received noninsulin treatments ($n = 728$) than basal insulin therapy ($n = 306$). We observed a significant reduction in A1C within the full cohort: from 10.1 ± 1.7 to $8.6 \pm 1.8\%$; $\Delta -1.5 \pm 2.2\%$ ($P < 0.001$). The largest reductions were seen in patients with a baseline A1C ≥12.0% ($n = 181$, A1C reduction -3.7%, $P < 0.001$). Significant reductions were seen in both treatment groups (basal insulin -1.1%, noninsulin -1.6%, both $P < 0.001$).

CONCLUSION | Prescription of the flash CGM system was associated with significant reductions in A1C in patients with type 2 diabetes treated with basal insulin or noninsulin therapy. These findings provide evidence for expanding access to flash CGM within the broader population of people with type 2 diabetes.

Large clinical trials have consistently demonstrated that maintaining near-normal glycemia can prevent or delay diabetes-related microvascular and macrovascular disease (1–4). However, suboptimal glycemic control using traditional blood glucose monitoring persists among a substantial number of patients with type 2 diabetes (5,6). As reported by Carls et al. (5), achievement of individualized targets declined from 69.8% in 2010 to 63.8% in 2014, and the percentage of individuals with an A1C >9.0% increased from 12.6 to 15.5% during the same time period. More recently, investigators estimated that more than half (51.5%) of adults with insulin-treated type 2 diabetes have an A1C level >8.0% (7).

Randomized controlled trials have demonstrated that use of flash continuous glucose monitoring (CGM) significantly lowers A1C (8), with reductions in hypoglycemia (9,10) and improved treatment satisfaction (8,9) in people with type 2 diabetes treated with a multiple daily injection (MDI) insulin regimen. However, use of flash CGM has not been well studied in individuals with type 2 diabetes who are treated with less intensive therapy.

The FreeStyle Libre 14-day flash CGM system and the recently cleared (cleared by the U.S. Food and Drug Administration on 15 June 2020) FreeStyle Libre 2 flash CGM system (both Abbott Diabetes Care, Alameda, CA) are the only flash CGM systems available in the United States. An earlier version (a 10-day system) was available from 2017 to 2019. These systems use a single-use, factory-calibrated sensor that continuously measures interstitial glucose levels. By scanning the sensor with a compatible reader or

Corresponding author: Eugene E. Wright Jr., eewright51@gmail.com

https://doi.org/10.2337/ds20-0069

smartphone, users can view their current glucose value, as well as their glucose pattern during the past 8 hours, along with trend arrows indicating the direction and velocity of changing glucose levels. The FreeStyle Libre 2 system functions similarly to the earlier FreeStyle Libre versions and has real-time optional alarms for low and high glucose levels but was not available during the study's observation period.

We evaluated changes in A1C levels after patients received a prescription for a flash CGM system in a large population of patients with suboptimally controlled type 2 diabetes who were treated with basal insulin or noninsulin therapy.

Research Design and Methods

Design

This retrospective, observational database analysis used a prespecified analysis scheme to assess the impact of a flash CGM system prescription in a large cohort of patients with type 2 diabetes and suboptimal glycemic control who were treated with basal insulin (defined in this study as long-acting, NPH, or a premixed insulin formulation) or non-insulin therapy. The primary outcome measure was change from baseline A1C levels after prescription of the flash CGM system. Secondary outcomes included A1C changes stratified by diabetes therapy and baseline A1C. Inclusion criteria were a diagnosis of type 2 diabetes, age <65 years, naive to any CGM, a baseline A1C ≥8.0%, prescription of a flash CGM system (10- or 14-day) between October 2017 and February 2020, no record of short- or rapid-acting insulin use, presence of baseline A1C test within the 180 days before or including the flash CGM prescription date, and presence of a post-observation A1C value between 60 and 300 days after the CGM prescription date.

Eligible patients were identified using data obtained from the IBM Explorys database, which includes de-identified electronic health record data that reside in a highly secure, Cloud-based, Health Insurance Portability and Accountability Act–enabled platform. The database contains underlying patient-level data for a defined population based on a set of selection criteria. Available data included demographic information, medical records, laboratory data, and pharmacy prescriptions. Available data were extracted for study on 29 April 2020.

International Classification of Diseases, 9th and 10th revisions (ICD-9 and ICD-10), billing codes and Systematized Nomenclature of Medicine–Clinical Terms (SNOMED CT) codes were used to identify patients with diagnosed type 2 diabetes. Diabetes type was determined from the closest relevant diagnosis before the flash CGM prescription. In

TABLE 1 Patient Characteristics (*N* = 1,034)

Age, years	51.6 ± 9.2
Male sex	50.9
Baseline A1C	
≥8.0 to <10.0% (*n* = 576, mean 8.8 ± 0.6%)	55.7
≥10.0 to <12.0% (*n* = 277, mean 10.9 ± 0.6%)	26.8
≥12.0% (*n* = 181, mean 13.1 ± 0.9%)	17.5
Baseline treatment type	
Basal insulin (long-acting, NPH, or premixed)	29.6
Noninsulin	70.4
Treatment regimens for noninsulin users	
No diabetes medications	22.4
1 diabetes medication	22.4
2 diabetes medications	27.0
≥3 diabetes medications	28.2
Comorbidities	
Lipid disorder	82.2
Hypertension	77.3
Obesity	62.1
Liver disease	16.3
Heart failure	7.7
Ethnicity*	
Hispanic	2.9
Non-Hispanic	68.4
Other	6.4
Unavailable or declined to answer	22.3
Race*	
African American	22.1
Asian	1.0
Caucasian	59.0
Hispanic/Latino	0.8
Multiracial	0.8
Other	1.8
Unavailable or declined to answer	14.5

Data are percentages, except age, which is mean ± SD. *Ethnicity and race were self-reported by patients.

the rare case that the closest encounter had codes related to both type 1 and type 2 diabetes, the patient was excluded. Patients with a gestational diabetes diagnosis in the 6 months before their flash CGM prescription were also excluded.

ICD-9, ICD-10, and SNOMED CT codes were also used to identify the prevalence of comorbidities within the study cohort. Comorbidities were identified by the presence of a related code in the medical encounters at any time from the beginning of each patient's data availability through the day of acquiring the prescription for flash CGM.

National Drug Code (NDC) data were used to identify patients who were treated with basal insulin or noninsulin therapy and who had a record of a flash CGM prescription in the same time period. Code sets were determined by medical expert review.

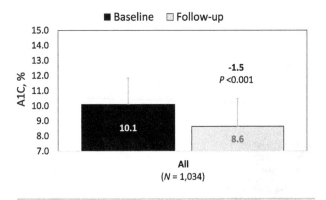

Statistical Analysis

The analysis was structured as patient-as-own-control. All changes in A1C values were evaluated with paired *t* tests, and changes in A1C categories were evaluated with χ² tests. Subgroup analyses are presented uncorrected for multiple comparisons. RStudio, v. 1.0.153 (Boston, MA), with R, v. 3.4.0, software was used for statistical analysis.

FIGURE 1 Change in A1C after flash CGM prescription.

Results

Patient Characteristics

From the IBM Explorys database, we identified a cohort of 1,034 patients with type 2 diabetes for assessment. Most patients were >50 years of age, had a baseline A1C of ≥8.0 to <10.0%, and were treated with noninsulin therapy. The majority of patients had hypertension and dyslipidemia, and more than half had a BMI >30 kg/m². Premixed insulin formulations were rare, with only 2.1% of patients using a premixed insulin as their only insulin therapy. Patient characteristics and diabetes medications are reported in Table 1.

To ensure that patients were naive to CGM, we excluded those with evidence of prior CGM prescription, including sensor, transmitter, or receiver, identified via either NDC codes or Healthcare Common Procedure Coding System codes. Prescriptions for the flash CGM system were identified through either the presence of associated NDC codes or the appearance of the system name in the prescription description field.

Outcomes

The primary outcome of the study was difference in A1C after acquisition of a prescription for a flash CGM compared with before receiving the prescription. Baseline A1C was defined as the value within 180 days pre-index closest to the flash CGM prescription date, including the CGM prescription date, and post-flash CGM A1C was defined as the value closest to 180 days post-prescription and within 60–300 days after the flash CGM prescription.

Secondary analyses included changes in A1C by treatment (insulin vs. noninsulin) and baseline A1C stratified into three subgroups: ≥8.0 to <10.0, ≥10.0 to <12.0, and ≥12.0%. An exploratory analysis was performed on the full spectrum of A1C baseline values, including people with A1C <8% who were excluded from the primary cohort analysis.

Outcomes

At study end point (mean follow-up 159 days), we observed a significant A1C reduction of 1.5 ± 2.2 percentage points within the full cohort (Figure 1).

In a subgroup analysis by insulin versus noninsulin therapy, patients treated with noninsulin therapy showed a notably greater A1C reduction (1.6 ± 2.3 percentage points) compared with those treated with basal insulin (1.1 ± 1.9 percentage points) despite starting at similar A1C levels before the flash CGM prescription (Figure 2).

The largest A1C reductions were observed in patients with a baseline A1C ≥12%, followed by those with a baseline A1C ≥10 to <12% (Figure 3).

An exploratory analysis was performed for the full spectrum of A1C baseline values, including people whose well-controlled A1C (<8%) excluded them from the primary cohort (n = 1,859)

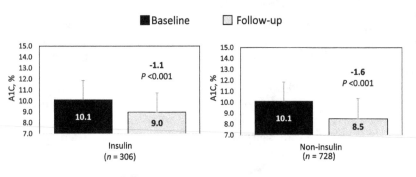

FIGURE 2 A1C changes by baseline treatment.

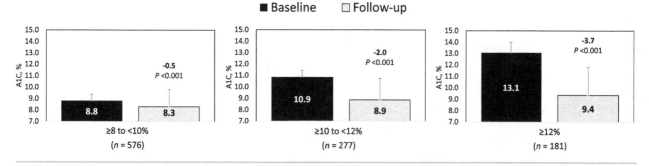

FIGURE 3 A1C changes by baseline A1C value.

(Figure 4). We observed a shift in the distribution of A1C values resulting in an increase in the percentage of patients who achieved A1C values <8.0% at end point (P <0.001). Reductions in the percentage of patients with an A1C ≥10.0 to <12.0 and ≥12.0% were also observed (both P <0.001). A narrower targeted comparison showed an increase in patients with an A1C <7%, from 21.7 to 32.2% (P <0.001).

Discussion

The use of flash CGM was recently shown to lower A1C in adults with type 2 diabetes treated with an MDI insulin regimen (8). To our knowledge, this is the first study to demonstrate the glycemic benefits of flash CGM use in a large population of people with type 2 diabetes treated with basal insulin or noninsulin therapies. Our findings showed a significant association between prescription of flash CGM and reductions in A1C. It was particularly interesting that patients treated with noninsulin therapies achieved notably greater A1C reductions compared with those on basal insulin therapy despite having similar baseline A1C levels.

As expected, patients with the highest A1C at baseline (≥12.0%) experienced the largest reduction in A1C; the percentage of patients with an A1C ≥12.0% at baseline

decreased by more than half after flash CGM prescription. We also saw a significant increase in the percentage of patients who achieved A1C levels <8 or <7%.

An important strength of our study was its use of the IBM Explorys database, which allowed us to track our cohort over time to detect changes in A1C levels before and after prescription of the flash CGM device without reliance on self-reported data. Moreover, our findings are potentially generalizable to the vast majority of individuals with type 2 diabetes who are treated with nonintensive therapy and have poorly controlled A1C. Recent data show that 14.1% of individuals with diabetes are treated with basal-only insulin, and more than half (51.7%) take oral or noninsulin injectable medications only (11).

A notable limitation is that the observational study design did not allow us to evaluate the degree or significance of A1C change compared with no CGM system prescription. Nor were we able to confirm acquisition of the system; the dataset only provided information on when patients received their prescriptions. Patients' A1C history outside our study window also was not captured. Additionally, we were not able to determine patients' persistence in monitoring or use of their glucose data. Moreover, our findings cannot be

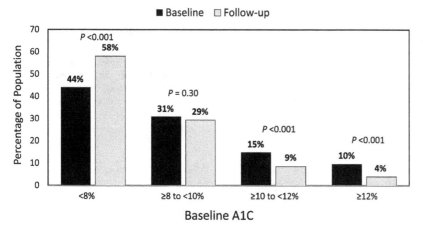

FIGURE 4 Change in A1C distribution after prescription of flash CGM.

generalized to elderly patients, a population that is at higher risk for severe hypoglycemia (12–14) and is less likely to use technology than younger patients with diabetes (15).

Nevertheless, our findings suggest that expanding insurance coverage of flash CGM to include patients with type 2 diabetes who are generally not considered to be eligible may help improve glycemic control within the larger type 2 diabetes population. However, changes in current eligibility criteria may occur sooner than expected. As a consequence of the coronavirus disease 2019 pandemic, an increasing number of clinicians are using telemedicine and digital diabetes technologies to provide essential care to minimize face-to-face clinic visits.

Flash CGM systems give patients the ability to automatically transfer glucose data to clinicians, who then use the data to provide guidance and therapy recommendations via remote clinical consults (16). Our findings of improved glycemic control and recent evidence demonstrating reductions in diabetes-related hospitalizations and health care resource utilization associated with flash CGM use (17) suggest that expanding CGM insurance coverage to type 2 diabetes patients treated with less intensive therapy would improve clinical outcomes.

Conclusion

In this real-world, retrospective, observational study, we observed significant A1C reductions within a large cohort of adult patients with type 2 diabetes who were treated with basal insulin or noninsulin therapy and had poorly controlled A1C at baseline after they received a prescription for a flash CGM system. Additional studies are needed to further elucidate patient behaviors relevant to monitoring persistence and use of data, as well as the impact of flash CGM on clinical outcomes and health care resource utilization within this population.

ACKNOWLEDGMENTS

The authors thank Chris Parkin of CGParkin Communications for providing medical writing support and Dr. Naunihal Virdi and Laura Brandner, both of Abbott Diabetes Care, for input and review of the manuscript.

FUNDING

This research was funded by Abbott Diabetes Care.

DUALITY OF INTEREST

E.E.W. has received consulting fees from Abbott, AstraZeneca, Bayer, Boehringer Ingelheim, Eli Lilly, Mannkind, Merck, Sanofi US, and Voluntis and has been a speaker for Abbott, Bayer, Boehringer Ingelheim, and Eli Lilly. M.S.D.K., I.J.R., and Y.N. are employed by Abbott. E.M. has received consulting fees from Abbott, AstraZeneca, Boehringer Ingelheim, Eli Lilly, Merck, Novo Nordisk, and Sanofi US and has been a speaker for Abbott, Boehringer Ingelheim, Eli Lilly, and Novo Nordisk.

AUTHOR CONTRIBUTIONS

All authors were responsible for designing the study. E.E.W. and E.M. wrote the manuscript. M.S.D.K., I.J.R., and Y.N. performed the data analysis. All authors reviewed/edited the manuscript. E.E.W. is the guarantor of this work and, as such, had full access to all the data in the study and takes responsibility for the integrity of the data and the accuracy of the data analysis.

PRIOR PRESENTATION

Portions of these data were presented as an abstract at the American Diabetes Association's virtual 80th Scientific Sessions, 12–16 June 2020.

REFERENCES

1. UK Prospective Diabetes Study Group. Intensive blood-glucose control with sulphonylureas or insulin compared with conventional treatment and risk of complications in patients with type 2 diabetes (UKPDS 33). Lancet 1998;352:837–853

2. Holman RR, Paul SK, Bethel MA, Matthews DR, Neil HAW. 10-Year follow-up of intensive glucose control in type 2 diabetes. N Engl J Med 2008;359:1577–1589

3. Nathan DM, Genuth S, Lachin J, et al.; Diabetes Control and Complications Trial Research Group. The effect of intensive treatment of diabetes on the development and progression of long-term complications in insulin-dependent diabetes mellitus. N Engl J Med 1993;329:977–986

4. Nathan DM, Cleary PA, Backlund JY, et al.; Diabetes Control and Complications Trial/Epidemiology of Diabetes Interventions and Complications (DCCT/EDIC) Study Research Group. Intensive diabetes treatment and cardiovascular disease in patients with type 1 diabetes. N Engl J Med 2005;353:2643–2653

5. Carls G, Huynh J, Tuttle E, Yee J, Edelman SV. Achievement of glycated hemoglobin goals in the US remains unchanged through 2014. Diabetes Ther 2017;8:863–873

6. Stone MA, Charpentier G, Doggen K, et al.; GUIDANCE Study Group. Quality of care of people with type 2 diabetes in eight European countries: findings from the Guideline Adherence to Enhance Care (GUIDANCE) study. Diabetes Care 2013;36:2628–2638

7. Lauffenburger JC, Lewey J, Jan S, Lee J, Ghazinouri R, Choudhry NK. Association of potentially modifiable diabetes care factors with glycemic control in patients with insulin-treated type 2 diabetes. JAMA Netw Open 2020;3:e1919645

8. Yaron M, Roitman E, Aharon-Hananel G, et al. Effect of flash glucose monitoring technology on glycemic control and treatment satisfaction in patients with type 2 diabetes. Diabetes Care 2019;42:1178–1184

9. Haak T, Hanaire H, Ajjan R, Hermanns N, Riveline JP, Rayman G. Use of flash glucose-sensing technology for 12 months as a replacement for blood glucose monitoring in insulin-treated type 2 diabetes. Diabetes Ther 2017;8:573–586

10. Haak T, Hanaire H, Ajjan R, Hermanns N, Riveline JP, Rayman G. Flash glucose-sensing technology as a replacement for blood glucose monitoring for the management of insulin-treated type 2 diabetes: a multicenter, open-label randomized controlled trial. Diabetes Ther 2017;8:55–73

11. American Diabetes Association. Fast facts: data and statistics about diabetes. Available from https://professional.diabetes.org/sites/professional.diabetes.org/files/media/sci_2020_diabetes_fast_facts_sheet_final.pdf. Accessed 20 May 2020

12. Meneilly GS, Cheung E, Tuokko H. Counterregulatory hormone responses to hypoglycemia in the elderly patient with diabetes. Diabetes 1994;43:403–410

13. Meneilly GS, Tessier D. Diabetes in the elderly. Diabet Med 1995;12:949–960

14. Schütt M, Fach EM, Seufert J, et al.; DPV Initiative and the German BMBF Competence Network Diabetes Mellitus. Multiple complications and frequent severe hypoglycaemia in 'elderly' and 'old' patients with type 1 diabetes. Diabet Med 2012;29:e176–e179

15. Czaja SJ, Charness N, Fisk AD, et al. Factors predicting the use of technology: findings from the Center for Research and Education on Aging and Technology Enhancement (CREATE). Psychol Aging 2006;21:333–352

16. Levine BJ, Close KL, Gabbay RA. Reviewing U.S. connected diabetes care: the newest member of the team. Diabetes Technol Ther 2020;22:1–9

17. Miller E, Kerr MSD, Roberts GJ, Souto D, Nabutovsky Y, Wright E Jr. FreeStyle Libre system use associated with reduction in acute diabetes events and all-cause hospitalizations in patients with type 2 diabetes without bolus insulin [Abstract]. Diabetes 2020;69(Suppl. 1):85-LB

Cannabidiol (CBD) Use in Type 2 Diabetes: A Case Report

Raymond G. Mattes,[1] Melchor L. Espinosa,[1] Sam S. Oh,[1] Elizabeth M. Anatrella,[2] and Elizabeth M. Urteaga[1]

[1]Feik School of Pharmacy, University of the Incarnate Word, San Antonio, TX; [2]Cleveland Clinic, Cleveland, OH

Cannabidiol (CBD) oil has been gaining popularity as a natural alternative for numerous disease states. CBD is a phytocannabinoid obtained from the *Cannabis sativa* plant. Unlike its relative tetrahydrocannabinol (THC), CBD does not activate CB_1 receptors in the brain and therefore lacks psychotropic effects (1). Instead, this substance is thought to work on the G-protein coupled receptor, endothelial cannabinoid receptor, and serotonin-1A receptors, among others.

Diabetes is the seventh leading cause of death and affects >30 million people in the United States (2). CBD has been investigated, mostly in animal models, for its ability to help treat diabetes. It is theorized that cannabis has desirable effects on hyperglycemia through its anti-inflammatory and antioxidant properties (3). The endocannabinoid system modulates food intake and energy homeostasis by activating cannabinoid receptors. Modulation of these receptors with CBD has the possibility to reduce body weight and A1C in people with diabetes.

In one study using mouse models, CBD was shown to significantly reduce the incidence of diabetes in these mice (4). This was shown by a significant decrease in pancreatic islets production of destructive insulitis and inflammatory cytokine production.

The potential to use CBD as a method to treat diabetes reveals the need for studies and case reports. The following case illustrates the initiation of CBD in a patient with type 2 diabetes.

Case Presentation

A 62-year-old Hispanic obese man (weight 113 kg, BMI 39 kg/m²) with a history of type 2 diabetes for 11 years began taking CBD oil to control his blood glucose in place of insulin degludec. Initiation of this product was independent of his clinician's recommendation and based on the patient's personal review of information that suggested CBD was beneficial for people with type 2 diabetes.

As shown in Table 1, the week before the patient's initiation of CBD, his A1C was 7.6%, and he was taking his currently prescribed medications: insulin degludec 32 units subcutaneously daily, metformin 1,000 mg orally twice daily, and empagliflozin 25 mg orally once daily. The patient reported adherence to his medications 6 days out of the week. Insulin degludec had been supplied as a sample, but his refill history suggested exceptional adherence to metformin and empagliflozin. His self-monitoring of blood glucose (SMBG) readings ranged from 124 to 176 mg/dL, with an average of 144 mg/dL. Because he was not meeting his goal A1C of <7.0%, he was prescribed saxagliptin 5 mg to be taken once daily. The patient had no macrovascular complications of diabetes and had normal liver and renal function but did have albuminuria.

One week later, the patient contacted his provider to report that he had self-discontinued insulin degludec after an episode of hypoglycemia and replaced his insulin therapy with 20 mg of oral CBD daily (SA Botanicals, San Antonio, TX). Given his history of side effects to glucagon-like peptide 1 receptor agonists and refusal to use insulin again because of concerns about hypoglycemia, the clinician agreed with his decision to discontinue insulin and suggested evaluating the patient's A1C on triple oral therapy plus CBD at his next visit.

At the next clinic visit 6 weeks after his CBD initiation, the patient's SMBG readings ranged from 122 to 158 mg/dL, with an average of 142 mg/dL. Based on his refill history and self-report, he had been adherent to his regimen of metformin, empagliflozin, saxagliptin, and CBD oil, and he reported no changes in diet or lifestyle. His weight remained stable at 112 kg.

Because his SMBG readings had not drastically changed with the discontinuation of insulin degludec, no medication

Corresponding author: Elizabeth M. Urteaga, montfort@uiwtx.edu

https://doi.org/10.2337/ds20-0023

TABLE 1 Patient's Blood Glucose Control and Medications During Case Timeline

	A1C, %	Preprandial Blood Glucose Range, mg/dL	Medications
Routine clinic visit	7.6	124–176	• Insulin degludec 32 units SQ daily • Metformin 1,000 mg PO twice daily • Empagliflozin 25 mg PO daily • Started saxagliptin 5 mg PO daily
1 week later: patient self-discontinued insulin degludec and started CBD 20 mg PO daily			
Week 6	NC	122–158	• Metformin 1,000 mg PO twice daily • Empagliflozin 25 mg PO daily • Saxagliptin 5 mg PO daily • CBD 20 mg PO daily
Week 11	7.6	130–177	• Metformin 1,000 mg PO twice daily • Empagliflozin 25 mg PO daily • Saxagliptin 5 mg PO daily • CBD 20 mg PO daily
Week 23	7.6	157–183	• Metformin 1,000 mg PO twice daily • Empagliflozin 25 mg PO daily • Saxagliptin 5 mg PO daily • CBD 18 mg PO twice daily
Week 56	7.7	127–184	• Metformin 1,000 mg PO twice daily • Empagliflozin 25 mg PO daily • Saxagliptin 5 mg PO daily • CBD 18 mg PO twice daily

NC, not collected; PO, orally; SQ, subcutaneously.

changes were made. After 4 months of using CBD oil, the patient increased his CBD dose to 18 mg twice daily and self-reported benefits for joint pain management. After 13 months of the patient's same medication regimen, his A1C remained stable at 7.7%, and his weight was 113 kg.

Discussion

CBD has become a popular substance since the Farm Bill was passed in 2018, removing hemp and cannabis from the Controlled Substance Act if they contain ≤0.3% THC (5). The U.S. Food and Drug Administration (FDA) has approved Epidiolex, a pharmaceutical-grade CBD, for treatment of seizures from Lennox-Gastaut syndrome; however, no other CBD products have been identified as safe and effective by the FDA. Despite this, several CBD products have been marketed for medical uses.

The literature regarding the use of CBD products as a medical treatment remains sparse. A meta-analysis published in 2015 in the *Journal of the American Medical Association* reviewed 79 studies that used CBD to treat various disease states (6). To date, promising results have only been demonstrated for the use of CBD as a treatment for severe forms of epilepsy, leading to the FDA's approval of Epidiolex (7,8).

With a deficit of studies on the use of CBD as a diabetes treatment, its effects in this regard have yet to be elucidated. One study of 62 patients with noninsulin-treated type 2 diabetes examined the effects of CBD 100 mg twice daily and tetrahydrocannabivarin (THCV) 5 mg twice daily for glycemic control (3). This study found a statistically significant reduction in resistin and an increase in glucose-dependent insulinotropic peptide compared with baseline but not compared with placebo, as well as surrogate outcomes suggesting a possible improvement in glycemic control. Beneficial effects on fasting plasma glucose levels and pancreatic β-cell function were only observed with THCV and not with CBD. The outcomes from this small study provide little confidence with regard to a benefit of CBD for people with type 2 diabetes.

In the case presented, several factors may have confounded the results in terms of efficacy, but useful conclusions may be drawn about the safety of CBD in people taking diabetes therapies. First, the nearly concurrent discontinuation of insulin degludec and initiation of both CBD oil and saxagliptin raises interest as to whether the CBD oil used had an appreciable effect on blood glucose and A1C. Saxagliptin has been proven in major clinical trials to reduce A1C for patients already on metformin therapy (9). Because the patient's A1C and SMBG remained stable when insulin degludec was replaced with CBD and saxagliptin was initiated, the saxagliptin may have masked a possible benefit from CBD. However, dipeptidyl peptidase-4 inhibitors such as saxagliptin reduce A1C by 0.7–0.8%, and it is unlikely that it had an equivalent A1C lowering to the dose of insulin degludec the patient had been taking previously. In addition, the patient used 20 mg of CBD oil daily, which may not have been a sufficient dose to receive the benefits mentioned in the aforementioned trial (3). Finally, the endocannabinoid system may vary among individuals, and CBD may be more effective in some patients.

The stable nature of the patient's A1C and SMBG readings and his general tolerability to this regimen does suggest that his use of CBD was safe, despite having questionable efficacy in this scenario. Additionally, his relatively stable A1C may have been attributable to the CBD. Most patients would have a significant increase in A1C after discontinuing insulin degludec at the dose the patient was taking. However, the insulinotropic effects of CBD may have maintained the patient's glycemic control by decreasing resistin. Increased resistin has been linked to insulin resistance and obesity, and because this patient was obese, it is reasonable to consider this as a possible mechanism for his stable A1C. In addition to its possible effects in improving glucose control, CBD may potentially have both macrovascular and microvascular benefits related to its anti-inflammatory effects (10–12).

No side effects were noted, including hypoglycemia or suspected CBD-induced hyperglycemia. The FDA and a meta-analysis have raised concerns that CBD products could cause liver injury, diarrhea, decreased appetite, male reproductive toxicity, irritability, agitation, and drowsiness (6,13). The potential for drug-drug interactions with CBD also exists. CBD is a strong cytochrome P450 inhibitor, as well as an inhibitor of UGT, and medications that are substrates of these enzymes may have decreased efficacy and safety when used in conjunction with CBD (14–16).

It should be reiterated that the risk of adverse effects may be heightened with the use of CBD products because of misbranding and adulteration (5). Risks may also be associated with patient nonadherence to guideline-recommended therapy in favor of CBD, as in this case. Widespread availability of CBD products and misleading marketing raise concern for unmoderated self-care of disease states that require professional intervention.

Summary

This case does not provide evidence for the use of CBD as an alternative treatment for uncontrolled type 2 diabetes. However, it does show that use of CBD did not cause harm or worsening of diabetes control. Regardless, health care providers should advocate for the continued use of proven therapies and monitor for harmful outcomes that may be associated with CBD should patients choose to use such therapy. Health care providers should be ready to discuss CBD and educate patients about the risks of CBD products and the potential for adulteration and misbranding in an effort to deliver the best care they can for their patients.

DUALITY OF INTEREST

No potential conflicts of interest relevant to this article were reported.

AUTHOR CONTRIBUTIONS

R.G.M. researched data and wrote and reviewed/edited the manuscript. M.L.E. and S.S.O. wrote the manuscript. E.M.A. researched data and wrote the manuscript. E.M.U. obtained case report data, contributed to discussion, and reviewed/edited the manuscript. E.M.U. is the guarantor of this work and, as such, takes responsibility for the integrity of the data presented and the accuracy of the data analysis.

REFERENCES

1. Mackie K. Cannabinoid receptors: where they are and what they do. J Neuroendocrinol 2008;20(Suppl. 1):10–14

2. Centers for Disease Control and Prevention. *National Diabetes Statistics Report, 2020*. Atlanta, GA, Centers for Disease Control and Prevention, U.S. Department of Health and Human Services, 2020

3. Jadoon KA, Ratcliffe SH, Barrett DA, et al. Efficacy and safety of cannabidiol and tetrahydrocannabivarin on glycemic and lipid parameters in patients with type 2 diabetes: a randomized, double-blind, placebo-controlled, parallel group pilot study. Diabetes Care 2016;39:1777–1786

4. Weiss L, Zeira M, Reich S, et al. Cannabidiol lowers incidence of diabetes in non-obese diabetic mice. Autoimmunity 2006;39: 143–151

5. U.S. Food and Drug Administration. FDA regulation of cannabis and cannabis-derived products, including cannabidiol (CBD). Available from https:// www.fda.gov/news-events/public-health-focus/fda-regulation-cannabis-and-cannabis-derived-products-including-cannabidiol-cbd. Accessed 27 March 2020

6. Whiting PF, Wolff RF, Deshpande S, et al. Cannabinoids for medical use: a systematic review and meta-analysis. JAMA 2015;313: 2456–2473

7. Pamplona FA, da Silva LR, Coan AC. Potential clinical benefits of CBD-rich cannabis extracts over purified CBD in treatment-resistant epilepsy: observational data meta-analysis. Front Neurol 2018;9:759

8. Epidiolex [package insert]. Carlsbad, CA, Greenwich Biosciences, 2018

9. Onglyza [package insert]. Princeton, NJ, AstraZeneca Pharmaceuticals, 2009

10. Rajesh M, Mukhopadhyay P, Bátkai S, et al. Cannabidiol attenuates high glucose-induced endothelial cell inflammatory response and

barrier disruption. Am J Physiol Heart Circ Physiol 2007;293: H610–H619

11. Rajesh M, Mukhopadhyay P, Bátkai S, et al. Cannabidiol attenuates cardiac dysfunction, oxidative stress, fibrosis, and inflammatory and cell death signaling pathways in diabetic cardiomyopathy. J Am Coll Cardiol 2010;56:2115–2125

12. Liou GI. Diabetic retinopathy: role of inflammation and potential therapies for anti-inflammation. World J Diabetes 2010;1:12–18

13. U.S. Food and Drug Administration. What you need to know (and what we're working to find out) about products containing cannabis or cannabis-derived compounds, including CBD. Available from https://www.fda.gov/consumers/consumer-updates/what-you-need-know-and-what-were-working-find-out-about-products-containing-cannabis-or-cannabis. Accessed 27 March 2020

14. Grayson L, Vines B, Nichol K, Szaflarski JP; UAB CBD Program. An interaction between warfarin and cannabidiol, a case report. Epilepsy Behav Case Rep 2017;9:10–11

15. Stout SM, Cimino NM. Exogenous cannabinoids as substrates, inhibitors, and inducers of human drug metabolizing enzymes: a systematic review. Drug Metab Rev 2014;46:86–95

16. Al Saabi A, Allorge D, Sauvage FL, et al. Involvement of UDP-glucuronosyltransferases UGT1A9 and UGT2B7 in ethanol glucuronidation, and interactions with common drugs of abuse. Drug Metab Dispos 2013;41:568–574

Beyond A1C—Standardization of Continuous Glucose Monitoring Reporting: Why It Is Needed and How It Continues to Evolve

Roy W. Beck[1] and Richard M. Bergenstal[2]

[1]Jaeb Center for Health Research, Tampa, FL; [2]International Diabetes Center, HealthPartners Institute, Minneapolis, MN

Continuous glucose monitoring (CGM) systems are becoming part of standard care for type 1 diabetes, and their use is increasing for type 2 diabetes. Consensus has been reached on standardized metrics for reporting CGM data, with time in range of 70–180 mg/dL and time below 54 mg/dL recognized as the key metrics of focus for diabetes management. The ambulatory glucose profile report has emerged as the standard for visualization of CGM data and will continue to evolve to incorporate other elements such as insulin, food, and exercise data to support glycemic management.

Continuous glucose monitoring (CGM) technology has evolved since it was first introduced about 20 years ago. Current systems include both real-time and intermittently scanned CGM devices. With both, glucose values are displayed for users to see their current glucose level and glycemic trend to assist in glucose management. Retrospective review of CGM data also is extremely valuable for quantifying the amount of time that glucose levels are in, above, or below the target range and the degree of glycemic variability, as well as for visualizing glucose patterns to enhance ongoing glucose management decisions.

For retrospective review, 10–14 days of CGM data provide a reasonably good representation of a patient's time in different glucose ranges, provided that there have been no major changes in diabetes management (e.g., the addition of a new glucose-lowering medication) or in life events affecting the patient's glycemia during this time period (1). Ten days of CGM data are usually sufficient for an estimate of mean glucose, time in the target range (i.e., 70–180 mg/dL), and time in hyperglycemia; however, ≥14 days of data may be needed to estimate hypoglycemia and glucose variability if glucose levels have considerable fluctuation.

As CGM technology has advanced, it has become in many cases the first advanced technology prescribed for diabetes management (before an insulin pump), and comparable outcomes are achieved in type 1 diabetes when CGM is used in conjunction with a pump or multiple daily injections of insulin (2). For the management of type 1 diabetes, CGM now should be considered part of standard care. Thus, there is an ever-growing need for standardization of glucose metrics and data visualization.

CGM Glucose Metrics

Because CGM use has expanded to the degree that it could be considered part of standard care, particularly in type 1 diabetes, the need for standardization of glucose metrics and data visualization has become more imperative. Several organizations have published consensus statements on the role of CGM and specific metrics to use for assessing overall glycemic management, hyperglycemia, hypoglycemia, and glycemic variability, and a conference was held with representatives of all organizations to reach a consensus on these matters (3–5). The American Diabetes Association's *Standards of Medical Care in Diabetes—2021* recommends CGM for all adults and children with type 1 or type 2 diabetes who are receiving insulin (6).

Standard metrics that were established by consensus include five ranges (>250, 181–250, 70–180, 54–69, and <54 mg/dL) and certain other metrics (i.e., mean glucose and coefficient of variation [CV] and SD [measures of glycemic variability]) (5). The percentage time in the range of 70–180 mg/dL is now commonly known as "time in range" (TIR). It is largely a measure of hyperglycemia in that, for most patients with diabetes, >90% of time outside of this range is >180 mg/dL. As such, TIR is highly correlated with the hyperglycemia metrics and with mean glucose (7). With respect to hypoglycemia, time spent with glucose <54 mg/dL has emerged as the most relevant CGM metric (8). Preventing glucose levels in the range of 54–69 mg/dL is

Corresponding author: Roy W. Beck, rbeck@jaeb.org

https://doi.org/10.2337/ds20-0090

important to minimize the risk of even lower glucose levels, but it is glucose levels <54 mg/dL that have been demonstrated to have deleterious physiologic effects, including the development of impaired glucose counterregulation and reduced hypoglycemia awareness (9–11), which has been associated with an increased risk of severe clinical hypoglycemic events (12); cognitive function impairment (13–16); an increase in cardiac arrhythmias (mortality) (17-22); adverse effects on quality of life, including sleep (17-22); reduced work productivity (23,24); and impaired driving, with an increase in car accidents (25–27). Additionally, CGM-measured hypoglycemia has been associated with a subsequent risk of a severe hypoglycemia event (28).

With respect to the two metrics of glycemic variability, SD is highly correlated with mean glucose, and CV is associated with the amount of hypoglycemia (29–31). Thus, in most cases, neither variability metric provides information that is impactful for diabetes management, since actionable management changes are to reduce hyperglycemia, which will decrease mean glucose and SD, and to reduce hypoglycemia, which will decrease the CV.

Among the eight standard CGM metrics, then, overall glucose control largely can be defined by one measure of hypoglycemia and one measure of hyperglycemia. Time <54 mg/dL clearly is the important metric for hypoglycemia. TIR has emerged as the preferred hyperglycemia metric instead of time >180 mg/dL or mean glucose.

Surveys have shown that TIR resonates with people with diabetes and is valued as important (32). There are several reasons for this finding. First, a change in the percentage of time in a range, which can be described in minutes per day, is more readily understood than a change in glucose level, which is expressed in mg/dL. Second, improvement represented by an increase in a metric is more motivating than improvement represented by a decrease (as is the case with mean glucose and time >180 mg/dL). Finally, seeing a picture of one's usual daily pattern of glucose values throughout the day and night is much more informative and likely more motivating to make needed adjustments in medications or lifestyle than just having a single number (A1C), which represents the percentage of one's glucose attached to hemoglobin in the red blood cells.

CGM Metric Targets

In addition to consensus having been achieved for a standard set of metrics, consensus also exists for goals or targets for these metrics (Table 1) (33). For TIR, a goal of >70% has been established for both type 1 and type 2 diabetes and equates on average with an A1C of ~7.0%.

TABLE 1 Targets for CGM Metrics	
CGM Metric	Target, %
TIR (70–180 mg/dL)	>70
Time >180 mg/dL	<25
Time >250 mg/dL	<5
Time <70 mg/dL	<4
Time <54 mg/dL	<1

Targets may differ for 1) older adults with diabetes or those considered at high risk for hypoglycemia, for whom a lower target may be the goal, and 2) pregnant women with diabetes, for whom the target may be 70% of values between 63 and 140 mg/dL.

Exceptions are for older adults with diabetes and those at high risk for hypoglycemia, for whom a lower target may be the goal, and for pregnant women with diabetes, for whom the target may be >70% of values between 63 and 140 mg/dL (7,34).

It is recognized, however, that many adults and children with diabetes have a TIR so far below this level that >70% is an unrealistic goal. As a result, in clinical care, emphasis should be placed on incremental improvements in TIR, with a 5% increase being a reasonable goal (33). Using Diabetes Control and Complications Trial (DCCT) data with standardized blood glucose measurements performed on 1 day every 3 months, Beck et al. (35) have shown that, for every 5% higher TIR, the risk of retinopathy was decreased by 22% and the risk of microalbuminuria by 15%, and for every 10% higher TIR, the risk decreases were 39 and 29%, respectively.

For time <54 mg/dL, the consensus target is <1%.

CGM Metrics and A1C

As CGM use has become widespread, there has been greater recognition of the limitations of A1C and the frequent discordance between laboratory-measured A1C and expected A1C based on mean glucose (36). Numerous studies have shown that there is a wide range of possible mean glucose levels for a given A1C level, meaning that for some people with diabetes, the laboratory-measured A1C may be an underestimate of mean glucose, and for others, it may be an overestimate. It is presumed that the discordance is often the result of red blood cell life span or other nonglycemic factors. The discordance is reflected in the correlation between mean glucose (or TIR) being only about 0.70 (7). Although this correlation may seem high, we would expect the correlation to be substantially higher if A1C was solely reflective of the level of glucose control.

Fabris et al. (37) demonstrated that, when hemoglobin glycation was modeled by a first-order differential equation driven by TIR, the A1C level estimated from TIR tracked closely with the laboratory-measured A1C, with the correlation between TIR and A1C increasing from about 0.70 to >0.90 (37). This analysis is important in terms of being able to extrapolate the strong association between A1C and vascular complications to also apply to CGM metrics of TIR and mean glucose.

An argument for continuing to rely on A1C for diabetes management has been that the level of A1C is associated with the risk for development of chronic diabetes complications. However, as CGM use has become more widespread, there are increasing data demonstrating an association between TIR and vascular complications. These studies primarily have been cross-sectional (38–44), although a recent study demonstrated the association of TIR and subsequent all-cause and cardiovascular disease mortality during median follow-up of 6.9 years (41). Additionally, the aforementioned analysis of DCCT data demonstrated a strong association between TIR and the development of microvascular complications (35).

In certain respects, A1C is a surrogate measure for mean glucose. Its availability had a transformative impact on diabetes management more than 25 years ago, long before CGM was available, and it became the gold standard for assessing hyperglycemia exposure over a 3-month period. Measurement of A1C to assess glucose control is particularly valuable for people with diabetes who are not using CGM. However, for those using CGM, the value of A1C, when the actual glucose concentrations can be continuously measured, must be questioned. Eventually, as CGM use becomes more readily available, particularly for people with type 2 diabetes, reliance on A1C may lessen. Until then, when CGM is available, there may be value in estimating A1C from CGM. This estimate of A1C from mean glucose is now known as the glucose management indicator (GMI) (45). This point was emphasized in a recent commentary by Battelino and Bergenstal (46) stating that, as we move from the A1C management era to the CGM management era, the GMI can be considered a bridge between A1C and TIR for clinical management.

Visualization of CGM Data

In using CGM to optimize diabetes management, the information available from CGM goes well beyond the metrics representing the amount of time in the different ranges. Viewing the pattern of glucose levels over a 24-hour day provides insights into when hyperglycemia and hypoglycemia tend to occur that are extremely valuable for adjusting basal and bolus insulin regimens. For many years, there was no standardized format for displaying CGM data irrespective of the CGM device, which likely in part stifled adoption of CGM by clinicians (47). Establishing common reporting metrics has helped substantially, and a standard format for displaying CGM data aggregated over a number of days has emerged as the ambulatory glucose profile (AGP) (46). The AGP was developed by Mazze et al. (48) in 1987 for use with self-monitoring of blood glucose data from glucose meters and was later refined for CGM data when Mazze joined the International Diabetes Center in Minneapolis, MN. The AGP gained traction in 2012, when Bergenstal et al. (49) of the International Diabetes Center held and then reported on the first CGM metrics and visualization expert panel (supported by the Leona M. and Harry B. Helmsley Charitable Trust), at which there was strong support to move to a standardized approach to the presentation of CGM data. Clinicians and researchers refined the AGP report with input from panel members, as well as industry and U.S. Food and Drug Administration regulatory observers. The expert panel consensus was presented to CGM manufacturing company representatives who, in subsequent years, began to incorporate the AGP into their CGM systems' reports.

The AGP has continued to evolve as there has been a coalescence of many different groups into an international consensus on refining CGM metrics and nomenclature. The core features of the AGP report (Figures 1 and 2) include a stacked bar showing the percentages of time in the different ranges specified in Table 1, the GMI, and a graphical display showing the distribution of glucose concentrations over each hour of the day. The distribution is depicted with a median line and the interquartile range (25th and 75th percentiles), which provides at a glance a sense of the patient's glycemic control and variability throughout the day, plus outlier cloud lines representing the 5th and 95th percentiles. The CGM metrics are useful as an overall summary of glucose levels and facilitate a quick assessment of the clinically important balance between TIR and time below range, while the graphical display is useful for identifying times of the day in which hypoglycemia or hyperglycemia tends to occur to target changes in diabetes management.

Future Directions

The AGP has undergone numerous enhancements during the past several years, but these are just a starting point for expanding this approach more broadly into diabetes management. In the next several years, we can expect the integration of insulin data from pumps and smart pens, as well as meal and exercise information (50). These additional

GLUCOSE STATISTICS AND TARGETS

August 10, 2018 - August 21, 2018   **12 Days**

% Time CGM is Active   **100%**

Ranges And Targets For	Type 1 or Type 2 Diabetes
Glucose Ranges	**Targets** % of Readings (Time/Day)
Target Range 70-180 mg/dL	Greater than 70% (16h 48min)
Below 70 mg/dL	Less than 4% (58min)
Below 54 mg/dL	Less than 1% (14min)
Above 180 mg/dL	Less than 25% (6h)
Above 250 mg/dL	Less than 5% (1h 12min)

Each 5% increase in time in range (70-180 mg/dL) is clinically beneficial.

Average Glucose	**175** mg/dL
Glucose Management Indicator (GMI)	**7.5%**
Glucose Variability	**45.5%**

Defined as percent coefficient of variation (%CV): target ≤36%

TIME IN RANGES

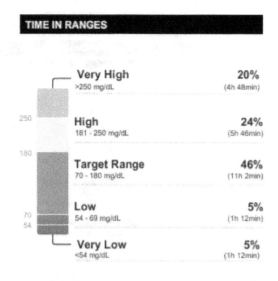

Very High	**20%**	
>250 mg/dL	(4h 48min)	
High	**24%**	
181 - 250 mg/dL	(5h 46min)	
Target Range	**46%**	
70 - 180 mg/dL	(11h 2min)	
Low	**5%**	
54 - 69 mg/dL	(1h 12min)	
Very Low	**5%**	
<54 mg/dL	(1h 12min)	

AMBULATORY GLUCOSE PROFILE (AGP)

AGP is a summary of glucose values from the report period, with median (50%) and other percentiles shown as if occurring in a single day.

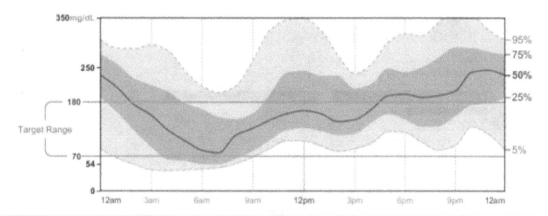

DAILY GLUCOSE PROFILES

Each daily profile represents a midnight to midnight period with the date displayed in the top-left corner.

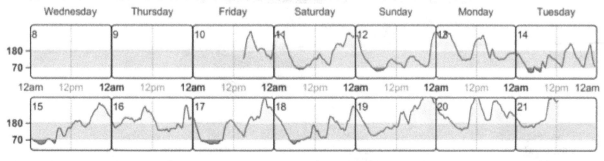

FIGURE 1 Case 1 AGP report interpretation. **Patient history:** Type 2 diabetes on metformin 1,000 mg twice daily, once-weekly glucagon-like peptide 1 receptor agonist, and 80 units insulin glargine at night. **Quick analysis:** *Panel 1.* Ask: Is action needed? Answer: Yes, both TIR and time below range (TBR) are not at target. TIR = 46% (target >70%); TBR (Low + Very Low) = 10% (target <4%); and TBR (Very Low) = 5% (target <1%). *Panel 2.* Ask: Where is action needed? Address hypoglycemia first. Note that from 4:00 to 8:00 a.m., 25% of values are <70 mg/dL, and from 3:00 to 6:00 a.m., 5% of values are <54 mg/dL. Note the classic "stair-step" pattern of postmeal elevations associated with overbasalization (continued titration of basal insulin without attaining glycemic targets). *Panel 3.* This graphic representation of data confirms low and high glucose occurring on both weekends and weekdays. **Plan:** Reduce basal insulin (we went to 36 units of glargine) and add premeal rapid-acting insulin (14 units at breakfast, 10 units at lunch, and 12 units at dinner). Also, work on consistency of food intake and exercise to address the considerable glucose variability.

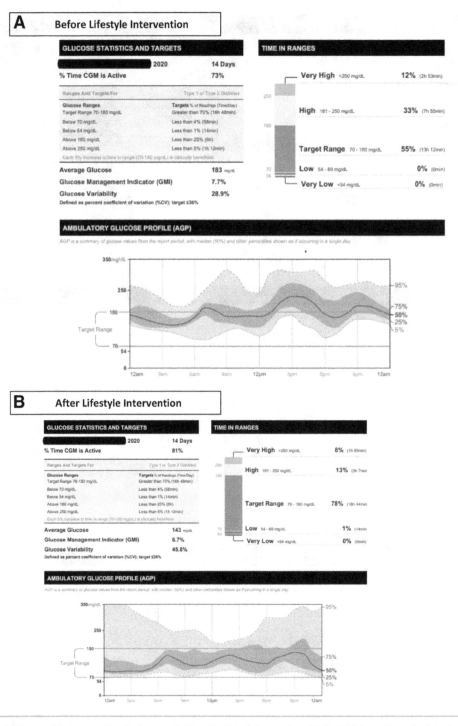

FIGURE 2 Case 2 AGP report interpretation before and after lifestyle intervention. **Patient history:** Type 2 diabetes with history of cardiovascular disease on metformin 1,000 mg twice daily and once-weekly glucagon-like peptide 1 receptor agonist. *A)* Initial AGP before lifestyle intervention. **Quick analysis:** *Panel 1.* Ask: Is action needed? Answer: Yes, TIR = 55% (target >70%), TBR = OK. *Panel 2.* Ask: Where is action needed? The entire glucose curve needs to shift down, and each postmeal excursion needs to be reduced, particularly after lunch. **Plan:** Initiation of a basal insulin was considered to shift the glucose curve down or the addition of a sodium–glucose cotransporter 2 inhibitor to minimize glucose excursions, but the patient wanted to try changing food intake. The patient was given the International Diabetes Center's CGM Lifestyle Choices guide (http://www.agpreport.org/agp/learning). *B)* Follow-up AGP after lifestyle intervention. Follow-up AGP was markedly improved. TIR increased from 55 to 78% with no hypoglycemia of concern. thepatient stated that he stopped drinking sugar-containing beverages (particularly at lunch), used the plate method of meal planning, and increased his daily walking, demonstrating that, with some guidance and support, CGM can facilitate helpful lifestyle changes.

enhancements will set the stage for incorporating decision-support tools using artificial intelligence to identify times of the day during which hyperglycemia or hypoglycemia tend to occur and provide additional guidance to patients and health care providers about how to optimally manage glucose levels.

More work is needed to fill the pressing need to standardize the incorporation of the AGP into electronic health records for ready access by providers at the time of a clinic visit, whether in person or virtual. The coronavirus disease 2019 pandemic has demonstrated the value of virtual telemedicine visits and has underscored the importance of ready access to CGM glucose data presented in a standardized format for review by health care providers and patients during virtual visits. Finally, striking a balance between comprehensive analysis with decision support and the need for a clear, simple understanding of the next steps to take to best address the needs of each person with diabetes is paramount.

Summary

Great advances have been made in CGM technology. CGM should be considered an integral part of diabetes management for all patients with type 1 diabetes and for many with type 2 diabetes. Metrics for summarizing CGM glucose data have been standardized, with TIR of 70–180 mg/dL and time <54 mg/dL recognized as the key metrics of focus for diabetes management. The AGP has emerged as the standard for visualization of CGM data. Future work is needed to seamlessly integrate the AGP report into electronic health records and to combine it with decision-support tools to guide changes in diabetes management.

DUALITY OF INTEREST

R.W.B.'s employer has received consulting fees, paid to his institution, from Bigfoot Biomedical, Eli Lilly, Insulet, and vTv Therapeutics; grant support and supplies from Dexcom and Tandem; and supplies from Ascenia and Roche. R.M.B.'s employer has received funds on his behalf for research support, consulting, or serving on the scientific advisory boards for Abbott Diabetes Care, Dexcom, Hygieia, Johnson & Johnson, Lilly, Medtronic, Novo Nordisk, Onduo, Roche, Sanofi, and UnitedHealthCare. No other potential conflicts of interest relevant to this article were reported.

AUTHOR CONTRIBUTIONS

R.W.B. and R.M.B. contributed equally to the writing of this article. Both authors are the guarantors of this work, and, as such, take responsibility for its content.

REFERENCES

1. Riddlesworth TD, Beck RW, Gal RL, et al. Optimal sampling duration for continuous glucose monitoring to determine long-term glycemic control. Diabetes Technol Ther 2018;20:314–316

2. Šoupal J, Petruželková L, Grunberger G, et al. Glycemic outcomes in adults with T1D are impacted more by continuous glucose monitoring than by insulin delivery method: 3 years of follow-up from the COMISAIR study. Diabetes Care 2020;43:37–43

3. Agiostratidou G, Anhalt H, Ball D, et al. Standardizing clinically meaningful outcome measures beyond HbA$_{1c}$ for type 1 diabetes: a consensus report of the American Association of Clinical Endocrinologists, the American Association of Diabetes Educators, the American Diabetes Association, the Endocrine Society, JDRF International, the Leona M. and Harry B. Helmsley Charitable Trust, the Pediatric Endocrine Society, and the T1D Exchange. Diabetes Care 2017;40:1622–1630

4. Beyond A1C Writing Group. Need for regulatory change to incorporate beyond A1C glycemic metrics. Diabetes Care 2018;41:e92–e94

5. Danne T, Nimri R, Battelino T, et al. International consensus on use of continuous glucose monitoring. Diabetes Care 2017;40:1631–1640

6. American Diabetes Association. 7. Diabetes technology: *Standards of Medical Care in Diabetes—2021*. Diabetes Care 2021;44(Suppl. 1):S85–S99

7. Beck RW, Bergenstal RM, Cheng P, et al. The relationships between time in range, hyperglycemia metrics, and HbA1c. J Diabetes Sci Technol 2019;13:614–626

8. International Hypoglycaemia Study Group. Glucose concentrations of less than 3.0 mmol/L (54 mg/dL) should be reported in clinical trials: a joint position statement of the American Diabetes Association and the European Association for the Study of Diabetes. Diabetes Care 2017;40:155–157

9. Clarke WL, Cox DJ, Gonder-Frederick LA, Julian D, Schlundt D, Polonsky W. Reduced awareness of hypoglycemia in adults with IDDM: a prospective study of hypoglycemic frequency and associated symptoms. Diabetes Care 1995;18:517–522

10. Cryer PE. Mechanisms of hypoglycemia-associated autonomic failure in diabetes. N Engl J Med 2013;369:362–372

11. Dagogo-Jack SE, Craft S, Cryer PE. Hypoglycemia-associated autonomic failure in insulin-dependent diabetes mellitus: recent antecedent hypoglycemia reduces autonomic responses to, symptoms of, and defense against subsequent hypoglycemia. J Clin Invest 1993;91:819–828

12. Weinstock RS, DuBose SN, Bergenstal RM, et al.; T1D Exchange Severe Hypoglycemia in Older Adults With Type 1 Diabetes Study Group. Risk factors associated with severe hypoglycemia in older adults with type 1 diabetes. Diabetes Care 2016;39:603–610

13. Heller SR, Macdonald IA. The measurement of cognitive function during acute hypoglycaemia: experimental limitations and their effect on the study of hypoglycaemia unawareness. Diabet Med 1996;13:607–615

14. Maran A, Lomas J, Macdonald IA, Amiel SA. Lack of preservation of higher brain function during hypoglycaemia in patients with intensively-treated IDDM. Diabetologia 1995;38:1412–1418

15. Mellman MJ, Davis MR, Brisman M, Shamoon H. Effect of antecedent hypoglycemia on cognitive function and on glycemic thresholds for counterregulatory hormone secretion in healthy humans. Diabetes Care 1994;17:183–188

16. van de Ven KC, Tack CJ, Heerschap A, van der Graaf M, de Galan BE. Patients with type 1 diabetes exhibit altered cerebral metabolism during hypoglycemia. J Clin Invest 2013;123:623–629

17. Chow E, Bernjak A, Williams S, et al. Risk of cardiac arrhythmias during hypoglycemia in patients with type 2 diabetes and cardiovascular risk. Diabetes 2014;63:1738–1747

18. Laitinen T, Lyyra-Laitinen T, Huopio H, et al. Electrocardiographic alterations during hyperinsulinemic hypoglycemia in healthy subjects. Ann Noninvasive Electrocardiol 2008;13:97–105

19. Novodvorsky P, Bernjak A, Chow E, et al. Diurnal differences in risk of cardiac arrhythmias during spontaneous hypoglycemia in

young people with type 1 diabetes. Diabetes Care 2017;40: 655–662

20. Pistrosch F, Ganz X, Bornstein SR, Birkenfeld AL, Henkel E, Hanefeld M. Risk of and risk factors for hypoglycemia and associated arrhythmias in patients with type 2 diabetes and cardiovascular disease: a cohort study under real-world conditions. Acta Diabetol 2015;52:889–895

21. Sanon VP, Sanon S, Kanakia R, et al. Hypoglycemia from a cardiologist's perspective. Clin Cardiol 2014;37:499–504

22. Stahn A, Pistrosch F, Ganz X, et al. Relationship between hypoglycemic episodes and ventricular arrhythmias in patients with type 2 diabetes and cardiovascular diseases: silent hypoglycemias and silent arrhythmias. Diabetes Care 2014;37:516–520

23. Brod M, Christensen T, Thomsen TL, Bushnell DM. The impact of non-severe hypoglycemic events on work productivity and diabetes management. Value Health 2011;14:665–671

24. Davis RE, Morrissey M, Peters JR, Wittrup-Jensen K, Kennedy-Martin T, Currie CJ. Impact of hypoglycaemia on quality of life and productivity in type 1 and type 2 diabetes. Curr Med Res Opin 2005; 21:1477–1483

25. Cox DJ, Gonder-Frederick L, Clarke W. Driving decrements in type I diabetes during moderate hypoglycemia. Diabetes 1993;42: 239–243

26. Cox DJ, Kovatchev B, Vandecar K, Gonder-Frederick L, Ritterband L, Clarke W. Hypoglycemia preceding fatal car collisions. Diabetes Care 2006;29:467–468

27. Cox DJ, Penberthy JK, Zrebiec J, et al. Diabetes and driving mishaps: frequency and correlations from a multinational survey. Diabetes Care 2003;26:2329–2334

28. Juvenile Diabetes Research Foundation Continuous Glucose Monitoring Study Group; Fiallo-Scharer R, Cheng J, Beck RW, et al. Factors predictive of severe hypoglycemia in type 1 diabetes: analysis from the Juvenile Diabetes Research Foundation continuous glucose monitoring randomized control trial dataset. Diabetes Care 2011;34:586–590

29. Gómez AM, Henao DC, Imitola Madero A, et al. Defining high glycemic variability in type 1 diabetes: comparison of multiple indexes to identify patients at risk of hypoglycemia. Diabetes Technol Ther 2019;21:430–439

30. Monnier L, Wojtusciszyn A, Molinari N, Colette C, Renard E, Owens D. Respective contributions of glycemic variability and mean daily glucose as predictors of hypoglycemia in type 1 diabetes: are they equivalent? Diabetes Care 2020;43:821–827

31. Rodbard D. Hypo- and hyperglycemia in relation to the mean, standard deviation, coefficient of variation, and nature of the glucose distribution. Diabetes Technol Ther 2012;14:868–876

32. Runge AS, Kennedy L, Brown AS, et al. Does time-in-range matter? Perspectives from people with diabetes on the success of current therapies and the drivers of improved outcomes. Clin Diabetes 2018;36:112–119

33. Battelino T, Danne T, Bergenstal RM, et al. Clinical targets for continuous glucose monitoring data interpretation: recommendations from the International Consensus on Time in Range. Diabetes Care 2019;42:1593–1603

34. Vigersky RA, McMahon C. The relationship of hemoglobin A1c to time-in-range in patients with diabetes. Diabetes Technol Ther 2019;21:81–85

35. Beck RW, Bergenstal RM, Riddlesworth TD, et al. Validation of time in range as an outcome measure for diabetes clinical trials. Diabetes Care 2019;42:400–405

36. Beck RW, Connor CG, Mullen DM, Wesley DM, Bergenstal RM. The fallacy of average: how using HbA1c alone to assess glycemic control can be misleading. Diabetes Care 2017;40: 994–999

37. Fabris C, Heinemann L, Beck R, Cobelli C, Kovatchev B. Estimation of hemoglobin A1c from continuous glucose monitoring data in individuals with type 1 diabetes: is time in range all we need? Diabetes Technol Ther 2020;22:501–508

38. Guo Q, Zang P, Xu S, et al. Time in range, as a novel metric of glycemic control, is reversely associated with presence of diabetic cardiovascular autonomic neuropathy independent of HbA1c in Chinese type 2 diabetes. J Diabetes Res 2020;2020:5817074

39. Lu J, Home PD, Zhou J. Comparison of multiple cut points for time in range in relation to risk of abnormal carotid intima-media thickness and diabetic retinopathy. Diabetes Care 2020;43: e99–e101

40. Lu J, Ma X, Zhou J, et al. Association of time in range, as assessed by continuous glucose monitoring, with diabetic retinopathy in type 2 diabetes. Diabetes Care 2018;41:2370–2376

41. Lu J, Wang C, Shen Y, et al. Time in range in relation to all-cause and cardiovascular mortality in patients with type 2 diabetes: a prospective cohort study. Diabetes Care 2021;44:549–555

42. Mayeda L, Katz R, Ahmad I, et al. Glucose time in range and peripheral neuropathy in type 2 diabetes mellitus and chronic kidney disease. BMJ Open Diabetes Res Care 2020;8:e000991

43. Ranjan AG, Rosenlund SV, Hansen TW, Rossing P, Andersen S, Nørgaard K. Improved time in range over 1 year is associated with reduced albuminuria in individuals with sensor-augmented insulin pump-treated type 1 diabetes. Diabetes Care 2020;43: 2882–2885

44. Yoo JH, Choi MS, Ahn J, et al. Association between continuous glucose monitoring-derived time in range, other core metrics, and albuminuria in type 2 diabetes. Diabetes Technol Ther 2020;22: 768–776

45. Bergenstal RM, Beck RW, Close KL, et al. Glucose management indicator (GMI): a new term for estimating A1C from continuous glucose monitoring. Diabetes Care 2018;41:2275–2280

46. Battelino T, Bergenstal RM. Continuous glucose monitoring-derived data report: simply a better management tool. Diabetes Care 2020;43:2327–2329

47. Rodbard D. Continuous glucose monitoring: a review of successes, challenges, and opportunities. Diabetes Technol Ther 2016; 18(Suppl. 2):S3–S13

48. Mazze RS, Lucido D, Langer O, Hartmann K, Rodbard D. Ambulatory glucose profile: representation of verified self-monitored blood glucose data. Diabetes Care 1987;10:111–117

49. Bergenstal RM, Ahmann AJ, Bailey T, et al. Recommendations for standardizing glucose reporting and analysis to optimize clinical decision making in diabetes: the ambulatory glucose profile (AGP). Diabetes Technol Ther 2013;15:198–211

50. Rodbard D. The ambulatory glucose profile: opportunities for enhancement. Diabetes Technol Ther. Epub ahead of print on 11 December 2020 (doi:10.1089/dia.2020.0524)

Exploring Why People With Type 2 Diabetes Do or Do Not Persist With Glucagon-Like Peptide-1 Receptor Agonist Therapy: A Qualitative Study

William Polonsky,[1] Cory Gamble,[2] Neeraj Iyer,[2] Mona Martin,[3] and Carol Hamersky[2]

[1]Behavioral Diabetes Institute, San Diego, CA; [2]Novo Nordisk, Plainsboro, NJ; [3]Health Research Associates, Inc., Mountlake Terrace, WA

OBJECTIVE | Despite the demonstrated benefits of glucagon-like peptide 1 (GLP-1) receptor agonist therapy, adherence and persistence with this therapy is often challenging. The purpose of this study was to expand current understanding of patients' experiences, motivations, and challenges relevant to their persistence with GLP-1 receptor agonist therapy.

DESIGN AND METHODS | This noninterventional, cross-sectional, qualitative study used face-to-face interviews with 36 adults with type 2 diabetes who had been treated with at least one GLP-1 receptor agonist medication. Inclusion criteria were: ≥18 years of age, diagnosed with type 2 diabetes, and currently treated with a GLP-1 receptor agonist for ≥1 month at the time of screening ("continuers") or discontinued use of a GLP-1 receptor agonist ≤1 year of screening but with a total ≥1 month of treatment ("discontinuers"). Interviews were conducted using a semi-structured qualitative interview guide that included open-ended questions and probes to obtain both spontaneous and prompted input from participants about their current and past treatment experiences with GLP-1 receptor agonist therapy.

RESULTS | Among continuers ($n = 16$), the most commonly identified facilitators supporting the decision to continue were the observations of improved glucose control (50%) and weight loss (55%). Among discontinuers ($n = 20$), the most commonly identified challenges leading to treatment discontinuation were side effects (55%) and high cost (50%). Continuers were more likely than discontinuers to receive clinically relevant information from their health care team, including facts about GLP-1 receptor agonist medications, likely treatment benefits, the importance of gradual dose titration, and the need to adjust diet after initiation.

CONCLUSION | Although cost is a major obstacle to treatment continuation, it can only be resolved through changes in ongoing reimbursement coverage and policies. However, many other obstacles could potentially be addressed (e.g., reducing side effects with gradual dosage titration and setting appropriate expectations regarding efficacy) through more collaborative patient-clinician interactions before initiating therapy.

Glucagon-like peptide 1 (GLP-1) receptor agonists are an innovative class of medications for people with type 2 diabetes that enhances glucose-dependent insulin secretion, suppresses pancreatic glucagon production, slows gastric motility, and reduces body weight by increasing satiety and decreasing appetite (1,2). Importantly, treatment with a GLP-1 receptor agonist confers a low risk of hypoglycemia when given as monotherapy or in the absence of sulfonylureas or insulin (2), and recent studies have linked certain GLP-1 receptor agonist formulations with cardiovascular (3–5) and renal (3,4,6,7) benefits, as well as cost savings (8–10).

Individuals who persist with GLP-1 receptor agonist therapy achieve significant A1C reductions, are more likely to achieve an A1C of <7%, and experience fewer hospitalizations and shorter hospital stays (8–10). As recently reported by Shah et al. (10), in individuals with type 2 diabetes and established cardiovascular disease (CVD) or elevated cardiovascular risk, treatment with a GLP-1 receptor agonist (liraglutide) was found to be a cost-effective and budget-neutral option with U.S. managed care plans. Recent guidelines from the American Diabetes Association recommend that a GLP-1 receptor agonist should be considered when atherosclerotic CVD, heart failure, or chronic kidney disease predominates, independent of A1C (11).

Despite the demonstrated benefits of GLP-1 receptor agonist therapy, adherence and persistence with therapy is

Corresponding author: Carol Hamersky, cahy@novonordisk.com

https://doi.org/10.2337/ds20-0025

frequently problematic, and discontinuation rates are high (12). As reported by Alatorre et al. (13), the proportion of people with type 2 diabetes who discontinued treatment during the first 6 months can range from 26 to 48%, depending on the formulation and/or required injection frequency (e.g., twice daily, once daily, or once weekly) (14). In a recent survey of 2,173 individuals with type 2 diabetes who discontinued GLP-1 receptor agonist therapy, respondents identified gastrointestinal side effects ("made me feel sick," 64.4%; "made me throw up," 45.4%) as their primary reason for discontinuation. Other reasons included "a preference for oral medications" (39.7%) and "inadequate blood glucose control" (34.5%) (15).

Although use of once-weekly formulations (e.g., semaglutide, extended-release exenatide, and dulaglutide) is associated with higher rates of adherence to GLP-1 receptor agonist therapy compared with once-daily formulations (16–18), there is limited evidence regarding other potential factors that may support or deter GLP-1 receptor agonist therapy adherence and/or persistence (e.g., psychosocial factors, drug cost, and clinician support). Understanding these factors may assist in formulating strategies that encourage therapy persistence, resulting in improved glycemic control, more efficient health care utilization, and costs savings over time.

This article reports findings from a recent qualitative study that investigated key contributors to continuation and discontinuation of GLP-1 receptor agonist therapy in adults with type 2 diabetes. Our aim was to uncover information that may point to practical guidance for clinicians when initiating GLP-1 receptor agonist therapy and when providing ongoing needed support in the pursuit of greater adherence and persistence with therapy.

Research Design and Methods

Research Design

This noninterventional, cross-sectional, qualitative analysis used face-to-face interviews with adults with type 2 diabetes who had been treated with at least one GLP-1 receptor agonist formulation. The objective of the analysis was to enhance current understanding of participants' experiences, motivations, and challenges relevant to their persistence with GLP-1 receptor agonist therapy.

Setting and Participants

The interviews were conducted between 24 January and 1 June 2018 at six clinical sites in the United States (in the states of Alabama, Indiana, North Carolina, Ohio, Texas, and Washington). Inclusion criteria were ≥18 years of age, diagnosed with type 2 diabetes, and currently treated with a GLP-1 receptor agonist for at least 1 month at the time of screening or discontinued use of a GLP-1 receptor agonist within 1 year of screening but with a total of at least 1 month of treatment. The study protocol was approved by a central institutional review board (Quorum Review, Seattle, WA) and performed in accordance with Good Clinical Practice and applicable regulatory requirements. All eligible participants provided written informed consent and demographic data before being scheduled for their interview visit.

Assessment Tool

Interviews were conducted using a semi-structured qualitative interview guide that included open-ended questions and probes to obtain both spontaneous and prompted input from participants about their treatment experiences with GLP-1 receptor agonist therapy. The guide included discussion items designed to elicit information regarding participants' reasons for treatment continuation, adherence/nonadherence, or discontinuation. Key items covered initiation of GLP-1 receptor agonist therapy, interactions with their health care team, and psychosocial contributors (facilitators) to continuing or discontinuing therapy. Table 1 presents a sample of the questionnaire items. In response to these questions, "spontaneous offered" was selected on the interview grid when participants offered a response concept on their own. "Recognized probe" was selected if the interviewer asked a probing, follow-up question to elicit a concept response. "No effect" was selected when participants stated that they had not experienced the response concept.

Tool Development and Interviewer Training

The interview tool was developed by an experienced qualitative research group (Health Research Associates, Inc. [HRA], Mountlake Terrace, WA) in collaboration with the study sponsor. Four interviewers reviewed the content of the interview guides and participated in mock interview sessions with each other (led by senior research staff) to test the flow of the questions to find any problematic, slow, or awkward areas and to test the general timing of the interview.

A training day of observed practice interviews was organized with the HRA and study sponsor team and the study interviewers. Willing volunteers with type 2 diabetes were recruited from a local volunteer list to take part in the training interviews; no participant information or results of the practice interviews were recorded or retained. After the practice interviews, the interview guide was finalized, and

---

TABLE 1 Sample Questions From the Interview Guide

Key: Main questions are shown in boldface; follow-up probes are listed with bullets.

How do you feel it went with your (first/second) GLP-1 receptor agonist medication?
- Was using this medication easier, more difficult, or about as much work as you expected? (describe)
- What could have helped you to be more successful with it when you were first getting started? (more information from the doctor, better instructions printed on the device itself, fewer administration times, fewer side effects, etc.?)
- Was there anything about the product that made it particularly easy or particularly difficult to use?

The challenges you have described that make it harder for you to use GLP-1 receptor agonist medications are: _____. (read back to patients what they have listed as challenges)

Now I'm going to read a list of challenges some people report when using GLP-1 receptor agonist medications. As I read this list, please tell me if you remember experiencing any of these.

(Interviewer: ONLY ask follow-up probes on challenges if they have not already been mentioned.)
- Interruption of daily activities
- Health care team was not accessible to answer questions
- Health care team did not provide enough education/information
- Insurance issues (lack of coverage/out-of-pocket costs are high)
- Insufficient instructions on use of injectable or pen device
- Limited or inadequate instructions around GLP-1 receptor agonist starting dose and the need for increases in the dose
- Side effects (make sure patients detail these)
- Having to make changes in diet
- Fear of needles/self-injection
- Burden of many medications to take
- Discomfort from being first time with injectable medication
- Sense that medication was not working
- Did not see a need to keep taking the medication
- Frustration or discouragement related to having diabetes in general
- Weight gain or lack of weight loss (specify)
- No instruction around importance of exercise and minimizing food volume and dietary fat at meals
- Disappointed that it did not work as well as I expected

Of all of the challenges we have just discussed, which ones were the most difficult for you to deal with? (describe why) **Which ones are the most important?**

[For patients who discontinued] **Which of these challenges was a part of the reason you discontinued the GLP-1 receptor agonist medication?**

Which were the most important contributors to why you discontinued?

---

changes were submitted to the institutional review board for approval.

Data Collection

Four trained HRA research staff members conducted the interviews in a private room at the enrolled clinic sites. Each interview visit was audio-recorded and lasted ~90 minutes. On arrival at the scheduled interview session, participants were given a brief introduction to the interview purpose and process. They were reassured about the confidential nature of the interview contents and the personal information they provided. All interviews were conducted in English and directed by the semi-structured qualitative interview guide.

Analysis

Digital audio files of subject interviews were transcribed and entered into the ATLAS.ti software program v. 7.1.0

(19) for coding. The coding process was structured for thematic analysis, identifying patients' expressions of concepts, highlighting quotations to tag them in the coding program, and assigning a code stem to them so the data could be organized by similar content and used to build thematic pictures of patients' responses. As new concepts appeared in patients' responses in the transcripts, new categories were made to capture them in the coding framework. Some sections of the interview were used to compile actual full responses from patients against specific questions in instances in which showing the spectrum of replies against a research question was important. The interviews included a few rating exercises for symptom severity or symptom-related bother, for which patients were asked to give a rating on a numerical scale ranging from 0 to 10. Data from these exercises were used to develop descriptive quantitative tables.

Methods:
1. Order transcripts in chronological sequence.
2. Evaluate new concept code appearance separately for each transcript group.
3. Compare each new transcript group to previous ones and identify newly appearing information.

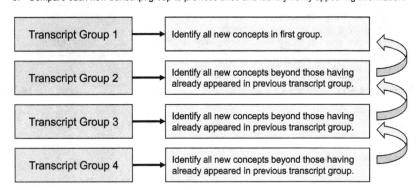

FIGURE 1 Method for evaluating saturation of concept.

Saturation of concept was assessed to determine whether a sufficient number of interviews had been conducted. Saturation of concept is reached when no new concepts are being identified in the interview data (20).

Transcripts were ordered chronologically based on interview completion date and then grouped into five groups of seven to eight transcripts each. Saturation was then evaluated by comparing the codes that were derived from the second transcript group with the codes that appeared in the transcripts from the first group to identify whether new information was still forthcoming. These evaluations and comparisons were repeated for each subsequent group. Once new information was no longer forthcoming, it was considered unlikely that further interviews with similar participants would have contributed any additional information or understandings (Figure 1).

Interrater agreement was used to assess consistency of code assignment. Two randomly selected interview transcripts were independently dual-coded and compared for percentage of agreement in the assignment of codes to concepts expressed by participants in the interview process.

Results

Thirty-six participants completed the qualitative interviews. Participants were predominantly older, female, and non-Hispanic White (Table 2). Participants who were currently on GLP-1 receptor agonist therapy at the time of the interviews (continuers) tended to have higher household incomes, shorter durations of diabetes, and lower A1C levels at the start of GLP-1 receptor agonist therapy than those who had stopped therapy (discontinuers). The 16 continuers were being treated with once-daily liraglutide, once-weekly exenatide, twice-daily exenatide, or once-weekly dulaglutide. Among the 20 discontinuers, which included discontinuation to one or more of all of the available GLP-1 receptor agonist formulations, 15 had discontinued GLP-1 receptor agonist therapy >6 months before their interview. The study did not include two recent additions to the GLP-1 receptor agonist class: once-weekly semaglutide and once-daily oral semaglutide.

Primary Facilitators Associated With GLP-1 Receptor Agonist Therapy Continuation

The number and percentages of continuers (*n* = 16) who identified primary facilitators for continuing GLP-1 receptor agonist use are presented in Table 3. The most commonly identified group of facilitators reflected participants' perception that the treatment was contributing to tangible, positive results (most importantly, glycemic control and weight loss). Some of the verbatim responses recorded during the interviews with GLP-1 receptor agonist therapy continuers are shown below.

"It helps my numbers so much, I don't want them to skyrocket again back above 8 [%]."

"What made it easier was I knew the benefits . . . . I saw the weight loss . . . . So, that was a positive on my end."

"The fact that it brought down my A1C would be the main thing."

"A lower blood sugar, and like I said, it feels like it stabilizes my sugars and stops them from yo-yoing."

"The knowledge of the cardiovascular benefit helped me stay on the GLP-1 [receptor agonist]."

TABLE 2 Demographic Characteristics

	Continuers (n = 16)	Discontinuers (n = 20)
Age, years	58.3 ± 8.5	58.3 ± 8.9
Sex		
Male	5 (31.2)	5 (20.0)
Female	11 (68.8)	16 (80.0)
Highest level of education completed		
Some high school	1 (6.3)	2 (10.0)
High school graduate	5 (31.3)	6 (30.0)
Some college	7 (43.7)	11 (55.0)
Bachelor's degree	3 (18.7)	1 (5.0)
Current employment outside the home		
Employed part-time or full-time	11 (68.8)	5 (25.0)
Retired	2 (12.5)	4 (20.0)
Not employed	3 (18.8)	11 (55.0)
Annual household income, $		
5,000–14,999	2 (12.5)	1 (5.0)
15,000–34,999	–	7 (35)
35,000–49,999	3 (18.8)	5 (25.0)
≥50,000	9 (56.3)	7 (35.0)
Racial group		
White or Caucasian	13 (81.2)	18 (90.0)
Black or African American	2 (12.5)	–
Other	1 (6.3)	1 (5.0)
Unknown	–	1 (5.0)
A1C at start of GLP-1 receptor agonist, %	7.7 ± 0.9	8.2 ± 1.4
	(n = 12)	(n = 10)
Most recent A1C, %	7.5 ± 1.3	7.9 ± 1.9
	(n = 16)	(n = 19)
Diabetes duration, years	12.7 ± 7.5	15.3 ± 8.4
Duration of current GLP-1 receptor agonist therapy, months		
>6	13 (81.3)	–
<6	3 (18.8)	–
Time since discontinuation, months		
>6	–	5 (25.0)
<6	–	15 (75.0)
Current GLP-1 receptor agonist therapy		
Once-daily liraglutide	5 (31.3)	–
Once-weekly exenatide	4 (25.0)	–
Twice-daily exenatide	2 (12.5)	–
Once-weekly dulaglutide	5 (31.3)	–

Data are mean ± SD or n (%).

The other major category of facilitators represented an appreciation of reduced or absent treatment burden (e.g., "no side effects," "available or low cost," and "ease of use").

"For me, personally, I feel [GLP-1 receptor agonists in general] have less side effects or problems with medications than some of the other diabetic medications that are on the market."

"The insurance factor's one of [the biggest factor in using it], because they cover it."

I didn't have any side effects from the medication."

Primary Challenges Associated With GLP-1 Receptor Agonist Therapy Discontinuation

The most commonly identified challenges leading to treatment discontinuation reflected participants' disappointment with the same two categories—in this case, lack of treatment efficacy and/or enhanced treatment burden (e.g., medication side effects or high costs) (Table 3).

TABLE 3 Primary Facilitators and Challenges to Continued Use of GLP-1 Receptor Agonist Treatment

Continuers (n = 16 [100%])		Discontinuers (n = 20 [100%])	
Primary facilitators that contributed to continued GLP-1 receptor agonist use		Primary challenges that contributed to discontinued GLP-1 receptor agonist use	
[Blood glucose] numbers improved	8 (50.0)	Side effects	11 (55.0)
Weight loss	4 (25.0)	High cost	10 (50.0)
[Blood glucose] numbers controlled	3 (18.8)	[Blood glucose] numbers did not improve	5 (25.0)
No side effects	3 (18.8)	High frequency of administration	1 (5.0)
Available or low cost	3 (18.8)	[Blood glucose] numbers worsened	1 (5.0)
Easy to use	3 (18.8)	Discomfort or fear of needles or self-injection	1 (5.0)
Long-term benefits	3 (18.8)	Pain or bruising with injection	1 (5.0)

Data are n (%).

"I was having nausea."

"The insurance coverage was [the] main reason I discontinued . . . . Insurance stopped covering [it]."

"It didn't work . . . [My A1C] didn't go back up, it just never really went down anymore . . . went down a couple of points, and that was it."

Influence of the Health Care Setting on GLP-1 Receptor Agonist Continuation and Discontinuation

In general, both continuers and discontinuers broadly reported supportive experiences with their health care provider team when initiating a GLP-1 receptor agonist. However, it appeared that continuers were more likely than discontinuers to receive clinically relevant information from their health care team, including facts about GLP-1 receptor agonist medications, likely treatment benefits (e.g., how the new treatment would contribute to better glucose control), the importance of gradual dose titration, and the need to adjust diet after initiation), as well as ongoing support (i.e., the health care team making proactive calls to check on their progress).

Table 4 presents the percentage of participants who confirmed specific statements included in the questionnaire. In most areas, the majority of continuers, in contrast to discontinuers, confirmed that they had good communication with their health care team and that their questions about medication were answered and they were provided information about the importance of gradual dosage titration.

Discussion

Although recent studies have provided initial insights regarding various reasons for discontinuation of GLP-1

receptor agonist therapy, the contributors to therapy persistence have not been well defined or understood (15). To our knowledge, this is the first qualitative exploration of factors that may affect an individual's decision to discontinue or continue GLP-1 receptor agonist therapy.

In this qualitative study, we interviewed 36 individuals with type 2 diabetes who shared personal accounts of their experiences with GLP-1 receptor agonist therapy. Despite the uniqueness of their individual circumstances, we identified two broad participant-perceived factors associated with medication persistence or nonpersistence: perceived treatment efficacy and perceived treatment burden.

Regarding the first factor, we see that the majority of participants who continued therapy cited aspects of treatment efficacy, including "numbers improved" (50.0%), "weight loss" (25.0%), and "numbers controlled" (18.8%) as primary facilitators of persistence with their therapy. Conversely, efficacy concerns appeared to influence discontinuation, with 25.0% of discontinuers reporting that "numbers did not improve." At the heart of this behavioral concept, it is apparent that, when individuals sense that their treatment is contributing to positive, tangible benefits, they are more likely to feel motivated to continue to use it (21).

Regarding the second factor, continuers reported a reduction or absence of treatment burden, with as many as 18.8% of participants citing such factors as "no side effects," "available or low cost," and "easy to use" as crucial to why they continued on GLP-1 receptor agonist therapy. Not surprisingly, we see the converse among discontinuers, with "side effects" (55.0%) and "high cost" (50.0%) as the most common primary challenges to therapy persistence.

TABLE 4 Comparison of Facilitating Experiences: Continuers Versus Discontinuers

Experiences	Continuers ($n = 16$)	Discontinuers ($n = 20$)
Good communication with health care team		
• My health care team explained that GLP-1 receptor agonist therapy would improve my blood glucose control.	13 (81.3)	12 (60.0)
• My health care team explained why my GLP-1 receptor agonist medication needs to be taken as an injectable.	12 (75.0)	15 (75.0)
• My health care team explained the importance of gradual dosage titration.	12 (75.0)	10 (50.0)
• My health care team explained how to manage food volume and fats.	7 (43.8)	7 (35.0)
Access to information		
• My questions about medications were answered by my health care team when I started on GLP-1 receptor agonist therapy.	15 (93.8)	15 (75.0)
• I was provided information about GLP-1 receptor agonist medications.	15 (93.8)	12 (60.0)
• I was provided general information about diabetes.	12 (75.0)	14 (70.0)
• My physician's office called to check on my progress and ask if I had any additional questions.	10 (62.5)	8 (40.0)

Data are n (%).

The interplay between the perceived value of a medication and the perceived concerns (or sense of burden) about that medication is a well-studied phenomenon in the medication adherence literature (22), and both of these factors are seen as crucially important. Although they are typically considered to be modifiable factors, it is well recognized that the biological response to GLP-1 receptor agonist therapy can vary significantly depending on individuals' unique physiological characteristics, current level of glycemic control, and specific drug formulation (23). Therefore, lack of glycemic improvement, lack of weight loss, and/or intolerability of side effects may simply be an unmodifiable class effect in some participants, which could explain why 25.0% of discontinuers reported "numbers did not improve" as their primary reason for discontinuation. Although "high cost" was reported as a primary factor affecting therapy persistence, this issue can only be resolved through changes in payer reimbursement policies.

Nevertheless, our results suggest that several of these other key issues could potentially be addressed through more collaborative patient-clinician interactions before initiating therapy. For example, it appears that participants who continued with GLP-1 receptor agonist treatment were more likely than discontinuers to receive more comprehensive preparation and instruction at the start of treatment. As reported, 93.8% of continuers (vs. 75% of discontinuers) confirmed receiving information about GLP-1 receptor agonist medications and having their questions answered when starting therapy. Importantly, only 50% of discontinuers versus 75% of continuers confirmed receiving

information about the importance of gradual dosage titration. This finding suggests that continuers may have been more likely than discontinuers to be started on a "low-dose" regimen at the time of initiation, which could account for the higher percentage of continuers versus discontinuers who reported "minimal or no side effects" with treatment: 87.5 versus 55.0%, respectively. Moreover, continuers were more likely than discontinuers (62.5 vs. 40%) to receive proactive phone contacts from their health care team during the first few months so that any concerns could be addressed. Through these interactions, participants likely received feedback on their progress, making them more aware of any tangible benefits (e.g., improved glycemic control, weight loss, cardiovascular benefits, and improved well-being) that might be accruing. It could also be that these patients were able to discuss with their health care team any issues they had with the therapy, which could have helped them overcome minor adverse effects.

This was an average sample size for qualitative research studies, and saturation of concept was achieved, indicating that a sufficient number of interviews had been conducted. However, given the large amount of individual variability found in this therapeutic area, the relatively small sample size limits the generalizability of these findings to the larger diabetes population. Additionally, participants' perceptions and continuation of therapy may have been affected by differences in GLP-1 receptor agonist formulations (e.g., frequency of administration and drug-specific side effects).

A key limitation is that no insurance coverage data were collected. Given that "high cost" was a common obstacle among discontinuers, it is reasonable to assume that more continuers versus discontinuers had insurance coverage for their medications. Additionally, because our population was heavily White/Caucasian, and there were no Black/African American participants in the discontinuer group, our findings cannot be generalized to the larger population of people with type 2 diabetes. Other limitations include self-selection for participation, dependence on participants' memories and/or articulation of their perceptions and experiences, and inability to exactly determine the range of previous GLP-1 receptor agonist medications that discontinuers may have tried.

Although larger, quantitative studies are clearly needed to confirm our findings and identify characteristics of each GLP-1 receptor agonist formulation that may affect treatment persistence, we believe the information and insights provided by the study participants may be useful to clinicians when initiating GLP-1 receptor agonist therapy, as these results point to strategies that could be adopted by health care providers to enhance perceived treatment efficacy while addressing and potentially resolving treatment burden issues. More specifically, these improvements could be accomplished by thoroughly informing patients about the potential benefits, limitations, and side effects of the medication. Doing this would prepare them with information and strategies to minimize any side effects that may arise. It would also provide ongoing support and feedback to highlight the tangible benefits of their therapy and help address any obstacles they may be encountering. Finally, these findings highlight the importance of insurance providers' coverage policies and ongoing access to GLP-1 receptor agonist medications, which will likely be a key driver of enhanced therapy persistence.

ACKNOWLEDGMENT

The authors thank Christopher Parkin, of CGParkin Communications, Inc., for editorial assistance.

FUNDING

Funding for this study was provided by Novo Nordisk.

DUALITY OF INTEREST

W.P. has served as a consultant for Astra Zeneca, Dexcom, Eli Lilly, Intarcia, Mannkind, Merck, Novo Nordisk, Onduo LLC, and Sanofi. M.M. is an employee of Health Research Associates, Inc. C.G., N.I., and C.H. are employees of Novo Nordisk.

AUTHOR CONTRIBUTIONS

All authors designed the study, reviewed the data, and wrote the manuscript. M.M. provided statistical analysis. W.P. is the guarantor of this work and, as such, had full access to all the data in the study and takes responsibility for the integrity of the data and the accuracy of the data analysis.

REFERENCES

1. Harris MI. Medical care for patients with diabetes: epidemiologic aspects. Ann Intern Med 1996;124:117–122

2. Nauck M. Incretin therapies: highlighting common features and differences in the modes of action of glucagon-like peptide-1 receptor agonists and dipeptidyl peptidase-4 inhibitors. Diabetes Obes Metab 2016;18:203–216

3. Mann JFE, Fonseca V, Mosenzon O, et al. Effects of liraglutide versus placebo on cardiovascular events in patients with type 2 diabetes mellitus and chronic kidney disease. Circulation 2018;138: 2908–2918

4. Leiter LA, Bain SC, Hramiak I, et al. Cardiovascular risk reduction with once-weekly semaglutide in subjects with type 2 diabetes: a post hoc analysis of gender, age, and baseline CV risk profile in the SUSTAIN 6 trial. Cardiovasc Diabetol 2019;18:73

5. Hernandez AF, Green JB, Janmohamed S, et al.; Harmony Outcomes committees and investigators. Albiglutide and cardiovascular outcomes in patients with type 2 diabetes and cardiovascular disease (Harmony Outcomes): a double-blind, randomised placebo-controlled trial. Lancet 2018;392:1519–1529

6. Bethel MA, Mentz RJ, Merrill P, et al. Renal outcomes in the EXenatide study of cardiovascular event lowering (EXSCEL) [Abstract]. Diabetes 2018;67(Suppl. 1):522-P

7. Gerstein HC, Colhoun HM, Dagenais GR, et al.; REWIND Investigators. Dulaglutide and renal outcomes in type 2 diabetes: an exploratory analysis of the REWIND randomised, placebo-controlled trial. Lancet 2019;394:131–138

8. Lin J, Lingohr-Smith M, Fan T. Real-world medication persistence and outcomes associated with basal insulin and glucagon-like peptide 1 receptor agonist free-dose combination therapy in patients with type 2 diabetes in the US. Clinicoecon Outcomes Res 2016;9: 19–29

9. Li Q, Ganguly R, Ganz ML, Gamble C, Dang-Tan T. Real-world clinical effectiveness and cost savings of liraglutide versus sitagliptin in treating type 2 diabetes for 1 and 2 years. Diabetes Ther 2018;9:1279–1293

10. Shah D, Risebrough NA, Perdrizet J, Iyer NN, Gamble C, Dang-Tan T. Cost-effectiveness and budget impact of liraglutide in type 2 diabetes patients with elevated cardiovascular risk: a US-managed care perspective. Clinicoecon Outcomes Res 2018;10: 791–803

11. American Diabetes Association. Summary of revisions: *Standards of Medical Care in Diabetes—2020*. Diabetes Care 2020;43(Suppl. 1):S4–S6

12. Yavuz DG, Ozcan S, Deyneli O. Adherence to insulin treatment in insulin-naïve type 2 diabetic patients initiated on different insulin regimens. Patient Prefer Adherence 2015;9:1225–1231

13. Alatorre C, Fernández Landó L, Yu M, et al. Treatment patterns in patients with type 2 diabetes mellitus treated with glucagon-like peptide 1 receptor agonists: higher adherence and persistence with dulaglutide compared with once-weekly exenatide and liraglutide. Diabetes Obes Metab 2017;19:953–961

14. Amblee A. Mode of administration of dulaglutide: implications for treatment adherence. Patient Prefer Adherence 2016;10: 975–982

15. Sikirica MV, Martin AA, Wood R, Leith A, Piercy J, Higgins V. Reasons for discontinuation of GLP1 receptor agonists: data from a real-world cross-sectional survey of physicians and their patients with type 2 diabetes. Diabetes Metab Syndr Obes 2017;10: 403–412

16. Nguyen H, Dufour R, Caldwell-Tarr A. Glucagon-like peptide-1 receptor agonist (GLP-1RA) therapy adherence for patients with type 2 diabetes in a Medicare population. Adv Ther 2017;34: 658–673

17. Johnston SS, Nguyen H, Felber E, et al. Retrospective study of adherence to glucagon-like peptide-1 receptor agonist therapy in patients with type 2 diabetes mellitus in the United States. Adv Ther 2014;31:1119–1133

18. Giorgino F, Penfornis A, Pechtner V, Gentilella R, Corcos A. Adherence to antihyperglycemic medications and glucagon-like peptide 1-receptor agonists in type 2 diabetes: clinical consequences and strategies for improvement. Patient Prefer Adherence 2018;12:707–719

19. Friese S. User's Manual for ATLAS.ti 7.1.0. Berlin, Germany, ATLAS.ti Scientific Software Development GmbH, 2013

20. Rothman M, Burke L, Erickson P, Leidy NK, Patrick DL, Petrie CD. Use of existing patient-reported outcome (PRO) instruments and their modification: the ISPOR Good Research Practices for Evaluating and Documenting Content Validity for the Use of Existing Instruments and Their Modification PRO Task Force Report. Value Health 2009;12:1075–1083

21. Polonsky WH, Skinner TC. Perceived treatment efficacy: an overlooked opportunity in diabetes care. Clin Diabetes 2010;28:89–92

22. Foot H, La Caze A, Gujral G, Cottrell N. The necessity-concerns framework predicts adherence to medication in multiple illness conditions: a meta-analysis. Patient Educ Couns 2016;99:706–717

23. Romera I, Cebrián-Cuenca A, Álvarez-Guisasola F, et al. A review of practical issues on the use of glucagon-like peptide-1 receptor agonists for the management of type 2 diabetes. Diabetes Ther 2019;10:5–19

CPSIA information can be obtained
at www.ICGtesting.com
Printed in the USA
BVHW082247260522
638162BV00005B/9